Whiplash Injuries

Although motor vehicle accidents with associated injuries are prevalent in today's society, a comprehensive text that incorporates a discussion on the biomechanics of an injury in conjunction with a discussion on the various injuries and their treatment is not available for the clinician. This text provides valuable information that hopefully will prove useful to those physicians who deal with the evaluation and treatment of patients who present with injuries after a motor vehicle accident, particularly those patients with legitimate injury after the so-called "low impact, rear end collision."

It is becoming increasingly difficult for patients to receive optimal treatment, and for clinicians to receive reimbursement for treatment of those patients injured in a motor vehicle accident where there has been little or no damage to their vehicle. Some of these patients present with a constellation of disabling symptoms ranging from neck and back pain to headaches to neurocognitive problems. However, in this scenario the personal injury automobile insurance carrier often fails to approve the recommended treatment using the argument that physical injuries cannot possibly occur without significant financial damage to the vehicle(s) involved in the accident. This bold arrogance on the part of the carrier is predicated upon their experience with the legal system, whereby juries are less inclined to recognize injuries sustained without significant physical damage to the vehicle. Why should they? Insurance company expert witnesses are very convincing in minimizing the forces involved in such collisions. A picture of an intact vehicle goes a long way. How could a person be injured by the collision when nary a scratch or a dent is present on the bumper? Insurance carriers are often inspired to refuse recommended treatment knowing the power of this argument. The result: patients do not receive the necessary evaluation and treatment, and providers are not reimbursed for their services.

In reality, a person can be injured in a low impact collision, and the forces that result in the injury are often significant. Many variables can play a role in patient injury including pre-existing physical condition of the passenger, trunk or head rotation at time of impact, movement of the vehicle after impact, size of the cars involved in the accident, to name a few. We as clinicians must evaluate and treat these patients optimally.

The following text begins with a chapter that discusses the biomechanics of low impact collisions. The focus of this chapter will be the rear end, low speed, motor vehicle collision. The injury potential of rear end collisions has been the topic of great controversy as to whether or not the event itself has a plausible mechanism to create acute or chronic pain. The practicing physician is often required to address the probability or possibility that the patient's reported injuries and symptoms are related to a specific traumatic event. The standard professional school education is inadequate at providing practicing physicians with the information that they need to evaluate these causation issues. Physicians have been trained to evaluate a new patient presenting after a trauma with a standard medical approach to guide the patient down an algorithm of diagnostic tests and care. This helps to ensure that all pathology is identified, and care is properly implemented. In this age of shrinking healthcare resources, physicians are often challenged with identifying not only the diagnosis and treatment plan, but they are also enlisted to aid in the responsibility of payment decisions. Due to the comprehensive and complex nature of this topic, this first chapter will be written with the practicing physician in mind to provide simple concepts that can be used to help the physician evaluate the injury mechanism and how it relates to the patient's reported symptoms and clinical profile. There are several references listed at the end of the chapter for the reader that is interested in pursuing a deeper understanding of biomechanics of the rear end collision.

Chapter 2 is an overview of the different types of pain syndromes that may occur after a motor vehicle accident (acute and chronic, soft tissue, bony, and neurogenic pain). This is followed by a discussion of the pathophysiology of pain (ascending and descending pain pathways in the peripheral and central nervous system).

In chapter 3, the reader is provided with information concerning gait abnormalities that can occur as result of injuries sustained in a motor vehicle accident. Over time, subtle gait abnormalities take their toll on the patient, often causing discomfort in distant locations (other than the lower extremities) due to alterations of normal body mechanics. In this chapter, there is discussion of the evaluation of patients suspected of having a gait deviation that may be contributing to their chronic pain. State-of-the-art technology is utilized to identify such gait deviations and appropriate treatment is discussed.

Chapter 4 reviews the various diagnostic tools available in working up the patient with a variety of pain complaints after a motor vehicle accident. This is followed by a series of chapters that describe the evaluation and management of common pain problems that can develop after a motor vehicle accident including: upper extremity pain (chapter 5); lower extremity pain (chapter 6); spine pain (chapter 7); headaches (chapter 8); neurogenic pain (chapter 10); and reflex sympathetic dystrophy (chapter 11). A separate chapter is devoted to a discussion of the management of those patients who suffer from a chronic pain syndrome (chapter 9).

Chapter 12 provides an overview of neuropsychological and psychological assessment of individuals who have sustained a whiplash induced Mild Traumatic Brain Injury (MTBI). Other topics reviewed include diagnostic criteria for Post Concussive Syndrome/ MTBI, mechanism of MTBI injury in low impact accidents involving whiplash, medical diagnostic techniques, common symptoms, co-morbid factors that should be considered during assessment, post trauma vision syndrome, and rehabilitation planning. A detailed case study is also presented.

Chapters 13–15 discuss various therapeutic modalities for patients who suffer injuries after a motor vehicle accident. For those patients who suffer unrelenting pain, chapters 13–15 describe more aggressive analgesic treatment techniques including the use of opioid analgesics (chapter 13), and the high technology options of spinal cord stimulation (chapter 14) and opioid pump implantation (chapter 15).

J.L.R

To my parents Lillian and Seymour, my wife Marlene,
and my children Alaina and Jordan—
for all of your love and support

Acknowledgments

Jack L. Rook, MD

Dick Maxwell and Mary Kirchner (librarians at Penrose Hospital, Colorado Springs, CO), and Karen Oberheim.

Scott Rosenquist, MS, DC

The author would like to thank all of the researchers who have dedicated the resources needed to improve our knowledge in this area.

Dennis A. Helffenstein, PhD, CRC and Robert Sokol, PhD

Drs Helffenstein and Sokol would like to express their appreciation to their wives, Diana and Mary, for their support during this project. They would also like to thank Vickie Novak for her help in editing the Reference section of their chapter.

Nicholas I. Sol, DPM, FACFAS, FACFAOM

The author would like to thank his wife Kelly and his son Spencer for their love, encouragement, and support.

The Biomechanics of Low Speed Rear End Collisions

Scott Rosenquist, Jack L Rook

Biomechanics is defined as how mechanical forces affect or alter living organisms. The field of biomechanics originated in 1917 with Hugh Dehaven, who survived a mid-air plane-to-plane collision. He noticed that the only reason that he survived, while the other pilot had been killed, was the maintenance of the occupant cage in his area. John Lane, an early biomechanics pioneer, also noted in 1942 that aircraft should be certified as being both airworthy and crashworthy. The application of crashworthiness was not applied to automobiles until 1962.

The field of biomechanics emerged from the science concepts of engineering, mathematics, physics, and medicine. Colonel John P Stapp, United States Air Force, was one of the first pioneers in the area of human crash testing. His famous sled test, where he detached his retina, is a good example of why clinical conclusions from non-live human volunteer crash testing cannot always be applied to the general population.

The area of biomechanics has far reaching effects on the medical community. The biomechanics expert works in several areas, which vary from automobile safety design to determining the likelihood of injury after a traumatic event. The latter has been the area that has stirred the most controversy and interest.

SALIENT TERMINOLOGY

Standardization is the formulation of standards for a given procedure. It is required by the medical community. Counting, measuring, and quantifying require standard (an established measure or model to which other similar things should conform) methodology. Such an approach gives physicians the ability to evaluate patient needs and assign medical resources. However, a standardized approach requires that the testing methods be sensitive, specific, reliable, and valid. These terms are defined as follows:

- *Sensitivity* means that the examiner is testing what they want tested and are obtaining data that they are seeking to measure
- *Specificity* refers to whether the test value obtained is specific to the item the clinician wanted to measure

- *Reliability* determines whether the examiner will get similar results when the same test or procedure is repeated
- *Validity* determines if the values obtained are accurate.

These concepts are vital in the evaluation of biomechanical data in low property damage, rear end collisions as the biomechanics expert often gives a value or number and then makes assumptions about injury causation and the patient's needs based upon those numbers. If those numbers do not follow the criteria listed above for being sensitive, specific, reliable, and valid, then false assumptions can be made and a patient's right to appropriate medical care can be restricted without merit. Unfortunately, standardized accuracy has, in many cases, eluded the area of low property-damage reconstruction.

HUMAN TISSUE TOLERANCE TO INJURY

Researchers have searched for a force value or number that can be used to determine the human tolerance to impact energy, or load, in the low- or no property-damage rear end collision. Such a value could be used to determine if injury did or could occur. This has been the elusive "golden goose" that biomechanics experts have attempted to quantify for years. The benefit of isolating this one human tolerance number would be far reaching. It would add standardization to the field of post-injury evaluation and management. Causation would now be an objective measurement and no longer part of provider bias, patient bias, payer bias, hidden agendas, or other inherent weakness in the system.

However, for any system to be standardized, one must standardize all of the variables. In the case of accident reconstruction and human tolerance in accidents, this would require that all of the people that drive on the roads do so in the exact same conditions, use the same type of car, all be the same height, weight, strength, age, and have the same medical history, level of function, systemic health status, etc. Standardization cannot have variance beyond acceptable levels and still be applicable to the entire population. Davis, Croft, Freeman, Bogduk, and others have published several articles on this problem of variability in accident reconstruction.[1–4]

Human tolerance is defined as the level of structural resistance that a human tissue has whereby:

- any load below that level would not be expected to cause tissue damage and injury
- with a load above that level, tissue damage and injury will ensue.

When tissue damage occurs, pain stimulation likely also occurs.[5–9]

The ability to evaluate a trauma from an objective perspective and state without controversy whether injury could or did occur has been the quest of several talented and well-funded organizations. The funding of any project of this magnitude does come with agendas and biases. Watts dealt with this bias in his textbook, which outlines the funding sources for some of the research that is commonly quoted in low property damage, rear end collision reconstructions.[10] This chapter discusses the problems with these methods, which often represent a type of "junk science" that has made its way into courtrooms and health care offices.

The basis of biomechanical research in the low property damage, rear end collision includes the kinematics of accidents, the common forces experienced in different types of traumas, and the evaluation of causation. The accident reconstructionist, biomechanics expert, or collision analysis expert does not always deal with low property damage biomechanics. However, a growing trend in biomechanics is the rear end, low speed, property damage collision reconstruction for determining issues of injury causation. The issue of causation is the area that is entering into physician's offices the most.

CAUSATION

Causation in any traumatic event determines who is responsible for the payment of the care and other medical-legal fees that are often attached to such cases. The practicing physician needs to know who to bill for his or her services. The likelihood that a traumatic event is the cause of the reported injuries and symptoms, and the long-term effect of those injuries, determines how financial resources are distributed.

The definition of causation is "the last act, contributory to an injury, without which such injury would not have resulted." In other words, if not for the trauma, would the patient have the reported injuries and the need for care? The court requires that the answer to this question be within medical probability, which is greater than a 50 percent chance of being accurate. There has been a gap in the education system, which has not prepared physicians to use scientific protocols in their evaluation methods related to causation.

The Daubert and Fry rules for court, which are commonly listed as rules 701 and 702 on the admissibility of expert testimony, are used to help determine the validity of scientific information. The 701-Fry ruling is the general acceptance test where the judge will rely on people in the profession. The 702-Daubert rule evaluates if the test, procedure, or method is reliable, if it has been tested, if it has been subjected to peer review, if the error rate is known, and if it is generally accepted. These are critical in disputing most low speed, property damage collision reconstructions that are performed with a bias or unscientific method.

There are a number of steps that the clinician can use in determining whether the causation of an injury is related to the motor vehicle accident in question. The first step in any causality determination is to establish the appropriate diagnoses. Next, the physician should define the injury exposure as comprehensively as possible, especially in the case of the low impact rear end collision. After establishing a diagnosis and defining the injury, the clinician should discuss any intervening factors that could have contributed to the development of the above-mentioned diagnoses. This would include any concurrent non-motor vehicle accident related injuries or disease processes, pre-existing impairment, or injuries related to avocational activities (sports, hobbies, etc.). Next, any scientific evidence that supports a cause and effect relationship between the diagnosis and the injurious exposure should be discussed. Lastly, the clinician needs to assign a medical probability level to the case in question (medically probable greater than 50 percent likely, medically possible less than or equal to 50 percent likely).

The method commonly implemented by physicians is to simply believe their patients and then expect to get reimbursed for their services. This is no longer acceptable in the medico-legal arena that requires a more accurate evaluation of causation. This is especially true in the often misunderstood and maligned evaluation and management of a rear end collision patient where there is little or no property damage. This has led to controversy, ignorance, and bias concerning whether the traumatic event was significant enough to cause injury and the need for care. The evaluation and management of all trauma patients require that the physicians involved keep accurate records, have thorough intake paperwork, and complete comprehensive exams with good documentation. These rules are even more pertinent if causation is being disputed, as is the case in some rear end collisions.

The establishment of a diagnosis requires that the clinician define the exposure or trauma, address any non-accident related factors that may be contributing to the symptoms, and then make a determination as to whether the reported trauma is the causal event. When causation is being disputed, these basic guidelines become even more important and the addition of information about the actual trauma becomes a focus of the investigation into causation.

Conventional professional schools do not educate health care providers in the concepts needed to properly evaluate a traumatic event from a biomechanical perspective. Conversely, engineering and physical science educations do not educate the biomechanical experts in the individuality and intricacies of the biomechanics of the human frame and how complex the nervous system is in relation to the pain experience. There is also a great divergence of literature in this area, which has allowed both sides to profess accuracy in their methods. This gap in training and the inability to define and identify the actual human tissue tolerance has left several opportunities for controversy, conflict, and propaganda.

The current total economic cost per year for motor vehicle accidents is estimated to be $170 billion with the rear end collision responsible for an estimated 60 percent of that value and low speed, property damage collisions accounting for 60 percent of the total rear end collision costs.[11,12]

Sturznegger documented that the rear end collision has an injury rate per collision that is twice as high as any other collision.[13] Even though the rear end collision garners a large percentage of the dollars spent on auto accident patients, the death rates of other collisions have focused the efforts of safety experts and legislators on those types of impacts. Table 1-1 documents the injury rates, and death rates based on the primary direction of force (PDOF) in motor vehicle accidents. As can be expected, head-on collisions cause the highest percentage of fatalities while rear end collisions lead to the highest percentage of injuries. This table explains why most vehicle safety features are designed to protect the occupant in a frontal collision. Rear end collisions account for the majority of the financial resources paid out for motor vehicle collisions yet they only account for a small percentage of the total collisions.

Table 1-1 Percentage of injuries and fatalities in automobile accidents per direction of force

Primary Direction of Force	Fatalities (%)	Injuries (%)
Frontal 12:00	49.1	20
Left Frontal 11:00	9.4	7.2
Right Frontal 1:00	14.9	10.4
Left Side 9:00	11.3	6.3
Right Side 3:00	9.9	7.0
Direct Rear 6:00	2.5	43.5
Left Rear 7:00	0.7	2.3
Right Rear 5:00	0.08	2.8

CONCEPTS USED IN BIOMECHANICS

To understand the biomechanics of the rear end, low property damage accident the reader must understand some basic biomechanic concepts and explore some of the emerging theories and research into rear end collisions. These theories are enlightening our understanding as to how and why patients get hurt in these events and not in ostensibly similar, impact loading events. There are several basic concepts that are used in the evaluation of rear end collisions. This chapter does not address low speed frontal, rollovers, side impacts, sideswipes, slip and falls, and other low speed events, as they do not garner the attention, financial resources, and demographics that rear end collisions do.

Collisions are categorized by the Primary Direction of Force (PDOF) imposed to the vehicle in question. This system uses the vehicle as a clock with 12 o'clock being a direct frontal impact and 6 o'clock a direct rear-end collision. Any collision in the 5 o'clock to 7 o'clock range is considered a rear impact with 6 o'clock being direct and the other values considered to be non-linear impacts.

The forces imposed on the car or the occupants are evaluated by the direction from which they are induced. For example, if a car with one occupant strikes a brick wall while traveling at 35 miles per hour, the occupants will follow the same motion patterns, barring any restriction, and continue to travel forward at 35 miles per hour until stopped. Conversely, if a stopped vehicle is rear-ended, the occupant will transfer backwards into the seat as the car moves out from under him or her.

Accident reconstructionists often attempt to indicate that a rear end collision occupant is unreliable if they state that their first motion in a rear end impact was forward (as the motion pattern is actually back towards the seat). The perceived forward motion is due to the fact that the car is moving forward, and if the occupant's eyes are focused outside the car on the horizon it may appear to them that they are actually moving forward. In contrast, if they are focused inside the vehicle, it will more likely appear that they are moving backward in the vehicle. Several researchers have documented that the rear end collision does not always create an extension-flexion of the head (the classical whiplash) beyond the normal range of motion, but rather causes an intersegmental problem where independent joints exceed their respective limits.[9–14]

The treating physician is often times presented with an accident report. The majority of accident reports have a diagram of the vehicle damage, the pertinent insurance facts, and a category of the damage (that varies from 1-slight, 2-moderate, and 3-extreme). The scene officer does have training in this system but the category into which the damage fits is still open to interpretation. Patient symptomatology will either be documented in this report or the ambulance report, if available. A physician's file should include all pertinent information. This avoids surprises later and allows the treating physician to review all documents.

A warning must be sounded prior to using this data. Physicians should not attempt to practice layperson biomechanics or engineering. However, engineering, biomechanics, and physics concepts are entering into the evaluation and management of injured patients. Therefore, physicians must have a basic understanding of these concepts to protect their patients' rights to care, prepare accurate reports and testimony, and properly evaluate injury causation.

Most biomechanics and engineering professionals use several basic concepts in accident reconstruction or collision analysis.

Acceleration is the change in velocity over the change in time or Delta-v divided by Delta-t. The formula is written:

$$A = \Delta v / \Delta t$$

This formula tells us that acceleration is related to time. The change in velocity of an object or the Δv is crucial in the area of automobile biomechanics. With mathematical manipulation reconstructionists can increase the estimated time factor of a collision, which will subsequently reduce the acceleration (of the target vehicle), and perceived severity of the collision.

Delta-v (Δv) or the change in velocity is measured as distance over time (meters per second, miles per hour, feet per second, etc.). The amount of time that it takes to change the acceleration of an object will determine the violence of the acceleration or deceleration experienced by the occupants of a vehicle.

Crashworthiness refers to how well a vehicle performs in a crash. The performance is based on multiple factors including the mass of the vehicle, rollover risk, restraint performance, antilock braking, traction control, and other factors.

Deformation refers to the relative movement of any two points on an object due to distortion of that object under load.

Displacement is the relative movement of any point on an object in relation to a fixed reference frame.

Energy is the ability to do work. In the case of motor vehicle accidents it is expressed in the form of strain energy and kinetic energy.[15–17]

G refers to the effect that the earth's gravity has on a structure and is defined mathematically by 9.8 meters per second squared. Reconstructionists will list the amount of estimated G-forces an occupant or vehicle sustains in an accident. This is done by converting the Δv of the collision to G values. As an example, consider a bullet vehicle traveling at five miles per hour that comes to rest after impact. Five miles per hour is 40 meters/second squared. This number is then divided by the known G value of 9.8 meters per second squared to arrive at 4.1 G in this example. This attempts to state that the target vehicle sustained a 4.1 G force. However, since a rear end collision occurs in 100 milliseconds or more, it is not a static loading condition. Therefore, the G-unit *is not* the best measurement for the motor vehicle collision.

Impulse is the change in momentum and is a relational factor for force and time. An example of this is an egg thrown against a hanging sheet that comes to rest on a cushion as opposed to an egg that hits a solid barrier and is instantaneously destroyed. In this example, increasing the time the force was distributed decreases the impulse.

Inertia is the tendency of an object to stay at rest and to resist change, or the tendency of an object to remain in motion and to resist change. An example is an occupant in a car traveling at 35 miles per hour that hits a brick wall. Because of inertia, the occupant will continue to move at 35 miles per hour until they are stopped by another more powerful force (e.g., the seat belt). The head and neck are good examples of bodily structures that will have a large amount of inertia in a motor vehicle collision.

Jolt and *Jerk* are terms commonly used in accident reconstruction papers. In general, a jolt is defined as an abrupt sharp blow or movement, knocking or shaking violently, and tending to unsettle or dislodge. A jerk is defined as a single quick motion of short duration. Jerk is feet per second, per second, per second. Acceleration is the rate of change over time. The differences between velocity, acceleration, and jerk define why occupants in auto accidents are injured.

Kinetic Energy is expressed mathematically as:

$$\text{Kinetic Energy} = \tfrac{1}{2} \text{ Mass} \times \text{Velocity Squared.}$$

$$\text{KE} = \tfrac{1}{2} Mv^2$$

The fact that the velocity is squared in this formula indicates that an error in the acceleration (change in velocity) calculation will quadruple the error on the product of kinetic energy.

Force is any action that tends to change the state of rest or motion of a body to which it is applied.

Load is a general term describing the application of a force to a structure.

Load Deformation is a graphical representation of the relationship between load on an object and the deformation of a given point on that object. (The load–deformation curve, also known as a stress–strain curve will be discussed in greater detail shortly).

Elasticity refers to the stiffness properties of a structure.

Momentum is an object's damage energy potential. It is mathematically expressed as:

$$\text{Momentum} = \text{Mass} \times \text{Acceleration.}$$

The greater the momentum, the greater the damage transfer potential from the bullet to target vehicle.

Plastic Deformation occurs when the structure is exposed to enough strain energy for the structure to undergo permanent deformation. If a vehicle experiences plastic deformation some of the energy will be transferred to the occupant cage, while most of the energy in the collision goes to deforming or destroying parts of the vehicle. As vehicles become stiffer, property damage costs go down but the potential for occupant injury increases (increased energy transferred to the occupant cage).

Shear occurs when two forces are imposed onto a structure at the same time from different directions. Several different independent research facilities have documented that inter-segmental spinal shear is the most likely cause of pain after the rear end collision.

Strain is defined as the change in length of a structure divided by the original length in response to a load. Some loads do not cause permanent deformation. The toughness of a structure can be determined by the structure's ability to withstand a load without any noticeable strain. The portion of a stress–strain curve where the structure has not deformed is known as the *elastic area* of the curve and the area where there is permanent strain is the *plastic area*. If a structure has a very small amount of plastic deformation prior to failure it is listed as being brittle. The larger the area of elastic stress in a stress–strain curve, the larger amount of energy that structure stored prior to failure.

An example of an energy transferring mechanism in the rear end collision is the bumper and the seat back. If they do not permanently deform, they store energy and then transfer that energy out to the occupant cage when the load is removed or vehicle separation occurs. As manufacturers make vehicles stiffer they reduce damage costs but increase the stored energy in the vehicle and the jolt and inertia transferred to the occupant cage. In contrast, the racecar that falls apart after impact minimizes the damage energy to the driver. In general, standard car bumpers are designed to avoid or reduce vehicle damage in a low speed collision, not to serve as a safety device to prevent or reduce injuries to people in the car. Rather the bumper is designed to protect sheet metal parts of the car as well as safety related equipment such as parking lights and headlamps.

Stress determines a structure's strain behavior. The ultimate stress is the failure point of a structure, or the point of no return.

Yield stress is the point at which the stress–strain curve goes from elastic to plastic.

Stress–Strain Curves are a graphical representation of the relationship between stress and strain. Another term for this graph is the *Load–Deformation graph*.

Torque is the force exerted by a lever. This can cause a small force to create a larger force at the base due to leverage. The head ramping over a headrest in a rear end collision can produce this effect.

A **vector** has three primary properties: length, magnitude, and direction. This is important in the reconstruction formulas as reconstructionists will often attempt to compare forces and they must be comparable in magnitude, direction, and the way they were generated to be accurate.

Whip implies two forces in different directions, opposing each other in a differential motion.

NEWTON'S LAWS OF MOTION

Newton's First Law of Motion

Newton's laws of motion are critical in the evaluation of all motor vehicle accidents. The first law states that every body preserves its state of rest or uniform motion in a straight line unless it is compelled to change that state by forces imposed thereon. Simply put, an object will continue in motion along a straight path at a constant velocity unless a non-zero resultant force acts upon it. This is a basic concept but it is critical to the evaluation of motor vehicle collisions. This first law introduces the concept of *inertia*.

If an automobile is suddenly stopped, the passengers inside the vehicle obey this first law and continue in motion with constant velocity until some external force changes their state of motion. The seat belt, the dash, airbag, steering wheel, and other secondary collisions or contact traumas can account for this. The violence of the deceleration force will determine the injury potential. Conversely, if a patient is in a vehicle that is not moving and the vehicle is induced to move as in the case of most rear end collisions, the patient will not move until acted upon. The seat acts upon the patient as the seat is bolstered to the frame of the car.

However, we now know that the laws of inertia allow different parts of the occupant to move at different times and in different directions. Logically this is a problem in that whenever you have one body part moving in one direction while another remains at rest or travels in another direction, you have shear and could also have torque, distraction, compression, tension, and other injurious forces imposed on the tissues at the same time. Biomechanics experts, as early as the 1950s, documented the lag time in the response of the head and neck relative to the other structures in low speed collisions.[18,19] The entire rear end accident occurs in approximately 0.1 seconds or 100 milliseconds. However, shoulder movement peaks at 150 milliseconds while head movement peaks at 250 milliseconds. The head reaches peak acceleration of around 15 G, the shoulder reaches peaks of around 6 G, and the car reaches peaks of around 4 G. This demonstrates the magnification of the accelerations transferred to the occupant.

The concept of inertia and Newton's first law is best exampled in the frontal motor vehicle collisions. If a vehicle is traveling at 35 miles per hour, its occupants have great potential for injury. The faster the deceleration occurs the more injurious it can be to the occupant.

Reconstruction experts will often attempt to indicate that if a collision occurred across a longer period of time, the injury potential is less. The current research indicates that the initial phase of the rear end collision creates a sigmoid (S-shaped) curve to the cervical spine inducing shear injury that reduces the spine's tolerance levels to load. Also the high property damage, rear end collision and the low property damage, rear end collision both present with different injury potentials. The Δt or time of a collision can determine the injury potential of some entities but is not of itself a variable that will determine if injury did or did not occur. Increasing the Δt does add a ride down benefit to the occupant in some cases. In conclusion Newton's first law states that a body at rest remains at rest and a body in motion remains that way until acted upon by an outside, external force.

Newton's Second Law of Motion

The second law states that Force = Mass × Acceleration. Simply put, if you increase the mass of an object that is traveling it will increase the force potential it has if a collision occurs. Also if you increase the acceleration of an object it will increase the force potential it has. These physical laws define how in motor vehicle accidents the mass of the striking vehicle and its acceleration at impact help to determine their energy transfer potential.

It is important for the practicing physician to have in their file a description of the violence of the collision. This relates to the mass and force potential of the bullet-striking car compared to the target-struck car. If a patient presents and states that they were in a compact car and were struck by a large sport utility vehicle (SUV) on wet pavement and there was no damage to their car, this must be well documented. The force potential of the SUV as the bullet car is much larger than the compact car and produces larger force transferability than if the opposite collision occurred.

It is also known from the law of conservation of momentum and energy equations that momentum and energy are always conserved. The conservation of momentum and energy equations were discussed by Smith in his article that addressed why property damage is a poor method for evaluating injury potential.[17] These laws describe how the energy or momentum prior to a collision between two objects must be the same as after the collision. Smith explained that the energy method is a better procedure in a no vehicle damage collision. *No vehicle damage does not mean low velocity or low energy.* This mechanism has a high potential for injury to the occupant if there is no residual crush damage to the car. Robbins also discussed this issue and plotted crush damage and the energy to the occupant (Figure 1-1).[20]

The momentum equation requires that all momentum prior to the collision equals all momentum after the collision. There is a small amount that is lost to heat energy, sound energy, braking, and other sources but these are universally accepted as not being significant enough to require addressing.[17]

Therefore, physicians need to document the types of vehicles involved in the crash and their estimated speeds in their paperwork. Physicians do not evaluate vehicles but are often asked to explain how the injuries occurred when there is little or no vehicle damage. An understanding of the Newtonian laws along with other mathematic, physics, and engineering concepts can assist the physician in this regard. It is important to remember that the energy of the collision or the momentum of a collision are conserved and not lost.

One of the most common approaches by reconstructionists is to use the Law of Momentum and known crash data in an attempt to obtain the estimated Delta-v of the accident. The Delta-v (Δv) which is the change in velocity that occurred to either the vehicle or its occupant are elusive numbers that reconstructionists attempt to derive from vehicle inspections, accident photos, and other data they obtain. This number is often changed to an estimated G-force number.

Physicians evaluating these reports must find out what data was provided, if the reconstructionists evaluated the vehicles, pictures, copies of pictures, speed estimates, actual skid marks or estimates, and any other data. Several experts believe that the Δv or the change in velocity is one of the best indicators of accident severity. Reconstructionists will often play with the Δt or change in time of a collision as acceleration is relative to the

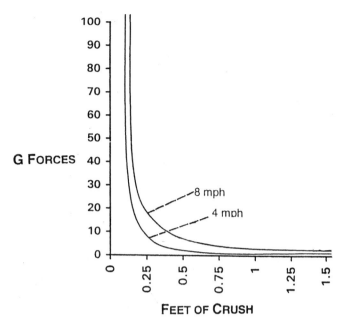

Figure 1-1 The graph demonstrates the relationship between crush distance and G-forces generated by impacts at 4 and 8 mph. As can be seen, vehicles that do not crush can experience very high G-forces. Thus, an occupant in a low speed collision with no damage to the vehicle may have a higher risk of injury than an occupant in a collision with a damaged vehicle. (Modified from Robbins MC: *The lack of relationship between vehicle damage and occupant injury,* SAE Pub 970494. Society of Automotive Engineers.

time of the collision, and altering the time of collision can reduce the values obtained in a reconstruction. If you increase the time of the collision you will reduce the acceleration factors calculated. This is deceptive and must be evaluated.

Quality reconstructionists will give a range of values and they will list what factors they used in their calculations. They will also list any complicating factors (out of normal body position, mass incompatibility, unprepared occupants, road conditions, skid mark estimates, damage deformation patterns, etc).

The calculation of Δv makes several assumptions. The first critical assumption is that the stopping force of the collision is a linear function of residual crush depth. However, some vehicles (those with sturdy metal frames or older cars made without crumple zones) have a large resistance to the initial amount of crush damage giving them a large initial energy storage capacity prior to permanent deformation. It is this stored energy that may traumatize the occupants.

The bumper standards are designed to reduce property damage in low speed events. The bumper has been documented as having a function of protecting the vehicle and has never been designed or proposed as an occupant safety device. The 2.5 or 5.0 mile per hour bumper standard simply implies that at these speeds no vehicle damage can occur. This does not imply that the speed to cause damage cannot be much higher. To clarify this means that no damage is allowed due to the bumper standard unless the impact speed is more than five miles per hour into a solid barrier. This is the goal of the manufacturers to lower the cost of property damage.

Experts often attempt to summarize that if no damage occurred, then the accident was below the five mile per hour standard when the opposite is actually true. Medical experts are often coerced into believing that a no property damage collision should mean that there is no injury potential. The opposite may be a more true statement in some cases. Szabo documented impact speeds as high as 18 miles per hour without damage,[21] and King and Bailey from MacInnis engineering documented speeds of 7.8–12.0 miles per hour with up to 100 impacts to the same vehicle in similar rear end crash tests with no vehicle damage.[22]

This concept is important as there is a misunderstanding that the bumper is a protective device for the occupant and that the bumper standard indicates that if no damage occurred, then the accident impact speed was less than the five mile per hour. Neither is true or accurate. The bumper standards are also established against an immovable barrier, which will increase the crush damage at lower speeds making these values a gross overstatement.

The momentum equation includes the known weights of the vehicles. Additional information required for this equation includes the crush depth of the vehicles, the drag factor or resistance of the road surface, and the skid marks. All of this information is required to properly determine the impact speed of the bullet car. In a low speed, property damage collision the variables required to obtain a product have an error factor that is too large to make causation determinations from these estimates.

There are several computer programs that make these calculations easier and they again are open to the expert plugging data into a particular equation until he or she obtains the number they like. One such equation measures the offending vehicle's speed prior to skidding. The equation reads:

$$S = \text{the square root of } (30 \times D \times F)$$

This equation is referred to as "speed from distance and drag". In this equation:

S = speed (mph) when brakes are first applied;
D = skid distance (feet); and
F = the "deceleration factor" or "road surface drag factor."

With regards to the road surface drag factor (F), different road surfaces (concrete, asphalt, wet, dry, etc) will have specific "F" values. In the equation, the speed prior to skidding (S) is equal to the square root of the product of 30, D, and F. For example, if there is a measured skid distance of 120 feet and the deceleration factor for the vehicle and road surface were 0.7 G, then according to this equation, the vehicle is calculated to have been going 50 miles per hour when the brakes were applied;

$$50.1 \text{ miles per hour} = \text{the square root of } [30 \times (120 \text{ feet}) \times (0.70 \text{ Gs})]$$

If the police officer at the accident scene does not obtain accurate data, then the product will be off. If the actual skid marks are not documented at the time of the accident, reconstructionists often just estimate this value and therefore the product is invalid. In the court setting, reconstructionists use these various techniques to determine occupant injury potential. Logically, human tolerance is still elusive and cannot be obtained from this data as the variability of each event precludes standardization, reliability, and validity that reach a level of significance. If scientific standards are applied to accident reconstruction of the low property damage accident, then evaluating the event instead of the patient should fall out of favor in the court systems.

If the car does permanently deform, then the collision damage would increase the Δt which could decrease the injury potential in a low speed event. New vehicles that have considered these concepts include energy-absorbing factors in their product design. If the energy of the collision does not go to crushing the vehicle, it can go into accelerating it and that force will transfer to the occupant cage. This is the reason why most safety devices for vehicles are designed to absorb energy (i.e. crumple zones, air bags, etc.). A racecar that crashes has a violent explosion of the vehicle parts; this is to dispense energy to the crushing, deforming, and flying parts and reduce the energy to the driver. This is done by increasing the time of the collision thereby increasing the survivability factors, as the occupant can manage the forces better across time.

There is also controversy on the basic dispute that all of the reconstructionist's tolerance or vehicle damage data is useless. In any scientific experiment or research project one of the primary goals is to reduce variance of all kinds. The reconstructionists must estimate at some point to come up with their product. Since the only known values are the vehicle masses and the stop distance, surface resistance and impact speed are often estimated. Considering that the accident reconstructionist is required to obtain values that are estimated, the variance rises to a level where scientific standards are not met.

Newton's Third Law of Motion

Newton's third law is the equal and opposite law. It states, to every action there is always opposed an equal reaction. If two bodies act upon each other a directly opposite action occurs. If A implies a force to B then it can be concluded "B returns a force to A." This is important as it lets us know that if a bullet car (the striking vehicle) hits a target car (the resting vehicle in a rear-end collision), there will not only be an effect from the striking car but also from the target car. Biomechanics experts use these concepts in the reconstruction and analysis of all traumas.

THE G-FORCE

The G-force is often the number listed in the accident reconstruction data. Allen,[23] and Rosenbluth[24] popularized the G-force calculation. Allen and Rosenbluth attempted to quantify the amount of G-force involved in standard activities of daily living events and then compare those to auto accidents (Table 1-2).[23,24]

However, there are numerous problems with their methodology and the G-force analysis should be considered invalid. G-forces are more appropriate for evaluating static

Table 1-2 Activities and associate G-forces

Activity	Reported G value (g)
Step off curb	8
Plop in chair	6
Stand up and sit down	2
Plopping backwards into a low back office chair	10.4
Bumper cars	6
Coughing	2–3.5
Skipping rope	4–6
Roller coaster	5
Laughing	2

The above values are simply numbers and should not be listed as tolerance levels for any tissue.[37,38]

conditions. Auto accident biomechanics demand that the concepts of kinetic energy, momentum, inertia, jolt and jerk be used. The rear end collision occurs in 1/10th of a second or 100 milliseconds, which makes it an event that is not conducive to the use of the G-force as the unit of impact severity.

Allen used eight subjects for his study, which automatically invalidates the applicability of his data to the general population due to the small sample size. In addition the test-to-test values had such a large mean and standard deviation that it again invalidates their data for use in the scientific community.

Prominent whiplash experts have published articles that address the problems with Allen's whiplash/biomechanics article.[25,26] The potential for injury is not only related to the total G-force exposure but also the duration of the exposure. The rear end collision is an event that is not conducive to the use of G-forces as a method of evaluating injury potential.

Allen, Rosenbluth, and others have used the G-force concept to compare a rear end collision to plopping into a chair, jumping rope, stepping off a curb, or other non-injurious activities of daily living. These articles attempted to document activities of daily living G-force values and then use these to conclude that these forces were similar to or greater than the ones experienced by occupants in rear end collisions.[23,24] Reconstructionists have then concluded that if the G value they calculate for a rear end collision is within the values of the activities of daily living events, that any injuries claimed in the accident were false. They have also attempted to compare listed tolerance levels that have no bearing on rear end collision mechanics, to rear end collisions for similar purposes. Accident reconstructionists commonly use tables that list these forces in their reports to compare them to the forces estimated from their reconstruction of an accident. This is a simple technique to attempt to reduce the perceived severity of the rear end impact.

Physicians must realize that the values listed are not comparable and should not alter their opinions on their patients' care needs. If the acceleration of an object and the mass of the object is known, the force of the object can be calculated. The rear end, low speed, property damage collision has many variables that are significant and are often not addressed in accident reconstruction reports.

The numbers listed in the accident reconstruction reports must be criticized for mathematical accuracy, scientific standards, and applicability to the area they are addressing. A simple G-force number is not sufficient to use as a comparative factor in injury potential. Human factors that can alter G-force tolerance include the occupant's age, height, weight, blood pressure, heart rate, and aerobic and strength conditioning.[27] Caution is advised to any physician who is interpreting accident reconstruction data that includes G-force values.

It should be noted that a 100 lb female exposed to 8 G has a force imposed onto her structures of 8×100 or 800 pounds. Forces exceeding 10 G have been documented repeatedly in crash tests where the impact speed was eight miles per hour or less. Additionally, the rear end collision is a multi-vector complicated loading event that occurs in a compromised position of energy transfer, which decreases tissue tolerance.

Cadaver studies have been performed to document load values after simulated collisions. It should be noted that live tissue is less tolerant to impulse loading. Compressive loads have been documented as high as 475–700 lb in a 21 mile per hour rear end collision. McConnell documented 35 lb of axial forces in a 5.7-mile per hour rear end reconstruction.[28,29] If the body is leaned forward, the tolerance will decrease further.

King *et al* has documented no damage to a vehicle that has an impact speed of 18 miles per hour.[30,31] Szabo has documented no damage with impact speeds of up to 10 miles per hour and documented no damage in crash tests as high as 8.5 miles per hour with as many as 100–150 impacts. Szabo has documented that a 9 mile per hour impact speed can cause an acceleration force to the head of the occupant of 17 G. This is equal to a force of 170 lb on the head. In a follow-up study, this same researcher found that under similar circumstances the occupant's head acceleration after impact was in the range of 12 G, a 30 percent variation from his earlier study. Other researchers have demonstrated similar variations.[21,32,33] The variance of the acceleration values recorded in controlled crash tests suggests that the information should not be used in a court setting.

McConnell, in two separate studies has demonstrated a head acceleration G-force variation of 4–14 Gs in individuals subjected to an impact velocity of five to six miles per hour. This represents a greater than 300 percent variation demonstrated in two separate similar studies by the *same* researcher.[28,29]

Therefore, when a reconstructionist estimates G forces of 2–4 G with an impact speed of five miles per hour, this data could be in error in excess of 300 percent. Since the court standards mandate that medical probability be within 51 percent or greater accuracy, this information places the reconstructionists' opinions in question. Other crash tests have documented similar variance with different subjects that have been exposed to the same crash tests in controlled circumstances. The amount of variance in the real world would be expected to be even greater.

The variability of the human frame is vast and cannot be evaluated in simple terms. For example, it has been demonstrated that neck circumference affects peak head acceleration (in Gs) after impact. It was demonstrated that a 20 percent reduction in neck circumference (from 15.7 inches to 12.6 inches) resulted in a peak head acceleration that was nearly 2.5 times higher. This higher acceleration occurred with the exact same impact speed and seating situation, and with proper head restraints.[34,35]

In conclusion on the issue of G-force data, there are several problems with the approach advocated by Allen, Rosenbluth and other similar authors.

1. The activities documented by Allen and others are not tolerance activities in that they are learned proprioceptive events that are not known to exceed the tolerance limits of the body. The forces imposed on the body in activities of daily living events are for the most part generated by the human and not from an outside force. The motion patterns are learned behaviors with a programmed neuroproprioceptive response that is also learned, making the injury potential minimal. In contrast, accidents are uncontrolled events with a primary outside generating force in a compromised mechanical position.

2. The forces documented by Allen were primarily in the x axis or the sagital plane and research indicates that the rear end collisions produce multi-vector planes which apply forces at different angles to the same body part at the same time.

3. Brault documented that there are 16 variables in human crash tests that when available and analyzed together can positively predict injury with an 80 percent accuracy rate. Many of these variables are not available in the average accident reconstruction.[36,37]

4. The Allen method also violates the known rules of force comparison. Comparing "plopping into a chair" to a rear end collision violates the laws of force comparison and makes this method invalid. The forces involved in activities of daily living are internally generated which are designed to produce a safe amount of tension, compression, distraction, etc, on the structure it affects. In contrast, accidents have forces that are produced from external sources. The body does not have a learned neuroproprioceptive memory of an accident, an activity that is not internally generated.

5. Crash tests with different subjects, in the same vehicles, with the same controlled conditions, have been shown to produce varied acceleration responses amongst the occupants.[38] This is another area of variability that removes accident reconstruction reports from being a valid method of determining injury potential.

6. The forces documented by Allen included a great variance with even the same person doing the same activity repeated times, which reduces the validity and reliability of the data and does not allow it to be compared to the general population.

7. The forces documented for plopping in a chair were as high as 10.1 G. That activity was performed without producing symptoms. In contrast, clinical studies of low speed, rear end collisions produced symptoms in healthy, primarily male subjects, that were in a safety enhanced environment. Siegmund, Brault and Wheeler documented symptoms in 29 percent of subjects tested with a Δv of 2.5 miles per hour and 39 percent tested at five miles per hour in a staged, safety-enhanced crash test.[36,37] Researchers from the University of Rochester School of Medicine documented that 38 percent of female drivers and 19 percent of male drivers reported neck pain lasting one day or more following low speed rear end collisions

where there was no damage reported. In one study, when the vehicle damage was listed as minor, 54 percent of female and 34 percent of male drivers reported neck pain lasting one day or more.[39]

8. The forces documented by Allen were done with the accelerometer or measurement tool on the top of a helmet that was not securely fastened to the subjects. He evaluated the peak acceleration in one plane. This represents only one variable. The Siegmund study documented that 16 distinct variables are required to reach an 80 percent predictive accuracy on whether symptoms would occur.

9. Since the Allen study did not produce injuries, there was clearly no threshold established for tissue injury.

10. In a study by Kumar it was documented that if a subject is prepared for a collision, the peak acceleration for men was reduced by 27–36 percent and for women it was reduced by 29–34 percent.[40] It can be assumed that the Allen study underestimated the significance of this variable. Ryan realized that the unprepared occupant increases the injury potential by up to 15 times.[41] Sturznegger listed this as one of the four most important complicating factors in a rear end collision.[42] Muhlbauer documented that there was a dramatic increase in the head acceleration in the rear impact volunteer studies if the head was away from the headrest at the time of impact. They documented a difference from 5 G when the headrest was effective and 12 G when it was not for an impact that was performed at a Delta-v of 10.5 km/hour.[43] The Allen study, and others like it are measuring acceleration values for prepared subjects, which is not comparable to real life events.

11. The G-force deals with forces of gravity in a single plane whereas recent literature indicates that *multi-vector* forces are the cause of injury in low speed rear end collisions.[17]

EVALUATING INJURY POTENTIAL

To adequately evaluate injury potential we must cause tissue damage. This commonly results in pain due to the mechanical, chemical, and physical stimulation of pain receptors. The most popular comparative methods to obtain data and use it in other event analysis are: hybrid dummy crash tests, animal testing, finite element modeling, cadaver studies, and human volunteer tests.

The *finite element modeling method* incorporates known values for certain structures and then has the computer run simulations to evaluate the potential outcomes. This of course is dependent on the initial information, which is not available on real life events and patients.

The *hybrid dummy crash tests* are helpful in evaluating the patterns of motion, deformation, and kinematics, but this does not evaluate the tolerance of human tissue. The data from these tests cannot be used to determine actual tissue damage caused by real life traumatic events. The studies by Davis, Siegmund, Nordhoff, and others documented that the variability of all of the factors used in accident reconstruction prohibits the use of these reports in the medical-legal arena.[44,45]

The *cadaver studies* do provide data on kinematics and tissue injury. This area of research has produced impressive rear end collision data.[34,46–54] These articles have also documented that biomechanically the rear end mechanism places the cervical spine in an injury position that is not encountered anywhere else.

The area that garners the most attention is the *human volunteer tests*. As with any test involving human subjects these studies must pass the scrutiny of a review board to ensure that the exposures that the volunteers must face are not harmful. These staged tests commonly use young healthy males that know that they are volunteering for a crash test, are aware of the impending collision, and also have the benefit of a safety-enhanced environment. Some authors of crash tests state that the occupants were unaware due to blinding techniques, but they still know what is about to happen. The human volunteer data is similar to the other methods in that it does derive some basic motion pattern information but does not have any validity as a tool for comparisons on human tissue tolerance to injury.

Animal studies may give insight into patterns of tissue deformation and injury, but the tissue tolerance levels are being established on animals and not humans.

Therefore, problems exist with each method of biomechanical testing, such as:

- the human population cannot be compared to animals due to differences in anatomy
- human test subjects cannot be loaded to cause any injury
- mathematical models are difficult to validate and there is a tendency to use the model beyond its validation boundaries
- hybrid dummy responses are different than humans.

The patients in real life motor vehicle collisions are not the same as the subjects in these tests. The vehicles have variability, the conditions have variability, and of course no two humans are alike. These factors make the comparisons academically interesting, but not valid for the medical-legal arena.

The Load–Deformation/Stress–Strain Graph

There are several problems with human volunteer tests when the expert attempts to use this data and make it relative to a real life traumatic event. To accurately evaluate injury and tissue damage, a stress–strain graph and/or a load–deformation graph documenting the point of permanent deformation must be obtained.[55,56] This is simple to do in a lab but difficult when you are evaluating a patient as you cannot use surgical investigation techniques to evaluate the tissue integrity. Cadaveric studies document lesions only via autopsy, and radiographic studies often are not sensitive and specific enough to confirm or deny injury.

The true evaluation of tolerance involves a stress–strain graph and also requires tissue deformation to the point where permanent tissue damage is sustained. Obviously, this cannot be accomplished with dummies, finite element modeling, and computer reconstructions. Human crash tests cannot set up a test where human injury is the goal, or any other postulation of what is a patient's tolerance. Cadaver tests have been the most revealing on the mechanisms involved in the rear end collision.[57] However, the cadaver tests may underestimate the forces and mechanisms involved in the rear end collision due to the complicating factors that can only be appreciated with live subjects in real life accidents.

In simple terms loading causes deformation, whether it be deformation of metal, plastic, glass, or human tissue (disc, bone, muscle, tendon, ligament, joint capsule, etc). If a load in a known direction is imposed on a structure, deformation of that structure can be measured and plotted on a load–deformation curve. Strength and stiffness and other mechanical properties of the structure can be gained by this curve.

In this graph, the load is on the vertical axis and deformation on the horizontal axis. The elastic region is the part of the curve where no deformation occurs with the progressively increasing load. The plastic region, plotted past the *yield point*, is where deformation occurs. The energy required to cause this deformation is the area under the curve. The ultimate failure point is where the structure cannot return to its pre-load state when the load is removed (Figure 1-2). This graph can be used to evaluate both organic and inorganic materials.

In the initial phase of the graph, the elastic portion, recovery of the material or tissue can occur; the elasticity of the tissues determines its capacity to return to its original shape when the load is removed. The yield point is the elastic limit of the structure or when plastic deformation occurs. Soft tissues are viscoelastic, and do not respond well to inertial loading or jolting forces like the ones experienced in a rear end collision.

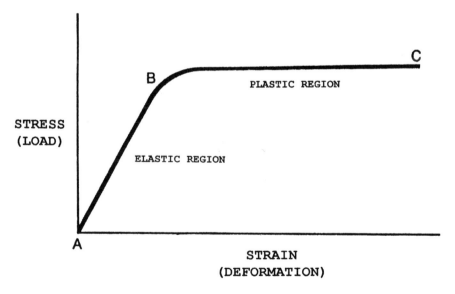

Figure 1-2 If a load is imposed on a structure, deformation of that structure can be measured and plotted on the stress–strain or load–deformation curve. In this graph, the load is on the vertical axis and deformation on the horizontal axis. The elastic region (AB) is the part of the curve where no deformation occurs with a progressively increasing load. The plastic region (BC), plotted past the yield point (B), is where deformation occurs. The energy required to cause this deformation is the area under the curve. The ultimate failure point (C) is where the structure cannot return to its pre-load state when the load is removed.

Therefore, the load–deformation curve provides the following information:

a. The load a structure can sustain before failure occurs
b. The deformation the structure can sustain before failing
c. Strength of a material or structure is determined by how much energy the structure or tissue can store and is indicated by the size of the area under the curve. The larger the area, the stronger the energy that builds up in the structure as the load is applied
d. The slope of the elastic region of the curve determines the stiffness of the structure. A steep slope indicates a stiff structure.

The load–deformation/stress–strain curve evaluates the different stiffness properties of different structures. For example, glass has no bend prior to breaking, so the yield point of glass is almost zero and there is a very small plastic region as it has little deformation prior to failure. Metal, conversely, deforms greatly prior to yielding so it will have a high plastic area on a stress–strain curve.

Structures can be evaluated in tension, compression, bending, shear, or torsion. The low speed, rear end collision creates several of these forces at the same time making the injury potential greater.

The techniques and studies used by accident reconstructionists and others to evaluate whether an injury did occur or if the tolerance for injury was exceeded, typically do not incorporate the load–deformation/stress–strain curve, so they cannot be evaluating the tolerance of any specific structure or tissue. Any comment on the injury potential to an occupant involved in a motor vehicle accident that does not use these methods is therefore invalid.

The ability of different structures to have different failure rates with similar loading conditions allows us to understand how one person can be injured in a traumatic event while another might not be. A recent article about a famous female model demonstrated a left frontal impact (11 o'clock) to a car where she was the front seat passenger. She sustained significant injuries including a liver laceration and near death. This accident caused only minor trauma to the driver of the car. The PDOF in that accident concentrated the seat belt loading across the area that caused the model's liver laceration. An exact opposite right frontal collision (1 o'clock) may have placed her spleen at risk for injury due to the altered motion and loading patterns. The injury to the model's liver was easily explained from a biomechanical loading perspective.

The biovariability of the population and the variability of most traumatic events make comparisons almost impossible when the issue is tissue tolerance or injury potential. The current available diagnostic tests are not adequate to isolate some of the common whiplash disorders.

Several cadaver studies on the whiplash injury mechanism have documented rim lesions in the discs, subchondral defects, fractures, bruising, damage, interarticular inclusions, hemarthrosis, facet capsule injuries, articular pillar injuries, and other injuries that were not appreciated on any of the diagnostic studies previously performed.[58–66] Lord and Bogduk documented that only four of the 73 lesions that were identified at autopsy were visualized on the standard diagnostic studies.

MECHANISMS OF INJURY IN THE LOW PROPERTY DAMAGE, REAR END COLLISION

This section will evaluate the proposed or validated methods of injury that have been documented to occur in the rear end collision. The goal of the biomechanics expert in this field is to explain the mechanism of injury, giving a plausible explanation for tissue injury based upon accepted tolerance values for those tissues. Any evaluation must include comprehensive knowledge of the pain sensitive structures and the distribution of the body that they express themselves.

Pain sensitive structures include the discs, facet joints, and their capsules. The facet joint, capsules, discs and other pain sensitive structures of the upper body are at risk for injury in the low speed, property damage collision primarily due to the altered loading that occurs early in this event. Early studies by Bogduk and others documented that during the rear end collision a change in the normal motion patterns in the cervical spine occurs.[67] The initial compression induced to the spine by the loading of the seatback and the inertia of the head and torso cause a reduction in the load bearing ability of the spine between the head and torso.[68,69]

The shear mechanism that occurs when the sigmoid curve or S-shaped curve is produced from the loading of the torso by the seat causes the lower cervical facets to go into relative hyperextension at the same time the upper cervical facets are in hyperflexion.[46,47] An S-shaped curve is produced from this differential motion (Figure 1-3) In a rear end collision the S-shaped curve induced by the differential forces occurring at the same time causes a gliding of the facets on top of each other that is not the natural motion of these intersegmental joints.[46] When this occurs, the posterior facets get "jammed together" and the gliding places increased stress on the anterior and posterior pain sensitive structures (the facets, facet capsules, discs, annulus, anterior and posterior longitudinal ligaments, meniscoid infolding). This causes increased injury potential. This also explains why the low speed, property damage collision can create symptoms when other ostensibly similar loading events do not.

The study by Kaneoka, documented that in a rear end collision the spine is altered where the vertebral facets cannot slide smoothly on top of each other but instead one vertebra rotates or spins on top of the other.[46] This causes tension on one part of the joint complex and compression on the other, both injury mechanisms in low impact collisions.

Van den Kroonenberg documented that the rear end low speed collision causes significant compression.[35] This article documented that the spine experiences 50 lb of compression at the same time it experiences a 22-lb shear load in a six mile per hour impact. This article also documented that a 20 percent reduction in the neck circumference resulted in an increase in head acceleration by 2.5 times which further documents the variance of loading tolerance in these rear end events. Yang documented that compression lowers the tolerance level to load or force in the cervical spine.[70,71] This load decreases the spine's ability to withstand shear by 73 percent at the C5-6 joint, 57 percent at the C4-5 joint, 50 percent at the C3-4 joints, and 50 percent at the C2-3 joint. The compression factor and shear has been documented as some of the most prevalent injury mechanisms in the low property damage, rear end collision. These two articles document

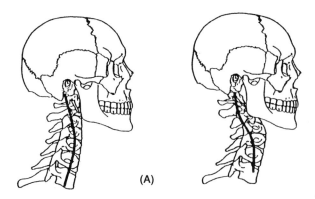

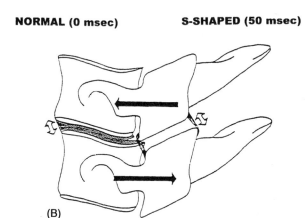

NORMAL (0 msec)   S-SHAPED (50 msec)

(A)

(B)

Figure 1-3 (A) The S-shaped curve occurs 50–75 milliseconds after impact. The curve is caused by early flexion of the upper cervical spine at the same time that the low cervical spine is undergoing extension. (B) The translating vertebra (dark arrows) will stress disc and ligament structures. (Modified from Grauer JN, Panjabi MM, Cholewicki J, Nibu K, Dvorak J. Whiplash produces an S-shaped curvature of the neck with hyperextension at lower levels. *Spine* 1997; 21:2489–2494.)

that even in a six mile per hour impact collision, several pain sensitive structures in the spine are at a compromised position for injury. The work by these, and other authors, outlines how the pain sensitive structures are injured in these rear end events.

This differential loading environment increases the likelihood of injury in the rear end collision and even in no property damage collisions. The values produced to the occupants are well above the reported tissue tolerance values due to these differential loading patterns. Damage to vehicles has been documented to be absent in impact speeds as high as 12–18 miles per hour.[72,73]

Boszczyk *et al* also documented that the facet capsule acts as a fibrocartilaginous wraparound ligament that withstands compression in addition to tension during torsional movements of the spine and helps to limit movement. This structure was also documented as having pain sensitive fibers histologicaly.[74] This work was further explored and validated by Cavanaugh who documented that stimulation of the facet capsule through distention or stretching fired the pain receptors locally and had a diffuse effect on the myofascial tissues in the same area across several levels.[75] This further documented how trauma to the disc and facet structures can contribute to the development of a diffuse myofascial pain syndrome, which is commonly encountered in patients that have had rear end collisions.

In addition, others have supported the sigmoid curve, and facet joint-capsule loading injury mechanisms documented by these authors. Panjabi and the authors of the other facet capsule and intersegmental axis of rotation articles noted that damage occurs in the early phase of the whiplash event. They use the term, *subcatastrophic capsule or joint failure*.[76–78] This term suggests that the pain sensitive facet capsule and joint structures (interarticular meniscoids, articular pillar, articular cartilage) are exposed to a loading trauma that does not create instability but does create tissue damage. Panjabi states that this could be one of the major contributing causes of the chronic pain syndrome as this sub-failure could lead to degeneration and instability syndromes later on.[79–81] These are the exact lesions documented on autopsy studies that were not identified on standard imaging and exam techniques.

Spinal injection studies have also documented pain referral patterns commonly encountered in the rear end collision patient.[82–84] Upper cervical level injections into pain sensitive structures have been documented to refer pain to the head, and lower level injections have been documented to refer pain to the posterior shoulder and upper back area.

This consistency of the research including autopsy studies, cadaver biomechanical experiments and human volunteer injection pain mapping studies give the whiplash event face validity. The sigmoid curve is not experienced in any other known loading event making it unique to the rear end collision. Cusick, Yogadan and Pintar reviewed the recent advances in the area of whiplash injury mechanisms. This addressed the vulnerability of several pain sensitive structures in the head and neck that are potential sites of pain after a rear end collision.[85] They concluded that:

> The nonphysiologic kinematic responses during whiplash impact may induce stresses in certain upper cervical neural structures or lower facet joints, resulting in possible compromise sufficient to elicit either neuropathic or nociceptive pain. These dynamic alterations of the upper level (occipit to C2) could impact potentially adverse forces to related neural structures, with subsequent development of neuropathic pain processes. The pinching of the lower facet joints may lead to potential for local tissue injury and nociceptive pain.

Bogduk[86,87] has commented that:

> Minor injuries of the cervical spine are essentially defined as injuries that do not involve a fracture. Some fractures that do not cause instability could be classified as minor injuries but are in a gray zone as is the fracture of the articular process or across the edge of the vertebral body. Archetypical of minor cervical injury is the whiplash injury. Among other reasons, neck pain after whiplash has been controversial because critics do not credit that an injury to the neck can occur in a whiplash event. In pursuit of the injury mechanism, bioengineers have used mathematical modeling, cadaver studies, and human volunteers to study the kinematics of the neck under the conditions of whiplash. Particularly illuminating have been the cinephotographic and cineradiographic studies of cadavers and normal volunteers.
>
> They demonstrate that externally, the head and neck do not exceed normal physiologic limits. However, the cervical spine undergoes a sigmoid deformation very early after impact. During this deformation, lower cervical segments undergo posterior rotation around an abnormally high axis of rotation, resulting in abnormal separation of the anterior elements of the cervical spine, and impaction of the zygapophyseal joints. The demonstration of a mechanism of injury of the zygapophyseal joints complements postmortem studies that reveal lesions in these joints, and clinical studies that have demonstrated that zygapophyseal joint pain is the single most common basis for chronic neck pain after injury.

OTHER INJURY MECHANISMS

Peripheral Myofascial Entrapment

The myofascial tissues of the upper quarter are for the most part viscoelastic tissues. As noted earlier, these tissues do not respond well to inertial loading conditions, which is what the rear end collision is. This indicates that the myofascial structures, which lay in close proximity to the neurovascular structures, could sustain sub-failure injuries.

The documented healing mechanism for these injuries is with type III collagen scar formation. Kellett, Oakes, Van der Meulen, Cohen, and others have documented that this healing tissue is less elastic, less mobile, and more sensitive than the original tissue.[88–91] Although most uncomplicated soft tissue injuries should heal in 6–8 weeks, not all do. One must keep in mind that scar tissue is never the same quality as the original tissue. Additionally, cervical spine structures are very pain sensitive and alterations of function will contribute to ongoing pain and possible migration of the pain process.

Rectus Capitis Posterior Minor Muscle

This muscle has been recently documented by Hack *et al.*, to have a fibrous band attachment to the outer layer of the dura matter.[92] This structure is located at the sub-occipital ridge and could logically be a large producer of cervicogenic head pain syndromes. McPartland documented that this structure shows atrophy characteristics in the posttraumatic whiplash head and neck pain population when compared to normal subjects.[93] Other authors confirmed this as well.[94] Vernon and others have documented that tension or stimulation of the dura can produce a diffuse head pain syndrome.[95]

Semispinalis Muscle

Magnusson performed surgical releases on 15 patients with intractable head pain after whiplash. He released the greater occipital nerve from the semispinalis muscle. This resulted in 72 percent of the patients reporting relief.[96]

Other articles have documented greater occipital, lesser occipital, and auricular peripheral entrapment syndromes.[97] Additionally, scar tissue surrounding the upper cervical nerve root(s) can cause peripheral nerve compression, and cervicogenic head pain, including vascular headache phenomena. These researchers operated on 16 patients, freeing the entrapped nerve roots. This resulted in 13/16 becoming pain free. The fact that this can be treated successfully in whiplash patients also validates the injury mechanism.

SCM and Other Myofascial/Myoneuronal Entrapments

McConnell documented that the head rotates around the Sternocleidomastoid (SCM) muscle during the low speed rear end collision.[98,99] McConnell listed this tensioning as an injury mechanism with an estimated impact speed tolerance to injury of five miles per hour. This was the tolerance for healthy male subjects in the crash test. This study was accepted as valid by the controversial and insurance funded Quebec whiplash study.[100] This mechanism explains some of the symptoms commonly associated with damage to the SCM muscle, which include head pain, dizziness, nausea, neck pain, restricted range of motion, and other upper quarter complaints.[97,101]

McConnell's work, quoted earlier, documented the SCM as a tissue that induces rotation due to its angular insertion. McConnell also found that tenderness in this muscle was one of the most common reported symptoms in test subjects after rear impact tests at less than eight miles per hour impact speeds.

Scalene, Pec Minor, Longus Coli, and Other Neurovascular Entrapments

Uhlig *et al.*, documented that cervical muscle biopsies in whiplash trauma patients demonstrated pathological changes in all tissue samples.[102] Sanders and Roo have also published several articles on the peripheral entrapment, Thoracic Outlet syndrome.[103] They stated:

> The soft tissue repair process has been documented by creating an area of type three collagen in the area of the tissue damage. This repair tissue is less elastic, more sensitive due to new pain fibers, and not as strong as the original tissue. If hypoxia and immobility occurs in the early phase of an injury this process may be extenuated.

The scalene, pec minor, first rib, and other structures have been documented by Roo, Sanders, and others as producing peripheral entrapment syndromes, including thoracic outlet syndrome. Controlled motion to break down the scar tissue cross fibers and enhance a good healing tissue is essential to help reduce the potential for long term soft tissue injury complications.[103,104]

Water Hammer Theory of Creating a Neuroma

Another possible injury mechanism proposed by Swedish researchers documented that an inertial jolt could cause a "water hammer" effect in the venous system of the cervical spine. They concluded that the inertial loading with associated spinal deformation causes a pressure pulse in the epidural venous plexus causing venous blood to be forced out of the veins in the intervertebral foramen. This causes a bruising injury to the spinal ganglion.[105–110] Bruising of the spinal nerve(s) could lead to neuroma formation. A neuroma is defined as a localized and painful nerve entrapment within scar tissue.

They further evaluated this theory by applying large doses of corticosteroids to a select group of patients presenting to an emergency room after a rear end collision and not to a control group. This study documented a statistically significant reduction in long-term disability and pain in the medicated group.[105] They concluded that the benefits of the corticosteroids were due to the alteration of the early changes associated with their proposed water hammer mechanism of injury, with prevention of the injury to the spinal ganglion. Their original studies included the verification of this phenomenon in low velocity whiplash simulations to animals and these lesions were documented upon autopsy. The studies quoted in the autopsy section also documented hematomas on the dorsal roots. Nerve root injury may also occur due to a pinching of the respective nerve root by bony structures in the IVF.

The abnormal motion induced to the cervical spine is certainly not experienced anywhere else that is known and especially cannot be compared to activities of daily living, bumper car rides, amusement park rides, or other safety enhanced or learned proprioceptive events.

Dorsal Root Ganglion (DRG), Discogenic Pain, and Other Pain Syndromes

The C2 dorsal root ganglion has been documented to be vulnerable to neurological compression syndromes. The C2 DRG occupies 76 percent of the space in the C2 IVF.[111] It was concluded that since entrapment of the C2 ganglion inevitably involves fibers that contribute to the greater occipital nerve, neurolysis of the greater occipital nerve by itself for treatment of post-traumatic headache syndromes would achieve limited success. Bogduk noted that during rotation combined with extension (e.g., whiplash injury) the posterior arch of the atlas and the superior articular process of the axis were approximated sufficiently to contact the C2 ganglion. Research by Muhle *et al.* documented that the neuroforaminal size decreased in extension by 20 percent.[112] This would imply that forced extension would decrease the C2 DRG space by up to 96 percent leaving little room for neural structures.

Further studies have documented a 90 percent success rate (average follow up 19.2 months) in a series of patients that underwent microsurgical decompression of the C2 ganglion for cervicogenic head pain.[113] Bogduk has documented success with neurotomy procedures for the upper cervical neurological structures in chronic head-neck pain syndrome patients.[114,115]

The dorsal root itself has been found to be both mechanically and chemically sensitive to changes in its environment and any deviation from the norm can produce increased firing of this pain sensitive structure. Leakage of chemicals from a traumatized disc could further irritate this structure.[116]

The intervertebral disc (IVD) has been documented as a source of central spine pain and extremity pain. Several articles have documented the mechanism of disc damage that occurs with concentrated force loading across the seat belt after a rear end collision. Changes in the lumbar and cervical lordosis can injure the disc. The initial flexed posture has been consistently documented as a pre-tensioning mechanism to the disc structures. Compression combined with the anterolateral loading causes significant forces across the outer annulus. An occupant with trunk rotation at time of impact is at great risk for an annular tear in a rear end collision. If the person is in a flexed and rotated position and is then rear-ended the vehicle moves out from under them and the mechanism for a disc injury to the annulus is established. Autopsy studies have documented rim lesions, herniations, and other discogenic damage to pain sensitive structures that were not evident on regular imaging techniques.[117–122] The advent of discography has identified several internally disrupted discogenic syndromes that do not refer pain in a classic radicular pattern.

Panjabi evaluated the vertebral artery and other vascular structures that have the potential for a vascular pain syndrome. The vertebral artery is a pain sensitive structure that when injured can cause a variety of vertebrobasilar neurologic syndromes (Wallenburg stroke, head pain, dizziness, nausea, vertigo, neck pain). Panjabi's work documented that the vertebral artery exceeded its elongation threshold or physiological limit in 2.5, 4.5, 6.5, and 8.5 G collision tests.[14] These load levels would be consistent with an impact speed that could leave a target vehicle with little or no property damage.

FACTORS THAT INCREASE INJURY IN REAR END LOW DAMAGE COLLISIONS

- As documented earlier, the rear end collision places the upper quarter in an injury prone position and therefore of itself is a risk factor for injury. Additionally, the rear end collision is a risk factor since treatment of injuries in this type of accident garners such a high percentage of the financial resources when compared to other impacts and it has been documented to produce an injurious force vector that is not identified in the other impacts.[123]
- Neck circumference is proposed as a risk factor for injury potential. A reduction in neck circumference by 20 percent increases the peak acceleration to the head and neck by 2.5 times.[35]
- There is a documented increased incidence of injury in females in the rear end collision.[13,41,42]
- *Mass of the target and bullet vehicles* has a direct relationship to injury. As explained earlier, if the mass of the bullet vehicle increases, its kinetic energy (KE) and momentum (*P*) follows suit. Therefore, damage energy increases if the bullet car is more hostile (larger) than the target vehicle. (KE $= \frac{1}{2}Mv^2$, and $P = Mv$).
- A greater impact speed of the bullet car increases its potential for damage according to the equation KE $= \frac{1}{2}Mv^2$. The velocity is squared, so if velocity increases the impact energy increases exponentially.
- *Drag factor of the road surface* will affect injury potential. If the road surface is dry the friction factor will increase. Anytime you increase friction in a low speed, property damage event you can increase the time of the collision. If the time of the collision increases, then the acceleration ($\Delta t/\Delta v$) increases, affecting injury potential. The opposite is also true. If the road surface is icy, wet, or has a reduced friction, then there is a higher likelihood that the energy of the collision will go to accelerating the target vehicle and not crushing it. This in turn will transfer more energy to the occupant cage (instead of the occupant). This concept must be reviewed with caution as it does not imply that the more damage that there is in a collision the less the injury potential. Once the damage threshold has been violated the injury potential changes due to the alteration of the mechanics. The low speed, property damage collision does however have a unique relationship to energy transfer as documented by Smith, Robbins, and others.
- *Body and head position at time of impact* directly affects injury potential. Flexion of the torso increases the tension across the lumbar disc structures and pre-disposes them to discogenic damage with loading.[118]
- Rotation of the neck increases the tension on one side of the neck and compression on the other thereby reducing the neck structures ability to withstand load. It has

been documented that abberant head position is a significant factor in the rear end collision prognosis.[41,42]

- The ability for the occupant to prepare for impact will affect injury potential. The study by Kumar documented that the peak acceleration to the head of a female was 29–34 percent higher in the unprepared female occupant and 27–34 percent higher for the unprepared male occupant. Sturzenegger documented this as one of four significant risk factors for chronic pain.[40]

- *Crashworthiness of the vehicles involved* in the collision directly affects injury potential. The hostility factor or mass-to-mass ratio and the bumper alignment of the target and bullet vehicles should be evaluated. The seat back was recently evaluated by Szabo and Welcher and they documented a dramatic difference in two different seat back designs.[21,32] The seat back, headrest, and overall crashworthiness of each vehicle do play a part in the injury potential. An SAE article documented the survivability of crashes per 1000 accidents for different makes of vehicles. This documented a variance that is up to 15 to 1.[124] It can easily be understood that an accident with an occupant in a large passenger car compared to a compact or sub-compact car will have a dramatically different injury potential.

- *Symptoms at the scene and within the initial 72 hours of the trauma* can be used to predict the chronicity of the injury. Loss or alteration of consciousness, dizziness, nausea, vision problems, bruises, cuts, abrasions, secondary collisions, and head pain post injury are all factors that can adversely affect recovery prognosis.

- *The Primary Direction of Force (PDOF)* will affect injury potential. The impact angle should be documented to see if a rotational component has been induced. The PDOF can tell the examiner which tissues were placed at compression or tension. For example, if the victim of an accident is subjected to forces that throw her forward and to the left, then the seat belt/chest restraint will create an area of load concentration on the liver.

CONCLUSIONS

The goal of documenting a human tolerance that is universally accepted will remain elusive due to the constraints of research that do not allow injury studies in laboratories on live volunteers to establish a database large enough to make it a valid tool for comparisons to the population. However, biomechanics is improving our understanding of the rear end injury mechanism, which could lead to increased safety standards and improved treatment outcomes.

The cadaver test, human pain mapping volunteer data, double blind injection studies, autopsy studies, and other studies have provided us with a better understanding of the pain mechanisms and pain producers in these low speed or low property damage, rear end collisions. However, these new techniques have not shown any promise in evaluating the individuality of the pain experience. Promising research by Kaneoka, Grauer, Ono, Panjabi, Bogduk, Lord, Taylor, Barnsley, Pintar, Yoganandan, and others has contributed greatly to our understanding of the unique nature of the loading that occurs in the rear end collision and why it is not comparable to other ostensibly similar loading events.

Brault *et al.*[36,37,125] has documented that the rear end collision has at least 16 factors that must be known to adequately evaluate the injury potential of any rear end traumatic event. The factors that Brault *et al.* required to adequately evaluate the injury potential of human crash test volunteers in a controlled environment cannot be obtained from an accident reconstruction that exists in real life. Studies by Szabo and King have documented that the damage threshold can be as high as 12 miles per hour for the impact speed, which is well above the level where symptoms have been documented in staged crash tests. This would suggest that the injury tolerance for actual accidents is much lower than the damage threshold. The five mile per hour healthy male threshold was upheld by the insurance funded Quebec study as a valid standard for the lower end of tolerance to impact for healthy males. This again would suggest that in the real world, the threshold for injury could be even lower. The Brault study documented symptoms in controlled labs at 2.5 and 5.0 miles per hour, both well below the expected level of property damage in most collisions. This data flies in the face of reconstructionists that state that a traumatic event was below the injury potential, their conclusions based only upon property damage and force estimates.

Brault, Davis, and others have also discussed the variability that is experienced in these staged crash tests when they use the same occupants and same vehicles at the same speeds.[36,37] Nordhoff has also discussed this variability, stating that the same crash tests on different occupants created a variance in the Δv values that varied from 6.7 to 12.0 G in a 5 mile per hour crash and 1.6 to 5.0 G for a 2.5 miles per hour crash.[126]

It stands to reason that if consistent force data cannot be produced on subjects under controlled circumstances with the same conditions in a lab, then the application of this data to the general population is invalid and does not meet the standards of the court system. The factors listed by these authors indicate that low speed, rear end collision reconstruction data in the real world may provide some information but is invalid in the use of injury causation, probability, or possibility.[36,37]

The area of biomechanics has made significant contributions to our knowledge of known risk factors for injury. In summary:

- Injury potential cannot be determined by an evaluation of the vehicle's property damage alone. In staged crash tests the variability of the acceleration values listed for different subjects indicates that the applicability of this data to the general population violates the laws of scientific study and basic logic. The diffuse variables that are present in all traumatic events make comparisons impossible. The most complex variable is the human tolerance to load and the pain experience.
- Reduced property damage in a rear end collision does not of itself validate that the event was low speed, low force, or that the injury potential was low. The national insurance databank indicates that most injuries occur in accidents where little or no property damage exists.
- Due to the storage and eventual transfer of kinetic energy and the failure of the vehicle structure to deform in low property damage accidents this energy is made available to create occupant injuries.[17,20]

- Energy and momentum in a collision are both conserved after the collision. Momentum is the damage potential of an object and is calculated by multiplying mass by velocity. If the energy of a collision does not cause crush damage the majority of the energy is transferred in the form of kinetic energy to the target vehicle.[17,20,33]
- The amount of energy that the occupant experiences has been consistently documented as being two to ten times that of the vehicle in low property damage, rear end collisions.[15,16,19]
- Conventional imaging methods do not appreciate the injuries that are commonly encountered in these low speed, rear end collisions and patients who have negative or inconclusive studies should not be listed as not being injured. Autopsy analysis of trauma patients has documented lesions only with microscopic analysis.[9,52,127,128]
- Recent research documents that the rear end collision creates a variety of unique injury mechanisms for the head and neck structures including the S-shaped curve, abnormal water hammer effect, and intersegmental axis of rotation changes.
- There are several pain sensitive structures that experience an overload stimulus in even no damage collisions to create pain in the structures in the upper quarter.
- Pain distribution studies have shown correlation with biomechanical cadaver and animal studies.
- There are several studies that document that the facet joints and capsules are a significant source of pain in the post motor vehicle accident, chronic pain population. They further document that these patients respond to double blind blocks, which further validates the injury mechanism. The facet joints of the cervical spine have to withstand 85 percent of the weight bearing force of the head. The facets' articular cartilage and cervical discs are avascular and require motion and osmosis for their nutrient and waste product exchange. The lack of cervical motion after injury prevents the healing nutrients from reaching these structures, further accelerating the degenerative process.
- Human tolerance to injury in rear end collisions is reduced with head rotation. Head rotation causes pre-tensioning of the cervical facet capsule and can predispose this very pain sensitive structure to sub-catastrophic failure or sub-failure.[5,6,14,41,42,76,77]
- The head restraints are not adequate in the majority of the cars on the road today. The average driver also does not sit in a safety-optimized position that would enhance the benefit of the headrest. If a patient is away from the headrest at impact the change in the acceleration factors to the head and neck are increased.
- The variability in the safety, mass, and quality of the vehicles today prohibits estimates of injury potential from simple photograph analysis or accident reconstructions.
- Accident reconstruction has several stages where an error in the factors used can result in a large error in the product. This value should always be a range and should only be used as additional information and not as an absolute evaluation of whether an injury did occur.
- The S-shaped curve, the change in the instantaneous axis of rotation, the decreased load tolerance with compression in the spine, the G-force alterations that occur with different neck circumferences, the pressure induced into the neural structures from the water hammer effect, the rectus capitis muscle injury, and other biomechanical research all support that the rear end collision has a unique injury mechanism.

Additionally, the biomechanical data, if interpreted properly, clearly supports several injury mechanisms in the low property damage rear end collision. To evaluate and manage low property damage, rear end collision patients, the physician must understand the pertinent research in this area and also have an up-to-date understanding of the pain syndromes and management tools available for these injuries.

- Vehicles are engineered to avoid crush in low speed events to reduce property damage costs. As described earlier, if the energy of the low speed crash does not go to crushing the vehicle (which increases the Delta-t or time of the collision), it will go to accelerating the vehicle and increase the kinetic energy of the target vehicle thereby increasing the damage potential. The mass of the striking vehicle and the immediate pre-impact velocity will determine the initial amount of energy available to cause injury to the occupant(s) of the target car.

There is no simple relationship between overall crash severity and the specific forces or tolerances experienced by the occupants. There is human variability, crash variability, scene condition variability, vehicle variability, subjective interpretation variability, and a multitude of other factors that preclude any traumatic event from being quantified, as they are all different. It is true that mathematics, physics, engineering, and other sciences can influence medicine in a positive way. However, this should be limited to evaluating if the injury patterns are consistent with the forces, not whether the injuries are consistent with the force values. The focus should be on making automobile travel safer, more efficient, and on innovation, not controversy and speculation.

The engineering world is not a perfect one. The prediction of an event retrospectively from a set of information that is proven to be inadequate is not only invalid, it violates the laws of our court systems and attempts to elevate engineers to the level of a treating physician (MD, DO, chiropracter). When an engineer's statements alter or direct patient care, it is the patient who potentially suffers. The practicing physicians should become familiar with these concepts to ensure that they do not induce bias into their decision-making due to the lack of information about the true kinematics and biomechanics of these low property damage, rear end collisions.

Physicians should not label patients with negative studies as having no injury. A thorough exam, history, subjective profile including pain distribution mapping, and evaluation of the biomechanics of the trauma can identify several factors that will not be appreciated on special studies. There are many reasons why acute pain becomes chronic. Some contributing factors include:

1. Poor evaluation and management (e.g., the prolonged use of a soft collar in the absence of instability, the overuse of potent medications, and the chronic use of passive modalities that establish provider-patient learned helplessness or dependency) can contribute to delayed recovery. The failure to properly workup a patient and obtain accurate diagnoses may ultimately contribute to the development of chronic pain. This problem can at times be avoided by involving other professionals at an early stage of delayed recovery or diagnosis. The physician is still responsible for educating patients on what they have, determining whether they are the right provider for them, and instructing the patient on self-management tools to promote

recovery. This will help calm the fears over hurt verses harm as they go through the rehabilitation process.

2. The system can also fail the patient. Frustration about perceived poor treatment and lack of improvement, medico-legal enticements, and other system failures can contribute to delayed recovery.
3. The patient may not have the psychological tools to recover. Some patients have sustained childhood or spousal abuse, or they may have other unresolved psychological traumas that contribute to the development of chronic pain.
4. The injuries sustained may be too great for our physical sciences and evaluation methods to cure. It is not inconceivable that the health care sciences simply cannot isolate and fix a posttraumatic problem. The intricacy of the nervous system and the personalized nature of the pain experience make this very possible.

A final warning is advised to all physicians and engineers to stay within the purview of their respective fields. Engineers should not practice medicine. There are several arguments that are still raised against the validity of the whiplash event including:

- without the potential for litigation in the system, the incidence of injury is reduced
- no property damage means no injury
- a rear end collision can be compared to other simple loading activities like plopping in a chair
- pathological tissue changes are not associated with simple soft tissue injuries.

The information provided in this chapter disputes these conclusions.

Physicians should take the time to evaluate the truly unique forces that are generated in the rear end collision and work to identify a model of care that works on results. The biomechanical information that has been obtained in the last 10 years will hopefully go to reducing the existence of these injuries through better design methods and enable physicians to explore new treatment paradigms to enhance patient care and safety at the same time.

REFERENCES

1. Davis C. Rear impacts: vehicle and occupant response. *J Manipulative Physiol Ther* 1998; 21(9): 629.
2. Davis CG. Injury threshold. Whiplash associated disorders. *J Manipulative Physiol Ther*, 2000; 23(6): 420.
3. Croft A. Practical auto crash reconstruction in LOSPIC Parts 1–5. *Dynamic Chiropractic* 1999–2000.
4. Bogduk N. Treatment of whiplash injuries. In Malaga GA (ed). *Cervical Flexion-Extension/Whiplash Injuries. Spine State of the Art Reviews*, pp 469–483. Philadelphia, Hanley and Belfus; 1998.
5. Panjabi M, Vasvada A, White A. Biomechanics of the cervical spine and whiplash injuries. *Sem Spine Surg* 1998, 10(2): 141.
6. Panjabi M, Cholewicki J, Nibu K, *et al.* Simulation of whiplash trauma using whole cervical spine specimens. *Spine* 1998; 23(1): 17.
7. Winkelstein B, Nightingale R, Richardson W, Myers B. The cervical facet capsule and its role in whiplash injury. *Spine* 2000; 25(10): 1238.
8. Winkelstein BA, McLendon RE, Babir A *et al.* An anatomic investigation of the cervical facet capsule quantifying muscle insertion area. *J Anatomy* 2001; 198(Pt4): 455.

9. Yoganandan N, Pintar F, Kleinberger M. Cervical vertebral and facet joint kinematics under whiplash. *J Biomech Eng* 1998; 120: 305

10. Watts AJ, Atkinson DR, Hennessy CJ. *Low Speed Automobile Accidents*, 2nd ed. Tucson, AZ, Lawyers & Judges Publishing Co., 1999.

11. Lord SM, Barnsley L, Wallis BJ, Bogduk N. Chronic cervical Zygapophyseal joint pain after whiplash. A placebo-controlled prevalence study. *Spine* 1996; 21: 1737.

12. Cervicogenic Headache Society Meeting. Presentation by Bogduk, N, Las Vegas, Nevada, 1998. http://www.cervicogenic.com

13. Sturzenegger M, DiStefano G, *et al.* SAE Pub 912913. Society of Automobile Engineers. SAE World Headquarters, 400 Commonwealth Drive, Warrendale, PA 15096; SAE Automotive Headquarters, 755 W. Big Beaver, Suite 1600, Troy MI 48084; SAE Washington Office, 1300 Eye Street N.W., Washington, DC 20005.

14. Panjabi M, Cholewicki J, Nibu K, Grauer J, *et al.* Mechanisms of whiplash injury. *Clin Biomech* 1998; 13: 239.

15. Croft A. Auto crash reconstruction in LOSRIC, Parts 1–5. Dynamic Chiropractic Archives. Part 1. Volume 17(12) 5/31/99, Part 2. Volume 17(14) 6/28/99, Part 3 Volume 17(16) 7/26/99, Part 4. Volume 17(18) 8/23/99, Part 5. Volume 17(20) 9/20/99. (no page numbers are given)

16. Foreman SM. Acceleration-deceleration injuries. In Foreman SM, Croft AC (eds). *Whiplash Injuries. The Cervical Acceleration Deceleration Syndrome*, 2nd Ed. Williams & Wilkins, Baltimore, MD, 1995.

17. Smith JJ, *Biomechanics, Statistics, of Automobile Rear Impact Collisions.* Auto Litigation-Colorado Chapter, June 1993.

18. Severy D, Mathewson J, Bechtol C. *Controlled automobile rear end collisions—an investigation of related engineering and medical phenomena.* Medical Aspects of Traffic Accidents, Proceedings of the Montreal Conference, 1955. 152.

19. Navin, Romilly. *An investigation into vehicle and occupant response to rear impacts.* Proceedings of the Multidisciplinary Road Safety Conference VI. June 5–7, 1989.

20. Robbins MC. *The lack of relationship between vehicle damage and occupant injury*, SAE Pub 970494. Society of Automotive Engineers. SAE World Headquarters, 400 Commonwealth Drive, Warrendale, PA 15096; SAE Automotive Headquarters, 755 W. Big Beaver, Suite 1600, Troy MI 48084; SAE Washington Office, 1300 Eye Street N.W., Washington, DC 20005.

21. Szabo T, Welcher J. *Dynamics of low speed crash test with energy absorbing bumpers*, SAE Pub 921573. New York, Society of Automotive Engineers, 1992.

22. King D, Siegmund G, Bailey M. *Automobile bumper behavior in low speed impacts*, SAE Pub 930211. Detroit, Society of Automotive Engineers, 1993.

23. Allen ME, Weir-Jones J, Motiuk DR, *et al.* Accelerations: perturbations of daily living. A comparison to whiplash. *Spine* 1994; 19(11): 1285.

24. Rosenbluth W, Hicks L. Evaluating Low Speed Rear Impact Severity and Resultant Occupant Stress Parameters. *J Forensic Sci* 1994 1393.

25. Freeman M, Croft A, Rossignol A, Weaver D, Reiser M. A review and methodological critique of the literature refuting whiplash syndrome. *Spine* 1999; 24(1): 86.

26. Freeman M, Croft C, Rossignol A. Whiplash associated disorders: Redefining whiplash and its management by the Quebec Task Force. *Spine* 1998; 23(9): 1043.

27. Sanders M, McCormick E. *Human Factors in Engineering and Design,* 7th ed. New York, McGraw Hill, 1993.

28. McConnell W, Howard R, Poppel J, *et al.* *Human neck-head kinematics after low velocity rear impacts. Understanding whiplash.* In. 29th Stapp Car Crash Conference Proceedings, 95274, pp. 215–238. 1995, Phoenix, AZ.

29. McConnell WE, Howard RP, Guzman HM, *et al.* SAE tech paper series, pp 21–31, SAE Pub 930889. Society of Automotive Engineers, 1993. SAE World Headquarters, 400 Commonwealth Drive, Warrendale, PA 15096; SAE Automotive Headquarters, 755 W. Big Beaver, Suite 1600, Troy MI 48084; SAE Washington Office, 1300 Eye Street N.W., Washington, DC 20005.

30. King, D, Siegmund G, Bailey M. *Automobile bumper behavior in low speed impacts*. SAE Pub 930211. Detroit, Society of Automotive Engineers. SAE World Headquarters, 400 Commonwealth Drive, Warrendale, PA 15096; SAE Automotive Headquarters, 755 W. Big Beaver, Suite 1600, Troy MI 48084; SAE Washington Office, 1300 Eye Street N.W., Washington, DC 20005.

31. Navin F, McNabb M. *An investigation into vehicle and occupant response subjected to low speed rear impacts*. Proceedings of the Multidisciplinary Road Safety conference June 5–7, 1989.

32. Szabo T, Welcher J, Anderson R, *et al*. *Human occupant kinematic response to low speed rear impacts*, SAE Pub 940532. New York, Society of Automotive Engineers, 1994.

33. Mellon M. *The Guide to Low Velocity Whiplash Biomechanics*. Olympia WA, Body Mind Publications, 1997.

34. Yang KH, Begeman PC, Muser M, *et al*. *On the role of cervical facet joints in rear end impact neck injury mechanisms*. Society of Automotive Engineers, 1997; SAE 970497.

35. van den Kroonenberg A, Philippens M, Cappon H, *et al*. *Human head–neck response during low speed rear end impacts*. 42nd Stapp Car Crash Conference Proceedings (P-337), SAE document number 983158. Society of Automotive Engineers, 1998.

36. Brault J, Wheeler J, Siegmund G, *et al*. Clinical response of human subjects to rear end automobile collisions. *Arch Physical Med Rehabil* 1998; 79: 72.

37. Siegmund GP, King DJ, Lawrence JM, *et al*. *Head and neck kinematic response of human subjects in low speed rear end collisions*, pp m 357–385, SAE Pub 973341. Warrendale, Society of Automobile Engineers, 1997. SAE World Headquarters, 400 Commonwealth Drive, Warrendale, PA 15096; SAE Automotive Headquarters, 755 W. Big Beaver, Suite 1600, Troy MI 48084; SAE Washington Office, 1300 Eye Street N.W., Washington, DC 20005.

38. Nordhoff LS. Motor vehicle collision injuries. Nordhoff LS (ed). *Mechanisms, Diagnosis, and Management*. Gaithersburg, Maryland, Aspen Publishers, Inc. 1996.

39. Rochester School of Medicine Lecture at the Society of Automotive Engineers Whiplash Conference 1998, Phoenix, AZ. SAE World Headquarters, 400 Commonwealth Drive, Warrendale, PA 15096; SAE Automotive Headquarters, 755 W. Big Beaver, Suite 1600, Troy MI 48084; SAE Washington Office, 1300 Eye Street N.W., Washington, DC 20005.

40. Kumar S, Narayan Y, Amell T. Role of awareness in head–neck acceleration in low velocity rear impacts. *Compendium of papers presented at the Traffic Safety and Auto Engineering Stream, World Congress on Whiplash Associated Disorders*. 1999; 276.

41. Ryan GA, Taylor GW, Moore VM, Dolinis J. Neck strain in car occupants. *Injury* 1994; 25: 533.

42. Sturzenegger M, DiStefano G, Radanov B, Schnidrig A. Presenting symptoms and signs after whiplash injury. The influence of accident mechanisms. *Neurology* 1994; 4: 688.

43. Muhlbaur M, Eichberger A, Geigl BC, Steffan H. Analysis of kinematics and acceleration behavior of the head and neck in experimental rear impact collisions. *Neuro Orthopedics* 1999; 25: 1.

44. Davis C. Injury threshold whiplash associated disorders. *JMPT* 2000; 23(6): 420.

45. Siegmund G, King DJ, Lawrence JM, *et al*. *Head/neck kinematic response of human subjects in low speed collisions*, SAE Pub 973341. SAE 41st Stapp Car Crash Conference Proceedings 1997.

46. Kaneoka K, Ono K, Inami S, Hayashi K. Motion analysis of cervical vertebrae during whiplash loading. *Spine* 1999; 8: 763.

47. Grauer JN, Panjabi MM, Cholewicki J, Nibu K, Dvorak J. Whiplash produces an s-shaped curvature of the neck with hyperextension at lower levels. *Spine* 1997; 21: 2489.

48. Ono K, Kaneoka K, Wittek A, and Kajzer J. *Cervical injury mechanism based on analysis of human cervical vertebral motion and head–neck-torso kinematics during low speed rear end impacts*, SAE Pub 973340. Detroit, Society od Automotive Engineers, 1997.

49. Stapp Car Conference 39th Proceedings. Sponsored by the SAE. SAE World Headquarters, 400 Commonwealth Drive, Warrendale, PA 15096; SAE Automotive Headquarters, 755 W. Big Beaver, Suite 1600, Troy MI 48084; SAE Washington Office, 1300 Eye Street N.W., Washington, DC 20005.

50. Panjabi M, Cholewicki J, Nibu K, *et al*. Mechanism of whiplash injury. *Clin Biomech* 1998; 13: 239.

51. Yoganandan N, Pintar F, Kleinberger M. Cervical vertebral and facet joint kinematics under whiplash. *J Biomech Eng* 1998; 120: 305.

52. Yoganandan N, Pintar FA, *et al.* Facet joint local component kinetics in whiplash trauma. *ASME Adv Bioeng* 1997; 36: 221.

53. Yang KH, Begeman PC. *A proposed role for facet joints in neck pain in low to moderate speed rear impacts.* Part I. Biomechanics 6th Injury Prevention Through Biomechanics Symposium, May 9–10, 1996.

54. Bogduk N. Acute and chronic whiplash. *Spineline* 2001. Volume 11, Issue 5: 8.

55. Nordin M, Frankel V. *Basic Biomechanics of the Musculoskeletal System,* 2nd ed. Philadelphia, PA, Lippincott Williams & Wilkins, 1989.

56. Whiting W, Zernicke R. *Biomechanics of Musculoskeletal Injury.* Human Kinetics, Publisher. 1st Ed, 1998.

57. Panjabi M, Cholewicki J, Nibu K, *et al.* Simulation of whiplash trauma using whole cervical spine specimens. *Spine* 1998; 23(1): 17.

58. Schonstrom N, Twomey L, Taylor J. The lateral Atlanto–Axial joints and their synovial folds. An in vitro study of the soft tissue injuries and fractures. *J Trauma* 1993; 35(6): 886.

59. Taylor JR, Twomey LT. Neck Injuries. *Lancet.* 1991, 338: 1343.

60. Taylor JR, Taylor MM. Cervical spinal injuries an autopsy of 109 blunt injuries. *J Musculoskeletal Pain* 1996; 4: 61.

61. Jonsson H, Bring G, Raushning W, *et al.* Hidden cervical spine injuries in traffic accident victims with scull fractures. *J Spinal Disord* 1991; 4:251.

62. Abel MS. Occult traumatic lesions of the cervical vertebrae. *Crit Rev Clin Radiol Nucl Med* 1975; 6(4): 469.

63. Twomey LT, Taylor JR, Taylor MM. Unsuspected damage to the lumbar zygapophyseal (facet) joints after motor-vehicle accidents. *Med J Aust* 1989; 151(4): 210, 215.

64. Rauschning W, McAfee P, Jonsson H. Pathoanatomical and surgical findings in cervical spinal injuries. *J Spinal Disord.* 1989; 2(4): 213.

65. Unterharnscheidt F. Pathological and neuroanatomical findings in Rhesus monkeys subjected to −*Gx* and +*Gx* indirect impact accelerations. In Sances A, Jr, Thomas DJ, Unterharnscheidt F, *et al. Mechanism of Head and Spine Trauma,* pp 565–663. Gosher NY, Aloray. 1982.

66. Davis D, Bohlman H, Walker AE, *et al.* The pathological findings in fatal craniospinal injuries. *J Neurosurg* 1971; 34: 603.

67. Bogduk N. Treatment of whiplash injuries. In Malanga GA (ed). *Cervical Flexion–Extension Injuries. Spine State of the Art Reviews,* pp 469–483. Philadelphia, PA, Hanley and Belfus, 1998.

68. Matsushita T, Sata T, Hiraboyashi K, *et al. X-ray study of the human neck motion due to head inertia loading,* SAE Pub 942208. Society of Automobile Engineers, 1994. SAE World Headquarters, 400 Commonwealth Drive, Warrendale, PA 15096; SAE Automotive Headquarters, 755 W. Big Beaver, Suite 1600, Troy, MI 48084; SAE Washington Office, 1300 Eye Street N.W., Washington, DC 20005.

69. Matsushiata T, Yamazak N, Sata T, *et al.* Biomechanical and medical investigations into human neck injury in low velocity collisions. *Neuro-Orthopedics* 1997; 21: 27.

70. Yang K, Begeman P. *On the role of cervical facet joints in rear impact neck injury mechanisms.* Society of Automotive Engineers, 1997. SAE World Headquarters, 400 Commonwealth Drive, Warrendale, PA 15096; SAE Automotive Headquarters, 755 W. Big Beaver, Suite 1600, Troy, MI 48084; SAE Washington Office, 1300 Eye Street N.W., Washington, DC 20005.

71. Yang K, Begeman P. *A proposed role for facet joints in neck pain in low to moderate rear impacts.* Biomechanics 6th Injury Prevention Through Biomechanics Symposium at WSU, May 9–10, 1996, pp. 59–62.

72. King D, Siegmund G, Bailey M. *Automobile bumper behavior in low speed rear end impacts,* SAE Pub 930211. Detroit, Society of Automotive Engineers, 1993.

73. Mellon M. *The Guide to Low Velocity Whiplash Biomechanics.* Olympia WA, Body Mind Publications, 1997.

74. Boszczyk BM, Boszczyk AA, Putz R, *et al.* An immunohistochemical study of the dorsal capsule of the lumbar and thoracic facet joints. *Spine* 2001; 26(15): E 338.

75. Cavanaugh JM. *A proposed role for facet joints in neck pain in low to moderate speed rear end impacts* Part II. Neuroanatomy and Neurophysiology 6th Injury Prevention through biomechanics symposium at WSU. May 9–10, 1996, pp. 65–71.

76. Panjabi M, Cholewick J, Nibu K, *et al.* Mechanism of whiplash injury. *Clin Biomech* 1998; 13: 239.

77. Panjabi MM, Cholewicki J, Nibu K, Grauer J, Vahldiek M. Capsular ligament stretches during in vitro whiplash stimulations. *J Spinal Disord* 1998; 11(3): 227.

78. Winkelstein BA, Nightingale RW, Richardson WJ, Myers BS. The cervical facet capsule and its role in whiplash injury. A biomechanical investigation. *Spine* 2000; 25(10): 1238.

79. Saal J. The role of inflammation in lumbar pain. *Spine* 1995; 20(16): 1831.

80. Chen C, Cavanaugh J, Ozaktay AC, *et al.* Effects of phospholipase A-2, on lumbar nerve root structure and function. *Spine* 1997; 22(10): 1057.

81. Gen-Zhe Liu, Ishihara H, *et al.* Nitric oxide mediates the change of proteoglycan synthesis in the human intervertebral disc in response to hydrostatic pressure. *Spine* 2001; 26(2): 134.

82. Lord SM, Barnsley L, Wallis BJ, *et al.* Chronic cervical zygapophyseal joint pain after whiplash. A placebo-controlled prevalence study. *Spine* 1996; 21(15): 1737.

83. Lord SM, Barnsley L, Wallis BJ, *et al.* Percutaneous radio-frequency neurotomy for chronic zygapophyseal joint pain. *New Eng J Med* 1996; 335(23): 1721.

84. Barnsley L, Lord SM, Wallis BJ, Bogduk N. The prevalence of cervical zygapophyseal joint pain after whiplash. *Spine* 1995; 20(1): 20.

85. Cusick J, Pintar F, Yoganandan N. Whiplash syndrome, kinematic factors influencing pain patterns. *Spine* 2001; 26(11): 1252.

86. Bogduk N, Mercer S. Biomechanics of cervical spine part 1. Normal kinematics. *Clin Biomech* 2000; 15: 633.

87. Bogduk N, Yoganandan N. Biomechanics of the cervical spine Part 3. Minor injuries. *Clin Biomech* 2001; 16: 267.

88. Kellett J. Acute soft tissue injuries—a review of the literature. *Med Sci Sports Exerc* 1986; 18(5): 489.

89. Oakes BW. Acute soft tissue injuries, nature and management. *Aust Fam Phys* 1981; 10(7 suppl): 3.

90. Muelen van der. Present state of knowledge on processes of healing of collagen structures. *Int J Sports Med* 1982; 3: 4.

91. Cohen K, Diegelmann RF, Lindblad WJ (eds). *Wound Healing: Biochemical & Clinical Aspects.* Philadelphia, PA, WB Saunders Co, 1992.

92. Hack GD, Koritzer RT, Robinson WL, Hallgren RC, Greenman PE. Anatomic relation between the rectus capitis posterior minor muscle and the dura mater. *Spine* 1995; 20(23): 2484.

93. Hallgren RC, Greeman PE, Rechtien JJ. Atrophy of suboccipital muscles in patients with chronic neck pain. A pilot study. *J Am Osteopath Assoc* 1994; 94(12): 1032.

94. McPartland JM, Brodeur RR, Hallgren RC. Chronic neck pain, standing balance, and suboccipital muscle atrophy—A pilot study. *J Manipulative Physiol Ther* 1997; 20(1): 24.

95. Vernon H. *Cervical factors in head pain.* Lecture from the Cervicogenic Head Pain conference 1998.

96. Magnusson T, Ragnarsson T, Bjornsson A. Occipital nerve release in patients with whiplash trauma and occipital neuralgia. Travel and Simmons myofascial pain patterns. *Headache* 1996; 36: 32.

97. Jansen J, Markakis E, Rama B, *et al.* Hemicranial attacks or permanent hemicrania—a sequel of upper cervical root compression. *Cephalgia* 1989; 9.

98. McConnell W, Howard R, Poppel JV, *et al. Human neck–head kinematics after low velocity rear impacts. Understanding Whiplash.* In. 39th Stapp Car Crash Conference Proceedings 95274, 1995, pp. 215–238.

99. McConnell WE, Howard, RP, Guzman HM, *et al. Analysis of human test kinematic responses to low velocity rear end impacts.* SAE Tech Paper Series, Pub 930889, pp. 21–31. Society of Automotive Engineers 1993.

100. Spine Supplement. Quebec Task Force. *Spine Ap* 15 1995, 20(8S) (Supplement).

101. Ommaya AK. The neck: classification, physiopathology and clinical outcomes of injuries to the neck in motor vehicle accidents. The biomechanics of impact trauma. In Aldman B, Chapon A (Eds). *The SCM, Semispinalis and Other Peripheral Myoneuronal Entrapment Syndromes*, pp 127–138. New York, Elsevier Science, 1984.

102. Uhlig Y, Weber BR, Grob D, Muntner M. Fiber composition and fiber transformations in neck muscles of patients with dysfunction of the cervical spine. *J Ortho Res* 1995; 13: 240.

103. Mellon M. *The Guide to Low Velocity Whiplash Biomechanics*. Olympia WA, Body Mind Publications, 1997.

104. Murphy D. *Whiplash Trauma Certification Seminar*. Denver, CO, Murphy Publications Seminar Notes, 1997.

105. Pettersson K, Toolanen G. High dose methylprednisone prevents extensive sick leave after whiplash. A prospective, randomized, double blind study. *Spine* 1998; 23(9): 984.

106. Jane JA, Steward O, Gennarelli T. Axonal degeneration induced by experimental non-invasive minor head injury. *J Neurosurg* 1985; 62: 96.

107. Norris SH, Watt J. The prognosis of neck injuries resulting from rear end collisions. *J Bone Joint Surg (Br)* 1983; 65: 608.

108. Svensson MY. *Neck injuries in rear end collisions*, Thesis. Goteborg, Sweden, Chalmpers University of Technology, 1993.

109. Unterharnscheidt F. Pathological and neuropathological findings in rhesus monkeys subjected to −Gx and +Gx indirect impact accelerations. In. Stances A, Jr, Thomas DJ, *et al. Mechanisms of Head and Spine Trauma*, pp 565–664. Deer Park, NY, Aloray, 1986.

110. Ortengren T, Hansson HA, Lovsund P, *et al.* Membrane leakage in spinal ganglion nerve cells induced by experimental whiplash extension motion. A study in pigs. *J Neurotrauma* 1996; 13(3): 171.

111. Lu J, Ebraheim N. Anatomic considerations of C2 nerve root ganglion. *Spine* 1998; 23(6): 649.

112. Muhle C, Resnick D, Sudmeyer M, *et al.* In vivo changes in the neuroforaminal size at flexion-extension and axial rotation of the cervical spine in healthy persons examined using kinematic magnetic resonance imaging. *Spine* 2001; 24: E287.

113. Pikus HJ, Phillips JM. Characteristics of patients successfully treated for cervicogenic headache by surgical decompression of the second cervical nerve root. *Headache* 1995; 35: 621.

114. Bogduk N, Lord S. The cervical synovial joints as sources of posttraumatic headache. *J Musculoskeletal Pain* 1996, 4(4): 81,.

115. Bogduk N, Anatomy and Physiology of Headache. *Biomed Pharmacother* (1995) 49: 435.

116. Takebayashi T, Cavanaugh J, *et al.* Effect of Nucleus Pulposus on Neural Activity of Dorsal Root Ganglion. *Spine* 2001, 26 (8): 940.

117. Neumann P. Nordwall A, *et al.* Traumatic instability of the lumbar spine. A dynamic in vitro study of the flexion-distraction injury. *Spine* 1995; 20(10): 1111.

118. Hedman T, Fernie G. Mechanical response of the lumbar spine to seated postural loads. *Spine* 1997; 22(7): 734.

119. McNally DS, Adams MS, Goodship AE. Can intervertebral disc prolapse be predicted by disc mechanics. *Spine* 1993; 18(11): 1525.

120. Mannion A, Adams, M, Dolan P. Sudden and unexpected loading generates high forces on the lumbar spine. *Spine* 2000; 25(7): 842.

121. Solomonow M, Zhou BH, Harris M, *et al.* The ligamento-muscular stabilizing system of the spine. *Spine* 1998; 23(23): 2552.

122. Edwards T, Ordway NR, *et al.* Peak stresses observed in the posterior lateral annulus. *Spine* 2001; 26(16): 1753.

123. Watanabe Y, Ichikawa H, Kayama O, *et al.* Influence of seat characteristics on occupant motion in low speed impacts. *Compendium of papers presented at the Traffic Safety and Auto Engineering Stream, World Congress on Whiplash Associated Disorders*, 1999. 297–324.

124. Eichenberger. *Soft tissue injury of the cervical spine in rear end and frontal crashes. Neck injury factor for various car models.* International Conference on the Biomechanics of impact 1995.
125. Siegmund GP, Brault JR, Wheeler JB. *The relationship between clinical and kinematic responses from human subjects testing in rear end collisions.* Traffic Safety and Automobile Engineering Stream of the World Congress on Whiplash Associated Disorders, 1999. 181–207.
126. Nordhoff L. *Motor vehicle collision injuries. Human volunteer studies in published literature on low velocity rear-end crashes and low velocity crashes,* Seminar Notes 1998–2000.
127. Yoganandan N, Pintar F. *Frontiers in Head and Neck Trauma*, pp 344–373. Amsterdam, IOS Press, 1998.
128. Yoganandan N, Kumaresan S, Pintar F. Biomechanics of the cervical spine part 2. Cervical spine soft tissue responses to biomechanical modeling. *Clin Biomech* 2001; 16: 1.

2

Pain

Jack L Rook

The taxonomy committee of the International Association for the Study of Pain considered definitions of pain and concluded: Pain is a "an unpleasant sensory and emotional experience associated with actual or potential tissue damage, or described in terms of such damage." They added crucial notes to this sentence:

- Pain is always subjective. Each individual learns the application of the word through experiences related to injury in early life. It is unquestionably a sensation in a part of the body but it is also always unpleasant and therefore also an emotional experience.
- Many people report pain in the absence of tissue damage or any likely pathophysiological cause. Usually this happens for psychological reasons. There is no way to distinguish their experience from that due to tissue damage, if we take the subjective report. If they regard their experience as pain and if they report it in the same ways as pain caused by tissue damage, it should be accepted as pain. This definition avoids tying pain to the stimulus.[1]

Pain is often described as being either acute or chronic. A distinction between the two is necessary both clinically (as treatment approach varies considerably) and from a litigation perspective. It seems immediately obvious and has long been recognized that acute pain enables the organism to sense impending tissue damage and thus avoid harm and prolong survival. In this sense, pain is usually thought of as a "warning signal" of potential injury. It may also aid in recovery by encouraging rest behavior in the injured individual in order to promote healing and recuperation. Thus, from the biomedical point of view, pain may be thought of as a sensation of actual or impending injury signals and as a "need-state" for rest.

These considerations, however, apply only to the conditions of acute, short-term pain. Injury signals may enable us to avoid burns or similar trauma, seek help for appendicitis or toothache, and enforce appropriate convalescence following sprains and surgery. Therefore, acute pain seems to serve to warn of impending tissue damage or the need for convalescent rest.

Chronic pain, on the other hand, seems to confer no clear biological service. The syndrome of chronic pain is characterized by the behaviors of chronic invalidism (decreased activity levels, polypharmacy, polysurgery, reduction of income, depression, disruption in family relationships). The pain complaint becomes an over-determined symptom highly resistant to change. These features are more often seen in "benign" or "chronic non-malignant" pain patients than in those with cancer or other malignant diseases.

Such patients also report that, with continued pain, they become less tolerant of any pain. Even minor injuries (stubbing a toe, bumping against furniture), which formerly would have been shrugged off, seem major calamities. Apparently, pain tolerance is lowered in association with longer-continued pain and inadequate sleep. In addition, a change in eating behavior often occurs, with some patients reporting a loss of appetite and weight loss, and others the opposite. A general decrease in motor activity often occurs, usually associated with fatigue, lack of energy and weight gain.

Although injuries are common, only a small subset of patients go on to develop chronic pain. However, it is those patients, although a small subset, which create the majority of financial costs to third-party payers in society. Although constituting only a small percentage of all patients with some sort of pain problem, they account for the vast majority of all medical costs that result from occupational injuries and motor vehicle accidents. It has been demonstrated in epidemiologic studies that individuals who remain off of work greater than six months will have a slim chance of returning to the work force in his or her lifetime. Therefore, there should be a sense of urgency with regards to aggressive early management of a painful injury with great effort made to return the patient to the work force as quickly as possible.

As noted, painful syndromes are often classified as being either acute or chronic. Acute traumatic pain implies that tissue injury is generating painful impulses to the central nervous system resulting in the perception of pain. Technically, as the body regenerates healthy tissue, the acute painful episode should subside over a relatively short (one to three months) period. This assumes that the degree of injury was such that normal tissue healing and regeneration can correct the underlying painful process.

A chronic painful condition lasts greater than three to six months and may be expected to be permanent. It occurs in one of two scenarios:

1. When the inciting injury is of such magnitude that a permanent structural abnormality occurs involving muscles, ligaments, joint structures, or bony tissue. For example, a severe whiplash injury could result in tearing of musculature, tendon, or ligamentous tissue. When such soft tissue structures are torn, healing occurs through scar tissue formation. Scar tissue, because of its disorganized microscopic structure, does not have the strength found in the carefully aligned parallel fibers of muscles, tendons, and ligaments. Injured muscle loses flexibility and strength, and repeated tearing within these muscles can occur with activities that previously were well tolerated, resulting in frequent episodes of ongoing pain. A similar scenario occurs with ligamentous injury. Ligamentous tissue consists of highly organized, parallel fibrils of collagen that collectively have great strength. The development of scar tissue within ligaments gravely compromises its strength, possibly leading to repeated tearing, potential instability of adjacent bones, and chronic pain. Tearing of ligaments about joints or involving a joint capsule could

impair the integrity of these joints resulting in instability, cartilage damage, and chronic osteoarthritic pain. Trauma to spinal ligaments may lead to segmental instability, herniation of the nucleus pulposus, nerve root irritation, and/or chronic back or neck pain.

2. Chronic pain could also occur as a result of physiologic changes within the nervous system without significant objective evidence of tissue pathology. The initial injury sets off a neurological chain of events that can result in "wind-up" of the pain transmission cells within the spinal cord and brain. It is the hyperactivity of these cells that is felt to contribute to the chronic pain syndrome in select individuals. For example, some of these patients may be classified as having fibromyalgia syndrome. These patients have a paucity of objective clinical findings, and the diagnosis is based upon a characteristic constellation of symptoms. However, these individuals suffer greatly, complaining of severe pain and functional limitations, despite normal x-rays and unrevealing laboratory data. Fibromyalgia syndrome is an example of an ongoing chronic pain syndrome that can occur after trauma, even relatively benign trauma, not associated with any obvious pathological damage to soft tissue structures. Changes within the central nervous system underlie the extreme perception of pain in these individuals.

PAIN PROBLEMS CAUSED BY MOTOR VEHICLE ACCIDENTS

A variety of pain problems may develop after a motor vehicle accident.

- With rear or front-end collisions, the patient's head may strike the windshield or headrest. With T-bone collisions, the patient's body or head could strike the side window or the doorframe. Unrestrained drivers, and/or those without a chest restraint or air bag may encounter a direct impact of the driver's trunk against the steering wheel resulting in trauma to the chest, ribs and sternum.
- Another common problem occurs when passengers strike their knees against the dashboard traumatizing the knee joint(s). People who have time to brace their arms prior to impact can develop a variety of upper extremity problems. The driver who grabs the steering wheel tightly, or the passenger who braces against the dashboard or back seat in anticipation of the impact, is prone to upper extremity joint injury. Hyperextension of the wrist(s) with forces transmitted through the arm(s) can occur. Lower extremity bracing against the floorboard could result in trauma to the feet or ankles. Such forces could also be transmitted up the leg resulting in indirect trauma to the knee, hip, sacroiliac joint, or even the spine.
- *Whiplash* refers to a hyperflexion-hyperextension injury that may disrupt soft tissue structures extending from the base of the skull to the low back region (spinal muscles, interspinous ligaments, ligaments at the base of the skull, spinal ligaments that surround the facet joints, the posterior longitudinal ligament, and fibers of the intervertebral disc).
- With a cervical hyperextension injury, there may be tearing of the anterior neck muscles (sternocleidomastoid and scalene muscles), the anterior longitudinal

ligament and anterior annulus fibrosis of the intervertebral disc. With trunk hyperextension, there may be tearing of abdominal musculature, or lumbar spinal structures including the anterior longitudinal ligament and anterior annulus fibers of the intervertebral disc.

- Upper extremity pain can occur secondary to bracing prior to impact. Hyperextension may ensue at the wrist, with forces spreading throughout the arm.
- Lower extremity pain problems may develop due to direct trauma of lower extremity structures against the floorboard, door, dashboard, or stick shift panel. With bracing of the lower extremities prior to impact, forces may pass through the joints of the lower extremity extending to the sacroiliac joint(s) of the pelvis.
- Torquing injuries may result from side impact collisions, or if the patient is turned even slightly to one side or the other at the time of a frontal or rear end collision. A torquing injury can result in rather severe spinal trauma due to tearing of facet joint capsule(s) and/or the outer layers of the intervertebral disc. The rotational forces associated with torquing injuries place greater stress on the spinal ligaments than do hyperflexion/hyperextension injuries of similar intensity. As a result, fairly significant injuries may occur after relatively minor impacts when rotational forces are experienced by the patient.

Bone Pain

Bony pain due to fractures may result from a motor vehicle accident. With lower extremity bracing prior to impact, foot and/or ankle fractures may occur, and the forces associated with the bracing could be referred through the leg resulting in a tibia, fibula, or femur fracture. Impact of the knees against the dashboard could result in a patella fracture. With severe motor vehicle accidents, pelvic or spinal fractures may occur. Spinal vertebral compression fractures occasionally result in retropulsion of bone and debris into the spinal canal. The principal complication of this scenario can be spinal cord injury. Sternal fractures may occur if there is impact of the chest wall against the steering wheel or a caught chest restraint. Cranial fractures may occur with head trauma against the doorframe, roof, window, or windshield.

Myofascial Pain Syndrome

A subset of patients develops chronic pain after a motor vehicle accident. Some patients develop a muscular condition known as a myofascial pain syndrome, characterized by chronic tender muscles that have "trigger points" within them. A trigger point is a hyperirritable band of muscle that refers pain to characteristic regions in distant parts of the body. These distant muscular regions may contain "latent" trigger points; potentially tender areas that have not yet become hypersensitive or activated. However, when pain is referred to these distant latent trigger points, they become sensitized and surrounding muscles may go into spasm. Therefore, pain will migrate to this new region and these new active trigger points may in turn refer pain to other areas, possibly causing further migration of the myofascial condition.[2]

Fibromyalgia Syndrome

Some patients go on to develop a diffuse myofascial condition known as fibromyalgia syndrome. This condition is not necessarily associated with muscle spasm or active trigger points. Rather, these patients suffer from chronically tender muscles throughout their bodies. The muscles have "tender points" rather than "trigger points," the differentiation being that pressure on tender points does not necessarily refer pain to other regions. The fibromyalgia patient has a characteristic constellation of symptoms including poor sleep, irritable bowels, chronic fatigue, headaches and depression. Fibromyalgia may result from an initially localized injury that impairs sleep. It might also result from a more severe traumatic injury that causes muscular and ligamentous disruption throughout the spine and extremities.[3,4]

Chronic Pain Syndrome

The inadequate management of pain early on may predispose an individual to develop a chronic pain syndrome. In certain individuals the pain impulses from the damaged tissues activate and sensitize pain cells in the spinal cord. These hypersensitive cells continue to fire pain impulses toward the brain, **even after the original injury has healed**. This phenomenon is known as *wind-up* of pain pathways. Therefore, aggressive management of discomfort early on is important in preventing the original injury from becoming a chronic pain problem in certain patients.

Temporomandibular Joint Dysfunction

Patients may develop temporomandibular joint problems after a motor vehicle accident. This occurs due to a number of reasons:

- Trauma to the joints may occur at the time of the original injury.
- Some patients with neck injuries have cervical myofascial trigger points that refer pain to latent trigger points in muscles surrounding the temporomandibular joints (the masseter and pterygoid muscles). Activation of these latent trigger points will produce myofascial pain surrounding the temporomandibular joint(s) with the development of joint discomfort.
- Lastly, patients with a sleep disturbance due to chronic pain of any etiology may suffer from bruxism, whereby the patient grinds his/her teeth at night. Bruxism may cause the development of jaw problems.

Headaches

Headaches are very common after motor vehicle accidents due to a variety of pathophysiological processes:

- Whiplash may cause injury to neck musculature producing muscle spasm that involves the paracervical suboccipital muscles (neck muscles at the base of the skull). This will cause irritation of four nerves in the back of the head known as the occipital nerves. Irritation of these nerves will cause headaches. Another term for this is occipital neuralgia. The four nerves include two greater occipital nerves and two lesser occipital nerves. Irritation of a greater occipital nerve typically refers pain to the ipsilateral forehead and behind the eye, while an irritated lesser occipital nerve refers pain to the base of the skull and behind the ear.

- Muscle spasm and trigger points in the cervical region occasionally refer pain to and activate trigger points within the temporalis muscle(s). Muscle contraction headaches occur due to muscle spasm of paracervical and temporalis musculature. This condition and occipital neuralgia may coexist after a whiplash injury.
- Vascular headaches occur due to neurological changes in the brain and brainstem after trauma.
- Headaches may also occur in conjunction with temporomandibular joint dysfunction.
- Headaches that persist after a motor vehicle accident are usually multifactorial (sometimes referred to as "mixed headaches") including a tension component associated with the development of vascular or migraine headaches.

Therefore, posttraumatic headaches may be a conglomeration of two or three different headache types including muscle tension, occipital neuralgia, vascular, and headache pain due to temporomandibular joint dysfunction. These will be further discussed in the chapter entitled headaches.

THE DIFFERENT TYPES OF PAIN

Different types of pain that can occur after motor vehicle accidents include soft tissue pain, bony pain, joint pain, and neurogenic pain.

Soft Tissue Pain

Strain

Different types of muscular pain syndromes can occur after a motor vehicle accident. Immediately after the accident, muscular pain is often labeled as being due to a "strain." This refers to the stretching and tearing of muscle fibers in the area of involvement. Normal muscle tissue is composed of highly organized parallel fibrils, oriented in such a way as to produce elasticity when relaxed and great strength when contracting. A relaxed muscle only allows a certain amount of movement before its fibrils are stretched to capacity and tearing ensues. A muscle that is contracting at the time of impact (perhaps due to bracing) will have a lessened ability to stretch before tearing. Pain is generated by the strained muscle tissue.

Whenever muscle tears, it heals by the development of scar tissue. The healed muscle tissues will never be as strong or elastic as the muscle fibers were prior to injury.

Muscle Spasm

Muscle spasm is a response to painful injury, a protective reflex that occurs after trauma. For example, if one were to break a bone, the muscles around that bone would go into spasm. This would help immobilize the underlying fracture. Unfortunately, the muscle spasm itself becomes a secondary focus of pain and discomfort aside from the fractured bone.

The muscle fibers involved in spasm are working very hard to maintain a chronically contracted state. The contracted muscle fibers generate toxic waste products of metabolism. Unfortunately, these waste products, which include carbon dioxide and lactic acid, are irritating to adjacent pain nerve endings. This produces more discomfort that further perpetuates the cycle of spasm and pain. The only way to stop this discomfort is to break the cycle of muscle spasm through therapeutic modalities and pharmacologic agents.

In addition to toxic metabolite production, when muscle fibers go into spasm, they contract very tightly compromising blood supply to the muscles. The capillaries permeating muscle fibers collapse under the pressure generated by muscle spasm. This causes a shortage of oxygenated blood and nutrients to the area of muscle spasm. The lack of oxygen (hypoxia) in conjunction with the generation of waste products further irritate nociceptors within the muscle spasm contributing to the painful state.

When muscle spasm persists for a long period of time, the respective muscle shortens and loses elasticity. In addition, any scar tissue formation further shortens the muscle tissue. When patients try to stretch out a shortened (tight) muscle, there can be further tearing of intact muscle fibers. This will further perpetuate the cycle of chronic pain, muscle spasm, production of toxic metabolites and chronic hypoxia of these tissues.

Myofascial Pain Syndrome

Over time, chronically tight muscle tissue may become a more permanent problem known as a myofascial pain syndrome. This type of muscular pain syndrome is characterized by chronically tender muscles, increased muscle tone, decreased length of the involved tissue and the presence of trigger points.

Different muscles may be injured with a whiplash injury. In the cervical area, the scalene and sternocleidomastoid muscles may be involved anteriorly, and the paracervical and trapezii posteriorly. The trapezii extend from the base of the skull to the mid back between the shoulder blades. Injured trapezii are common causes of neck pain, shoulder pain, or upper back pain.

With cervical muscular injury, a variety of other problems can evolve over time. Occasionally, patients with paracervical muscle spasm develop dizziness due to a phenomenon known as cervical vertigo. The dizziness occurs as a result of disruption of proprioceptors (position receptors) that are normally present within neck musculature. This condition is not due to an inner ear or brain injury.

A myogenic thoracic outlet syndrome occurs frequently in whiplash patients due to myofascial pain involving scalene or pectoral muscles. This causes irritation of the underlying brachial plexus contributing to upper extremity pain and paresthesias post motor vehicle accident.

Myofascial pain syndrome in the suboccipital region could cause irritation of occipital nerves. This will generate headaches labeled as occipital neuralgia. In addition, paracervical trigger points may refer pain to the temporalis muscle(s), causing reactive spasm with the development of muscular tension headaches.

Paracervical myofascial pain referred to the pterygoid or masseter muscles could result in temporomandibular joint discomfort. Pain may also be referred to the mid and lower back musculature with the development of reactive discomfort or spasm in this region.

Ligament Injury

Ligamentous trauma may also contribute to acute pain after a motor vehicle accident. A ligament is a firm fibrous tissue that connects adjacent bones, providing support and controlled movement between the articulations. Although ligamentous tissue has a poor blood supply, it has a rich neural innervation. When injured, ligaments can generate significant pain due to:

- irritation of nerves within the torn ligament
- the instability that develops as a result of the ligamentous disruption
- and/or as a result of the inflammation associated with the torn tissue.

Over time, torn ligamentous tissue will repair itself by the production of scar tissue. Scar tissue is highly disorganized and often has inadequate strength to provide the necessary support between bony structures.

In the lower extremity, strained ligaments may involve the ankle, knee or hip joint. This may occur as a result of impact of a braced leg against the floorboard, or after direct impact of the leg with the door, stick shift, or dashboard.

The sacroiliac joint is involved in weight-bearing activities and change of position of the trunk. The ligaments that stabilize this joint may be torn during a motor vehicle accident, usually due to an extreme hyperflexion/hyperextension injury to the trunk, or as a result of transferred forces through the leg braced against the pedal or floorboard immediately prior to impact. Strain of these ligaments could result in chronic low back/pelvic pain.

An extensive series of ligaments span the entire vertebral column. Between the vertebral bodies are the intervertebral discs that are bounded by the annular ligament fibers. Anterior and posterior to the vertebrae are the anterior and posterior longitudinal ligaments that extend from the base of the skull to the sacrum. Lining the facet joints are ligaments that make up the facet capsule. Interspinous ligaments between all of the spinous processes add further stability. The intactness of these various ligaments contribute to spinal stability, and their disruption could result in a chronic painful condition.

Commonly injured ligaments in the upper extremities include those ligaments that lend support to the base of the thumb, and ligaments of the wrists, elbows, and shoulder joint complex. The thumb ligaments may be injured due to hyperextension of that joint against the steering wheel after a collision. Likewise, the wrist, elbow and shoulder may be injured with a braced extremity. Shoulder ligaments may also be compromised as a result of direct impact of the shoulder joint against a lap belt that has caught. Occasionally, it is the opposite shoulder joint that is affected as a result of excessive movement since it is not stabilized by the lap belt post impact.

Tendon Injury

A tendon is a fibrous structure that attaches muscle to bone. The fibers that make up a tendon have a parallel organization, thereby giving them great strength. Although their blood supply is limited, they are highly innervated by nerve endings and are potential generators of pain. Tendons can cause pain due to tearing or inflammation of their fibers.

Lower extremity tendons that may be injured in a motor vehicle accident include the Achilles tendon (which attaches the calf musculature to the calcaneus bone of the foot), the hamstring tendons (which connect the hamstring musculature to the tibia), and the quadriceps tendon (which extends over the patella and connects the quadriceps muscle group to the tibia anterior and inferior to the knee joint).

In the upper extremity, tendon injury may involve the biceps tendon, rotator cuff tendon and tendons about the wrist and elbow. At the level of the wrist, two commonly strained tendons are those that connect the abductor longis and extensor digitorum brevis muscles to the thumb joint. These may be traumatized as a result of forceful gripping of the steering wheel prior to impact. The inflammation of these tendons is known as DeQuervain's tenosynovitis. Elbow pain may occur with tendonitis involving the wrist flexor and extensor tendons, which insert at the medial and lateral epicondyles of the humerus, respectively. They may be injured as a result of bracing against the steering wheel, dashboard, or back seat at time of impact. The biceps tendon may be traumatized when the shoulder joint directly impacts against a caught shoulder harness. A similar injury mechanism could result in the development of rotator cuff tendonitis. The rotator cuff conjoined tendon connects the rotator cuff muscles (supraspinatus, infraspinatus, teres major, and subscapularis) to the head of the humerus. Rotator cuff tendonitis is a common cause of shoulder pain after a motor vehicle accident. Excessive movement of the shoulder joint contralateral to the shoulder harness could also precipitate a shoulder tendinitis.

Bursitis

Bursas occur around most major joints of the body. These are lubricated tissues whose principal purpose is to facilitate joint motion. These tissues are highly vascularized and innervated by nerve fibers. They are therefore, significant potential foci of both pain and inflammation. Bursitis commonly occurs around the ankle, knee, hip and shoulder regions.

The Achilles bursa may be traumatized due to bracing the leg against the floorboard or brake prior to impact. Such patients develop pain and inflammation around the posterior ankle joint. Knee trauma may result in patella bursitis or pes anserine bursitis. The passenger whose hip impacts against a caught seat belt, another passenger, the door or stick shift may develop a trochanteric bursitis with acute severe hip pain. The most commonly injured bursa is under the acromion of the shoulder joint. Subacromial bursitis is characterized by sharp pain at the tip of the shoulder that worsens with any movement of the arm, particularly overhead movement.

Bony Pain

Bone trauma is another cause of pain after an accident. In the feet, phalangeal, metatarsal, or tarsal fractures may result from direct trauma of the foot against the floorboard or foot pedal. With bracing of the lower extremity prior to impact, an ankle fracture may occur. In more severe accidents, fractures of the tibia, fibula, kneecap, or femur could occur due to bracing, or if the leg strikes against the dashboard, stick shift panel, door frame or back seat. Fractures of the bony pelvis would result in acute pelvic pain.

There are several types of spinal fractures that can cause discomfort after an accident. With hyperflexion injury, cervical, thoracic and/or lumbar compression fractures may develop. Compression fractures are graded as I through IV with a grade I fracture representing compression of up to 25 percent of the height of the vertebral body, a grade II fracture up to 50 percent compression, grade III up to 75 percent, and grade IV greater than 75 percent compression. Aside from causing severe pain, this type of fracture also poses the risk of retropulsion of vertebral bone with the potential for spinal cord injury. Likewise, fracture(s) of the spinous processes and/or the posterior vertebral arch will also cause back pain with the potential for spinal cord injury. Upper extremity fractures (small bones of the hand and/or wrist, radius, ulna, humerus) may occur due to bracing against the steering wheel, dashboard or back seat prior to impact. Lastly, skull fractures may result from head trauma.

Joint Pain

Discomfort may also emanate from the numerous joints within the human body. A joint refers to an articulation between two adjacent bones. There are different types of joints within the body, classification being based upon the amount of movement involved in the articulation and the type of capsule surrounding the joint. Joints with little movement (synarthrodial joints) are found within the spine (the intervertebral disc) and pelvis (the pubic symphysis and the sacroiliac joints). An even tighter joint, known as a suture, is found connecting the multiple bones that make up the skull. These joints do not allow any motion.

The classical movable joint is the diarthrodial or synovial joint. This type of joint articulates two bones that move one against the other. A capsule holds the joint together, and each bone of the articulation is lined by smooth cartilage that assists with gliding movement of one bone upon the other. In addition, the intra-articular joint capsules have a synovial lining made up of cells that secrete a lubricating substance for the joint.

Therefore, the typical synovial joint has a capsule (made up of firm ligaments that add stability to the joint), a cartilaginous lining of the articulating bones (which promotes smooth movement) and a synovial lining (specialized cells that add lubrication). There are numerous synovial joints throughout the body including all small joints of the hands and feet, the elbows, shoulders, hips, knees, ankles, part of the sacroiliac joints, and the posterior facet joints of the spine. The joints of the human body have varying degrees of motion depending on the degree of ligamentous support and the orientation of the opposing bones that make up the joint.

Degrees of Motion

The *human shoulder joint* has the greatest range of motion of any joint within the body. It has six planes of motion including flexion, extension, abduction, adduction, and internal and external rotation. The shoulder joint is a ball and socket joint. The large ball shaped head of the humerus inserts into a rather shallow cup known as the glenoid fossa. This orientation contributes to the great movement found within this joint. However, this great movement occurs at the expense of stability, and, with sufficient stressors, there can be subluxation of the shoulder joint.

In contrast, the *hip joint*, which is also a ball and socket joint, involves a round femoral head articulating with a rather large cup known as the acetabulum, which is part of the pelvis. The cup surrounds the majority of the ball lending great stability to this joint. Hip motion includes flexion, extension, abduction, and adduction. However, the range of motion is not nearly as great as the shoulder joint because of the great stability afforded by the femoral head/acetabulum complex.

The *knee joint* only has two ranges, flexion and extension, due to the orientation of the bones that make up the joint, as well as the extensive system of ligaments surrounding and within it. The knee joint gets its medial and lateral stability from the medial and lateral collateral ligaments, respectively. Anterior and posterior stability is afforded by the hamstring muscles and their tendons posteriorly, the quadriceps mechanism anteriorly, and the anterior and posterior cruciate ligaments within the joint.

The *elbow joint* moves in only flexion and extension due to the orientation of bones and ligaments surrounding it. The *wrist and ankle joints* each have four planes of motion. The wrist has flexion, extension, inversion, and eversion while the ankle has dorsi flexion, plantar flexion, inversion and eversion. Except for the thumb, which has three planes of motion (flexion, abduction, extension), the small joints of the fingers and feet have only two planes of motion, flexion and extension.

Joints can be a significant focus of pain. The surrounding ligaments, tendons and synovial tissue, as well as the bones of the articulation are highly innervated by pain fibers. Joint pain may occur due to ligament tearing, instability, and degeneration of cartilage. The cartilage itself does not have neural innervation. Nevertheless, as the cartilage degenerates (a phenomenon known as chondromalacia), there is irritation of the underlying bone with associated pain. Cartilage fragments that have broken off may add to joint discomfort.

Commonly Traumatized Joints

Joints commonly traumatized in motor vehicle accidents include the ankle, knee, and hip in the lower extremities, the first carpometacarpal joint, wrist, and shoulder joints in the upper extremities, and the sacroiliac joint, spinal facet joints and thoracic costochondral joints in the spine or trunk.

Within the *shoulder joint* impingement may occur when soft tissues within the joint press against the overlying acromion, or a bone spur emanating from it. Impingement involves compression of the subacromial bursa and the musculotendinous insertion of the rotator cuff within the shoulder joint complex. This condition is characterized by pain at the tip of the shoulder, difficulty lifting the involved arm, and performing over the shoulder activities without experiencing shoulder joint discomfort.

The *knee joint* may sustain trauma due to direct impact against the dashboard, back seat, doorframe, or stick shift. Knee joint pathology might include a ligamentous or meniscal tear, chondromalacia, or the development of instability. A common phenomenon, the so-called "dashboard knee" occurs due to direct impact of the patella against the dashboard. This can result in chondromalacia, the degeneration of cartilage underlying the patella. Chondromalacia can cause persistent knee discomfort after a motor vehicle accident.

The *hip joint* may be injured as a result of forces transmitted through a braced leg. Significant compression of the hip within the acetabulum may traumatize the blood supply to the femoral head resulting in a painful condition known as aseptic necrosis. Aseptic necrosis, a rare occurrence, refers to a premature degeneration of the joint due to loss of blood supply.

Sacroiliac joint injury may occur due to a motor vehicle accident either as a result of a flexion-extension or torquing injury to the trunk, or due to bracing one or both legs against the floorboard or brake prior to impact. The sacroiliac joint, a critical structure involved in trunk movements and weight-bearing activities, has both a fibrous and a capsular component. Both portions could be damaged as a result of an accident.

Spinal facet joints may be injured in a motor vehicle accident. With a hyperflexion injury or side impact collisions, cervical and lumbar facet joint capsules are stressed and can tear. The hyperextension component of a whiplash injury will cause the facet joints to impact against each other. This can cause acute trauma to the bones of the joint with the development of joint pain and reactive muscle spasm. Therefore, motor vehicle accidents can result in both stretching/tearing of facet joint capsules, as well as compression of the bony components of the joint itself.

The *thoracic costochondral joints* may be traumatized as a result of direct impact of the chest against the steering wheel, air bag, or a chest restraint that has caught after the impact. Pressure against the anterior chest wall may disrupt the costochondral cartilaginous/bony articulations causing chest pain that typically worsens with deep inspiration and/or localized pressure.

In the *upper extremities*, joint injuries commonly involve the hands, wrists and shoulders. With forceful gripping of the steering wheel at time of impact, hyperextension of the thumb may injure the first carpal/metacarpal joint causing pain at the base of the thumb. Hyperextension of the wrist due to bracing against the steering wheel, dashboard, or back seat, may strain or disrupt ligaments within the wrist joint causing persistent wrist discomfort and/or instability. The shoulder joint may be injured by an overlying chest restraint that catches after impact. Pressure from this restraint may traumatize anterior shoulder joint structures causing inflammation of the bicipital tendon (which courses anteriorly through the bicipital groove of the humerus). The humeral head may be forced into the shoulder joint producing impingement of the rotator cuff tendon and the subacromial bursa as they press against the bony shelf of the acromion. This could result in chronic pain from tendonitis and bursitis, respectively. Muscle spasm involving musculature about the shoulder could contribute to shoulder discomfort and cause irritation of the underlying brachial plexus.

Neurogenic Pain

Neurogenic pain occurs due to injury of the peripheral or central nervous system (CNS). The CNS refers to the brain and spinal cord whereas the peripheral nervous system refers to all nerves that emanate from the CNS, providing motor, sensation, and autonomic function for the human body.

Peripheral nervous system injury may occur as a result of a motor vehicle accident causing pain when peripheral nerve fibers are either bruised or transected. Some patients develop hypersensitive regions (neuromas) around partially injured nerves. A neuroma may generate considerable discomfort, both lancinating and/or persistent in quality. Nerve entrapments may develop as a result of direct trauma to a nerve at a susceptible location (such as the median nerve at the wrist, ulnar nerve at the elbow or tibial nerve at the ankle), or as a result of chronic muscular tightness entrapping an underlying nerve (such as the median nerve through the pronator mass or the brachial plexus through thoracic outlet musculature).

Whenever nerves are transected or damaged, the possibility for a severe pain syndrome exists. Peripheral nerves do have the ability to regenerate, as individual axon fibers can grow at a rate varying from 1 to 10 mm per week. However, if there has been damage to the sheaths that encase the axons themselves, the regrowth process could be disrupted leading to neuroma formation, and other neurogenic pain problems. Nerve injury may predispose some patients to develop the reflex sympathetic dystrophy syndrome, a severely painful condition.

Symptoms of neurogenic pain include discomfort out of proportion to the degree of injury, extreme skin hypersensitivity such that non-noxious stimuli is perceived as being noxious (allodynia), lancinating pain that emanates from the site of nerve injury, paresthesias (pins and needles, tingling, numbness) and night time awakening due to pain and/or paresthesias (nocturnal paresthesias).

Physical signs consistent with nerve injury include sensory, motor, and/or reflex changes in the distribution of the injured peripheral nerve. With the reflex sympathetic dystrophy syndrome, there may be skin color and/or temperature changes, along with extreme hypersensitivity with light palpation (allodynia).

There are numerous neurogenic pain diagnoses that the clinician might encounter after a motor vehicle accident. Peripheral nerve entrapments occur in both the upper and lower extremities. In the upper extremities, the median nerve can be entrapped at the wrist (carpal tunnel syndrome) or within volar forearm muscles (pronator syndrome), the radial nerve may be entrapped within dorsal forearm muscles (radial tunnel syndrome), and proximal spasm involving pectoral and scalene muscles may result in a thoracic outlet syndrome (due to irritation of the underlying brachial plexus).

A number of lower extremity nerve entrapments can occur after a motor vehicle accident. With trauma to the ankle, there can be irritation and/or damage to three nerves, the tibial nerve (adjacent to the medial malleolus), the superficial peroneal nerve (which courses anterior to the ankle), and the sural nerve (behind the lateral malleolus). The most common of these three nerves to become entrapped is the tibial nerve at the medial ankle (the tarsal tunnel syndrome). More proximally, the peroneal nerve adjacent to the fibular head may be injured due to direct trauma of this region against the door or stick shift panel. Some patients who traumatize their feet may develop entrapment of an interdigital nerve (interdigital neuritis or a Morton's neuroma). Such patients may develop significant foot pain, particularly with weight-bearing.

Lastly, some patients develop a piriformis syndrome due to entrapment of the sciatic nerve as it passes through the two heads of the piriformis muscle in the gluteal region. Acute or chronic spasm of the piriformis muscle may entrap the sciatic nerve causing symptomatology that mimics the sciatica normally experienced with lumbar radiculopathy.

A cervical or lumbar radiculopathy refers to peripheral nerve entrapment at the level of the spinal nerve root. In such a case, a bone spur or soft tissue structure (such as a herniated intervertebral disc) may apply pressure to a cervical or lumbar nerve root resulting in pain, paresthesias and weakness in the extremity involved by the radicular process. Such patients complain of extremity pain, motor weakness and sensory abnormalities. Some patients who sustain cervical flexion and extension injuries develop chronic headaches due to irritation of the occipital nerves. The four occipital nerves originate from the C1 through C3 sensory nerve rootlets. They course up the back and sides of the head. Two greater occipital nerves supply sensation to the top of the head while the lesser occipital nerves supply the occipital region and around the ears. Entrapment, irritation, or damage to these nerves can refer pain to the front or side of the head resulting in headaches after a motor vehicle accident, a phenomenon known as occipital neuralgia.

THE PATHOPHYSIOLOGY OF PAIN

Most patients with acute injury after a motor vehicle accident recover with rest, analgesics, physical therapy, and appropriate restrictions. Occasionally, a worst-case scenario develops characterized by a progressively worsening or migrating pain syndrome that evolves despite aggressive therapeutic interventions. Diffuse pain in association with headaches, depression, and sleep disturbance are symptoms commonly seen in chronic pain syndromes. This section will review the neuroanatomy of pain pathways.

Ascending Pain Pathways

Pain Fibers

Painful impulses are transmitted from the periphery to the central nervous system (CNS) via nociceptive C- and A-delta afferent nerve fibers.[5–8] Musculoskeletal structures presumed to be innervated by primary nociceptors include joint capsules, ligaments, tendons, muscles, periosteum and bone.

Activation of C- and A-delta Fibers

The C-fiber (unmyelinated) nociceptor responds to noxious thermal, mechanical, and chemical stimuli. A-delta (thin myelinated) nociceptors are of two types, the A-delta mechanical nociceptors, which are particularly sensitive to sharp, pointed instruments, and A-delta mechanothermal nociceptors, which respond to heat.[9,10]

The function of a sensory receptor is to respond to a particular type of stimulus while remaining relatively insensitive to all other types. For example, C- and A-delta nociceptors are sensitive to intense mechanical and thermal stimuli and to irritant chemicals. Somehow, the presence of such stimuli leads to the generation of nociceptive nerve impulses. The process by which noxious stimuli depolarize the nociceptor is called transduction. It is not known exactly how transduction occurs.[11] Possibly, the nociceptor terminals are chemosensitive in that they are activated by pain-producing substances that accumulate near the terminals following tissue injury. At least three sources of these noxious compounds are known:

1. they may leak out from damaged cells
2. they may be synthesized locally by enzymes – either those released by cell damage or those that enter the damaged area from the bloodstream
3. they may be released by activity in the nociceptor itself.[11]

Damaged tissue cells will produce leakage of the intracellular contents. Released chemicals that either activate or sensitize nociceptors include acetylcholine, serotonin, adenosine triphosphate, potassium and histamine.

Transducing or sensitizing agents synthesized by enzymes in the area of the tissue damage include bradykinins and metabolic products of arachidonic acid (prostaglandins and leukotrienes). Several of the prostaglandins sensitize primary afferent nociceptors.

In addition to chemical mediators that are released from damaged cells or synthesized in the region of the damage, the nociceptors themselves release a substance or substances that enhance nociception. Substance P, an 11-amino acid polypeptide, is believed to be a likely constituent. Substance P, a potent vasodilator, causes the release of histamine from mast cells and promotes the formation of edema. Histamine, which activates nociceptors, also can produce vasodilatation and edema.[12–15]

Thus, tissue damage results in transduction of the nociceptive stimuli. There is subsequent transmission of these impulses to the CNS. Without appropriate treatment, there may be further sensitization and spread of this nociceptive process.

Peripheral Nerves

Major peripheral nerves are made up of different types of afferent and efferent nerve fibers. Afferent fibers (fibers that carry impulses towards the spinal cord) include C- and A-delta nociceptors and large myelinated A-alpha mechanoreceptor sensory fibers.

The majority of peripheral nerve axons are primary afferents and, of these, three-fourths are unmyelinated C-fibers. Thus, C-fiber afferents are the most common element in most peripheral nerves, and the overwhelming majority of C-fibers are believed to be nociceptors.[16,17] Nociceptive impulses are transmitted by A-delta and C-fibers into the dorsal horn of the spinal cord.

Dorsal Horn

Rexed divided the gray matter of the spinal cord into ten laminae on the basis of the microscopic appearance of the neurons (their size, orientation, and density) (Figure 2-1).[18] He had numbered the laminae sequentially from dorsal to ventral. Important layers with respect to ascending pain pathways include layers I, II, and V. In layer I is the nociceptor-specific pain transmission cell (NSPTC). In layer II, there are interneurons that project to other layers. In layer V are the large wide dynamic-range neurons (WDRN). The second-order pain transmission cells (NSPTCs and WDRNs) in layers I and V project to the thalamus.

A-delta and C-fibers terminate in the dorsal horn. The NSPTC in layer I responds maximally to noxious stimuli and tends to have a smaller receptive field than the WDRN. It receives input from the A-delta fibers and from C-fibers. The NSPTC projects to the thalamus. The WDRN in layer V receives both nociceptive (A-delta and C) and non-nociceptive (A-alpha) afferent information. The WDRN responds to both noxious and non-noxious stimuli. The WDRN has a larger receptive field than does the NSPTC. Stimulation of this cell ultimately results in poorly localized pain. The WDRN also projects to thalamic nuclei.[19]

Spinothalamic Tract and Anterolateral Quadrant

Axons from each class of second-order projection neuron cross to the contralateral anterolateral quadrant, forming the spinothalamic tract (STT), the major pathway for the ascending nociceptive fibers that travel to target nuclei in the brainstem and thalamus (Figure 2-2).[19–23]

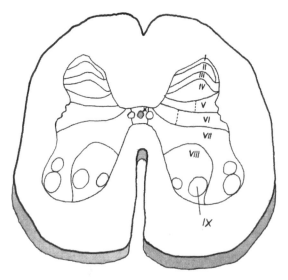

Figure 2-1 Rexed[18] divided the spinal cord gray matter into ten laminae, on the basis of the microscopic appearance of the neurons. Reprinted by permission from Rook JL: Neuroanatomy: ascending pain pathways and the descending pain modulatory system. In Cassvan A, Rook JL, Mullens SU, *et al.* (eds): *Cumulative Trauma Disorders*, p 20, Fig 3-3. Boston, Butterworth-Heinemann, 1997.

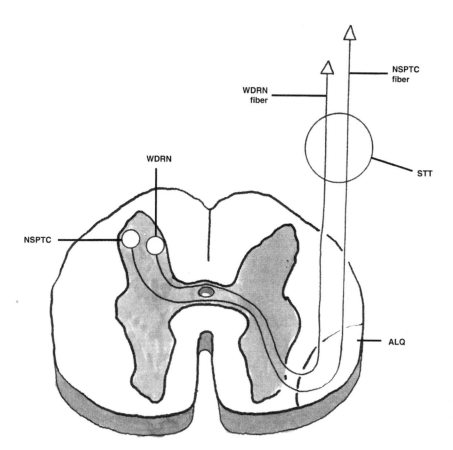

Figure 2-2 Axons from second-order pain transmission cells cross to the con-
tralateral anterolateral quadrant (ALQ) to form the spinothalamic tract (STT). The
STT is somatotopically organized, with wide dynamic-range neuron (WDRN) fibers
occupying a more medial position than nociceptor-specific pain transmission cell
(NSPTC) fibers. Reprinted by permission from Rook JL: Neuroanatomy: ascend-
ing pain pathways and the descending pain modulatory system. In Cassvan A,
Rook JL, Mullens SU, *et al.* (eds): *Cumulative Trauma Disorders*, p 22, fig 3-5.
Boston, Butterworth-Heinemann, 1997.

Pain Pathways Within the Brain

Within the STT, two distinct pathways have been identified anatomically and are
believed to have evolved phylogenetically. A medial, more primitive pathway, the
paleospinothalamic tract, courses to the medial thalamic nuclei stimulating third-order
cells, which project to the frontal cortex, limbic system, and reticular formation of the brainstem.[22,24,25] Activity in this pathway leads to poorly localized pain (WDRN contribution),
with emotional connotations, depression, anxiety, sleep disturbance and other features
characteristic of the chronic pain syndrome.

The lateral pathway, which projects to lateral thalamic nuclei, is known as the
neospinothalamic tract. Input to lateral thalamic third-order neurons comes principally

from the NSPTCs in layer I of the contralateral spinal cord. These third-order cells have smaller receptive fields and help to localize the noxious input. The lateral thalamic nuclei give rise to a dense projection restricted to the somatosensory cortex (Figure 2-3).

The striking differences in receptive field organization of the neurons in these two regions, and their distinct efferent projections, suggest that the paleospinothalamic and neospinothalamic tract pathways make functionally distinct contributions to nociception.[22]

Descending Pain Modulatory Pathways

The concept of an independent and specific CNS network that modified pain sensation was first suggested by the observation that electrical stimulation of the midbrain in rats, selectively repressed responses to painful stimuli.[26,27] This phenomenon, termed stimulation-produced analgesia, was confirmed in humans when neurosurgeons placed electrodes in homologous midbrain sites and demonstrated that stimulation produced a striking and selective reduction of severe clinical pain.[28-30] Stimulation-produced analgesia is elicited by stimulation of the midbrain in the region of the peri-aqueductal gray matter (PAG) and the rostroventral medulla (RVM).[31-34]

The analgesic effect of midbrain stimulation is due to activation of a pain-modulating circuit that projects to the spinal cord dorsal horn. This descending pain modulatory circuit, which contains high concentrations of endogenous opioid peptides, can be activated by opiate analgesics. Major sources of the input to the PAG come from frontal cortical, hypothalamic, and limbic system structures, suggesting that cognitive and emotional input plays a role in pain modulation.

The RVM gives rise to a major projection to the spinal cord via the dorsolateral funiculus (DLF). The terminals of the DLF fibers concentrate in dorsal horn laminae I, II, and V, where there are synaptic connections with terminals of nociceptive primary afferents, opioid-secreting interneurons, and cell bodies of STT neurons (the second-order pain transmission cells). Stimulation of either the PAG or RVM inhibits nociceptive neurons in these laminae.[35]

Another major brainstem projection to the spinal cord via the DLF arises from the dorsolateral pons. These spinally projecting neurons are noradrenergic.[36-38] Application of norepinephrine directly to the spinal cord selectively inhibits nociceptive dorsal horn neurons (Figure 2-4).[39,40]

In contrast to this noradrenergic system, the RVM contains a high percentage of spinally projecting serotoninergic neurons. Serotonin inhibits dorsal horn nociceptive neurons including STT cells.[41,42]

Hence, there are two descending pain modulatory pathways, one (noradrenergic) originating from the dorsolateral pons and the other (serotoninergic) from the RVM. Both travel via the DLF to the superficial layers of the spinal cord, where there is inhibition of nociceptive transmission.

Opiate Activation of the Descending Pain Modulatory System

Opiates produce analgesia by directly affecting the CNS. The injection of small amounts of opiates directly into the brain can produce potent analgesia.[43,44] The brainstem regions

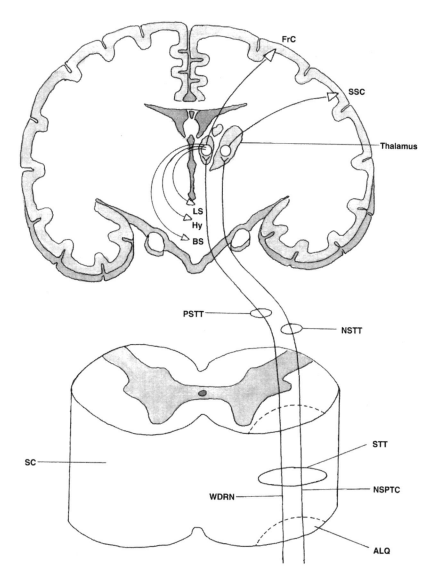

Figure 2-3 Somatotopic fiber organization continues at the brainstem level. The paleospinothalamic tract (PSTT) courses to medial thalamic nuclei, stimulating third-order cells, which project to the frontal cortex (FrC), limbic system (LS), hypothalamus (Hy), and reticular formation of the brainstem (BS). This paramedian pathway, with its diffuse projection to the limbic system and frontal lobe, subserves the affective-motivational aspects of pain. The lateral pathway, which projects to lateral thalamic nuclei, is known as the *neospinothalamic tract* (NSTT). The lateral thalamic nuclei give rise to a dense projection restricted to the somatosensory cortex (SSC). (STT = spinothalamic tract; SC = spinal cord; ALQ = anterolateral quadrant; WDRN = wide dynamic-range neuron; NSPTC = nociceptor-specific pain transmission cell.) Reprinted by permission from Rook JL: Neuroanatomy: ascending pain pathways and the descending pain modulatory system. In Cassvan A, Rook JL, Mullens SU, *et al.* (eds): *Cumulative Trauma Disorders*, p 23, fig 3-6. Boston, Butterworth-Heinemann, 1997.

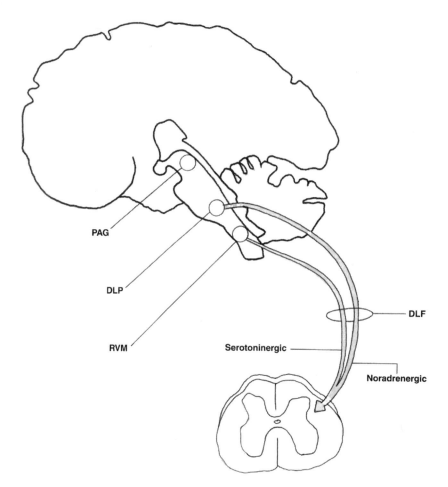

Figure 2-4 The dorsolateral funiculus (DLF). The rostroventral medulla (RVM), which gives rise to a major projection to the spinal cord via the DLF, contains a high percentage of spinally projecting serotoninergic neurons. Another major brain-stem projection to the spinal cord via the DLF arises from the dorsolateral pons (DLP). These spinally projecting neurons are noradrenergic. (PAG = peri-aqueduc-tal gray matter.) Reprinted by permission from Rook JL: Neuroanatomy: ascending pain pathways and the descending pain modulatory system. In Cassvan A, Rook JL, Mullens SU, et al. (eds): *Cumulative Trauma Disorders*, p 26, fig 3-8. Boston, Butterworth-Heinemann, 1997.

that produce analgesia when electrically stimulated largely overlap those at which opiate microinjection produces analgesia. It has been possible to map the distribution of opiate receptors in the brain using radioactively labeled opiates. Dense concentrations of opiate binding sites have been localized to the midbrain PAG, the RVM, and the superficial dorsal horn of the spinal cord.[45–48]

Once the opiate receptor had been identified, researchers began searching for the endogenous opioid ligands to bind at these highly specific receptor sites. The first major breakthrough occurred when Hughes et al.[49] reported that they had isolated two endogenous opioids from the brain, the enkephalins. Since the discovery of the enkephalins, a number of the other endogenous opioid peptides have been discovered, including the endorphins, and the dynorphin peptides.

The enkephalins, beta-endorphin, and the dynorphins are all present in the PAG. The enkephalins and dynorphins are also present in the RVM and in regions of the spinal dorsal horn involved in nociception. Thus, all the known opioid peptide families are present in structures identified with nociceptive modulation, and it is believed that they normally function to relieve pain.[50,51] Furthermore, systemically administered narcotic analgesics produce analgesia by mimicking the action of the endogenous opioid peptides in the PAG, RVM, and spinal cord.

The patient who is immediately post motor vehicle accident and who has fairly localized or even diffuse chronic pain, has activity principally emanating from layer I and the NSPTC. This second order pain transmission cell projects to the lateral thalamus and the somatosensory cortex, localizing pain from the area of injury. However, since the patient has not yet developed a chronic pain situation, there is less activity in the more midline pathways (WDRNs, medial thalamus, limbic system, frontal cortex, brainstem), structures involved in the affective component of pain. However, as the pain persists, patients may develop a chronic pain syndrome with symptoms including sleep disturbance, depression and anxiety. By this time, there is greater activity in these midline pathways. This shift of pain impulses through the more primitive paleospinothalamic tract accounts for the chronic pain symptomatology.

Therefore, there is a pathophysiological model that accounts for the transition of acute, post-motor vehicle accident pain into a more complex chronic pain syndrome with emotional and affective components. Understanding these pathways helps the practitioner to better manage both acute and chronic pain syndromes.

REFERENCES

1. Merskey H, Bogduk N. *Classification of Chronic Pain: Descriptions of Chronic Pain Syndromes and Definitions of Pain Terms*, 2nd edition. Seattle, IASP Press, 1994.
2. Harden RN, Bruehl SP, Gass S, *et al*. Signs and symptoms of the myofascial pain syndrome. A national survey of pain management providers. *Clin J Pain* 2000 March; 16 (1): 64.
3. Millea PJ and Holloway RL. Treating fibromyalgia. *Am Fam Physician* 2000; 62(7): 1575, 1587.
4. Aaron LA, Burke MM, Buchwald D. Overlapping conditions among patients with chronic fatigue syndrome, fibromyalgia, and temporomandibular disorder. *Arch Intern Med* 2000; 160(2): 221.
5. Freeman MAR, Wyke B. The innervation of the knee joint. An anatomical and histological study in the cat. *J Anat* 1967; 101: 505.
6. Langford LA, Schmidt RF. Afferent and efferent axons in the medial and posterior articular nerves of the cat. *Anat Rec* 1983; 206: 71.
7. Stacey JJ. Free nerve endings in skeletal muscle of the cat. *J Anat* 1969; 105: 231.
8. Adriaensen H, Gybels J, Handwerker HO, *et al*. Response properties of thin myelinated (A delta) fibers in human skin nerves. *J Neurophysiol* 1983; 49: 111.
9. Georgopoulos AP. Functional properties of primary afferent units probably related to pain mechanisms in primate glabrous skin. *J Neurophysiol* 1974; 39: 71.
10. Fields HL. The peripheral pain sensory system. In Fields HL (ed). *Pain*, p 13. New York. McGraw-Hill, 1987.

11. Juan H, Lembeck F. Action of peptides and other algesic agents on paravascular pain receptors of the isolated perfused rabbit ear. *Naunyn Schmiedebergs Arch Pharmacol* 1974; 283: 151.

12. Chahl LA, Ladd RJ. Local edema and general excitation of cutaneous sensory receptors produced by electrical stimulation of the saphenous nerve in the rat. *Pain* 1976; 2: 25.

13. Chapman LF, Ramos AO, Goodell H, *et al.* Neurohumoral features of afferent fibers in man. *Arch Neurol* 1961; 4: 617.

14. Otsuka M, Konishi S, Yanagisawa M, *et al.* Role of substance P as a sensory transmitter in spinal cord and sympathetic ganglia. *Ciba Found Symp* 1982; 91: 13.

15. LaMotte RH, Thalhammer JG, Robinson CJ. Peripheral neural correlates of magnitude of cutaneous pain and hyperalgesia. a comparison of neural events in monkey with sensory judgments in human. *J Neurophysiol* 1983; 50: 1.

16. Ochoa J, Mair WGP. The normal sural nerve in man. I. Ultrastructure and numbers of fibers and cells. *Acta Neuropathol* 1969; 13: 197.

17. Torebjork HE. Afferent C units responding to mechanical, thermal, and chemical stimuli in human nonglabrous skin. *Acta Physiol Scand* 1974; 92: 374.

18. Rexed B. A cytoarchitectonic atlas of the spinal cord in the cat. *J Comp Neurol* 1952; 96: 415.

19. Willis WD. *The Pain System.* Basel, Switzerland. Karger, 1985.

20. Willis WD, Kenshalo DR Jr, Leonard RB. The cells of origin of the primate spinothalamic tract. *J Comp Neurol* 1979; 188: 543.

21. Willis WD, Trevino DL, Coulter JD, *et al.* Responses of primate spinothalamic tract neurons to natural stimulation of hindlimb. *J Neurophysiol* 1974; 37: 358.

22. Fields HL. Pain pathways in the central nervous system. In Fields HL (ed). *Pain*, p 41. New York. McGraw-Hill, 1987.

23. Albe-Fessard D, Berkley KJ, Kruger L, *et al.* Diencephalic mechanisms of pain sensation. *Brain Res Rev* 1985; 9: 217.

24. Jones EG, Leavitt RY. Retrograde axonal transport and the demonstration of non-specific projections to the cerebral cortex and striatum from thalamic intralaminar nuclei in the rat, cat, and monkey. *J Comp Neurol* 1974; 154: 349.

25. Kaufman EFS, Rosenquist AC. Efferent projections of the thalamic intralaminar nuclei in the cat. *Brain Res* 1985; 335: 257.

26. Fields HL, Basbaum AI. Brainstem control of spinal pain transmission neurons. *Annu Rev Physiol* 1978; 40: 217.

27. Mayer DJ, Price DD. Central nervous system mechanisms of analgesia. *Pain* 1976; 2: 379.

28. Baskin DS, Mehler WR, Hosobuchi Y, *et al.* Autopsy analysis of the safety, efficiency, and cartography of electrical stimulation of the central gray in humans. *Brain Res* 1986; 371: 231.

29. Hosobuchi Y, Adams JE, Linchitz R. Pain relief by electrical stimulation of the central gray matter in humans and its reversal by naloxone. *Science* 1977; 197: 183.

30. Richardson DE, Akil H. Pain reduction by electrical brain stimulation in man. *J Neurophysiol* 1977; 47: 178.

31. Abols IA, Basbaum AI. Afferent connections of the rostral medulla of the cat. a neural substrate for midbrainmedullary interactions in the modulation of pain. *J Comp Neurol* 1981; 201: 285.

32. Beitz AJ. The organization of afferent projections to the midbrain periaqueductal gray of the rat. *Neuroscience* 1982; 7: 133.

33. Mantyh PW. The ascending input to the midbrain periaqueductal gray of the primate. *J Comp Neurol* 1982; 211: 50.

34. Zorman G, Hentall ID, Adams JE, *et al.* Naloxone-reversible analgesia produced by microstimulation in the rat medulla. *Brain Res* 1981; 219: 137.

35. Fields HL, Heinricher MM. Anatomy and physiology of a nociceptive modulatory system. *Philos Trans R Soc Lond B Biol Sci* 1985; 308: 361.

36. Westlund KN, Bowker RM, Ziegler MG, *et al.* Descending noradrenergic projections and their spinal terminations. *Prog Brain Res* 1982; 57: 219.

37. Westlund KN, Bowker RM, Ziegler MG, *et al.* Origins and terminations of descending noradrenergic projections into the spinal cord of the monkey. *Brain Res* 1984; 292: 1.
38. Reddy SVR, Yakah TL. Spinal noradrenergic terminal system mediates antinociception. *Brain Res* 1980; 189: 391.
39. Belcher G, Ryall RW, Schaffner R. The differential effects of 5-hydroxytryptamine, noradrenaline, and raphe stimulation on nociceptive and non-nociceptive dorsal horn interneurons in the cat. *Brain Res* 1978; 151: 307.
40. Duggan AW. Pharmacology of descending control systems. *Philos Trans R Soc Lond B Biol Sci* 1985; 308: 375.
41. Bowker R, Westlund KN, Coulter JD. Origins of serotonergic projections of the spinal cord in rat. An immunocytochemical retrograde transport study. *Brain Res* 1981; 226: 187.
42. Jordan LM, Kenshalo DR, Martin RF, *et al.* Depression of primate spinothalamic tract neurons by iontophoretic application of 5-hydroxytryptamine. *Pain* 1978; 5: 135.
43. Leavens ME, Hill CS Jr, Cech DA, *et al.* Intrathecal and intraventricular morphine for pain in cancer patients: initial study. *J Neurosurg* 1982; 56: 241.
44. Nurchi G. Use of intraventricular and intrathecal morphine in intractable pain associated with cancer. *Neurosurgery* 1984; 15: 801.
45. Fields HL. Central nervous system mechanisms for control of pain transmission. In Fields HL (ed), *Pain*, p 99. New York, McGraw-Hill, 1987.
46. Chang KJ. Opioid receptors. multiplicity and sequelae of ligand-receptor interactions. In Conn PM (ed), *The Receptors*, vol 1, p 1. Orlando, FL. Academic, 1984.
47. Martin WR. Pharmacology of opioids. *Pharmacol Rev* 1984; 35: 283.
48. Snyder SH, Matthysse S. Opiate receptor mechanisms. *Neurosci Res Prog Bull* 1975; 13: 1.
49. Hughes J, Smith TW, Kosterlitz HW, *et al.* Identification of two related pentapeptides from the brain with potent opiate agonist activity. *Nature* 1975; 258: 577.
50. Khachaturian H, Lewis ME, Watson SJ. Enkephalin systems in diencephalon and brainstem of the rat. *J Comp Neurol* 1983; 220: 310.
51. Palkovits M. Distribution of neuropeptides in the central nervous system. a review of biochemical mapping studies. *Prog Neurobiol* 1984; 23: 151.

3

Gait Pattern Considerations in Whiplash Injuries

Nicholas I Sol

Gait analysis is a recent but not widely practiced clinical consideration in the evaluation and care of acceleration injuries of the cervical spine. When practiced, visual gait analysis is usually performed by the "trained" observer despite the lack of a permanent record for review. This is unfortunate because the value of video records is widely accepted in a wide spectrum of differing activities. Despite the wide availability and decreasing cost of the equipment, video gait analysis is not yet widely practiced. Table 3-1 outlines the many advantages of video gait analysis in comparison to observational gait analysis. It is the

Table 3-1 Comparison between video gait analysis and observational gait analysis

Video Taped Gait Analysis	Observational Gait Analysis
Permanent record	No permanent record
Can be reviewed	Cannot be reviewed
Can be reproduced	Cannot be reproduced
Multiple perspectives	Single perspective
Can view multiple images from differing vantages on a single frame	Observer can only view one image from one perspective at a time
An event can simultaneously be observed on several planes	An event can be observed in one plane only
Higher and variable resolution	Lower and static resolution
From 30 frames/second (standard video) to 240 frames/second (high speed video)	Approximately 15 frames/second
Timing is variable	Timing is static
Slow motion	
Pause	
Jog & shuttle	
Functional relationships can be measured	Functional relationships can only be estimated

author's experience that video analysis is invaluable as a clinical tool that renders observational gait analysis increasingly obsolete.

Computerized motion capture and analysis (CMCA) has been available for many years but the price of the equipment and the training necessary for operation and data interpretation have generally been prohibitive to the individual clinician. As computer hardware and video equipment become more powerful and less expensive, increasingly sophisticated CMCA applications are finding wider clinical use. These systems use digital video to capture the motion of multiple markers placed on anatomical landmarks. Once captured, the data is then analyzed by sophisticated software. In most cases the analysis is based on the motion itself. As generalized use of this technology expands, so will the library of both normative and pathological data. Hopefully it will become standard practice both to capture motion digitally and then compare it to an extensive reference library of benchmarked data based on sophisticated software modeling. The increasing acceptance of technology based biomechanical analysis is encouraging. Byproducts include the aforementioned wealth of new data and the reshaping of accepted biomechanical tenets. Until recently, most of the CMCA applications captured data from only the pelvis and lower extremities. In response to the emerging data and the ongoing evolution in biomechanical theory, these applications increasingly include kinematic modeling of data captured from the motion of the spine, shoulders, upper extremities, neck, and head. Contemporary gait analysis now includes every segment of the kinetic chain.

THE KINETIC CHAIN

The basic unit of kinetic modeling is the "segment."[1] Each segment is assumed to be a rigid structure. Since living tissue has mechanical properties (e.g., elasticity, deformability, volumetric changes), this assumption of rigidity is fundamentally invalid. To nullify this assumption, kinetic modeling attempts to increase validity and reliability by increasing the number of segments modeled. For example, a spine modeled with three segments (cervical, thoracic and lumbar) is more valid and the data more reliable than a spine modeled as a single solid unit. Likewise, a seven-segment model of the cervical spine (a segment for each vertebrae) is more valid and the data more reliable than a single segment model of the cervical spine. The assumption that each segment is rigid puts practical limits on how many segments to model. As the number of segments increases, the validity of the model and the reliability of the data become proportionately more dependent on the mechanical characteristics of the individual tissues (e.g., elasticity, deformability, volumetric changes). In contemporary CMCA, the 14-segment model has become widely accepted (Figure 3-1).

This model of the kinetic chain includes the cervical spine, shoulders, upper arms, lower arms, torso, lumbar spine, pelvis, hips, upper legs, lower legs, and feet. Note that the torso and shoulders are modeled as a single segment. In short, the kinetic chain includes any body segment that is in motion during gait. Therefore the timing, amplitude, direction, and duration of the motion can have both a cause and effect relationship with gait.

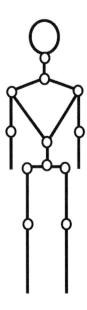

Figure 3-1 14-segment kinematic model. Note that the torso is modeled as a single segment.

GAIT AND THE SPINE

Lumbar spine pathology has undergone intense investigation, in part, because of its widespread epidemiology and enormous economic impact. The lower incidence of cervical spine pathology has resulted in a relative paucity of published references. There are few, if any, that specifically examine the relationships between gait and the cervical spine.

Porterfield and DeRosa contend that there are "marked similarities" between the lumbar and cervical spine with regard to anatomy and biomechanics.[2] They go on to say that the etiology, pathogenesis, and prognosis for mechanical low back pain are similar to the etiology, pathogenesis, and prognosis for mechanical neck pain. Like low back pain patients, the largest share of medical resources are consumed by the relatively small group of cervical spine pain patients that do not respond to conservative and/or surgical management.

Shoulder-pelvis counter-rotation is a visually observable phenomenon demonstrating one relationship between gait and the spine (Figure 3-2).[3] This phenomenon can be likened to "pendulums in a coupled system."[4] In this model, kinetic energy from counter-rotation of the two horizontal pendulums (shoulder and pelvis) creates potential energy in the form of axial torque and deformation of the vertical connecting rod (spine). The potential energy is stored in the form of stretching and tension of connective and viscoelastic tissues (e.g., thoracolumbar fascia, intervertebral ligaments, intervertebral discs). Potential energy is then converted back into kinetic energy as the counter-rotation changes direction. This is an energy conserving system. In one study, researchers found that subjects required 10 percent more oxygen to walk a given path with their trunks immobilized compared to the same subjects walking the same path without trunk immobilization.[5]

The anatomic curvature of each spinal segment (cervical, thoracic, and lumbar) offers mechanical advantage. Lovett first coined the term "coupled motion" in his examination of

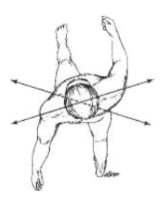

Figure 3-2 Shoulder-pelvis counter-rotation. Reprinted by permission from Valmassy RL: *Clinical Biomechanics of the Lower Extremities*, p 36. St. Louis, Mosby, 1996.

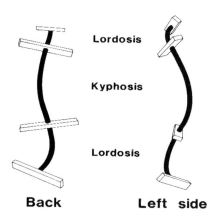

Lordosis

Kyphosis

Lordosis

Back   **Left side**

Figure 3-3 The lordosis-kyphosis-lordosis orientation of the spine segments maximizes shoulder-pelvis coupled motion while stabilizing the cervical spine and head. Reprinted by permission from Gracovetsky S: *The Spinal Engine*. New York, Springer-Verlag, 1988.

spinal mechanics. This examination demonstrated that a lateral bending force applied to one end of an inherently curved segment produced axial torque at the opposite end.[6] Gracovetsky further examined the relationship between gait and the spine and coined the term "the spinal engine."[4] In his book by the same name, Gracovetsky likened the three curved spinal segments (cervical, thoracic, and lumbar) to spinal building blocks. He demonstrated that the orientation and combination of lordosis-kyphosis-lordosis curves enabled the spine to maximize the axial torque created at the pelvis by lateral bending of the shoulders while simultaneously stabilizing and minimizing axial motion of the cervical spine and head (Figure 3-3). Interestingly, Gracovetsky concluded that gait function was inseparable from spinal function.

REPETITION AND SYMMETRY

Human gait can be divided into three phases: development, rhythmic, and decay.[7,8] While energy use during the development and decay phases is high, energy expenditure during rhythmic gait is relatively low. Energy during this phase comes increasingly from momentum, gravity, and the elastic tissue response and decreasingly from direct muscle activity. Although reports vary, the normal range of human cadence during rhythmic gait is 90 to 120 steps per minute.[9,10] On an hourly basis, that is 5400 to 7200 steps per walking hour. Table 3-2 delineates the total number of cycles (steps) based on walking hours. It is intuitive that patients with more cycles (steps) and/or greater degree of asymmetric function will be more likely to be affected by their gait style. One of the most potentially strenuous phases in the gait cycle is limb lift. Dananberg demonstrated that each lower extremity weighs approximately 15 percent of total body weight. Table 3-3 demonstrates the lower extremity weight of each lower extremity for individuals of varying total body weight. In the consideration of lower extremity lifting load during ambulation, Table 3-4 outlines the cumulative lift per side for an individual with a total body weight of 160 pounds. While the number of cycles can be quantified, the degree of asymmetric function cannot. It is the author's experience that asymmetric function is most frequently a compensation strategy for assisting dysfunctional limb lift and less frequently a compensation strategy for single limb support on an unstable limb. The quantification and classification of functional asymmetry may someday be predictive of the role of gait style in mechanical musculoskeletal pain including whiplash injuries. Perhaps this will become possible with careful analysis of objective data from the wider clinical use of CMCA.

Casual observation of gait styles demonstrates an almost infinite number of combinations of functional asymmetries. When recognizing the "walk" of a friend, what

Table 3-2 Total steps on an hourly basis

Walking Hours	Total Steps @ 90/minute	Total Steps @ 120/minute
1	5 400	7 200
2	10 800	14 400
3	16 200	21 600
4	21 600	28 800
5	27 000	36 000
6	32 400	43 200
7	37 800	50 400
8	43 200	57 600

Table 3-3 Each lower extremity weighs approximately 15 per cent of total body weight

Body Weight (lbs)	Lower Extremity Weight (lbs)
120	18
140	21
160	24
180	27
200	30

Table 3-4 Cumulative lifting per minute per side for a 160 lb patient with 24 lb limbs

Walking Minutes	Cumulative Lift/Side (lbs) @ 90 steps/min	Cumulative Lift/Side (lbs) @ 120 steps/min
1	1 080	1 440
10	10 800	14 400
20	21 600	28 800
30	32 400	43 200
60	64 800	86 400
120	129 600	172 800

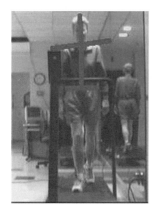

Figure 3-4 Lateral torso bending or lateral carriage.

is really recognized is their pattern of asymmetry—their limping pattern. This pattern may be divided into two categories: postures and movements. Postures are characteristically present during 100 percent of the gait cycle and movements are phasic and described in relation to when they occur (i.e., during initial swing).

Postures of the upper portion of the kinetic chain include lateral carriage, forward carriage, shoulder tilt and head tilt. When phasic, lateral carriage is termed lateral torso bending and forward carriage is termed forward torso bending (Figures 3-4 and 3-5). Other phasic movements of the upper kinetic chain include unequal shoulder rotation, head tilting, shoulder tilting, and cervical bending. Since human cadence is 90 to 120 steps per minute, unilateral phasic movements occur 45 to 60 times each walking minute. Figure 3-6 demonstrates several compensatory postures and movements of the upper kinetic chain. In each case, the muscle group undergoing repetitive contraction is indicated.

BALANCE

Maintaining erect posture during static stance and both single and double limb support phases during gait is a multi-sensory task. The hallmarks of functional development from

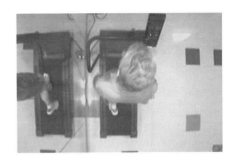

Figure 3-5 Forward torso bending or forward carriage.

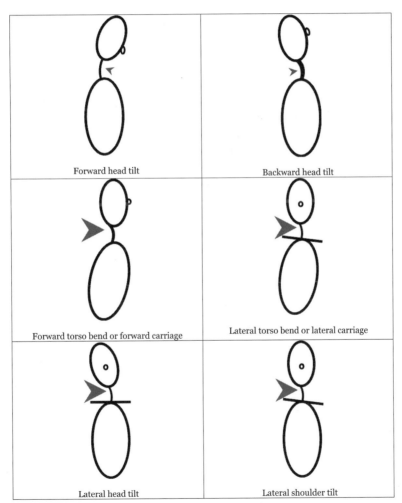

Forward head tilt

Backward head tilt

Forward torso bend or forward carriage

Lateral torso bend or lateral carriage

Lateral head tilt

Lateral shoulder tilt

Figure 3-6 Various postures and movements. Arrows indicate muscle group contraction.

toddling to mature gait include the increase in single limb support duration, decrease in the base of gait (ankle span narrower than pelvic span), shoulder-pelvis counter-rotation and consistency in motion.[11] These hallmarks reflect improving balance from developing vestibular, somatosensory and visual mechanisms. It is beyond the scope of this chapter to examine the mechanisms of balance in depth. Instead, the author will briefly discuss the vestibular and neck proprioceptive systems in relation to balance, posture and gait.

The vestibular mechanism monitors position and movement of the head. The input to this mechanism is from five organs: saccular, urticular and the cristae of the three semicircular canals.[12] The otoliths (saccular and urticular) sense linear acceleration of the head. Rotational acceleration is sensed by the three cristae of the semicircular canals. Interestingly, all five organs are within the temporal bone although the significance of this is undefined. In a landmark study, Zangemeister, *et al.* found a functional linkage between otolith signals and activity in lower extremity muscles during gait. In particular, they found a generalized increase in tibialis anterior and vastus medialis activity while subjects walked with posterior head tilt. This head posture resulted in significantly increased peak ground reactive forces. The most notable result, though, was the detection of an additional phasic burst of activity from the tibialis anterior.

Other authors have found that positional changes of the trunk in relation to the head evokes tonic neck reflexes.[13,14] Vestibulospinal reflexes are evoked by positional changes of the trunk in relation to the movements of the body in space. In the simplest model, these reflexes target a "straight and level" head position relative to gravity. Hence, the neck musculature functions in both sensory and motor roles as the proprioceptors send continuous information to the brainstem which sends efferent signals back to the muscles to maintain, change and/or correct head position.

Whiplash injuries disrupt the normal sensory data from neck proprioceptors.[15] Following the application of both neuropsychological and otoneurological tests to whiplash patients, Gimse, *et al.* concluded that injuries of the neck from whiplash disorganizes normal neck proprioceptive activity. In support of this finding, Heikkila and Wenngren concluded that restricted cervical motion due to acute acceleration injury (i.e., whiplash) causes proprioceptive dysfunction in the cervical spine.[16]

The same injury disrupts the ability of the neck musculature to effectively maintain, change and/or correct head position.[17] Loudon, *et al.* demonstrated that whiplash patients were unable to consistently reproduce a target head position with respect to body or environment. Taguchi, *et al.* found that subjective vertical shifted toward the affected side in subjects with unilateral vestibular dysfunction.[18] They also found a clinically significant relationship between body sway and the degree that subjective vertical deviated from true vertical.

Pozzo is one of the most widely published investigators into the relationship between postural control, balance, vision, and head position. He was a member of the team that made an unusual examination of the role of vision to control upside-down standing posture.[19] They concluded that visual references help to maintain fine balance control by conveying the optimal zone for the center of gravity. In an examination of the relationship between balance and movements of the head and trunk, Pozzo, *et al.* concluded that complex equilibrium tasks require head angular stabilization.[20] They postulated that angular stabilization of the head provides the central nervous system with essential visual and vestibular references. In a two-part examination of locomotor tasks, Pozzo, *et al.* described head stabilization as a basis for inertial guidance in normal subjects.[21] In their examination of patients performing locomotor tasks in darkness, they found decreased head rotations in normal subjects while the head rotation of patients with bilateral vestibular deficits increased.[22]

Grossman and Leigh have also collaborated on several investigations. One study examined the frequency and velocity of rotational head movement during locomotion in normal subjects.[23] They found that the head was stabilized incompletely but adequately during locomotion and concluded that that did not saturate the vestibular-ocular reflex. In a later study, they evaluated gaze stability of normal subjects during various locomotor activities including standing, walking in place and running in place.[24] Interestingly, they found that gaze was stable within 0.4 degrees vertically and horizontally during all activities.

There appears to be a pattern of increased reliance on vision in patients who have suffered whiplash injuries. Rubin, *et al.* suggested that these patients increasingly use visual data for postural stability and that they cannot use their vestibular orienting data to resolve conflicts between visual and somatosensory systems.[25] This seems to confirm the necessity of adequate head and visual stability during locomotion.

CONCLUSION

Fluid posture and balance control is a function of continuous sensory and motor activity. In patients with acceleration injury to the cervical spine (i.e., whiplash), both sensory and motor activity becomes dysfunctional. Posture and balance suffer predictably making efficient, purposeful, and stable gait more difficult. Increased asymmetric load is placed on the kinetic chain by gait pathomechanics that place additional functional demands on acutely injured tissues.

Restoring symmetric, efficient, purposeful and stable gait becomes an important clinical consideration to move these patients from slips, trips and falls toward improved recovery, stability and function.

REFERENCES

1. Seliktar R, Bo L. The theory of kinetic analysis in human gait. In Craik RL, Oatis CA (eds): *Gait Analysis Theory and Application*, pp 223–238. St. Louis, Mosby, 1995.
2. Porterfield JA, DeRosa C. Principals of mechanical neck disorders. In Porterfield JA, DeRosa C. *Mechanical Neck Pain: Perspectives in Functional Anatomy*, pp 1–20. Philadelphia: WB Saunders, 1995.
3. Wernick J, Volpe RG. Lower extremity function and normal mechanics. In Valmassy RL (ed). *Clinical Biomechanics of the Lower Extremities*, p 36. St Louis, Mosby, 1996.
4. Gracovetsky S. The theory of the spinal engine. In Gracovetsky (ed). *The Spinal Engine*, pp 286–315. Vienna, Springer-Verlag, 1988.
5. Ralston HJ. Effects of immobilization of various body segments on the energy cost of human locomotion. *Ergonomics* 1965; suppl: 53

6. Lovett AW. A contribution to the study of the mechanics of the spine. *Am J Anat* 1903; 2:457–462.

7. Lettre C, Contine R. Accelerographic analysis of pathological gait. *New York University School of Engineering and Science Technical Report 1368.01*. New York, New York University Press, 1967.

8. Sutherland DH, Kaufman KR, Moitoza JR. Kinematics of normal human walking. In Rose J, Gamble JG (eds). *Human Walking*, pp 23–44. Baltimore, Williams & Wilkins, 1994.

9. Dananberg HJ. Gait style as an etiology to chronic postural pain. Part 1. Functional hallux limitus. *J Am Podiatr Med Assoc* 1993 Aug; 83(8): 433–441.

10. Dananberg HJ. Gait style as an etiology to chronic postural pain. Part 2. Postural compensatory process. *J Am Podiatr Med Assoc* 1993 Nov; 83(11): 433–441.

11. Skinner S. Development of gait. In Rose J, Gamble JG (eds). *Human Walking*, pp 123–138. Baltimore, Williams & Wilkins, 1994.

12. Zangemeister WH, Bulgheroni MV, Pedotti A. Normal gait is differentially influenced by the otoliths. *J Biomed Eng* 1991; 13: 451–458.

13. Grossman GE, Leigh RJ, Bruce EN, Huebner WP, Lanska DJ. Performance of the human vestibuloocular reflex during locomotion. *J Neurophysiol* 1989 Jul; 62(1). 264–721.

14. Demer JL, Oas, JG, Baloh RW. Visual-vestibular interaction in humans during active and passive vertical head movement. *J Vestib Res* 1993 Summer; 3(2): 101–114.

15. Gimse R, Tjell C, Bjorgen IA, Saunte C. Disturbed eye movements after whiplash due to injuries to the posture control system. *J Clin Exp Neuropsychol* 1996 Apr; 18(2): 178–186.

16. Heikkila HV, Wenngren BI. Cervicocephalic kinesthetic sensibility, active range of cervical motion and oculomotor function in patients with whiplash injury. *Arch Phys Med Rehabil* 1998 Sep; 79(9): 1089–1094.

17. Loudon JK, Ruhl M, Field E. Ability to reproduce head position after whiplash injury. *Spine* 1997; 22(8): 865–868.

18. Taguchi K, Sakaguchi S, Ishiyama T, Sato K. Clinical significance of the subjective vertical in patients with unilateral vestibular disorders. *Acta Otolaryngol (Stockh)* 1997; Suppl 528: 74–76.

19. Cl'ement G, Pozzo T, Berthoz A. Contribution of eye positioning to control of the upside-down standing posture. *Brain Res* 1988; 73(3): 569–576.

20. Pozzo T, Levik Y, Berthoz A. Head and trunk movements in the frontal plane during complex dynamic equilibrium tasks in humans. *Brain Res* 1995; 106(2): 327–338.

21. Pozzo T, Berthoz A, Lefort L. Head stabilization during various locomotor tasks in humans. 1. Normal subjects. *Brain Res* 1990; 82(1): 97–106.

22. Pozzo T, Berthoz A, Lefort L, Vitte E. Head stabilization during various locomotor tasks in humans. 2. Patients with bilateral peripheral vestibular deficits. *Brain Res* 1991; 85(1): 208–217.

23. Grossman GE, Leigh RJ, Abel LA, et al. Frequency and velocity of rotational head perturbations during locomotion. *Brain Res* 1988; 70(3): 470–476.

24. Grossman GE, Leigh RJ, Bruce EN, et al. Performance of the human vestibuloocular reflex during locomotion. *J Neurophysiol* 1989 Jul; 62(1): 264–272.

25. Rubin AM, Woolley SM, Dailey VM, Goebel JA. Postural stability following mild head or whiplash injuries. *Am J Otol* 1995; 16(2): 216–221.

4

Diagnostic Workup

Jack L Rook

BLOOD TESTS

A number of serologic studies are available to help the clinician rule out various systemic disorders that can contribute to chronic pain states. Included would be the connective tissue profile, thyroid studies, and evaluation of endogenous steroid production.

The connective tissue profile includes testing to rule out rheumatoid arthritis, systemic lupus erythematosus, and ankylosing spondylitis. The serological test for rheumatoid arthritis is the rheumatoid factor, a test that identifies the IgM antibody, one of several classes of antibodies (also including IgG and IgA) that attack normal joint tissue contributing to the pathophysiological changes seen in this arthritic disorder. Patients with rheumatoid arthritis complain of diffuse joint arthralgias with an early predilection for small joints of the hands and feet.

Systemic lupus erythematosus (SLE) is a connective tissue disorder whereby the body's own immune system attacks organs and tissues throughout the body. One of the symptoms of this disorder is diffuse joint arthralgias. The principal serological test for detection of SLE is the antinuclear antibody (ANA). High ANA titers are consistent with this diagnosis.

Patients with ankylosing spondylitis (AS) can develop diffuse spinal pain and stiffness. There are characteristic x-ray changes that can be seen as this disorder progresses. However, the serological marker the HLA B27 antigen may aid in early detection of AS.

A nonspecific test for connective tissue diseases is the erythrocyte sedimentation rate (ESR), which tends to be elevated whenever a systemic inflammatory process contributes to a chronic pain situation. The ESR is the rate at which erythrocytes settle out of anticoagulated blood in one hour. This test is based on the fact that inflammatory processes cause an increase in blood proteins that attach themselves to red blood cells (RBCs), causing the red cells to aggregate. This makes them heavier and more likely to fall rapidly when placed in a special vertical test tube; the faster the settling of cells, the higher the ESR. The sedimentation rate is a nonspecific diagnostic laboratory finding that is indicative of some disease process that must be investigated further.

To perform the test, anticoagulated blood is suctioned into a graduated sedimentation tube and is allowed to settle for exactly one hour. The amount of settling is the patient's ESR. Normal Westergren ESR values for men are 0 to 15 mm/hr and in women 0 to 20 mm/hr.[1]

Patients who are hypothyroid may complain of generalized fatigue and diffuse body aches, similar symptoms to those experienced by the fibromyalgia patient. The serological tests used to evaluate for hypothyroidism are the T3, T4, and TSH (thyroid stimulating hormone). The T3 and T4 refer to actual thyroid hormone in the blood stream. These hormones emanate from the thyroid gland in response to another hormone generated by the pituitary known as thyroid stimulating hormone (TSH). In the hypothyroid state, the pituitary works extra hard in an effort to try to get the thyroid gland to liberate thyroid hormone. The serological result is a very high TSH value along with low T3 and T4 levels.

Patients who have hypoactive adrenal glands may also complain of generalized lethargy and discomfort. Endogenous steroids can be detected in the blood with serum cortisol level, and in the urine with a quantitative 24-hour urine study for cortisol. In addition, the cortisol stimulation test is used to assess how well the adrenal glands respond to a bolus injection of the pituitary trophic hormone, ACTH.

RADIOGRAPHY (X-RAY)

Radiography (roentgenography, x-ray) is the oldest method of body imaging, having been used to demonstrate bony and soft tissue pathology since the discovery of x-rays by Wilhelm Roentgen in 1895. Since then, it has continued to be useful diagnostically in every branch of medicine. More recently-developed imaging techniques, such as radionuclide scanning, ultrasonography, computerized tomography, and magnetic residence imaging, are complementing, and, in some instances, replacing long-established conventional x-ray techniques.

X-rays are electromagnetic waves with wave lengths that are only 1/10,000 the length of visible light rays. Because of this short wave length, x-rays can penetrate very dense substances to produce images or shadows that then can be recorded on photographic film placed behind the subject. The basic principle of radiography rests with the fact that differences in density between various body structures produce images of varying light or dark intensity on the x-ray film. Dense structures appear white, air-filled areas are black, and various tones of gray represent varying degrees of tissue density through which the x-ray beams have passed. A radiopaque contrast medium is frequently employed to help distinguish separate structures, thus making x-rays easier to interpret. Roentgenography is safe when properly used by trained personal.

Radiography produces excellent anatomic images of almost any body part. Costs of equipment and examinations are considerably less than compared to those of most other imaging systems. Space requirements for ordinary radiographic equipment are not excessive, and, because there are a great many specialists exclusively trained in radiography, its use is not confined to large medical centers.

The major disadvantage of radiographic imaging is its fundamental basis in ionizing radiation. Exposure of the human body to x-rays carries with it certain risks. Genetic alterations (mutations) may occur in the exposed person's offspring if reproductive organs are exposed to radiation. Somatic mutations (those that occur in body tissue other than reproductive cells) may also occur in tissues receiving excessive or repeated doses of radiation. For example, radiation can be the cause of cancer that develops many years after exposure. During the first trimester of pregnancy, the fetus is especially at risk for genetic alterations. Precautions must be taken to prevent or minimize radiation exposure to the pregnant uterus.

The dangers of exposure to radiation arise from both the absorption of relatively large amounts of radiation over a short time period, and also from the cumulative effects of smaller amounts received over longer time periods. More over, the cumulative effects of radiation may not become evident for several years.

Common x-ray films obtained after a motor vehicle accident correspond to areas of pain or suspected pathology. Cervical, thoracic, and lumbar films are frequently obtained to evaluate for acute fractures, the development of instability, and the presence of underlying degenerative arthritis (which may have become symptomatic as a result of forces generated in the accident).

Shoulder x-rays can be obtained to evaluate for the presence of bone spurs (which contribute to shoulder pain due to impingement), underlying degenerative arthritis, and to determine if there has been a traumatic glenohumeral or acromioclavicular joint separation. Rib, pelvic, and extremity x-rays can be obtained to evaluate for acute fractures.

Specialized cervical and lumbar x-ray techniques are available to assess for spinal pathology. Cervical oblique films can be obtained to evaluate for bony compromise of neuroforamina. Flexion and extension views help to evaluate for cervical spine instability. Open mouth views are obtained to assess the integrity of the dens of the axis (fracture with displacement of this bone is potentially lethal). Lumbar x-ray oblique views are used to check for the vertebral arch defect known as spondylolysis, whereas flexion and extension views are used to assess for lumbar spine instability.

COMPUTERIZED TOMOGRAPHY (CT, CAT SCAN)

Computerized tomography, also called CT scanning or computerized axial tomography (CAT), produces x-rays similar to those used in conventional radiography, but taken with a special scanner system.

Conventional x-ray machines produce a flat picture with the body's organs superimposed over one another. The result is a two-dimensional image of a three-dimensional body. With CT scanning, an interconnected x-ray source and detector system is rapidly rotated around a supine patient within a gantry. Detectors record the number of transmitted x-rays during the scan period. Digital computers integrate the collected information, which is reconstructed into a cross-sectional image (tomogram) that is displayed directly on a television screen. The image can be photographed or stored for later retrieval. Therefore, CT produces cross-sectional images (slices) of anatomic structures without superimposing tissues upon one another. Additionally, CT can differentiate tissue characteristics within a particular solid organ.

Radiograms and CT scans are reflections of the amount of x-rays passing through the body tissues and reaching the respective detectors. Tissues which absorb much of the x-ray beam (e.g., bone) will appear as white (radiopaque) shadows on the CT scan, just as they do on conventional x-rays; tissues that absorb little photon energy (e.g., fat and gas) record as black (radiolucent) shadows; soft tissues record as various shades of gray. Body tissues of varying density have their own radioattenuating values, which are denoted by CT numbers. Water has been assigned a CT number of zero; fat and gas have negative CT numbers; bone and metal have positive CT numbers; and soft tissues have varying positive CT numbers greater than zero (the CT number of water), but less than the CT number of bone. Any tissue on the CT slice can easily be assigned a CT number by the machine.

The advantages of CT scanning are that it demonstrates organ morphology exceptionally well, is relatively easy to interpret, and can be done on an outpatient basis. Its disadvantages are its basis in ionizing radiation, the size and immobility of the equipment, and cost of the studies.

To perform the procedure, the patient lies supine, without moving, on a motorized couch that moves into a donut-shaped gantry. X-ray tubes within the gantry move around the patient generating pictures that are projected onto a monitor screen at the same time. The patient needs to remain still during the procedure so that serial images can be adequately obtained. Sedation and analgesics may help the uncooperative or anxious patient lie quietly during the test.

During the examination, should a questionable area need further clarification, iodine contrast substance can be injected intravenously and more pictures taken, assuming there is no allergy to iodine (a contraindication to its use). Hypersensitivity reactions may occur when contrast materials are injected. The patient may experience warmth, flushing of the face, salty taste, and nausea with IV injection of contrast material. An emesis basin should be available as a precaution. After injection of the contrast, the patient must be monitored for untoward signs and symptoms such as respiratory difficulty, heavy sweating, palpitations, or progression to an anaphylactic reaction. Resuscitation equipment and drugs should be readily available.[2]

Common CT films that can be obtained after a motor vehicle accident include scans of the head, spine, pelvis, and the abdomen.

- CT scan of the head can be obtained to rule out a skull fracture, subdural hematoma or intracerebral bleed. The CT scan is the best test available to evaluate for a basilar skull fracture (fracture of the skull at the base of the brain).
- CT scans can be obtained of the cervical, thoracic, and lumbar spine to evaluate for acute pathology such as fracture or subluxation, degenerative changes, herniated discs, and for spinal cord and/or nerve root injury.
- CT scan of the pelvis can be obtained to rule out intrapelvic organ damage and to evaluate for fracture(s) of the pelvis or sacroiliac joint(s).
- CT scan of the abdomen can be utilized to evaluate for intra-abdominal trauma (e.g., ruptured spleen). CT abdominal examination is often preceded by having the patient

drink a contrast preparation that helps outline the bowels so it can be readily differentiated from other structures during the study. Pelvic CT examinations may require colorectal (barium enema) contrast administration. Female patients undergoing pelvic CT scans may require insertion of a vaginal tampon to help delineate the vaginal wall.

MRI SCANNING

It is generally agreed that magnetic resonance (MR) is probably the most powerful and versatile imaging technique in medicine. Clinical MR imaging has its basis in the nuclear properties of hydrogen atoms within the body. The nucleus of a hydrogen atom consists of a single proton. Any atom containing an odd number of protons has the nuclear property of spin, with its nucleus behaving like a tiny magnet. Ordinarily, the axis of spin of each hydrogen nucleus within the body is randomly oriented. However, if the whole body or part of it is placed in a strong magnetic field (like that produced by the large magnets housed in MR imagers), the hydrogen nuclei of the body part within that field will wobble like a top around the lines of magnetic force. If these nuclei are then additionally stimulated by short pulses of radio waves of appropriate frequency, they absorb the energy and invert their orientation within the magnetic field (they are elevated to a state of higher energy). Once the short radio frequency pulse terminates, the hydrogen nuclei return at various speeds (depending on the density of the tissues they reside in) to their original low-energy orientation in the magnetic field. Energy is emitted in the form of radio waves as this process occurs, a phenomenon called nuclear magnetic resonance (NMR). The emitted radio wave energies from the resonating hydrogen nuclei are collected by the MR units, converted to digits, coded spatially, and the information is reconstructed into tomographic body images that resemble CT scans. In other words, when the radio waves generated by the MR scanner are discontinued, the protons within the body rapidly return to a lower energy state producing a signal (tiny radio waves) that a computer can detect and covert into an image.

MR tomographic images are reflections of the varying hydrogen densities in different body organs and diseased tissues. Rigidly bound hydrogen nuclei, such as those in compact bone and calcified structures, register as black zones on the MR image. They are said to be MR silent (they do not generate radio wave energy). Hydrogen nuclei that move too rapidly are also MR-silent and register as black zones on the imaging. Thus, moving blood, for example, is imaged in various shades of black depending on the rate of blood flow. Loosely bound hydrogen nuclei within fat generate stronger radio waves during MR testing and will appear white on the MR scan. Thus, fat is demonstrated by MR as a bright, intense white image, the opposite of the black image it gives on radiograms and CT scans. Tissues of the brain, spinal cord, viscera, and muscles produce MR signals of intensities between the brightest white images of fat and the black images of cortical bone.

There are many advantages to MR imaging: it uses no ionizing radiation; no harmful genetic effects have been attributed to the energy ranges used for MR imaging; no bowel preparation or fluid/food restrictions are necessary; contrast media are not required to distinguish the gastrointestinal tract or vascular structures; and the images produced by MR give better information about soft tissues than any other method of imaging.

Disadvantages of MR imaging include:

- the equipment is very large and expensive, resulting in studies that cost more than other imaging procedures
- patients with metallic implants including surgical clips, joint replacements, pacemakers, spinal cord stimulators, cardiac defibrillators, and morphine pumps cannot be exposed to the powerful magnetic field used in MR imaging
- respiratory motion causes severe artifacts in abdomen and thoracic imaging
- severely obese persons may not fit into the gantry opening
- claustrophobic patients may be unable to tolerate MR imaging.

Although there is no special patient preparation required before an MRI, there are numerous safety factors that must be considered. Absolute contraindications to MRI include the presence of implanted devices, pacemakers, cochlear implants, some prosthetic devices, drug infusion pumps, neurostimulators, bone growth stimulators, certain intrauterine contraceptive devices, and internal metallic objects (metallic fragments, bullets, shrapnel, and surgical clips, pins, plates, screws, metal sutures, or wire mesh). Electronic implants are at risk of damage from both magnetic fields and the radio frequency pulses. Pregnancy and epilepsy are relative contra-indications.

Before entering the MR suite, patients should be advised to remove dental bridges, hearing aids, credit cards, keys, hair clips, shoes, belts, jewelry, clothing with metal fasteners, hairpins, wigs, and hairpieces. Fasting or drinking clear liquids several hours before examination for abdominal or pelvic MR may be necessary.

When performing the MR examination, the patient is positioned on a moveable examination couch, which is moved into the tunnel-shaped gantry. The patient is asked to remain still during the procedure. The gantry is narrow and sedation may be required if the patient is claustrophobic or otherwise unable to hold still during the procedure. In some instances, gadolinium DPTA, a non-iodinated contrast, will be injected into a vein for better visualization of anatomy. Gadolinium has very low toxicity and fewer side effects than x-ray contrast agents. Throughout the procedure, the patient will hear a rhythmic knocking sound. There is no discomfort associated with the MR examination.[3,4]

Common films obtained after motor vehicle accidents include MR scans of the head, cervical, thoracic, or lumbar region, abdomen, pelvis, and shoulder joints.

- MRI scans of the head are useful in ruling out intracerebral bleed, subdural hematoma, and skull trauma.
- MRI scans of the cervical, thoracic, or lumbar region are useful in determining the presence of degenerative changes, herniated discs, acute spinal fractures, and spinal cord or nerve root compression.

- MRI scans of the abdomen and pelvis can be useful in determining intra-abdominal trauma such as a splenic rupture, intrapelvic trauma, pelvic fracture, and/or sacroiliac joint disruption.

MRI scans of the shoulder are useful in delineating shoulder capsular tears, bursitis, tendonitis, and rotator cuff tears.

RADIONUCLIDE IMAGING (NUCLEAR IMAGING)

Nuclear imaging is obtained by means of intravenous infusion of a radionuclide tracer substance. A radionuclide is an atom with an unstable nucleus within its orbital electrons. In an attempt to reach stability, the radionuclide emits radiation, the most common types being alpha, beta, and gamma electromagnetic radiation particles. In nuclear medicine, gamma radiation is used in diagnostic procedures, as it is easy to detect, and is the least ionizing type.[4,5]

Computerized scintillation detectors detect gamma radiation by giving off a light flash or scintillation. Collectively, the scintillations will appear on the imaging device, outlining the organs under study, providing information on their size, shape, position, and functional activity.[5]

The radioactive materials used in nuclear medicine diagnostic imaging are called radiopharmaceuticals.[4] The most common radiopharmaceuticals are technetium 99M diethylenetriamine pentaacetic acid (DTPA), and technetium 99M dimercaptosuccinic acid (DMSA).

Several types of imaging devices are used in the field of nuclear medicine. The most basic is the gamma camera, an instrument placed over the target area that it views in two dimensions. The major limitation of the gamma camera is that it is two-dimensional, and lacks depth perception. Today, through single photon emission computed tomography (SPECT), gamma cameras have achieved the third dimension, increasing the diagnostic ability of nuclear medicine imaging.[5]

The major disadvantage of radionuclide studies is the radiation hazard to the patient, who retains the radioactivity for relatively short periods until it either dissipates on its own and/or is eliminated in urine and feces. These tests may be harmful to a fetus or infant and will be contraindicated during pregnancy or lactation. Advantages of these procedures include the fact that, in almost all instances, radionuclide imaging exposes the patient to less radiation than would be received if he/she were undergoing more traditional diagnostic x-ray studies. In addition, the test is safe and painless, and side effects, such as nausea, are minimal.

The radiopharmaceutical is administered intravenously to the patient, the quantity calculated based upon the age and weight of the individual. A sufficient time interval is allowed for the radioactive material to concentrate in the specific tissue to be studied. An imaging device then records the position and concentration of the radiation that emerges from the radionuclide, and a computer processes the recorded radiation.[5]

Abnormal results could indicate an occult fracture that was too small to be picked up on conventional radiography. Bone scanning techniques are also useful in helping to make the diagnosis of reflex sympathetic dystrophy (RSD). For that, the triple-phase bone scan is required. Triple-phase bone scanning will demonstrate blood flow abnormalities, providing further supporting objective documentation of the diagnosis, though such scans may be negative in up to 40 percent of patients in whom RSDS is clinically diagnosed.[6,7] Triple-phase scanning employing radiopharmaceutical technetium coupled with a phosphate complex has been used to help facilitate the diagnosis of RSD. However, many different conditions can produce bone demineralization (common with RSD), and a triple-phase bone scan does not distinguish between causes of bone demineralization. In general, then, triple-phase bone scanning may be considered a highly sensitive but not very specific tool. Though it will help to support the diagnosis, clinical acumen and correlation ultimately are required to diagnose RSD.[8]

Clinical information can be derived from each of the three phases of the triple-phase bone scan after injection of the radiopharmaceutical agents. First is the angiogram phase, as the compound remains intravascular for one to two minutes immediately following the injection. Serial images are recorded rapidly. Over the next five to ten minutes, the radiopharmaceutical compound diffuses into the extracellular fluid spaces of the body. This period reflects soft-tissue distribution of the compound and is referred to as the blood pool phase (phase 2). After two or three hours, the tracer is maximally bound to bone and will increase in areas where there is stimulus of bone turnover. It is during this time (phase 3) that images of skeleton or bone are obtained.

In early (stage 1) RSD, uptake of the tracer during phases 1 and 2 is increased. However, in RSD stages 2 and 3, uptake during these phases can actually be decreased. During phase 3, one will see diffuse bony uptake in the involved limb, reflecting bone turnover secondary to focal osteoporosis.[9–19]

THERMOGRAPHY

Thermography, an infrared imaging technique that can measure very subtle temperature differences between involved and uninvolved regions, might provide objective documentation of autonomic dysfunction, as seen with RSD. Temperature differences are seen as different colors on the thermographic images. Serial thermograms can be used to help determine the effectiveness of treatment over time.[20] Thermography is most useful in identifying early cases of RSD and, for this purpose, is actually better than triple-phase bone scanning, the sensitivity of which is in the range of 50 to 70 percent. Infrared stress studies significantly improve sensitivity and the specificity of standard thermographic procedures by challenging the integrity of the autonomic nervous system. The cold-water stress test is performed as follows:

- A baseline quantitative thermal emission of the symptomatic extremity is obtained.
- After baseline imaging, the contralateral or asymptomatic extremity is immersed for five minutes in a cold-water bath.

- At the end of the five-minute session, a quantitative thermal image of the symptomatic extremity is obtained.
- The quantitative pre- and post-test-image changes in temperature are calculated. Post-test cooling of the non-immersed extremity is the expected result. Paroxysmal warming is strongly suggestive of vasomotor instability.

The warm-water stress test is performed in a similar fashion but with opposite results expected. Physiologic thermovascular challenges may demonstrate decreased autonomic function in suspected cases of sympathetically mediated pain. An asymmetrical thermovascular rate of change in involved extremities has been deemed clinically useful in the study of RSD.[21–28]

ELECTRODIAGNOSTIC TESTING (EMG/NCV)

Electrodiagnostic testing is a helpful adjunct to the clinical examination. It provides the most accurate physiological information available concerning peripheral nerve damage. The typical electrodiagnostic study consists of an initial assessment of how well each nerve conducts electrical impulses followed by a needle examination of muscles that may be involved in the nerve damage process. The nerve conduction velocity study (NCV) is used to assess how well nerves conduct electricity. This information can be compared with normal values of the general population. The electromyogram (EMG) is performed by inserting needles into different muscles and looking for abnormal electrical potentials consistent with nerve damage.

The electrodiagnostic study is performed with an EMG machine. To perform a motor NCV study, the examiner uses a two-pronged electrical stimulator to stimulate the nerve that is to be studied. After stimulation of a motor nerve, the impulse travels along the nerve and causes a muscle contraction in the muscle at the end of the nerve. This response is recorded by an active electrode taped to the muscle being studied (Figure 4-1). The response of the muscle contraction can be recorded on an oscilloscope screen on the EMG machine. This response is known as the Compound Motor Action Potential (CMAP) (Figure 4-2). The amount of time it takes for the impulse to reach the muscle and cause the CMAP is known as the latency. If a nerve is stimulated at two different points, and if the examiner knows the distance between the two points, then the examiner has all the information necessary to calculate a motor NCV (Figure 4-3). Upon completion of the motor nerve conduction study, the examiner has information concerning the distal latency of the nerve and how well it conducts the electrical impulse (NCV). This information is then compared with normals.

The sensory NCV is performed in a similar fashion. However, it is not based on a muscle contraction. Rather, the electrical potential is recorded as it passes under an active electrode (Figure 4-4). The response, known as the Sensory Nerve Action Potential (SNAP), is recorded on the oscilloscope. Amplitude, latency, and nerve conduction velocity (NCV) can be calculated from this response and compared to normal values (Figure 4-5).

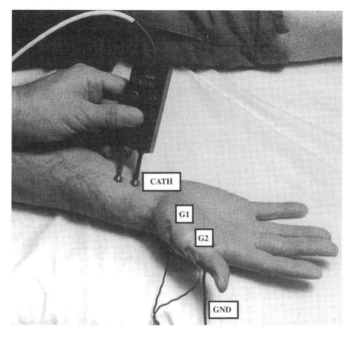

Figure 4-1 Motor conduction study setup. Median motor study, recording the abductor pollicis brevis muscle, stimulating the median nerve at the wrist. In motor studies, the "belly-tendon" method is used for recording. The active recording electrode (G1) is placed on the center of the muscle, and the reference electrode (G2) is placed distally over the tendon. Reprinted by permission from Preston DC, Shapiro BE (eds): *Electromyography and Neuromuscular Disorders—Clinical-Electrophysiologic Correlations*. Boston, Butterworth-Heinemann, 1998.

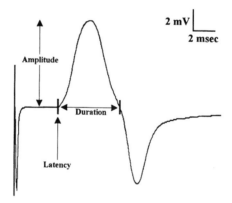

Figure 4-2 Compound muscle action potential (CMAP). The CMAP represents the summation of all the underlying muscle fiber action potentials. The CMAP is a biphasic potential with an initial negative deflection. Latency is the time from the stimulus to the initial negative deflection from baseline. Amplitude is most commonly measured from baseline to negative peak, but can also be measured peak to peak. Duration is measured from the initial deflection from baseline to the first baseline crossing (i.e. negative peak duration). Latency reflects only the fastest conducting motor fibers. All fibers contributed to amplitude. Reprinted by permission from Preston DC, Shapiro BE (eds): *Electromyography and Neuromuscular Disorders—Clinical-Electrophysiologic Correlations*. Boston, Butterworth-Heinemann, 1998.

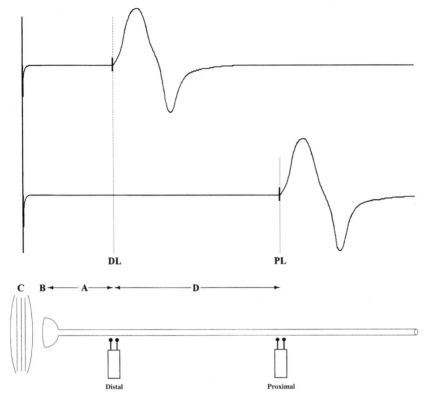

DL   PL

C B◄——A——►◄————————D————————►

Distal   Proximal

Figure 4-3 Motor conduction velocity calculation. Median motor study, recording abductor pollicis brevis, stimulating wrist and elbow. The proximal latency is longer than the distal. Distal motor latency (DL) cannot be used alone to calculate a motor conduction velocity. Two stimulations are necessary. The proximal motor latency (PL) includes the distal nerve conduction time as well as the nerve conduction time between the proximal and distal stimulation sites. The distance between those two sites can be measured, and the conduction velocity can be calculated (distance divided by time). Conduction velocity reflects only the fastest fibers. Reprinted by permission from Preston DC, Shapiro BE (eds): *Electromyography and Neuromuscular Disorders—Clinical-Electrophysiologic Correlations.* Boston, Butterworth-Heinemann, 1998.

To perform the EMG, needle electrodes are inserted into the muscles to be studied in the involved extremity. If a nerve leading to the muscle is damaged, abnormal wave potentials will be seen on the oscilloscope screen (Figure 4-6). The examiner can then determine what nerves are actually damaged based upon the distribution of muscles showing abnormalities.

The major advantage of electrodiagnostic testing is that it provides very accurate physiologic information concerning potential nerve damage. It can determine if a nerve is irritated, chronically compressed, slightly damaged, or profoundly damaged. In contrast, imaging studies such as MRI or CAT scans provide only pictures of the anatomy.

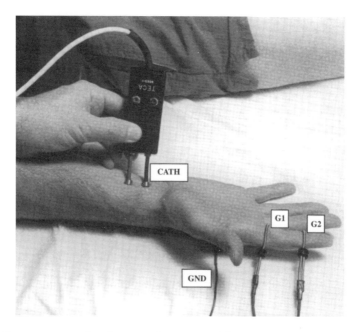

Figure 4-4 Sensory conduction study setup. Median sensory study, antidromic technique. Ring electrodes are placed over the index finger, 3 to 4 cm apart. The active recording electrode (G1) is placed more proximally, closest to the stimulator. Although the entire median nerve is stimulated at the wrist, only the cutaneous sensory fibers are recorded over the finger. Reprinted by permission from Preston DC, Shapiro BE (eds): *Electromyography and Neuromuscular Disorders—Clinical-Electrophysiologic Correlations.* Boston, Butterworth-Heinemann, 1998.

The electrodiagnostic study is a physiologic test that will demonstrate the sequela of the abnormal anatomical or clinical findings.

The major disadvantage of this procedure is that it is uncomfortable for the patient. The nerve conduction studies involve repetitive electrical stimulation that some patients perceive as an extremely noxious experience. Likewise, insertion of needles into multiple sites is both painful and anxiety provoking for the patient who undergoes this procedure.

Electrical studies are indicated for all patients suspected of having a neurologic injury involving the peripheral nervous system (PNS). The typical clinical presentation of the patient with a PNS injury may include symptoms of extreme pain, numbness, tingling, or weakness in a nerve's distribution. Nocturnal awakening with paresthesias suggests a peripheral nerve entrapment. Pain that radiates from the neck or low back into the upper or lower extremities respectively may indicate a proximal (root level) lesion perhaps due to a herniated disc or bony spinal pathology.

The procedure is indicated whenever there is a question of a neurological injury contributing to the patient's symptomatology. After motor vehicle accidents, this test is commonly used to rule out nerve entrapment or radiculopathy. Peripheral nerve entrapments in the upper extremity that can be ruled out through electrodiagnostic testing

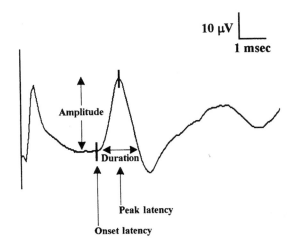

Figure 4-5 Sensory nerve action potential (SNAP). The SNAP represents the summation of all the underlying sensory fiber action potentials. The SNAP is usually biphasic or triphasic in configuration. Onset latency is measured from the stimulus site to the initial negative deflection. Onset latency represents nerve conduction time from the stimulus to the recording electrodes for the largest cutaneous sensory fibers. Peak latency is measured at the mid-point of the negative peak. Amplitude is most commonly measured from baseline to negative peak, but can also be measured from peak to peak. Duration is measured from the initial deflection from baseline to the first baseline crossing (i.e. negative peak duration). Only one stimulation site is required to calculate a sensory conduction velocity, because sensory onset latency represents only nerve conduction time. Reprinted by permission from Preston DC, Shapiro BE (eds): *Electromyography and Neuromuscular Disorders—Clinical-Electrophysiologic Correlations.* Boston, Butterworth-Heinemann, 1998.

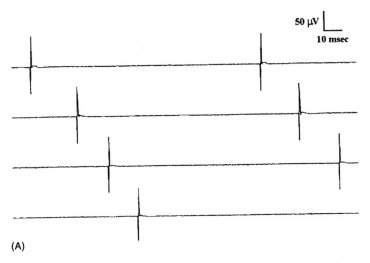

(A)

Figure 4-6 (A). Fibrillation potential (rastered traces). Note the regular firing pattern, which helps identify the potential as a fibrillation.

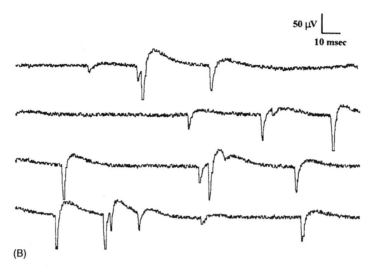

(B)

Figure 4-6 (continued) (B). Positive waves (rastered traces). Positive waves have the same significance as fibrillation potentials. They represent the spontaneous depolarization of a muscle fiber. Note the initial positive deflection and the slow negative phase. Reprinted by permission from Preston DC, Shapiro BE (eds): *Electromyography and Neuromuscular Disorders—Clinical-Electrophysiologic Correlations.* Boston, Butterworth-Heinemann, 1998.

include carpal tunnel syndrome, ulnar nerve entrapment at the wrist or elbow, pronator syndrome, radial tunnel syndrome, thoracic outlet syndrome, or cervical radiculopathy. In the lower extremities, peripheral nerve entrapment as well as lumbosacral radiculopathy may also be detected with this technique.

There are several relative contraindications to the performance of electrical testing including the presence of a pacemaker, anticoagulation, and severe peripheral vascular disease. Lastly, patients who are severely debilitated should not have this test performed until their condition improves.

COGNITIVE AND PSYCHOLOGICAL TESTING

The neuropsychological assessment for evaluation of cognitive complaints after a motor vehicle accident, and screening tools available to assess for depression are addressed in Chapter 12.

REFERENCES

1. Fischbach F. Blood studies. In Fischbach F (ed). *A Manual of Laboratory and Diagnostic Tests,* 5th edition, pp 23–146. Philadelphia, Lippincott-Raven, 1996.
2. Fischbach F. Blood studies. In Fischbach F (ed). *A Manual of Laboratory and Diagnostic Tests,* 5th edition, 683–743. Philadelphia, Lippincott-Raven, 1996.

3. Palubinskas AJ. Imaging of the urinary tract. In Smith DR (ed). *General Urology*, 11th edition, pp 55–108. New York, Lange Medical Publications, 1984.
4. Gray M. Diagnostic procedures. In Gray M (ed). *Genitourinary Disorders*, pp 32–51. St. Louis, Mosby, 1992.
5. Fischbach F. Blood studies. In Fischbach F (ed). *A Manual of Laboratory and Diagnostic Tests*, 5th edition, pp 617–682. Philadelphia, Lippincott-Raven, 1996.
6. Schwartzman RJ, McLellan TL. Reflex sympathetic dystrophy—a review. *Arch Neurol* 1987; 44: 555.
7. Kozin F, Soin JS, Ryan LM, *et al.* Bone scintigraphy in the reflex sympathetic dystrophy syndrome. *Radiology* 1981; 138: 437.
8. Rook JL. Reflex sympathetic dystrophy syndrome. In Cassvan A, Rook JL, Mullens SU, *et al* (eds). *Cumulative Trauma Disorders*, p 160. Boston, Butterworth Heinemann, 1997.
9. Tietjen R. Reflex sympathetic dystrophy of the knee. *Clin Orthop* 1986; 209: 234.
10. Markoff M, Farole A. Reflex sympathetic dystrophy syndrome: case report with a review of the literature. *Oral Surg Oral Med Oral Pathol* 1986; 61: 23.
11. Weiss L, Alfano A, Bardfeld P, *et al.* Prognostic value of triple phase bone scanning for reflex sympathetic dystrophy in hemiplegia. *Arch Phys Med Rehabil* 1993; 74: 716.
12. Davidoff G, Werner R, Cremer S, *et al.* Predictive value of the three-phase technetium bone scan in diagnosis of reflex sympathetic dystrophy syndrome. *Arch Phys Med Rehabil* 1989; 70: 135.
13. Intenzo C, Kim S, Millin J, *et al.* Scintigraphic patterns of the reflex sympathetic dystrophy syndrome of the lower extremities. *Clin Nucl Med* 1989; 14: 657.
14. Constantinesco A, Brunot B, Demangeat J, *et al.* Three-phase bone scanning as an aid to early diagnosis in reflex sympathetic dystrophy of the hand: a study of 89 cases. *Ann Chir Main Memb Super* 1986; 5: 93.
15. Greyson N, Tepperman P. Three-phase bone studies in hemiplegia with reflex sympathetic dystrophy and the effect of disuse. *J Nucl Med* 1984; 25: 423.
16. Demangeat J, Constantinesco A, Brunot B, *et al.* Three-phase bone scanning in reflex sympathetic dystrophy of the hand. *J Nucl Med* 1988; 29: 26.
17. Berstein BH, Singsen BH, Kent JT, *et al.* Reflex neurovascular dystrophy in childhood. *J Pediatr* 1978; 93: 211.
18. Laxer RM, Malleson PN, Morrison RT. Technetium 99m–methylene diphosphonate bone scans in children with reflex neurovascular dystrophy. *J Pediatr* 1985; 106: 437.
19. Holder LE, Mackinnon SE. Reflex sympathetic dystrophy in the hands: clinical and scintigraphic criteria. *Radiology* 1984; 152: 517.
20. Rowlingson JC. The sympathetic dystrophies. *Int Anesthesiol Clin* 1983; 21(4): 117.
21. Hobbins WB. Differential diagnosis of painful conditions and thermography. In Parris WCV (ed). *Contemporary Issues in Chronic Pain Management*, p 251. Boston, Kluwer Academic, 1991.
22. Hobbins WB. Pain management in thermography. In Raj PP (ed). *Practical Management of Pain*, 2nd edition, p 181. St. Louis, Mosby, 1992.
23. Green J. A preliminary note: dynamic thermography may offer a key to the early recognition of reflex sympathetic dystrophy. *J Acad Neuromusc Thermogr* 1989; 8: 104.
24. Green J. The pathophysiology of reflex sympathetic dystrophy as demonstrated by dynamic thermography. *J Acad Neuromusc Thermogr* 1989; 8: 121.
25. Green J. Tutorial 12: thermography medical infrared imaging. *Pain Dig* 1993; 3: 268.
26. Uematsu S, Jankel WR. Skin temperature response of the foot to cold stress of the hand: a test to evaluate somatosympathetic response. *Thermology* 1988; 3: 41.
27. Feldman F. Thermography of the hand and wrist: practical applications. *Hand Clin* 1991; 7: 99.
28. Karstetter KW, Sheran RA. Use of thermography for initial detection of early reflex sympathetic dystrophy. *J Am Podiatr Med Assoc* 1991; 81: 198

5

Upper Extremity Pain

Jack L Rook

THE HAND AND WRIST

Anatomy

There are 27 bones within the human hand. The thumb (finger one) consists of two bones, the distal and proximal phalanges. The index, middle, ring and small fingers (fingers two through five) each consist of three bones, the proximal, middle, and distal phalanges. Within the substance of the hand are five metacarpal bones (which articulate with the respective proximal phalanges), and eight carpal bones. The carpal bones (the proximal row contains the scaphoid, lunate and triquetrum—the distal row contains the trapezium, trapezoid, capitate, hamate, and pisiform) articulate with the metacarpals distally, and with the radius and ulna at the wrist joint (Figure 5-1).

There are multiple joints within the hand and wrist, each named by the bones involved in the articulation. The thumb has two joints, the distal interphalangeal joint, and the metacarpal phalangeal joint. Fingers two through five each have a distal interphalangeal joint, proximal interphalangeal joint, and a metacarpal phalangeal joint. At the base of the thumb is the first carpometacarpal joint. The carpal bones articulate with the radius and ulna to form the wrist joint.

Strong ligaments occur between wrist and carpal bones providing stability. Ligaments are strong fibrous bundles that articulate between two bones. Ligamentous fibers are composed of a parallel arrangement of collagen fibrils. This orientation affords tremendous strength to each ligament. When a ligament is torn, altered mechanics at the wrist joint may produce instability and pain. Naming of carpal ligaments is based on the bones with which they articulate (e.g., Lunotriquetral, pisohamate, pisometacarpal).

Four nerves course over the wrist joint and enter the hand. Two, the median and ulnar nerves have both motor and sensory fibers. The superficial radial and dorsal ulnar cutaneous nerves are purely sensory. The sensory distribution of the median nerve encompasses the thumb, index, middle, and the radial half of the ring finger. The ulnar nerve sensory distribution includes the ulnar half of the ring finger and the small finger. The superficial radial nerve distribution encompasses the dorsum of the thumb and the

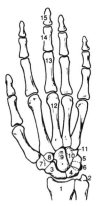

Figure 5-1 Bones of the hand and wrist: 1. Distal radius; 2. Ulnar styloid process; 3. Scaphoid; 4. Lunate; 5. Triquetral; 6. Pisiform; 7. Trapezium; 8. Trapezoid; 9. Capitate; 10. Hamate; 11. Hook of hamate; 12. Metacarpal shaft; 13. Proximal phalynx; 14. Middle phalynx; 15. Distal phalynx. Reprinted by permission from Unwin A, Jones K (eds). *Emergency Orthopaedics and Trauma*, p 103 (fig 11.3). Oxford, Elsevier Science Ltd, 1995.

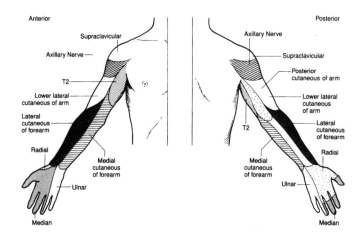

Figure 5-2 Peripheral nerve sensory supply to the upper limb. Reprinted by permission from Unwin A, Jones K (eds). *Emergency Orthopaedics and Trauma*, p 105 (fig 11.6). Oxford, Elsevier Science Ltd, 1995.

web space between thumb and index finger. The dorsal ulnar cutaneous nerve divides into two dorsal branches that supply skin overlying the dorsum of the hand, the fifth digit, and half of the fourth digit (Figure 5-2). The motor distribution of the median nerve includes the muscles of the thenar eminence (abductor pollicis brevis, flexor pollicis brevis, opponens pollicis), while the ulnar motor distribution innervates muscles of the hypothenar eminence (abductor, opponens, and flexor digiti quinti, third and forth lumbricals, palmar and dorsal interossei, adductor pollicis, and flexor pollicis brevis).

After the median nerve passes through the carpal tunnel, it breaks into a motor branch that supplies muscles of the thenar eminence, and sensory branches known as the digital nerves. Likewise, the ulnar nerve passes through its own tunnel (Guyon's canal) where it breaks up into motor and digital sensory branches (Figure 5-3).

The carpal tunnel is bounded superiorly by the transverse carpal ligament and inferiorly by the carpal bones. Through this anatomic structure pass all of the finger flexor tendons

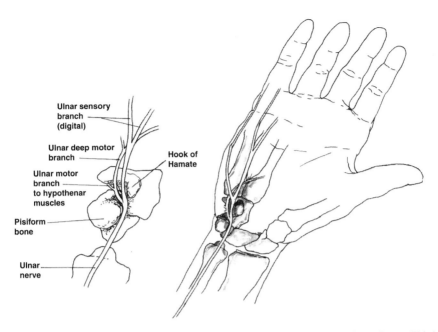

Figure 5-3 Anatomy of Guyon's canal. Reprinted by permission from Weiss LD. Occupation-related cumulative trauma disorders. In Cassvan A, Weiss LD, Weiss JM, Rook JL, Mullens SU (eds). *Cumulative Trauma Disorders*. Boston; Butterworth-Heinemann, 1997.

and the median nerve. Therefore, a lot of anatomy passes through this relatively confined space and there is not much room for additional inflammation (which could precipitate the carpal tunnel syndrome) (Figure 5-4).

At the wrist, the ulnar nerve enters the hand in a shallow trough between the pisiform bone and the hook of the hamate bone (Guyon's canal). Its roof is the volar carpal ligament and the palmaris longus muscle. Upon distal emergence through this tunnel, the ulnar nerve gives off cutaneous branches that supply sensation to the ulnar palm, and the fourth and fifth fingers. A deep motor branch innervates muscles of the hypothenar eminence, the third and fourth lumbricles, all of the interossei, the adductor pollicis, and the flexor pollicis brevis.[1] This tunnel can be a site of ulnar nerve entrapment. (See Figure 5-3.)

Lastly, multiple tendons (fibrous structures which interpose between bone and muscle) pass across the wrist joint and enter the substance of the hand. On the palm side of the hand lie the finger flexor tendons that pass through the carpal tunnel. They originate in the forearm as terminations of the finger flexor muscles and insert upon the proximal and distal interphalangeal joints of the fingers. On the dorsum of the wrist pass the extensor tendons, which originate in the forearm as terminations of wrist and finger extensor muscles. They connect at the wrist and proximal and distal interphalangeal joints of the fingers, promoting wrist and finger extension, respectively. Two additional tendons pass along the radial forearm to the base of the thumb. They are the abductor pollicis longus and extensor pollicis brevis tendons. When inflamed, these tendons can cause a painful syndrome known as DeQuervain's tenosynovitis (Figure 5-5).

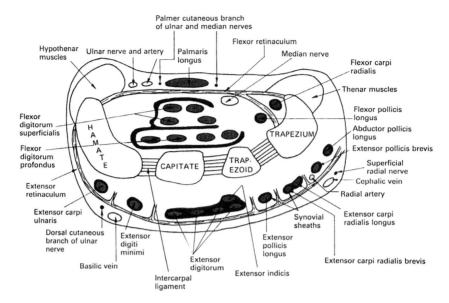

Figure 5-4 Transverse section through the wrist region showing the relationships of the various structures which pass into the hand. Reprinted by permission from Palastanga N, Field D, Soames R (eds). *Anatomy and Human Movement—Structure and Function*, 3rd ed. p 225 (fig 3.104b). Oxford, Elsevier Science Ltd, 1998.

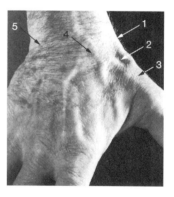

Figure 5-5 Tendons involved in DeQuervain's Tenosynovitis (*arrows 1, 2*). Reprinted by permission from Apley AG, Solomon L (eds). *Concise System of Orthopaedics and Fractures*, 2nd ed. p 132 (fig 15.1). London, Hodder Arnold, 1994.

Mechanism of Injury

Wrist or hand pain may occur after a motor vehicle accident due to a variety of mechanisms. The person who grips the steering wheel forcefully prior to impact will be prone to hand and wrist injuries. Hyperextension at the base of the thumb may lead to the development of tendonitis or a ligament tear. There may also be a sudden, direct impact of the base of the hand against the steering wheel, perhaps setting the stage for the development of a post-traumatic carpal tunnel syndrome.

Hyperextension at the wrist will strain wrist ligaments and acutely increase pressure within the carpal tunnel. Therefore, acute hyperextension of the wrist could both tear wrist ligaments and predispose to the development of carpal tunnel syndrome. For the passenger within the involved vehicle, an acute hyperextension injury to the wrist could occur if the individual braces against the back seat or dashboard prior to impact.

Common Hand and Wrist Injuries Caused by Motor Vehicle Accidents

A number of pathological conditions can involve the upper extremities after a motor vehicle accident. Some of the more common ones include:

- tendonitis
- development of a hand or wrist ganglion
- the development of a trigger finger
- wrist or thumb ligamentous strain
- bony fractures
- wrist ligament tear
- nerve injury with causalgia and/or the reflex sympathetic dystrophy syndrome (see Chapter 11).

Tendonitis

The patient with tendonitis complains of hand or wrist discomfort that increases with use of the extremity. There may or may not be visible inflammation. However, increased pain is usually associated with forceful gripping, torquing activities, or lifting. The physical examination will demonstrate palpatory tenderness of the involved tendon with increased pain in association with forced resistance against the muscle whose tendon is involved in the inflammatory process.

Diagnostic testing is not helpful in diagnosing tendonitis. Because this is a soft tissue problem, x-rays do not show any abnormalities. The diagnosis is principally a clinical one, based on the history and physical examination findings.

Treatment of tendonitis includes anti-inflammatories, rest (perhaps via immobilization), and application of ice. Once the inflammation subsides, progressive range of motion and reconditioning of involved muscles become part of the treatment protocol. If the tendonitis seems particularly severe, occupational therapy should be ordered for appropriate modalities, which may include iontophoresis, ultrasound, and immobilization via splinting. Different splints can be fabricated depending on which tendon or tendons are involved in the tendonitis. If the patient fails to improve with these conservative measures, he or she may benefit from a steroid injection into the region of the inflamed tendon. Steroids are potent anti-inflammatories that can reduce the degree of inflammation so as to accelerate recovery. Oral anti-inflammatories are also a useful adjunct, assuming the patient can tolerate the potential GI side effects of these medications. Topical creams may provide some symptomatic relief. Application of ice also decreases pain and acute inflammation. Therefore, the hallmarks of treatment for tendonitis include:

- relative rest of the muscles involved in the tendonitis
- immobilization via splinting (absolute rest)
- use of anti-inflammatories
- and ultimately a reconditioning program for involved muscles.

Surgery is usually not indicated in the management of tendonitis.

Long-term complications of tendonitis include chronic wrist and hand pain, weakness due to the chronic pain, and contractures and/or decreased range of motion due to prolonged immobilization with inadequate therapy.

DeQuervain's Tenosynovitis

As noted above, DeQuervain's tenosynovitis is an inflammation of the abductor pollicis longus and extensor pollicis brevis tendons. These tendons are located at the radial aspect of the wrist. When the thumb is fully abducted, they can be seen outlining the anatomical "snuffbox" (Figure 5-5). Patients with this diagnosis complain of pain at the radial aspect of the wrist.

Physical examination will demonstrate tenderness and possibly swelling in this region, and there will be a positive Finkelstein's test. The Finkelstein's test is done by asking the patient to grip their thumb underneath the other fingers and to ulnar deviate their wrist (Figure 5-6). If the patient complains of increasing pain, they most likely have a DeQuervain's tenosynovitis. Since this is a soft tissue process, diagnostic workup is unrevealing. The diagnosis is a clinical one based on history and physical examination.

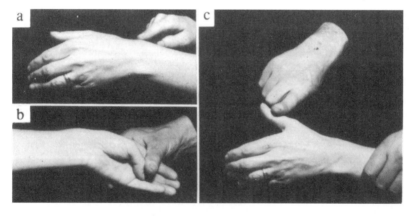

Figure 5-6 DeQuervain's disease. (a) The patient can point to the painful area; (b) forced adduction is painful (the Finkelstein test); (c) pain on active extension against resistance. Reprinted by permission from Apley AG, Solomon L (eds). *Concise System of Orthopaedics and Fractures*, 2nd ed. p 137 (fig 15.10a–c). London, Hodder Arnold, 1994.

The treatment of DeQuervain's tenosynovitis includes:

- occupational therapy for appropriate modalities
- immobilization via splinting using a thumb spica
- use of anti-inflammatories
- application of topical creams for symptomatic relief
- if necessary, a steroid injection.

In some cases, the pain is unrelenting despite conservative care. These patients may benefit from a surgical procedure known as a first dorsal compartment tenovaginectomy. This procedure involves a release of constricting tendon sheaths and scar tissue surrounding the inflamed tendons, helping to promote reduction of pain and inflammation.

A Ganglion

A ganglion is a potentially painful fluid collection that can develop within a joint capsule or tendon sheath. It is seen most commonly on the back of the wrist (Figure 5-7). It arises from cystic degeneration of the joint capsule or tendon sheath. The distended cyst contains fluid.

The patient presents with a painless lump, usually on the back of the wrist. Occasionally there is a slight ache. The symptomatic ganglion will cause hand and/or wrist discomfort. As this is a soft tissue problem, x-rays do not assist in making the diagnosis, which is principally a clinical one based on the history and physical examination.

Physical examination will demonstrate the small localized swelling, which may be accentuated by flexing or extending the hand or wrist. The lump is well defined, cystic, and usually non-tender. Palpation of the ganglion may elicit discomfort. A symptomatic ganglion is usually visible due to fluid build-up within the ganglion. This fluid can be aspirated by insertion of a small needle. If needle aspiration is done, it is frequently helpful

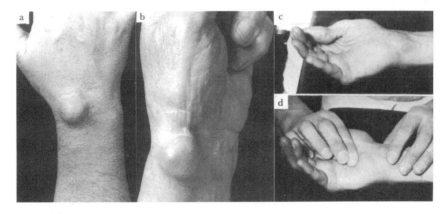

Figure 5-7 Wrist ganglion. Reprinted by permission from Apley AG, Solomon L (eds). *Concise System of Orthopaedics and Fractures*, 2nd ed. p 137 (fig 15.9a). London, Hodder Arnold, 1994.

to follow the aspiration with an infusion of a steroid solution that might help reduce inflammation and possibly eliminate the ganglion. Repeated aspirations may be necessary to fully obliterate the ganglion. The patient might also benefit from occupational therapeutic modalities to reduce inflammation, including splinting and iontophoresis. Anti-inflammatory medications and topical creams may also prove helpful. If the patients fail to improve with these modalities, surgical intervention to remove the ganglion may prove necessary.

Complications related to the presence of a ganglion, include persistent pain and swelling, decreased grip strength and dexterity as a result of the pain, decreased range of motion, and recurrence despite apparently successful aspiration or surgery. Recurrence necessitates further treatment.

Trigger Finger

The term "trigger finger" refers to a condition whereby the patient's finger locks in a flexed position after it is flexed, and the patient is then either unable to extend it or experiences a sudden snapping sensation of the finger during re-extension (Figure 5-8). This occurs most frequently in the middle or ring fingers and is attributed to direct, severe trauma to the flexor portion of the fingers. The injury occurs as the flexor tendon pinches between the head of the metacarpal and the bruising object (e.g., steering wheel, dashboard). The tendon enlarges into a fusiform swelling and forms a nodule that may get stuck within its synovium-lined sheath.[2]

Physical examination may demonstrate a palpable swelling and/or bump at the palmar base of the finger involved with the triggering. This represents the localized tendonous swelling which is precipitating the triggering phenomenon. This swollen area may or may not be tender to palpation. As with the other soft tissue conditions, diagnostic workup such as x-rays is of limited value.

Treatment of this problem might include occupational therapeutic modalities to reduce inflammation. The patient might benefit from a steroid injection or a series of injections. If the patient fails to improve, a surgical procedure to release the tendon from its sheath may become necessary.

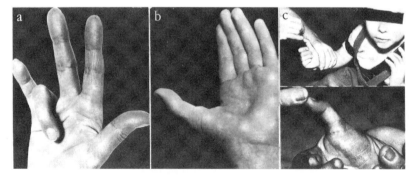

Figure 5-8 Stenosing tenovaginitis/trigger finger. Reprinted by permission from Apley AG, Solomon L (eds). *Concise System of Orthopaedics and Fractures*, 2nd ed. p 145 (fig 16.9a). London, Hodder Arnold, 1994.

If left untreated, the patient may develop more severe triggering and possibly a locking of that finger in a nonanatomical position. There may be chronic pain associated with this problem, as well as decreased dexterity and grip strength as a result of the anatomical abnormality and any associated pain.

Strained Ligaments

Hand and wrist ligaments can be strained during a motor vehicle accident usually by forceful gripping of the steering wheel or wrist hyperextension by the passenger bracing against the dashboard or seat. The most common ligaments strained are at the base of the thumb or the wrist. These patients complain of thumb/wrist pain that worsens with forceful gripping, repetitive activities, or range of motion of the involved joint(s).

Physical examination reveals tenderness of the involved ligaments. There may or may not be associated inflammation. The patient will have discomfort with range of motion of the thumb or wrist.

The diagnostic workup for this soft tissue condition is usually unrevealing. X-rays are unremarkable unless there is a fracture associated with the strained ligament. The diagnosis is based on the history of the trauma, the symptomatology, and the physical examination.

Treatment for a strained wrist or thumb ligament is similar to treatment for tendonitis, including immobilization, management of inflammation, and occupational therapy modalities. Splinting (absolute rest) of the thumb or wrist is often indicated, as well as relative rest for the hand and wrist. Steroid injections may be necessary if the more conservative treatment does not help. Oral anti-inflammatories and topical creams may be helpful. In general, surgery is not indicated for strained ligaments but rather is reserved for torn ligaments with chronic pain and instability.

Complications of ligamentous strains would include chronic pain in the thumb or wrist, contractures and/or decreased range of motion due to prolonged immobilization or lack of appropriate therapy, decreased dexterity and decreased grip strength.

Torn Wrist Ligaments

In contrast to a strained ligament, the ligaments of the wrist may actually be torn as a result of trauma from a motor vehicle accident. Wrist ligaments that commonly tear include the scapholunate and lunotriquetral. Patients with wrist ligament tears complain of pain within the wrist, which worsens with use of the hand, and there may be "popping" within the joint, suggesting instability. Directed physical examination will demonstrate localized tenderness overlying the tear, and provocative maneuvers will demonstrate excessive laxity of the wrist joint.

Plain x-rays may not reveal anything, but stress x-rays, whereby the wrist joint is stressed in a particular direction during imaging, may demonstrate a pathological increase in distance between normally opposed bones, indicative of a torn ligament. In addition to stress x-rays, an arthrogram (injection of dye under pressure into the wrist joint), may demonstrate the tear as the dye extrudes abnormally through the torn ligamentous fibers.

Treatment of a torn wrist ligament depends on the severity of the tear and its associated symptomatology. For mild or relatively asymptomatic tears, conservative care should be employed. Strengthening of forearm musculature may help to provide some degree of stability across the wrist to help compensate for the torn ligaments. Splinting or bracing of the wrist may be necessary particularly if the patient is performing activities that strain the joint. Anti-inflammatories may be needed to reduce inflammation associated with chronic subluxation. For severe pain, analgesics including mild opioids may be necessary. Some patients benefit from steroid injections. A prolonged period of casting is helpful occasionally in initiating some degree of scar tissue formation within the torn ligament, which may help strengthen the joint. However, with severe tears, surgery to repair the tear or fuse the joint may be the only option to eliminate pain and improve stability of the joint.

Complications of torn ligaments include chronic wrist pain either due to the tear itself or the intermittent instability associated with it. With chronic pain and immobilization, there may be decreased range of motion over time. Certainly, after total or partial fusion of the wrist joint there will be a concomitant decrease in range of motion. Additionally, chronic pain contributes to decreased dexterity and decreased grip strength.

Fractures

A fractured bone may cause hand or wrist discomfort after a motor vehicle accident. Bones within the hand that may be fractured include the phalanges, metacarpals, and carpal bones. Patients with fractures complain of pain in the region of the traumatized bone. Physical examination demonstrates swelling and inflammation around the fracture, and acute tenderness with palpation. With complicated fractures, there may be distortion of normal anatomy.

Fractured bones are usually seen on conventional x-rays. For very small or occult fractures, bone scanning may be necessary. A bone scan involves the injection of a radioactive substance that has an affinity for the metabolically active region of the fractured bone(s). It is more sensitive than conventional x-rays in demonstrating an occult fracture. It is particularly useful for patients who have scaphoid fractures. This bone does not image well on conventional x-rays and the scaphoid fracture is frequently missed on the initial radiographic examination. The patient with a scaphoid fracture presents with pain, tenderness and swelling in the region of the anatomic "snuff box." If conventional x-rays are negative, the diagnosis of a scaphoid fracture may not be made until bone scanning is performed.

Treatment of a fractured bone requires immobilization (splint or cast). For more severe fractures, surgery may be necessary to reduce the bones, and for open reduction and internal fixation utilizing plates, pins, and/or screws. Anti-inflammatories and other analgesic medications are frequently necessary to alleviate discomfort particularly in the acute phase immediately post accident, or after surgery.

After a cast is removed, occupational therapy is indicated for progressive range of motion and strengthening as contractures and weakness are common after prolonged immobilization. Complications of fractured bones might include ongoing pain, contractures/decreased range of motion, decreased dexterity and decreased grip strength.

Causalgia and Reflex Sympathetic Dystrophy

Any traumatic event, particularly if it involves injury to a peripheral nerve, may precipitate the development of a neurologic phenomenon known as causalgia, reflex sympathetic dystrophy syndrome, or chronic regional pain syndrome (type I or type II). This neurological condition is characterized by severe pain and vascular abnormalities. The topic of reflex sympathetic dystrophy will be discussed in a separate chapter.

THE ELBOW

Anatomy

The radius, ulna, and humerus articulate to form the elbow joint (Figure 5-9). These bones are surrounded by ligaments that allow motion in four planes: flexion, extension, pronation, and supination.

The elbow joint is surrounded by nerves, muscles, and tendons, which pass from the proximal arm to the forearm. The volar elbow region is known as the antecubital fossa. The tip of the elbow is known as the olecranon. Surrounding the olecranon is a superficial bursa known as the olecranon bursa.

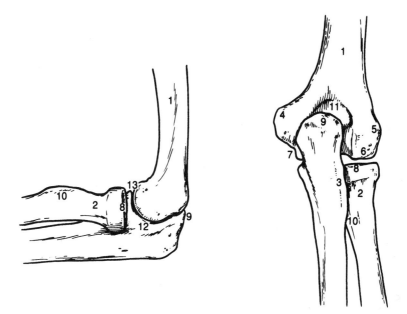

Figure 5-9 AP and lateral views of the elbow: 1. Shaft of humerus; 2. Radial neck; 3. Ulna; 4. Medial epicondyle; 5. Lateral epicondyle; 6. Capitellum; 7. Trochlea; 8. Radial head; 9. Olecranon; 10. Radial tuberosity; 11. Olecranon fossa; 12. Trochlea notch within ulna; and 13. Coronoid process of ulna. Reprinted by permission from Unwin A, Jones K (eds). *Emergency Orthopaedics and Trauma*, p 102 (fig 11.2). Oxford, Elsevier Science Ltd, 1995.

Four major nerves cross the elbow joint. Medially, traveling through the ulnar groove is the ulnar nerve. On the dorsal forearm is the radial nerve, which passes through a soft tissue passageway known as the radial tunnel. Through the anticubital fossa and volar forearm courses the large median nerve, which supplies much of the sensory and motor innervation of the hand and forearm, and the lateral antebrachial cutaneous nerve, an extension of the musculocutaneous nerve, that supplies the volar and radial half of the forearm to the level of the wrist.

Muscles of the volar forearm include the wrist and finger flexor muscles and the pronator muscle. On the radial forearm is the brachioradialis muscle. On the dorsal forearm are the wrist and finger extensor muscles and the supinator muscle.

The wrist extensor muscles join to form a common tendon that inserts into the lateral epicondyle of the humerus. In contrast, the wrist flexor muscles join to form a common tendon that inserts upon the medial elbow at the site known as the medial epicondyle of the humerus.

In the proximal forearm, the radial nerve passes through the radial tunnel. The radial tunnel is bounded by the supinator muscle inferiorly and a fibrous band superiorly, the proximal ligamentous arch at the origin of the supinator muscle, known as the "arcade of Frohse." The ulnar nerve travels through a groove at the medial elbow known as the "ulnar groove." The ulnar groove is located adjacent to the medial epicondyle of the humerus. The ulnar nerve is very superficial as it passes through this groove, and it is prone to entrapment at this site (Figure 5-10).

Mechanism of Elbow Injury

The elbow region may be injured in a motor vehicle accident. This may occur if the driver braces prior to impact with arms outstretched against the steering wheel. Likewise, a passenger might brace against the dashboard or back seat. When the arms are braced like this, forces after impact will be transferred from the hand or wrist, proximally to involve the elbow. The elbow may also sustain direct trauma as a result of impact against a door, adjacent car seat, stick shift, or another passenger within the vehicle.

Common traumatic conditions that can involve the elbow region after a motor vehicle accident include:

- forearm myofascial pain
- medial/lateral epicondylitis
- bursitis
- fracture
- nerve entrapment syndrome
- ligamentous strain
- development of neurogenic pain.

Forearm Myofascial Pain

In the volar forearm are a number of muscles that could be traumatized in a motor vehicle accident. The volar forearm muscles include the wrist and finger flexors, and the pronator

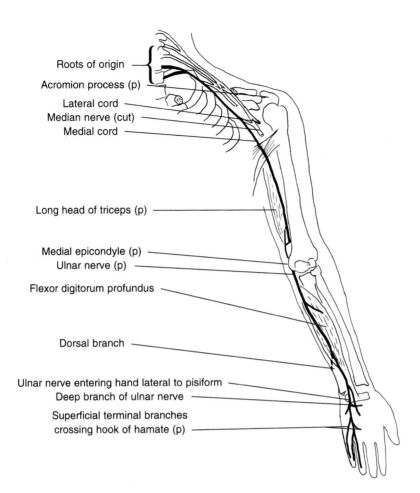

Roots of origin
Acromion process (p)
Lateral cord
Median nerve (cut)
Medial cord

Long head of triceps (p)

Medial epicondyle (p)
Ulnar nerve (p)

Flexor digitorum profundus

Dorsal branch

Ulnar nerve entering hand lateral to pisiform
Deep branch of ulnar nerve
Superficial terminal branches
crossing hook of hamate (p)

Figure 5-10 Course of the ulnar nerve. The ulnar nerve is superficial as it courses around the elbow adjacent to the medial epicondyle. Reprinted by permission from Field D (ed). *Anatomy: Palpation and Surface Markings*, 2nd ed. (fig 2.23c,d—schematic figure to right). Boston, Butterworth-Heinemann, 1997.

muscles. An initial strain of these muscles may occur at the time of impact due to extreme hyperextension of the wrist or direct trauma. This may initiate a myofascial condition characterized by chronic muscular tenderness and spasm. Forearm myofascial pain could refer discomfort back to the elbow region or distally to the hand. In addition, the median nerve courses through these muscles as it travels through the forearm and into the hand. Chronic spasm of these muscles could result in median nerve irritation with referred pain.

The extensor muscle mass and the supinator muscle on the dorsal forearm could also be traumatized during a motor vehicle accident. The extensor muscles, when in spasm, place stress on their common tendon at the lateral epicondyle. This could result in a tendonitis known as lateral epicondylitis. In addition, chronic muscle spasm involving this mass of muscles could irritate the underlying radial nerve.

The patient with forearm myofascial pain describes forearm discomfort that worsens with use of the hand and/or wrist. In severe cases, the pain occurs even without upper extremity usage. Physical examination will demonstrate tenderness of the forearm flexor and/or extensor muscles. Diagnostic workup in general is not very helpful since this is a soft tissue condition. X-rays will be unrevealing. With severe forearm myofascial pain, there may be entrapment of underlying nerves and electrodiagnostic studies may prove helpful in determining if a neurological condition exists in conjunction with the myofascial one.

The treatment of forearm myofascial pain includes relative rest with restrictions for the patient, and, if the patient does not improve, he or she should be referred for occupational therapy. Therapy should include modalities to decrease muscle spasm, gentle stretching, and progression to an exercise program to normalize tone of the involved muscles. Wrist splints are helpful in taking some stress off the involved forearm musculature. A wrist cockup splint is helpful for patients with forearm extensor muscle spasm or lateral epicondylitis. This type of splint shortens the wrist extensor muscles, taking pressure off the muscle bellies and their common tendon. Trigger point injection therapy may accelerate recovery from a forearm myofascial condition. Analgesics for pain, muscle relaxants, anti-inflammatories, topical creams, and a TENS unit may prove helpful. Rarely is surgery indicated for a myofascial condition unless there is an associated entrapped nerve or a persistent epicondylitis. In such cases, surgery to free the entrapped nerve, or an epicondylectomy may be indicated, respectively.

Complications of this condition include chronic myofascial pain involving the forearm muscles. As a result of the pain, there may be decreased forearm strength, decreased dexterity in the hand, and decreased grip strength. If there is involvement of underlying nerves, patients may experience paresthesias or dysesthesias involving their hand. When the forearm myofascial condition becomes chronic, it is very difficult to treat and principally requires symptomatic care.

Epicondylitis

A medial or lateral epicondylitis could result from chronic muscle spasm involving the forearm flexor or extensor muscles, or as a result of a direct blow to the medial or lateral elbow after impact. Some patients with chronic forearm myofascial pain and spasm will develop an epicondylitis. The forearm flexor mass when chronically in spasm will irritate its common tendon, which inserts onto the medial epicondyle causing a medial epicondylitis. The forearm extensor muscle mass when in chronic spasm will place stress on the common extensor tendon that inserts onto the lateral epicondyle contributing to a lateral epicondylitis. An epicondylitis refers to inflammation of the tendon insertion onto either the medial or lateral epicondyles of the humerus.

The history for these diagnoses includes pain in the region of the involved medial or lateral epicondyle. For medial epicondylitis, the pain worsens with flexion activities of the wrist, and, for lateral epicondylitis the pain worsens with extensor activities of the wrist joint (hitting a backhand in tennis, forceful gripping, writing, typing).

The physical examination for these diagnoses may reveal point tenderness at the medial or lateral epicondyles and possibly some associated inflammation. For medial epicondylitis, the pain may worsen with resisted wrist flexion. For lateral epicondylitis, the pain worsens with resisted wrist extension. Since this is a soft tissue condition, x-rays are usually non-revealing. The diagnosis is principally made from the history and physical examination.

With regards to treatment modalities, initially, rest, application of ice, and oral anti-inflammatories may prove helpful. If the patient fails to improve, occupational therapy for modalities and splinting may become necessary. Modalities such as ultrasound for deep heating and iontophoresis to reduce inflammation may prove helpful. Stretching exercises to alleviate spasm in the wrist flexor and extensor muscles may help in decreasing stress applied to the respective common tendons. Stretching exercises and a home exercise program should be initiated as part of the occupational therapy regimen. However, in the early stages of occupational therapy, immobilization via appropriate splinting will be indicated. By immobilizing the wrist, the patient with medial epicondylitis will not be able to produce the flexion movements that aggravate the medial epicondylitis. This would allow the flexor tendon inflammation to subside. Likewise, immobilization of the wrist would prevent repeated extension of the joint, which would take some pressure off the wrist extensor muscles and their common tendon, which inserts into the lateral epicondyle.

Occasionally, patients require surgical intervention to treat the chronic pain of medial or lateral epicondylitis. When it is necessary, the surgical procedure performed is a medial or lateral epicondylectomy with reinsertion of the common tendon at a different site.

Patients who have severe pain as a result of epicondylitis may benefit from anti-inflammatories and appropriate analgesics. Topical creams such as Zostrix cream or anesthetic/anti-inflammatory creams may prove helpful in decreasing some of the pain. Therefore, the hallmarks of conservative treatment include:

- relative rest through modification of activities
- absolute rest with splinting
- application of ice
- use of anti-inflammatories and analgesics.

If the patient fails to improve steroid injections or surgery may be necessary.

Long-term complications include chronic pain due to a non-healing inflammatory condition. There may be an overall decrease in strength, particularly of wrist extensors, wrist flexors, or grip with chronic epicondylitis. With decreased use of the elbow and relative immobilization, there may be some loss in range of motion.

Bursitis

Occasionally, patients with a traumatic injury to the elbow develop an olecranon bursitis characterized by swelling and pain at the tip of the elbow. Physical examination will demonstrate tenderness at the tip of the elbow with swelling that can be quite significant when effusion is present. Diagnostic workup is unrevealing as this is a soft tissue process. X-rays may demonstrate the soft tissue swelling, but usually there are no bony abnormalities.

With regards to treatment, needle aspiration of a fluid filled bursa may prove necessary to initiate the healing progress. After aspiration, a steroid injection should be performed to reduce inflammation and promote recovery. Application of ice, gentle compression via elbow straps, and use of anti-inflammatories may help reduce inflammation and prevent swelling at the tip of the elbow. Referral for occupational therapy modalities to reduce swelling (e.g., iontophoresis) may prove helpful. In rare cases, surgery may be necessary to remove the chronically swollen bursa. Complications of this condition include chronic pain at the tip of the elbow with associated swelling that waxes and wanes over time.

Fracture

With severe trauma to the elbow region, there may be a fracture of the radial head, the ulnar bone, or the distal humerus. Immediately after the accident, such patients will have severe localized pain. Physical examination for a closed fracture will demonstrate extreme tenderness and swelling in the region of the elbow. An open fracture will penetrate through the skin. X-rays are usually sufficient in demonstrating the fracture and its severity. Occasionally, for smaller fractures undetected by conventional x-rays, bone scanning may be necessary to demonstrate the lesion.

Treatment of a fracture includes immobilization with appropriate casting. For less complicated fractures, closed reduction with casting may be all that is necessary. For complicated or open fractures, surgery for open reduction and internal fixation is needed. After the patient comes out of the cast, occupational therapy is indicated to work on range of motion of the elbow joint and progressive strengthening of surrounding muscles.

Complications of fractures include chronic elbow pain that does not resolve despite adequate bone healing, and decreased strength associated with the chronic pain. Deformity, contractures, and limited elbow range of motion may also complicate a fractured bone in this region.

Nerve Entrapment Syndromes

A number of nerves pass over the elbow joint. Across the antecubital fossa are the median and lateral antebrachial cutaneous nerves. Around the medial elbow, passes the ulnar nerve and on the dorsal forearm is the posterior interosseous branch of the radial nerve. All of these nerves can become irritated, entrapped, or damaged as a result of trauma to the elbow region. A discussion of the various nerve entrapment syndromes in the region of the elbow is given later in this chapter.

Strain

Moderate trauma to the elbow region may strain ligaments that surround the joint. Patients with strained elbow ligaments complain of elbow discomfort that increases with activity of the respective extremity. Physical examination will demonstrate tenderness about the elbow that may or may not be associated with inflammation. There should not be any instability of the elbow joint. Diagnostic workup is generally unrevealing. Since this is a soft tissue process, x-rays are usually negative. Magnetic resonance imaging (MRI) may demonstrate torn ligaments.

Treatment includes use of appropriate analgesics and anti-inflammatories. Occupational therapy usually proves helpful for modalities to reduce inflammation, splinting to promote immobilization, and eventually range-of-motion exercises to correct any losses that may have resulted from prolonged immobilization. Steroid injections may prove helpful to reduce inflammation associated with the strain. Surgery is rarely indicated unless there is obvious instability due to ligament tearing at the level of the elbow. Complications include chronic elbow pain, decreased arm strength, and loss of range of motion.

Neurogenic Pain

As noted above, there are several different nerves that pass over the elbow region. With trauma to any of these nerves, a patient may develop neurogenic pain symptomatology (numbness, tingling, burning pain, and hypersensitivity) involving the forearm and hand. Patients may complain of awakening at night with paresthesias in a particular distribution (nocturnal paresthesias). A more complete discussion of the signs, symptoms, diagnostic workup, and treatment of neurogenic pain related to particular nerve injuries, as well as a chapter on reflex sympathetic dystrophy (another type of neurogenic pain) is forthcoming.

SHOULDER JOINT

Anatomy

The shoulder joint is the most complicated joint in the human body. Under normal conditions, this joint has the greatest mobility. The principal bony components of the shoulder joint include the head of the humerus, which has a rounded or ball-like appearance, and the shallow cuplike portion of the scapula that it articulates with (Figure 5-11). It is the arrangement of the ball-like humeral head articulating with the shallow cuplike portion of the scapula which contributes to the great mobility of this joint. In order to stabilize this inherently unstable arrangement, there is a complicated series of tendons and ligaments that surround the shoulder joint complex.

Around the shallow cup portion of the scapula bone is a fibrocartilaginous rim of tissue known as the "glenoid labrum." This tissue enlarges the cuplike surface with which the humeral head articulates. This concavity is known as the glenoid fossa (Figure 5-12).

The capsule of the glenohumeral joint is an extremely thin walled, spacious container that attaches around the entire perimeter of the glenoid rim. The capsule arises from the glenoid fossa and inserts around the anatomical neck of the humerus. There is a synovial lining throughout. The anterior portion of the capsule is reinforced by the superior, middle, and the inferior glenohumeral ligaments.[3] The shoulder joint capsule is the principal stabilizer of the joint. Other ligaments about the shoulder joint include the coracoacromial ligament, and the coracohumeral ligament (Figure 5-13).

Several tendons pass over the shoulder joint. The long head of the bicipital tendon runs anterior to the shoulder joint, through a groove in the head of the humerus known as the bicipital groove. It inserts into the supraglenoid tubercle of the scapula. The bicep has a

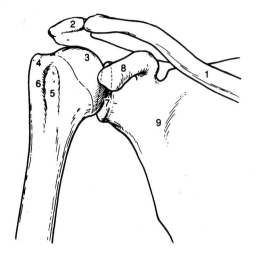

Figure 5-11 AP view of the shoulder region: 1. Clavicle; 2. Acromion; 3. Humeral Head; 4. Greater Tuberosity; 5. Lesser Tuberosity; 6. Bicipital Groove; 7. Glenoid Fossa; 8. Coracoid; 9. Scapula. Reprinted by permission from Unwin A, Jones K (eds). *Emergency Orthopaedics and Trauma*, p 101 (fig. 11.1). Oxford, Elsevier Science Ltd, 1995.

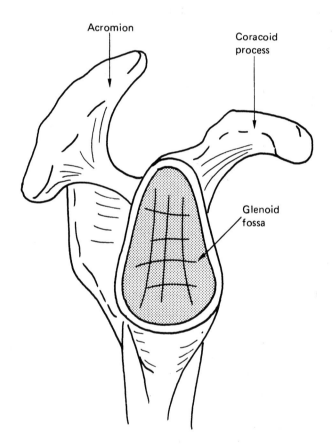

Figure 5-12 The glenoid fossa—the articular surface of the scapula bone. Reprinted by permission from Palastanga N, Field D, Soames R (eds). *Anatomy and Human Movement—Structure and Function*, 3rd ed. p 163 (fig 3.62a). Oxford, Elsevier Science Ltd, 1998.

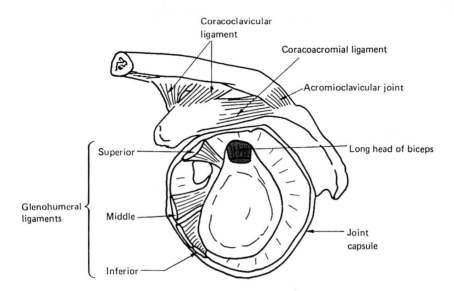

Figure 5-13 The shoulder joint capsule, glenohumeral and coacoacromial ligaments. The capsule of the glenohumeral joint arises from the glenoid fossa. The anterior portion of the capsule is reinforced by the superior, middle, and the inferior glenoid humeral ligaments. Reprinted by permission from Palastanga N, Field D, Soames R (eds). *Anatomy and Human Movement—Structure and Function*, 3rd ed. p 165 (fig 3.63a). Oxford, Elsevier Science Ltd, 1998.

second, short-head tendon that passes medial to the longhead tendon and inserts upon the coracoid process of the scapula (Figure 5-14). Another tendon that passes over the shoulder joint is the common tendon of the rotator cuff muscles. The rotator cuff muscles (supraspinatus, infraspinatus, teres major) work together to initiate abduction. The conjoined tendon of these muscles lies superior to the shoulder joint and inserts onto the greater tuberosity of the humerus (Figure 5-15). These various tendons provide additional limited stability for the shoulder joint complex.

Immediately above the rotator cuff tendon lies the subacromial bursa. This tissue generates a fine fluid film that helps lubricate the shoulder joint during motion. The rotator cuff tendon and the subacromial bursa can become inflamed foci of significant discomfort after trauma.

The rotator cuff muscles originate from the scapula and form a common tendon that passes over the shoulder joint and inserts onto the greater tuberosity of the humerus. When these muscles contract, they work to pull the humeral head into the glenoid fossa, which initiates abduction of the arm. Without the rotator cuff, arm abduction could not be completed. The initiation of abduction allows the deltoid muscle (the major arm abductor) to be in a position where it can complete the abduction process. Without the initial rotation provided by the rotator cuff, contraction of the deltoid muscle would simply pull the humerus upwards in a vertical fashion, into the acromion, without actually abducting the arm.[3] A traumatized or damaged rotator cuff will contribute to shoulder pain and impaired glenohumeral motion.

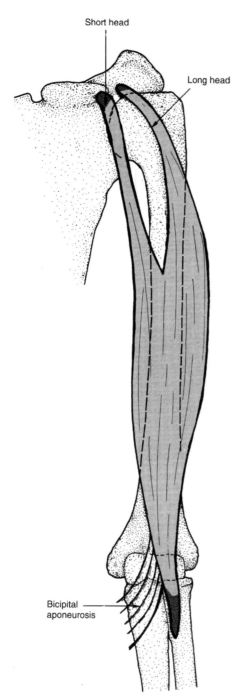

Figure 5-14 The attachments (shaded) of biceps brachii, anterior view. Reprinted by permission from Palastanga N, Field D, Soames R (eds). *Anatomy and Human Movement—Structure and Function*, 3rd ed. p 97 (fig 3.24). Oxford, Elsevier Science Ltd, 1998.

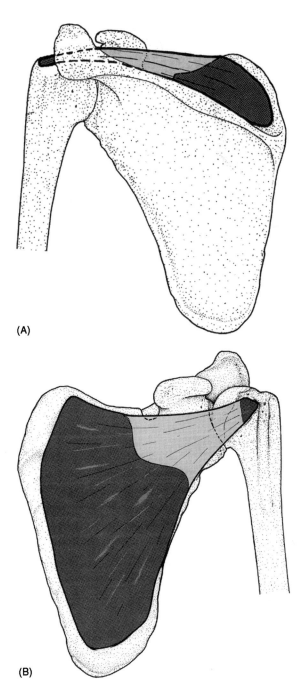

(A)

(B)

Figure 5-15 The common tendon of the rotator cuff muscles passes over the shoulder joint. The rotator cuff muscles (supraspinatus, infraspinatus, teres major) work together to initiate abduction. The conjoined tendon of these muscles lies superior to the shoulder joint and inserts onto the greater tuberosity of the humerus. (A) The attachments (shaded) of the supraspinatus. (B) The attachments (shaded) of subscapularis, anterior view.

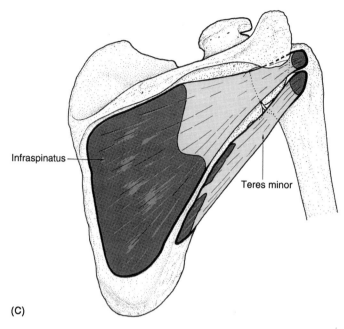

(C)

Figure 5-15 (continued) (C) The attachments (shaded) of infraspinatus and teres minor, posterior view. Reprinted by permission from Palastanga N, Field D, Soames R (eds). *Anatomy and Human Movement—Structure and Function*, 3rd ed. p 83 (fig 3.16a), p 93 (fig 3.22), p 95 (fig 3.23). Oxford, Elsevier Science Ltd, 1998.

As noted before, when operating properly the shoulder is the most mobile joint in the body. Full shoulder motion occurs due to a combination of movement involving both the scapula against the posterior thoracic cage and the humeral head within the glenoid fossa. The scapula rotates 45 degrees as the shoulder abducts fully. This is known as scapulothoracic motion whereas movement of the humeral head within the glenoid fossa is known as scapulohumeral movement (Figure 5-16). The planes of movement for the shoulder joint include flexion (0 to 180°), extension (0 to 50°), adduction (0 to 50°), abduction (0 to 180°), internal rotation (0 to 90°), and external rotation (0 to 90°).

Muscles around the shoulder joint include the rotator cuff muscles, the pectoral group, the latissimus dorsi, and the deltoid. The rotator cuff muscles originate from the scapula and have a common tendon that inserts onto the greater tuberosity of the humerus. Anterior to the shoulder joint are the pectoralis major and minor muscles. The pectoralis major muscle is a large fan shaped muscle with an extensive origin from the clavicle, the sternum, and the upper 6 costal cartilages and insertion into the proximal humerus. It flexes, extends, adducts, and medially rotates the arm. The pectoralis minor muscle is a flat triangular muscle that lies immediately deep to the pectoralis major. It arises from the third, fourth, and fifth ribs and inserts on the coracoid process of the scapula. It stabilizes the scapula by drawing it forward and downward and elevates the ribs from which it arises. The pectoral muscles also provide stability anterior to the shoulder joint.

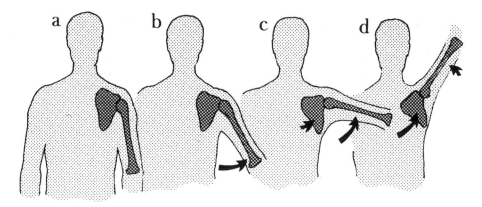

Figure 5-16 Scapulohumeral movement: during the early phase of abduction, most of the movement takes place at the glenohumeral joint (a–c). As the arm rises, the scapula begins to rotate on the thorax (c). In the last phase of abduction, movement is almost entirely scapulothoracic (d). Reprinted by permission from Apley AG, Solomon L (eds). *Concise System of Orthopaedics and Fractures,* 2nd ed. p 113 (fig 13.2). London, Hodder Arnold, 1994.

The latissimus dorsi provides some degree of stability posterior to the joint, and the deltoid muscle provides some lateral stability.[4]

The shelf of bone immediately above the humeral head is known as the acromion. The acromion is part of the scapula. It articulates with the clavicle at the acromioclavicular joint. Bone spurs may emanate from this joint, occasionally causing "impingement" upon underlying soft tissue structures.

Mechanism of Injury

Shoulder trauma may occur during a motor vehicle accident through a variety of mechanisms. The shoulder may strike directly against a door or another passenger at time of impact. This could cause acute impingement if the humeral head is pushed into the acromion. Impingement is more likely if a bone spur protrudes from the acromioclavicular joint. As described previously, an individual who braces themselves prior to impact, with arms extended against the steering wheel, dashboard, or back seat, will have forces transmitted up their arm(s) at time of impact. These forces could strain shoulder structures.

Some patients develop shoulder injuries as their shoulders impact against a caught shoulder harness after impact. For the driver, or passenger on the driver's side, the shoulder harness will pass over the left shoulder joint. The opposite occurs for those individuals on the passenger side of the vehicle. When the shoulder harness catches directly over the joint, there will be an acute, intense compression occurring at the shoulder. This may result in acute inflammation of the bicipital tendon, straining or tearing of the anterior shoulder capsular ligaments, and impingement. Therefore, appropriate functioning of the shoulder harness immediately post impact could traumatize the shoulder joint. In contrast, the contralateral, unrestrained shoulder will experience excessive anterior movement possibly straining or tearing its capsular ligaments.

Pathological Shoulder Conditions

A number of pathological conditions can involve the shoulder joint after a motor vehicle accident:

- shoulder bursitis
- rotator cuff or bicipital tendonitis
- capsular strains
- capsular tears
- subluxation of the shoulder
- fracture
- acromioclavicular joint separation/strain
- impingement
- rotator cuff tear
- surrounding myofascial pain
- development of a frozen shoulder.

Shoulder Bursitis

A patient with subacromial bursitis complains of shoulder joint pain that worsens with any activities above shoulder level. The pain is usually of a constant throbbing nature with sharp acute pain experienced with attempts to elevate the arm. Physical examination will demonstrate tenderness of the subacromial space and pain with elevation of the arm above shoulder level (positive impingement sign). There may be some boggy inflammation adjacent to the shelf of the acromion.

Diagnostic x-rays may be unrevealing, or may demonstrate an acromioclavicular bone spur protruding into the subacromial space. MRI scanning will demonstrate the inflamed bursal tissue within the shoulder joint. A subacromial anesthetic/steroid injection may be both diagnostic and therapeutic. If an anesthetic injected into the subacromial space provides the patient with resolution of symptomatology, it indicates that a nociceptive process exists in the subacromial region, usually a combination of bursitis and rotator cuff tendonitis. When a steroid is also infused, the injection may provide therapeutic benefit.

Treatment of acute shoulder bursitis includes relative rest, application of ice and use of oral anti-inflammatories. If the patient fails to improve, physical or occupational therapy should be initiated for modalities to reduce inflammation (ultrasound, iontophoresis), followed by progressive shoulder range of motion and strengthening. If the patient fails to improve, a subacromial steroid injection would be indicated. Occasionally, a series of two or three injections are necessary. If the steroid injections provide only temporary relief, further workup including MRI and referral to an orthopedic surgeon may be indicated to determine if arthroscopic surgery to decompress the shoulder joint is indicated. The surgical procedure for chronic bursitis would be a subacromial arthroscopy with subacromial decompression (removal of any bone spur impinging upon the bursa), and a bursectomy. Complications of chronic bursitis include chronic shoulder pain, loss of range of motion, and if the range of motion loss becomes severe, the patient may develop a frozen shoulder (adhesive capsulitis).

Rotator Cuff Tendonitis

The patient with rotator cuff tendonitis also complains of pain at the tip of the shoulder that worsens with over-the-shoulder activities. When severe, the tendonitis pain may refer down the arm, and proximally along the trapezius to the ipsilateral neck. On physical examination, there will be tenderness of the subacromial space and a positive impingement sign. There may be reactive muscle spasm in the shoulder girdle and neck region.

The diagnosis is based principally on the history and physical examination. X-rays often demonstrate a bone spur protruding from the acromion. MRI scanning is very sensitive for inflammation of the rotator cuff and its use is indicated if patients continue to have pain despite therapeutic measures. Arthrograms and MRI arthrograms may be helpful in delineating a rotator cuff tear. Lastly, a diagnostic injection with anesthetic may help confirm a nociceptive focus within the subacromial space. When steroids are included in the injection, the diagnostic injection may also be therapeutic.

The initial treatment of rotator cuff tendonitis should be conservative including several days of relative rest for the arm, application of ice and use of anti-inflammatories. If the patient fails to improve, occupational therapy for modalities (ultrasound and iontophoresis) to reduce inflammation, with gradual progression to shoulder range of motion and strengthening exercises will be needed. If the patient fails to improve with therapy, intra-articular steroid injections should be considered. A series of two or three injections may be required. However, a single injection may be all that is necessary to get the patient on the road to recovery. If the patient only gets short-term relief with the steroid injections, and if they have already failed a course of conservative measures including rest, medications and therapy, then a surgical evaluation with an orthopedic specialist would be indicated. If workup demonstrates a source of impingement with inflammation of the rotator cuff tendon, then arthroscopic subacromial arthroplasty is the procedure of choice. This procedure usually includes decompression of the subacromial space (grinding down the acromial bone spur, removal of part of the distal clavicle and the coracoacromial ligament, and a bursectomy). Ideally, this decompression will enable the tendonitis to heal over time. The patient may require postoperative therapy to improve shoulder strength and range of motion of the joint.

Complications of chronic tendonitis include loss of range of motion or even a frozen shoulder (if the patient immobilizes their joint due to fear of increased pain). Ongoing discomfort may be associated with decreased range of motion and weakness of the shoulder joint, even after an arthroplasty procedure. Surrounding muscle spasm may contribute to neck and shoulder girdle pain, and if the scalene and pectoral muscles are tight, there can be entrapment of the underlying brachial plexus with referral pain into the respective extremity (myogenic thoracic outlet syndrome).

Bicipital Tendonitis

The patient with bicipital tendonitis complains of anterior shoulder pain that worsens with flexion and supination activities of the involved extremity. Physical examination will demonstrate tenderness and possibly some inflammation of the long head of the bicipital tendon as it passes through the bicipital groove of the proximal humerus. The pain will increase with forearm flexion against resistance, and with supination (with the arm outstretched) against resistance.

Diagnostic workup is usually unrevealing. Because this is a soft tissue process, x-rays tend to be negative. An MRI scan may demonstrate inflammation of the bicipital tendon. However, usually the diagnosis can be made through the history and physical examination. Lastly, a diagnostic injection with anesthetic may help confirm the diagnosis of bicipital tendonitis. Infusion of a steroid with the anesthetic may prove therapeutic and diagnostic.

Initial treatment of bicipital tendonitis is conservative with application of ice, relative rest and use of anti-inflammatories. If the patient fails to improve, he/she should be referred to physical or occupational therapy for appropriate modalities (iontophoresis or ultrasound) with gradual progression to range of motion and strengthening exercises once the inflammation has subsided. If the patient fails to improve with conservative measures, steroid injection(s) as outlined above would be appropriate. If the pain persists, an orthopedic procedure to release pressure about the bicipital tendon may be necessary.

Complications of persistent bicipital tendonitis include ongoing shoulder pain, progressive loss of range of motion and weakness. If there is surrounding muscle spasm, patients may develop thoracic outlet symptomatology.

Shoulder Capsule Strain

The shoulder capsule may be strained after a motor vehicle accident as a result of impact against the door, steering wheel, another passenger, or the shoulder harness. Occasionally, it is the shoulder that is not restrained by the harness that may excessively stretch during the accident due to the forces produced.

The patient with a strained shoulder complains of shoulder pain with range of motion. Physical examination will demonstrate tenderness along the shoulder capsule. Impingement sign may be negative while the "apprehension sign" (forced shoulder abduction and external rotation) may be positive. There may be reactive muscle spasm in adjacent musculature. Shoulder range of motion may be limited by pain.

Diagnostic x-rays tend to be unrevealing since this is a soft tissue condition. If the fibers are strained and not torn, arthrography will not demonstrate any significant pathology. However, an MRI scan is more sensitive in demonstrating strains and inflammation of the shoulder capsule. A diagnostic injection with anesthetic may help confirm the location of pathology. Addition of steroids to the anesthetic may prove to be both diagnostic and therapeutic.

Early treatment of a severely strained shoulder includes sling immobilization for a few days post injury, anti-inflammatories and application of ice. As the pain subsides, progressive ranges of motion exercises are important so as to prevent the development of adhesive capsulitis and frozen shoulder. A referral for physical or occupational therapy may be needed for adequate modalities (ultrasound and iontophoresis), and progression to a more formal range of motion and strengthening program. Steroid injections may help promote recovery. Surgery is generally not indicated for severe strains, unless the patient loses shoulder range of motion as a result of inactivity. In such cases, manipulation of the joint under anesthesia can be performed to improve range of motion.

Inadequate treatment of a shoulder strain could result in chronic complications including adhesive capsulitis with loss of range of motion, chronic pain as a result of the fibrous contracture, weakness of surrounding musculature, and if there is spasm of surrounding musculature, thoracic outlet symptomatology may ensue.

Shoulder Capsule Tear

When forces to the shoulder are significant, capsular fibers can tear and the shoulder joint may sublux, usually in an anterior or inferior direction. A shoulder subluxation refers to the humeral head coming out of the glenoid fossa. A severe subluxation will not reduce itself and the patient will require skilled intervention to reduce the shoulder joint via a variety of orthopedic maneuvers. Less severe subluxations will reduce themselves and the patient will experience a transient popping within the shoulder as the humeral head goes out of position and then returns itself to normal alignment within the glenoid fossa.

The history for a patient with a capsular tear and subluxation is one of popping of the shoulder joint occurring with range of motion, associated with discomfort that may linger even after the joint pops back into place. Physical examination demonstrates tenderness of the torn ligament, loss of range of motion, surrounding muscle spasm, and a positive "apprehension sign." Conventional x-rays may demonstrate the subluxation when capsular tears are severe. An arthrogram with infusion of radiographic dye will demonstrate leakage of the dye through the torn capsule. MR imaging can also confirm the tear.

With regards to treatment, if the tear is small, physical or occupational therapy may be all that is necessary to help the patient stabilize the shoulder joint. The initial treatment usually requires modalities to reduce inflammation. Over time, range of motion and strengthening exercises are added. If the muscles around the shoulder joint can be strengthened sufficiently, it may provide for adequate stabilization of the joint. However, if the intermittent subluxations do not resolve, surgery to strengthen the joint capsule may be the only alternative. This can be done by a variety of orthopedic approaches designed to repair and strengthen the torn joint capsule. For small tears, arthroscopic techniques can be utilized. However, for larger tears, open repairs are usually required. The surgical techniques are beyond the scope of this text. Postoperatively, the patient will require therapy for progressive range of motion and strengthening of the shoulder musculature. Complications of capsular tears include persistent shoulder subluxation and pain. After shoulder surgery, loss of range of motion may occur, especially without adequate rehabilitation. A frozen shoulder is the worst-case scenario. With repeated subluxations, there may be stretching of the axillary nerve or the brachial plexus with associated injury. This can cause weakness or sensory abnormalities throughout the arm. Surrounding muscle spasm may contribute to thoracic outlet symptomatology.

Shoulder Fracture

The patient with a humeral head fracture after a motor vehicle accident will complain of sharp shoulder pain. Physical examination will demonstrate swelling, ecchymoses, and tenderness of the joint with gentle palpation. The diagnosis is confirmed through x-ray evaluation.

Appropriate treatment may range from putting the patient in a sling to surgical intervention for open reduction and internal fixation for more complicated fractures. After the fracture heals, the patient will require a course of therapy for progressive range of motion of the shoulder joint and strengthening of surrounding muscles. If the shoulder joint loses significant range of motion (due to the development of scar tissue and/or adhesive capsulitis), the patient may need to undergo manipulation under anesthesia (once the fracture heals appropriately), to help normalize range of motion.

Complications of a humeral head fracture include frozen shoulder, loss of range of motion, ongoing shoulder pain, and weakness of shoulder musculature. Chronic spasm of muscles in the shoulder region may contribute to the development of a myogenic thoracic outlet syndrome.

Acromioclavicular Joint Strain

The acromioclavicular (AC) joint may be strained after a motor vehicle accident, usually as a result of forces generated by the shoulder harness as it catches over the shoulder joint. The fibers that hold the AC joint intact may be torn and there could be actual separation of that articulation.

Patients with an acromioclavicular joint strain or separation, complain of pain at the tip of the shoulder that worsens with shoulder range of motion. Some patients may complain of a visible deformity at the tip of the shoulder. On physical examination, there may be deformity of the shoulder joint due to protrusion of the distal clavicle. There will be tenderness of the acromioclavicular joint, and shoulder range of motion will be limited by pain.

X-rays may demonstrate a frank separation. However, if the acromioclavicular fibers are torn, the presence of a separation may not be evident without stress views. With this technique, the patient has initial x-rays taken without any stress, and then he or she repeats the x-rays while holding a 10- or 20-pound weight, which will apply traction to the shoulder joint. This will accentuate any separation that may be present as a result of acromioclavicular joint fiber tear. MRI of the shoulder may also demonstrate the torn ligaments. An anesthetic/steroid injection is potentially both diagnostic and therapeutic. The acromioclavicular joint, which is relatively subcutaneous, is injected with the anesthetic/steroid solution. If the patient has pain relief, this indicates a strain or tearing of acromioclavicular joint fibers. The steroids may prove therapeutic in reducing inflammation and decreasing pain.

Treatment for an acromioclavicular strain depends on its severity. For a mild strain, conservative measures including relative immobilization of the shoulder joint with a sling, application of ice, and oral anti-inflammatories may be all that is necessary. A steroid injection might prove helpful in reducing inflammation and accelerating recovery. However, when the strain is more severe or when there is an actual tearing of acromioclavicular joint fibers with separation of the joint, more aggressive conservative measures or even surgery may prove necessary. A special sling can be ordered to immobilize the acromioclavicular joint, approximating the acromion with the clavicle.

It may need to be worn for three to six weeks. Physical or occupational therapy to reduce inflammation and maintain range of motion of the shoulder may be necessary. Occasionally, surgery is necessary to treat this problem. In general, there are no good surgical approaches to repair a torn and subluxated acromioclavicular joint. Usually, a distal clavicle excision is required to help reduce pain in these patients.[5]

Complications of acromioclavicular joint strain or separation include chronic subluxation with shoulder pain, loss of range of motion, weakness of surrounding musculature, and chronic deformity. If shoulder musculature goes into spasm, the patient may develop thoracic outlet symptomatology.

Rotator Cuff Tear

Acute shoulder impingement during a motor vehicle accident may result in tearing of the rotator cuff at its musculotendinous junction. This area, known as the critical zone, has a tenuous blood supply, which limits its ability to heal after trauma. The history of a patient with a rotator cuff tear includes severe pain within the shoulder joint or at the tip of the shoulder. Patients may have weakness with a partial tear, and, with a complete tear of the rotator cuff, he or she may be unable to initiate abduction of the arm.

On physical examination, there will be tenderness of the subacromial space, and weakness of shoulder movements, particularly internal and external rotation and abduction. There may be a positive "drop arm test." To perform this test, the patient fully abducts his/her involved arm and then slowly lowers it to their side. With a rotator cuff tear, the arm will drop to the patient's side from a position of about 90 degrees. If the patient is able to hold his/her arm in abduction, then a gentle tap on the forearm will cause the arm to fall.[6] Impingement sign is usually positive.

With regards to diagnostic workup, conventional x-rays may demonstrate a subacromial bone spur. Shoulder arthrography will demonstrate the perforation through the rotator cuff as contrast material leaks from the subacromial space, through the tear, to the inferior surface of the rotator cuff. MRI scanning is also highly sensitive for rotator cuff tear. A diagnostic anesthetic injection may relieve pain, but it really cannot be used to differentiate between rotator cuff tendonitis and a rotator cuff tear. The best procedures to demonstrate tearing are arthrography or MRI scanning.

Early treatment for a rotator cuff tear includes conservative measures, particularly if the tear is partial. This would include relative rest, application of ice, use of a sling, and anti-inflammatories. Physical or occupational therapy should be initiated for modalities to reduce inflammation, and progression to a range of motion and exercise program. The goals of therapy are to strengthen the remaining muscles of the rotator cuff to compensate for the torn tissues, and maintenance of shoulder strength and range of motion. Steroid injections may be helpful to reduce inflammation and pain associated with the tearing.

However, if pain persists with a partial tear or if a patient has a complete rotator cuff tear, surgical intervention may be the only alternative to correct the situation. This can occasionally be done arthroscopically, but often requires an open approach to the shoulder joint. Postoperatively, the patient will require physical or occupational therapy to improve shoulder range of motion, and to strengthen surrounding musculature and the repaired rotator cuff.

Complications of a rotator cuff tear include persistent shoulder pain and weakness and decreased range of motion, which when most severe may leave the patient with a frozen shoulder. If there is surrounding muscle spasm, the patient may develop thoracic outlet symptomatology due to pressure on the underlying brachial plexus.

Myofascial Pain Syndrome

Myofascial pain syndrome in the shoulder region will cause shoulder discomfort, as well as pain referred up to the neck and down the arm. Shoulder musculature can be injured directly after a motor vehicle accident, or it may go into reactive spasm as a result of pain generated from within the shoulder joint. Muscles that surround the shoulder joint include the pectoralis major and minor anteriorly, the deltoid laterally, the trapezius superiorly, and the scapula muscles (supraspinatus, infraspinatus, teres minor, subscapularis) and rhomboids posteriorly.

The patient with chronic myofascial pain in the shoulder region will complain of discomfort and tenderness of the involved muscles. Physical examination will demonstrate tenderness, increased muscle tone, and trigger points. Range of motion may be limited or painful. If there is irritation of the underlying brachial plexus, the patient may have positive provocative testing suggesting thoracic outlet syndrome (positive Adson's maneuver or a positive hyperabduction test). Diagnostic workup would be unrevealing for this soft tissue condition. The diagnosis is based on the history and physical examination.

Treatment for myofascial pain syndrome requires a therapy program that helps to minimize spasm and improve range of motion and strength of the involved musculature. Physical or occupational therapy is often necessary for appropriate modalities to decrease pain, spasm and inflammation, followed by stretching and strengthening exercises for the involved musculature. Surgery is not indicated for this condition. If the patient has discrete trigger points, they may respond favorably to trigger point injection therapy (injection of an anesthetic/steroid derivative into small, tender muscle bundles in an effort to break the cycle of pain and spasm).

Complications of chronic myofascial pain include ongoing discomfort, limitations of range of motion, thoracic outlet symptomatology, and weakness of shoulder muscles due to chronic inactivity.

Frozen Shoulder/Adhesive Capsulitis

Limitations of range of motion may occur with any acute injury to the shoulder. It occurs due to relative inactivity of the shoulder joint during the acute and subacute phase of injury. This, in conjunction with inadequate physical therapy to optimize range of motion after the acute injury has healed, can lead to range of motion loss. In the extreme case, a patient may develop a severe range of motion loss known as a frozen shoulder or adhesive capsulitis. In these cases, range of motion deficit is extreme and the patient holds his/her arm close to their body. The only range of motion that can occur is due to rotation of the scapula. Range of motion at the glenohumeral joint is severely disrupted.

Historically, a patient with adhesive capsulitis experiences shoulder pain after an initiating trauma that limits shoulder mobility, and, over time leads to a gradual loss of range of motion. The patient will state that range of motion is severely limited and any attempt at range of motion is extremely uncomfortable. There may be complaints of periarticular muscle spasm.

On physical examination, the patient will have limited shoulder range of motion, diffuse tenderness of shoulder structures (bicipital tendon, rotator cuff, subacromial space, and the shoulder capsule), and there may be surrounding muscle spasm (pectoral, trapezius, and scapular muscles). If the patient chronically wears a sling to keep the shoulder immobilized, he/she can develop a flexion contracture at the elbow. Upper extremity motor strength may be compromised because of muscle atrophy that develops over time. However, sensory examination and reflexes would be normal as this is not a neurological lesion.

Diagnostic workup including x-rays, arthrography, and MRI scan may all be normal, unless there is an underlying orthopedic problem (bone spur, bursitis, tendonitis, capsular tear, fracture) precipitating the development of the frozen shoulder. MRI and arthrography may demonstrate a rotator cuff tear and stress x-rays may demonstrate an acromioclavicular joint or shoulder separation. However, a frozen shoulder is a soft tissue condition and conventional imaging studies are often unrevealing.

Treatment of this condition should begin with a conservative program to attempt to improve range of motion. This would include either physical or occupational therapy for modalities (ultrasound or hot packs) to help loosen up the collagen fibers that contribute to the adhesions, followed by progressive range of motion exercises. Occasionally, a patient will benefit from a steroid injection to decrease inflammation within the joint. This may help facilitate the therapy. When conservative treatment fails to improve range of motion, the patient will require manipulation of the shoulder joint under anesthesia. To perform this, the patient goes under general anesthesia, and the orthopedic surgeon manipulates the shoulder joint, trying to achieve optimal range of motion. This procedure will result in tearing of scar tissue and adhesions that contribute to the frozen shoulder. Postoperatively, the patient may be in extreme pain and appropriate analgesics are necessary. After this procedure, the patient must engage in aggressive physical therapy to maintain and further improve range of motion. A home exercise program should be performed on a daily basis so as to maintain range of motion.

The principal complication of a frozen shoulder is ongoing pain and limited range of motion. Those patients with proximal muscle spasm may develop thoracic outlet symptomatology (paresthesias and weakness in the involved extremity).

UPPER EXTREMITY NERVE ENTRAPMENTS

After a motor vehicle accident, a patient may develop upper extremity pain due to nerve injury and/or irritation. There are multiple sites of potential nerve entrapment extending from the neck to the hand. Understanding upper extremity anatomy is important for the clinician who is trying to localize the site(s) of entrapment so that appropriate therapeutic measures can be instituted.

All upper extremity peripheral nerves emanate from motor and sensory cervical nerve roots levels C4 through T1. Following the exit of these nerve roots from their respective neural foramina they coalesce into a complex arrangement of nervous tissue in the supraclavicular region known as the brachial plexus (Figure 5-17). Nerve fibers within the brachial plexus pass through or under a number of structures where entrapment can occur causing a thoracic outlet syndrome.

Within the brachial plexus, nerve fibers rearrange into the major upper extremity peripheral nerves (axillary, musculocutaneous, radial, ulnar, and median. The axillary nerve is a sensory and motor nerve. It supplies sensation to the skin overlying the deltoid muscle and has motor innervation of the deltoid. The musculocutaneous nerve provides motor control of the biceps muscle, and then further courses into the forearm as the lateral antebrachial cutaneous nerve, which supplies sensation to the volar and radial half of the forearm to the level of the wrist. The radial nerve has motor supply to the triceps, and the wrist and finger extensor muscles. It courses around the humerus through a groove known as the radial groove following which it branches into the superficial radial nerve (a sensory nerve) and the posterior interosseous nerve (the motor branch of the radial nerve which supplies dorsal forearm musculature). Sensory innervation of the radial nerve includes the dorsum of the hand. (See Figure 5-2.) The ulnar nerve courses medially down the arm passing through a groove at the elbow (the ulnar groove). It passes into the hand

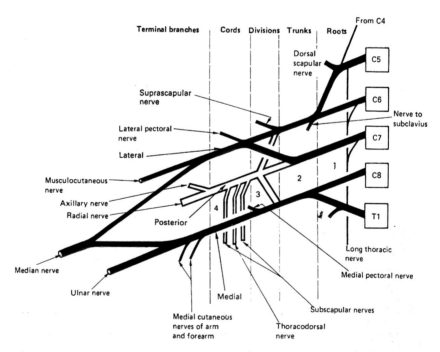

Figure 5-17 Schematic diagram of the brachial plexus. Reprinted by permission from Palastanga N, Field D, Soames R (eds). *Anatomy and Human Movement—Structure and Function*, 3rd ed. p 263 (fig 3.126). Oxford, Elsevier Science Ltd, 1998.

through Guyon's canal at the ulnar wrist. (See Figure 5-3.) The median nerve is the largest peripheral nerve in the upper extremity. It courses through the volar forearm into the hand through the carpal tunnel at the wrist (Figure 5-18).

There are multiple potential sites of entrapment for these various nerves:

- The median nerve can be entrapped at the level of the wrist (carpal tunnel syndrome) and in the forearm underneath the pronator mass (pronator syndrome).
- The ulnar nerve can be entrapped at the elbow (cubital tunnel syndrome) or at the level of the wrist as it passes through Guyon's canal.
- The radial nerve has three potential sites of entrapment including the radial groove of the humerus, the radial tunnel on the dorsal forearm, and its superficial radial branch can be entrapped along the radial distal forearm just above the wrist.
- Lastly, the brachial plexus can be irritated or entrapped at the level of the thoracic outlet. Such entrapment can occur through one of a number of anatomic structures

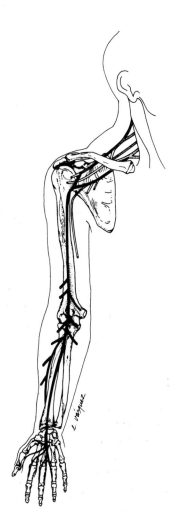

Figure 5-18 The median nerve. Reprinted by permission from Rosenbaum RB, Ochoa JL (eds). *Carpal Tunnel Syndrome and Other Disorders of the Median Nerve*, p 2 (fig 1.1). Boston, Butterworth-Heinemann, 1993.

(the scalene muscles, an accessory rib that occurs in a small subset of the population, between the first rib and the clavicle, and/or under the pectoralis minor muscle).

The Electrodiagnostic Study

For patients with persistent neurologic complaints, the most appropriate physiologic test available to evaluate for nerve injury is the electrodiagnostic study, or electromyography/nerve conduction velocity study (EMG/NCV).

EMG equipment has changed significantly over the past 50 years. As can be expected, with the advent of microcircuitry, the size of the machinery has decreased. Today's equipment is also capable of printing out reports and graphic information, calculating nerve conduction velocities as the test is performed, and various other functions.

Indications for the study include persistent signs and symptoms consistent with possible nerve irritation or injury including numbness, tingling, burning pain, and other paresthesias, weakness of a particular muscle group, reflex abnormalities, night-time awakening with pain or paresthesias (nocturnal paresthesias), neck pain with radicular symptomatology, persistent extremity pain without a formal diagnosis, and functional loss within the extremity.

There is an optimal time frame for some electrical studies to be performed. If one is trying to confirm a radiculopathy, it is doubtful that worthwhile findings will be seen within the first four weeks after the motor vehicle accident. On the other hand, many post-traumatic nerve entrapments can be detected in this early period. There are two different types of tests performed during the typical electrodiagnostic study, the NCV study and needle EMG.

The concept behind NCV studies is that damaged or entrapped nerves will not conduct electrical impulses optimally and there will be slowing of conduction velocities as compared to expected normals. Each peripheral nerve within the body conducts electrical impulses. The velocity with which these impulses travel is known as the NCV. Upper extremity NCVs tend to be a bit faster than lower extremity velocities. Normal upper extremity NCVs are usually greater than 50 m/sec, whereas lower extremity velocities are usually greater than 40 m/sec. In addition to the nerve velocities, the electromyographer also looks at distal latencies, the amount of time that the impulse takes to get from the point of stimulation to the muscle where the response is measured. If there is a distal entrapment (e.g., carpal tunnel syndrome), the distal latency of the respective nerve may be slower than the expected norms, or the value from an asymptomatic contralateral extremity.

The EMG study is performed utilizing very small needles that are inserted into different muscles of the extremity. A particular nerve supplies each muscle. The purpose of the EMG is to determine if there has been a more severe type of nerve injury, whereby the nerve fibers are actually transected as a result of the trauma. In such cases, there would be characteristic waveform abnormalities seen on the machine's oscilloscope that would indicate denervation (loss of nerve supply to the muscle being studied).

To perform NCVs, the EMG machine has a stimulation device that generates transient electrical pulses used to stimulate motor and sensory nerves. Responses (waveforms) that are generated by the electrical stimulation are picked up on the EMG machine's video screen. From these waveforms, the electromyographer can calculate nerve conduction velocities, distal latencies, and the amplitude of motor and sensory responses. The patient is hooked up to three electrodes (ground, active, and reference) (Figure 5-19). The electrodes come as discs, clips, or rings that can be taped to the skin or wrapped around a finger. Needle electrodes are utilized for the EMG portion of the evaluation.

Nerve conduction studies can be performed on every major upper extremity nerve that can potentially be entrapped including the median, ulnar, radial, axillary and musculocutaneous. With proximal stimulation techniques and utilization of F-waves, the brachial plexus can also be evaluated. All nerves within the body have been assigned a range of normal values for their nerve conduction velocity. Upper extremity nerves conduct electrical impulses at a velocity of approximately 50 to 70 m/sec.

F-waves are frequently used to rule out problems at the proximal root or plexus level (e.g., thoracic outlet syndrome [TOS] or radiculopathy). When performing F-waves, the electrical impulse is directed towards the spinal cord. Whenever a nerve is stimulated, the electrical impulse travels in two directions: orthodromic conduction towards the muscle, which is innervated, and antidromic conduction away from the muscle and towards the spinal cord. For calculation of F-waves, there is an antidromic electrical impulse that travels towards the spinal cord. Within the spinal cord, the nerve impulses

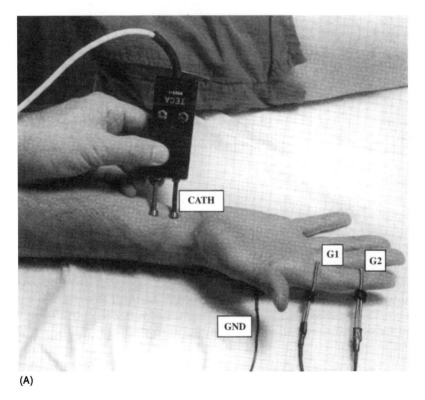

(A)

Figure 5-19 (A) Median sensory study. Stimulation site over the median nerve at the wrist, recording the index finger using ring electrodes (G1, G2). (GND = ground electrode, CATH = cathode of stimulator).

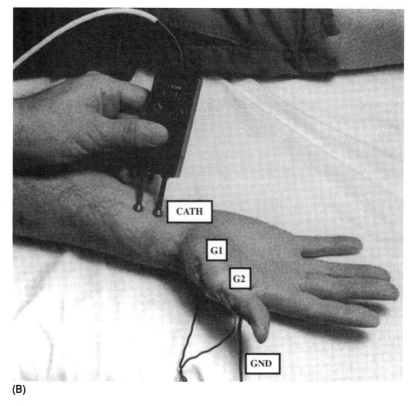

(B)

Figure 5-19 (continued) (B) Median motor study. Stimulation sites over the median nerve at the wrist, recording the abductor pollicis brevis muscle using disk electrodes (G1, G2). Reprinted by permission from Preston DC, Shapiro BE (eds). *Electromyography and Neuromuscular Disorders—Clinical-Electrophysiologic Correlations* (fig 9.3), (fig 9.2). Boston, Butterworth-Heinemann, 1998.

activate motor neurons that in turn generate orthodromic impulses that travel down the arm, causing a contraction in a distal muscle. The contraction is recorded as the F-wave (Figure 5-20). This technique provides information about the entire course of a nerve, including the thoracic outlet and proximal nerve roots.

When a motor nerve is stimulated, the electromyographer looks for information about its distal latency and the amplitude of the response. The motor response seen on the oscilloscope is known as the compound motor action potential (CMAP). (See Figure 4-2.) Its amplitude is a reflection of the number of muscle fibers that contract in response to the stimulation and the synchrony with which they respond.

Sensory nerve conduction studies are performed differently utilizing ring electrodes on the fingers. To perform a sensory NCV study, the sensory nerve that is stimulated generates an electrical impulse that passes under the ring electrodes. This generates a wave on the machine's oscilloscope known as a sensory nerve action potential (SNAP). (See Figure 4-5.) The latency and amplitude of this response are compared with normal values.

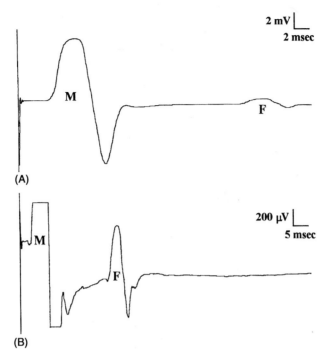

2 mV
2 msec

(A)

200 μV
5 msec

(B)

Figure 5-20 Normal F responses. (A) Stimulating median nerve at the wrist, recording abductor pollicis brevis. (B) To accurately measure the F response, the gain must be increased to 200 mcV and the sweep to either 5 or 10 msec. With these settings, the F response is well seen, but the M response saturates the amplifier and becomes distorted. (M = direct motor response/compound muscle action potential; F = F response.) Reprinted by permission from Preston DC, Shapiro BE (eds). *Electromyography and Neuromuscular Disorders—Clinical-Electrophysiologic Correlations* (fig 4.1). Boston, Butterworth-Heinemann, 1998.

Motor NCVs can be calculated after stimulation of the motor nerve at two different spots within the arm. This will generate two CMAP responses (Figure 5-21). The electromyographer then measures the distance between the points of stimulation. By knowing the distance and the amount of time between the CMAP responses, the electromyographer can calculate velocities in m/sec. Sensory velocities are calculated in a similar fashion. However, only one stimulation site is necessary. The sensory NCV is also measured in m/sec.

If there is a nerve injury somewhere along the course of a nerve, the electromyographer may witness a conduction block with neuropraxia. This refers to abnormally small amplitude of the CMAP response with associated temporal dispersion after stimulation proximal to the site of entrapment (Figure 5-22).

Carpal Tunnel Syndrome

Carpal tunnel syndrome is probably the most common nerve entrapment that a clinician will face. It involves entrapment of the median nerve, a large nerve that courses through

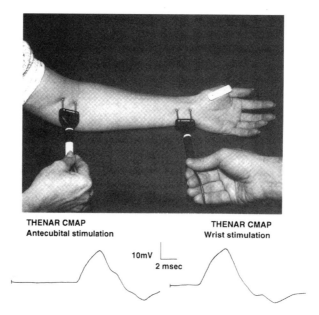

THENAR CMAP
Antecubital stimulation

THENAR CMAP
Wrist stimulation

10mV

2 msec

Figure 5-21 Motor NCVs can be calculated after stimulation of the motor nerve at two different spots within the arm. This will generate two CMAP responses. The CMAPs obtained over the thenar muscles from stimulation at the wrist and at the antecubital space are shown. Reprinted by permission from Rosenbaum RB, Ochoa JL (eds). *Carpal Tunnel Syndrome and other Disorders of the Median Nerve* (fig 7.1). Boston, Butterworth-Heinemann, 1993.

the arm and forearm into the hand through a passageway known as the carpal tunnel. The median nerve is a critical nerve and it has a huge representation within the cerebral cortex. It supplies sensation to the first three and one-half fingers of the respective hand, and provides motor control of the thumb. It originates from cervical nerve roots C4 through T1 that then coalesce within the brachial plexus to form the median nerve. The median nerve then courses through the arm and forearm and as noted above, enters the hand through the tunnel formed below by the carpal bones and above by the transverse carpal ligament. The finger flexor tendons also reside within this tunnel. In general, there is a very limited amount of space for all of these structures as they course through this small anatomic passageway. (See Figure 5-4.)

Carpal tunnel syndrome may occur after a motor vehicle accident due either to direct trauma or as a secondary response to a more proximal entrapment. A direct trauma may occur as the driver of a vehicle braces him/herself against the steering wheel prior to impact, or when the passenger braces against the dashboard or back seat. In contrast to direct trauma, when a nerve is compressed at a proximal site, its distal nerve fibers may become hypersensitive. In such cases, a mild asymptomatic entrapment distal to the site of injury might become symptomatic because of this hypersensitivity phenomenon.

Carpal tunnel symptomatology includes paresthesias (numbness, tingling, or burning pain) in a median nerve sensory distribution (thumb, index finger, middle finger, and the radial half of the fourth finger). The patient with carpal tunnel syndrome may complain of

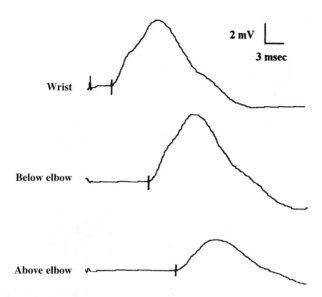

Figure 5-22 Conduction block at the elbow. If there is a nerve injury somewhere along the course of a nerve, the electromyographer may witness a conduction block with neuropraxia. This refers to abnormally small amplitude of the CMAP response with associated temporal dispersion after stimulation proximal to the site of entrapment (in this case at the elbow). Reprinted by permission from Prest-on DC, Shapiro BE (eds). *Electromyography and Neuromuscular Disorders—Clinical-Electrophysiologic Correlations* (fig 17.8). Boston, Butterworth-Heinemann, 1998.

hand weakness with frequent dropping of objects. The motor branch of the median nerve supplies the muscles of the thenar eminence of the palm. With advanced disease, there may be muscle atrophy and wasting of the thenar eminence. Frequently, patients complain of waking up at night with numbness, tingling, or pain in their hand. This phenomenon is known as nocturnal paresthesias. During the day they may complain of wrist or hand pain, decreased grip strength, decreased dexterity, and hand fatigue while writing.

Physical examination of the patient with carpal tunnel syndrome may demonstrate a positive Tinel's sign at the level of the transverse carpal ligament. To perform this, the examiner taps the wrist over the transverse carpal ligament. A positive Tinel's sign occurs when the patient develops an electrical radiating pain that follows a median distribution. Another provocative test for median nerve entrapment at the wrist is the Phalen's maneuver. To perform this test, the patient is asked to flex both hands together at the wrist (Figure 5-23). If the hand(s) develop numbness in a median distribution within a 60 second time frame, the patient is said to have a positive Phalen's test, which is consistent with median nerve compression at the wrist.

Sensory testing of the hand (light touch, pinprick, and two-point discrimination) may demonstrate abnormalities in a median nerve distribution. Normal two-point discrimination is less than 6 mm in the digits. Greater than 6 mm of two-point discrimination

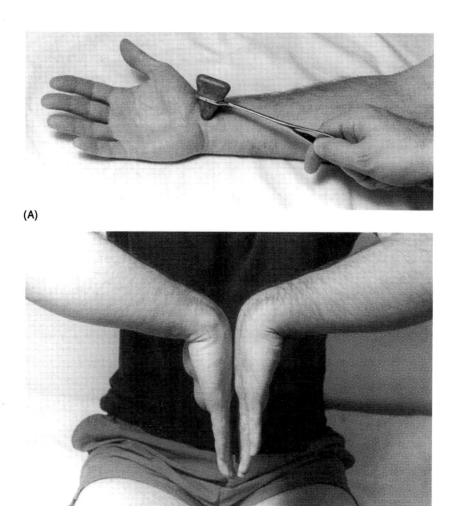

(A)

(B)

Figure 5-23 Provocative test for carpal tunnel syndrome. (A) Tinel's sign is elicited by tapping over the median nerve in the center of the wrist. If abnormal, the patient will report paresthesias radiating into median-innervated digits. (B) Phalen's maneuver is performed by passive wrist flexion. This position increases pressure within the carpal tunnel and it may provoke paresthesias radiating into median-innervated digits in patients with carpal tunnel syndrome. Reprinted by permission from Preston DC, Shapiro BE (eds). *Electromyography and Neuromuscular Disorders—Clinical-Electrophysiologic Correlations* (fig 16.5A & B). Boston, Butterworth-Heinemann, 1998.

indicates some sensory loss. Sensory abnormality in fingers one, two, three, and the radial half of the fourth finger occur in carpal tunnel syndrome. On motor assessment, the examiner looks for muscle atrophy in the abductor pollicis brevis muscle, and checks for weakness of thumb abduction.[7,8]

The most common diagnostic test for carpal tunnel syndrome is the electrodiagnostic study. The NCV study of carpal tunnel syndrome will demonstrate prolonged distal latencies of the median motor and sensory nerves as compared to the ulnar motor and sensory nerves on the same side. When the data is equivocal, there are a number of more sensitive tests that can be performed including the Ernest Johnson Fourth Finger Test, the Bactrien test, and conduction velocities across the wrist. For the Ernest Johnson Fourth Finger Test, ring sensory electrodes are placed on the fourth finger, a finger that has dual innervation by both the median and the ulnar nerves. Stimulation is done above the wrist at equal distances from the active electrode to each nerve. Johnson has found that in asymptomatic patients, when comparing the median sensory latency to the ring finger with the ulnar sensory latency to the same digit, that the difference in latency was 0.3 msec or less in 93 percent of the hands. Hence, if the median nerve conducts greater than 0.4 msec slower than the ulnar nerve, the test is considered positive for a mild carpal tunnel syndrome.[9]

Another provocative electrophysiologic technique is the Bactrien test. Here, sensory electrodes are placed on the thumb, which also has dual innervation by both median and superficial radial nerves. Each nerve is stimulated simultaneously, above the wrist (at a point midway between the two nerves). Excessive delay of the median potential produces a SNAP with two negative peaks, the so-called "double hump" known as the Bactrien sign (named after the Bactrien camel which has two humps on its back).[10–12]

Lastly, the examiner may wish to perform conduction velocities directly across the wrist by performing stimulation both distal and proximal to the carpal tunnel. Latency across the wrist greater than 1.5 msec is considered positive for carpal tunnel syndrome.[13] Kimura has extended this idea by stimulating the median nerve at 1 cm intervals across the wrist area while recording antidromically from the digital nerves. With this segmental stimulation technique it is possible to find a localized area where most of the slowing is concentrated. Kimura has found that in carpal tunnel syndrome this area of focal slowing is usually 2 to 4 cm distal to the wrist crease.[13] (See Figures 5-24 and 5-25.) Although the electrodiagnostic study is the most sensitive tool for diagnosing carpal tunnel syndrome, a small subset of patients has the disease without positive electrical findings.

Other techniques that can be used to help make the diagnosis of carpal tunnel syndrome include MR imaging of the carpal tunnel and thermography. MRI scan of the hand may demonstrate distortion and/or inflammation of the median nerve as it courses within the carpal tunnel. Thermography may demonstrate autonomic vasomotor abnormalities in a median nerve distribution. The median nerve is a mixed nerve containing motor, sensory, and autonomic nerve fibers. With compression, there may be damage to autonomic fibers that control the vasomotor tone of blood vessels. Damage to autonomic fibers will produce abnormalities of blood flow to the hand which can be picked up on thermographic studies, a technique that displays temperature gradients of the subject as a series of different colors.

If a patient is diagnosed as having carpal tunnel syndrome, treatment is critical to prevent a worsening of the disease. Treatment can be broken down into conservative measures, semi-invasive techniques, and surgical intervention. For patients who have been found to have mild to moderate carpal tunnel syndrome, conservative treatment

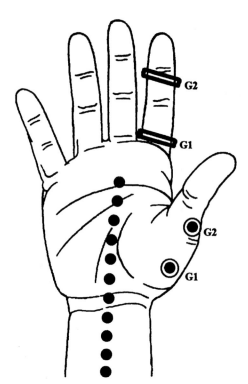

Figure 5-24 Motor and sensory inching across the wrist. The median nerve is stimulated at successive 1 cm increments from 4 cm proximal to the wrist crease to 6 cm distal to the wrist. Compound muscle action potential (CMAP) latency and amplitude of the abductor pollicis brevis can be measured by recording electrodes (G1 = active, G2 = reference), or a sensory nerve action potential (SNAP) latency and amplitude can be measured over the 2nd digit (G1 = active electrode, G2 = reference electrode.) Any significant increase in CMAP or SNAP amplitude signifies conduction block; any abrupt latency shift signifies focal slowing. Reprinted by permission from Preston DC, Shapiro BE (eds). *Electromyography and Neuromuscular Disorders—Clinical-Electrophysiologic Correlations* (fig 16.9). Boston, Butterworth-Heinemann, 1998.

should be tried initially. Most patients are referred for occupational therapy for initiation of a program that includes immobilization and modalities. Usually, the therapist fabricates a splint which keeps the wrist in a neutral position.[14] Such splints can also be obtained off the shelf at a surgical supply store or a pharmacy. Modalities such as iontophoresis can be used to reduce inflammation within the carpal tunnel. Tendon and nerve gliding exercises should also be employed. Other conservative measures include the use of anti-inflammatories, appropriate ergonomic changes at the work place and at home, and use of a TENS unit.

Patients who fail to improve with conservative measures may benefit from a steroid injection into the carpal tunnel. This technique may need to be repeated on one or two occasions assuming the patient is improving with each injection.[15]

For the patient who fails to improve with conservative and semi-invasive techniques, or for the patient who has severe changes both clinically and on electrodiagnostic studies, he or she will need to strongly consider surgical intervention. Surgery for carpal tunnel syndrome can be performed as an open procedure, (incision of the transverse carpal ligament and neurolysis of the underlying median nerve), and/or endoscopically which may be associated with a faster recovery time.[16]

Complications of carpal tunnel syndrome, even if treated with surgery, may include ongoing pain, paresthesias, and weakness. Whenever there is nerve injury, the patient may develop chronic neurogenic pain or causalgia/reflex sympathetic dystrophy. This type of pain is more intense, characterized by burning, hypersensitivity, and occasional

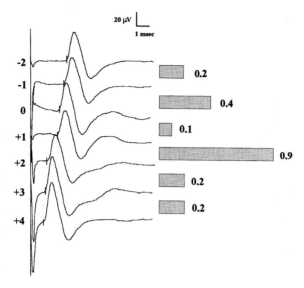

Figure 5-25 Focal sensory slowing: inching across the wrist (Kimura's method). *Left.* Stimulating the median nerve at 1 cm increments from 2 cm proximal to the wrist crease to 4 cm distal into the wrist, recording digit 2 sensory nerve action potential. *Right.* Relative change in latency between stimulation points is plotted on the right. Note the abrupt change in latency of the sensory nerve action potential between +1 and +2 cm distal to the wrist crease, signifying the area of focal slowing. Reprinted by permission from Preston DC, Shapiro BE (eds). *Electromyography and Neuromuscular Disorders—Clinical-Electrophysiologic Correlations* (fig 16.10). Boston, Butterworth-Heinemann, 1998.

lancinating (electrical shooting) pain. Patients who develop chronic neurogenic pain usually have associated symptoms including sleep disturbance, depression, and altered quality of life.

Pronator Syndrome

The median nerve courses through the pronator teres muscle in the proximal forearm (Figure 5-26). Compression of the median nerve can occur at this site when the patient has chronic myofascial forearm pain and spasm. This syndrome may occur after upper extremity trauma from a motor vehicle accident. Anatomically, the median nerve courses through the pronator muscle as it enters the forearm. Upon leaving the pronator teres, the median nerve gives rise to the anterior interosseous nerve. It then runs between the flexor carpi radialis and the palmaris longus to reach the carpal tunnel. In the forearm, the median nerve branches multiple times to supply all wrist and hand flexors except the flexor carpi ulnaris and the ulnar portion of the flexor digitorum profundus. Prior to entering the carpal tunnel, the median nerve gives rise to the palmaris branch, which pierces the forearm fascia to innervate the thenar eminence and the radial aspect of the wrist.[17] The sensory supply of the median nerve is the first three and one-half digits of the involved hand.

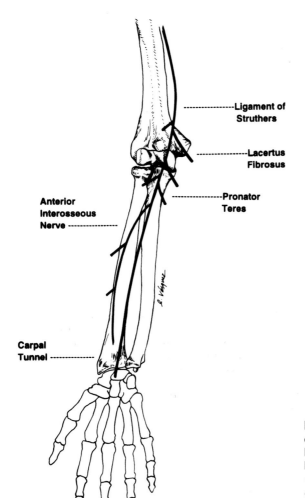

Figure 5-26 Potential sites of
compression of the median nerve.
Reprinted by permission from
Rosenbaum RB, Ochoa JL (eds).
*Carpal Tunnel Syndrome and
other Disorders of the Median
Nerve* (fig 17.1). Boston,
Butterworth-Heinemann, 1993.

Injury to this nerve may occur acutely when direct forearm trauma causes acute inflammation and swelling in the flexor forearm compartment. Chronic forearm myofascial spasm after a less severe injury may, over time, cause compression of the median nerve as it courses through the pronator muscle.

The clinical history of a patient with pronator syndrome is similar to the symptomatology seen with carpal tunnel syndrome, including paresthesias, numbness, and tingling in a median nerve distribution. Because of the more proximal entrapment there is weakness of finger and thumb flexor muscles, as well as the abductor pollicis brevis muscle within the thenar eminence. The weakness contributes to decreased grip and dexterity. The patient may have nocturnal paresthesias in a median nerve distribution. With pronator syndrome, patients frequently complain of pain in the volar forearm.

Physical examination will demonstrate irritation of the median nerve at the level of the pronator mass, and distally. There may be a positive Tinel's sign with tapping over the pronator mass and the pronator muscle itself will be extremely tender. Pressure on the pronator muscle may cause numbness and tingling in a median nerve distribution.[18] There may be surrounding myofascial tenderness and spasm involving the pronator and flexor muscles of the forearm. There may be weakness of pronation, finger flexion, and thumb movement.[17]

Electrodiagnostic findings with pronator syndrome includes slowing of the median NCV in the forearm, and decreased amplitude with temporal dispersion of the median CMAP with stimulation above the level of the pronator mass. This phenomenon, known as neurapraxia is consistent with an advanced pronator syndrome. Other findings include prolongation of the median F-wave (when compared to the contralateral median F-wave and the ipsilateral ulnar F-wave), a decrease in the median SNAP amplitude and slowing of the sensory NCV. On EMG testing, there may be acute denervation or membrane instability seen in the forearm flexors, pronator quadratus, and abductor pollicis brevis muscles, with sparing of the pronator and flexor carpi radialis muscles.

Treatment for pronator syndrome is geared towards relieving the nerve entrapment at the level of the pronator mass. Conservative treatment includes occupational therapy for modalities (iontophoresis, ultrasound, massage, stretching, electrical stimulation) and myofascial release techniques for tight forearm musculature.

Medications that may be helpful include anti-inflammatories, analgesics and muscle relaxants. A TENS unit may help. The patient may benefit from a steroid injection into the pronator mass. However, surgery may be required for pronator syndrome in the face of severe unrelenting clinical symptoms and positive electrodiagnostic findings. The surgical procedure includes a decompression of the median nerve as it courses through the pronator muscle.

Complications of pronator syndrome include ongoing pain, weakness, numbness, and nocturnal paresthesias. Neurogenic pain with a burning and/or lancinating component may occur in severe cases. Some patients go on to develop reflex sympathetic dystrophy.

Ulnar Nerve Entrapment

Guyon's Canal Syndrome

The ulnar nerve may be entrapped at the level of the wrist or elbow. At the wrist, the nerve can be entrapped as it passes through a bony canal known as Guyon's canal. Guyon's canal is formed by carpal bones (pisiform, hook of the hamate) and an overlying ligament. Through this anatomic structure courses the ulnar nerve. (See Figure 5-3.) This relatively small anatomical space may be a site of entrapment of the ulnar nerve with appropriate injury. During a motor vehicle accident, there can be injury to the wrist as a result of bracing the upper extremities prior to impact (against the dashboard, steering wheel, or back seat). There may also be direct trauma to the ulnar portion of the wrist unrelated to bracing at time of impact.

The patient with ulnar nerve entrapment through Guyon's canal will complain of ulnar wrist pain along with paresthesias, pain, and numbness in an ulnar distribution (fifth finger and the ulnar half of the ring finger). With advanced entrapment, there may be atrophy of the hypothenar muscle (abductor digiti quinti minimi), and the interosseii.

On physical examination, the patient will have a positive Tinel's sign with tapping over Guyon's canal. Sensory testing may demonstrate decreased sensation to light touch and pinprick in an ulnar distribution. Motor assessment may demonstrate weakness or atrophy of the abductor digiti quinti minimi, the interosseous muscles, and the first dorsal interosseous. There will be weakness of the ability to pinch with the index finger and thumb. The patient can be asked to try to hold a piece of paper while pinching with the index finger and thumb. If the patient is unable to maintain a pinch on this strength test, this indicates weakness of the first dorsal interosseous and is suggestive of ulnar nerve injury (Figure 5-27).[19]

Diagnostic workup includes the electrodiagnostic study. With Guyon's canal syndrome there will be prolongation of the ulnar motor and sensory distal latencies as compared to the uninvolved side or the ipsilateral median nerve. Along with this slowing, there may be a decrease in the amplitudes of the ulnar SNAP and CMAP. EMG examination may demonstrate membrane irritability and denervation potentials in the first dorsal interosseous and abductor digiti quinti minimi, with sparing of forearm ulnar innervated muscles.[19]

Treatment for this condition includes occupational therapy for appropriate splinting, modalities, and iontophoresis. A steroid injection into the region of Guyon's canal is often helpful. Use of anti-inflammatories, ergonomic modifications, and analgesics for more severe pain may also help. For the patient who fails to improve, surgical intervention to release the nerve within Guyon's canal may be the only alternative. Complications of Guyon's canal entrapment include ongoing symptomatology despite treatment and, in more severe cases, symptoms of neurogenic pain (as outlined previously).

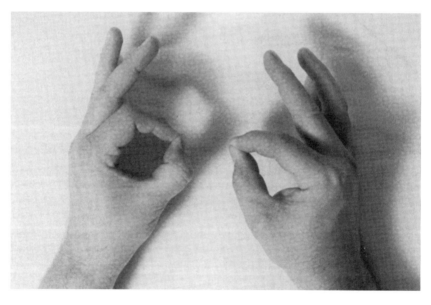

Figure 5-27 Froment's sign. Weakness of pinch with ulnar nerve injury. Reprinted by permission from Preston DC, Shapiro BE (eds). *Electromyography and Neuromuscular Disorders—Clinical-Electrophysiologic Correlations* (fig 17.5). Boston, Butterworth-Heinemann, 1998.

Cubital Tunnel Syndrome

The ulnar nerve may also be entrapped at the level of the elbow as it passes through a groove adjacent to the olecranon and the medial epicondyle known as the ulnar groove. The ulnar nerve originates from the C8 and T1 nerve roots, which coalesce within the lower cord of the brachial plexus to form the ulnar nerve. The ulnar nerve then courses through the proximal arm, passing around the elbow through the ulnar groove and into the ulnar portion of the forearm. (See Figure 5-10.) It has motor supply to the flexor carpi ulnaris in the forearm (a wrist flexor muscle), to the flexor digitorum profundus to digits IV and V, and to hand intrinsic muscles (interosseii, first dorsal interosseous, flexor pollicis brevis, adductor pollicis, and the abductor digiti quinti minimi). After the ulnar nerve courses through the ulnar groove at the elbow, it passes under the flexor carpi ulnaris muscle. This region can be a potential site of entrapment when there is chronic myofascial spasm involving that forearm muscle (Figure 5-28).

The ulnar nerve is very superficial as it courses through the ulnar groove and it can be easily traumatized after a motor vehicle accident. Injury to the ulnar nerve at the elbow could occur due to bracing prior to impact. Extreme hyperextension of the wrist at time of impact will stretch the ulnar nerve, possibly causing nerve irritation through the ulnar groove. In contrast to this indirect type of trauma, there may be a direct blow to the elbow region and the ulnar nerve at this superficial site. Additionally, ulnar nerve injury may occur as a result of extreme soft tissue swelling or bony distortion after a fracture in the elbow region.

The clinical history of a patient with ulnar nerve entrapment at the elbow includes complaints of elbow, forearm, and hand pain; paresthesias and/or numbness in an ulnar

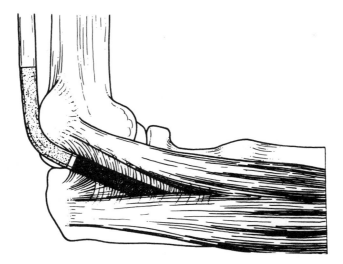

Figure 5-28 The ulnar nerve at the elbow and the region in which the nerve may be damaged in cubital tunnel syndrome (dark shading). Reprinted by permission from Osselton JW, Binnie CD, Cooper R, *et al.* (eds). *Clinical Neurophysiology—Electromyography, Nerve Conduction and Evoked Potentials* (fig 2.6.9). Boston, Butterworth-Heinemann, 1995.

distribution (ulnar forearm, wrist, hand, and fingers four and five); hand weakness; decreased grip strength; decreased dexterity; and nocturnal paresthesias in an ulnar distribution. There may be an electrical shooting-type pain that occurs with any contact of the ulnar groove.

Physical examination of these patients will demonstrate a positive Tinel's sign with tapping over the ulnar groove. Sensation may be diminished in an ulnar distribution. Motor testing will demonstrate weakness of ulnar innervated hand intrinsic muscles (abductor digiti quinti minimi, first dorsal interosseous, interossei) and the flexor carpi ulnaris (a wrist flexor). An inability to grasp a piece of paper between the outstretched index finger and thumb is indicative of ulnar nerve injury. This is known as a positive Froment's sign, and it is consistent with weakness of the adductor pollicis, flexor pollicis brevis, and the first dorsal interosseous. While having the patient hold a piece of paper between the thumb and index finger, the physician will observe compensation by the flexor pollicis longus muscle. Thus, the interphalangeal joint of the thumb will be held in flexion.[17] As the patient attempts to pinch harder to overcome the weakness, the deformity will increase. Owing to loss of the first dorsal interosseous muscle, abduction of the index finger is impaired, which further aggravates the pinch mechanism.[20] (See Figure 5-27.) Power grasp may be decreased if there is muscle loss due to involvement of the interosseous muscles and the flexor digitorum profundus to the fourth and fifth digits. Grasp may fall to as little as 20 to 25 percent of normal in severe cases.[20]

Diagnostic workup includes electrodiagnostic studies that will demonstrate slowing of motor and sensory NCV across the cubital tunnel. There may be a decrease in amplitude of the CMAP with stimulation above the ulnar groove. This phenomenon, known as neurapraxia, occurs due to demyelinization at the level of the elbow. With more advanced ulnar nerve injury at the level of the elbow, there will be slowing of the SNAP distal latency with decreased amplitude and temporal dispersion of the SNAP response. Additionally, there will be prolongation of the ulnar F-wave as compared to the contralateral ulnar F-wave and the ipsilateral median F-wave. The EMG examination will demonstrate membrane irritability or denervation in ulnar innervated hand intrinsic muscles along with the flexor carpi ulnaris and flexor digitorum profundus (IV, V).[20]

Treatment for cubital tunnel syndrome includes both conservative and invasive measures. Occupational therapy should be ordered for the symptomatic patient. Therapy should include splinting, modalities to reduce inflammation (iontophoresis), and nerve-gliding exercises to try to improve mobility of the ulnar nerve as it passes through the ulnar groove. Massage and myofascial release techniques for forearm muscles may help to decrease myofascial pain and spasm that is associated with or contributing to the cubital tunnel syndrome.

The patient may benefit from a steroid injection to help reduce inflammation of the ulnar nerve as it courses through the ulnar groove. This may help accelerate recovery. If the patient is in significant discomfort, appropriate analgesic medications will be necessary. Nonsteroidal anti-inflammatories, opioids, medications for neurogenic pain, topical creams, and trial of a TENs unit may also play a role in modulating chronic forearm discomfort.

For the patient who fails to improve with conservative measures, surgical intervention for neurolysis of the ulnar nerve followed by transposition of the ulnar nerve to the volar forearm may be necessary. Complications of chronic ulnar nerve entrapment include ongoing pain and paresthesias in an ulnar distribution. Some patients go on to have more severe neurogenic pain, causalgia, and/or reflex sympathetic dystrophy.

Superficial Radial Nerve Entrapment

Just distal to the elbow, the radial nerve bifurcates to form motor and sensory branches (posterior interosseous and superficial radial nerves, respectively). The superficial radial nerve courses along the radial forearm to enter the hand and supply sensation to the first web space and part of the thumb. This nerve is superficial as it crosses the wrist. It may be injured due to direct impact after a motor vehicle accident. Injury may also occur with chronic inflammation of the wrist after hyperextension due to bracing prior to impact.

The patient with a superficial radial nerve entrapment usually complains of wrist pain along the radial aspect of the joint. There may be numbness and tingling in the nerve's distribution (web space between the thumb and index finger). Some patients complain of an electrical shooting pain within this distribution. Since this is a sensory nerve there is no associated motor weakness, other than that associated with wrist pain. On physical examination, the patient with superficial radial nerve entrapment will demonstrate decreased sensation in a superficial radial nerve distribution. There will be a positive Tinel's sign with tapping of the nerve just above the radial styloid.

Diagnostic workup includes electrodiagnostic studies that will demonstrate a decrease in the conduction velocity of the superficial radial nerve on the involved side, along with temporal dispersion and decreased amplitude of the SNAP response when compared to the asymptomatic side. As this is a purely sensory nerve, EMG examination for this condition will be normal.

Treatment for superficial radial nerve entrapment should include conservative measures initially. Occupational therapy can be ordered for appropriate splinting and modalities. Other conservative measures include a trial of anti-inflammatories, topical creams, and/or a TENS unit. If the patient fails to improve, subcutaneous steroid injection into the region of the superficial radial nerve may help accelerate recovery. The patient who fails to improve despite these conservative measures will require surgical intervention for neurolysis of the superficial radial nerve. Complications of this disorder include ongoing symptoms (pain and paresthesias in a superficial radial nerve distribution), and occasionally more severe neurogenic pain or causalgia.

Radial Tunnel Syndrome

Cervical nerve roots C5 through T1 coalesce within the brachial plexus to form the radial nerve. This nerve courses through the arm by winding around the humerus through the radial groove. As the radial nerve is about to enter the forearm, it breaks into two branches, the superficial radial nerve (a purely sensory nerve), and the posterior interosseous nerve (principally a motor nerve). The posterior interosseous nerve passes through the supinator muscle under a fibrous band of tissue known as the Arcade of Frohse. Prior to passing through the supinator mass, the radial nerve gives off motor branches to the brachioradialis and wrist extensor muscles. After passing through the supinator mass, the nerve gives off motor branches to the supinator, the abductor pollicis longus, finger extensors, and all of the extensor muscles in the forearm.

The posterior interosseous branch of the radial nerve may be injured after a motor vehicle accident. This injury can occur as a result of direct trauma to the forearm, or secondary to reactive forearm muscle spasm involving wrist extensor and supinator muscles following a chronic hand or wrist injury. Radial nerve distortion and damage may result from fractures of bones around the elbow region, due to bone malalignment, and/or extreme inflammation and swelling.

The clinical history of the patient with radial tunnel syndrome includes pain in the region of the wrist extensor and supinator muscles. Occasionally, the pain will mimic that experienced with a lateral epicondylitis. With advanced nerve injury, there will be weakness of finger and wrist extension strength. As the posterior interosseous branch of the radial nerve is principally a motor nerve, patients typically do not complain of numbness.

Physical examination will demonstrate tenderness of the posterior interosseous nerve as it courses through the radial tunnel. There will also be tenderness of the supinator muscle and wrist extensor muscles. The patient will complain of increased pain with resisted supination (with the elbow bent). Sensory examination will be normal. With advanced disease, motor examination will demonstrate sparing of the triceps, the brachioradialis, and partial weakness of wrist extensors (branches to the extensor carpi radialis longus and brevis are spared) with weakness involving the finger extensor musculature. The patient may have tenderness of the lateral epicondyle if chronic myofascial spasm involving the wrist extensors causes a lateral epicondylitis.[21]

Electrodiagnostic studies may be abnormal for patients who have radial tunnel syndrome. Specifically, there may be slowing of posterior interosseous nerve conduction as the nerve courses through the supinator muscle. The SNAP for the superficial radial nerve will be normal since radial tunnel syndrome does not involve this nerve. Provocative NCS testing that may help demonstrate this nerve entrapment involves stimulation of the posterior interosseous nerve or radial nerve above the site of suspected entrapment while the patient supinates against resistance, or the examiner applies pressure to the supinator forearm mass. To perform this test, the active electrode is placed on the extensor indicis proprius (EIP) muscle and stimulation is performed below and above the radial tunnel. After a baseline proximal stimulation CMAP is obtained, the proximal stimulation is repeated, this time with the examiner applying downward pressure on the supinator mass or with the patient supinating against resistance by the examiner. A positive provocative test will demonstrate prolongation of the latency and a decrement in the amplitude of the EIP CMAP response. Lastly, electromyographic testing will demonstrate sparing of the triceps, brachioradialis, extensor carpi radialis longus, and supinator muscles, with abnormalities found in the extensor carpi ulnaris, extensor digitorum communis, extensor indicis proprius, abductor pollicis longus and brevis, and extensor pollicis longus.[21]

Treatment for radial tunnel syndrome includes both conservative measures and when necessary, surgery. Occupational therapy can be ordered for appropriate modalities, myofascial release techniques, and splinting. Medications for pain, muscle spasm, neurogenic pain, inflammation, and topical creams may prove helpful. Trial of a TENS unit may also be indicated. When conservative measures fail, a steroid injection may accelerate recovery by decreasing inflammation in the region of the radial tunnel. As a last resort, and in cases where obvious nerve damage is present both clinically and electrically, surgical intervention for neurolysis of the posterior interosseous nerve with transection of the arcade of Frohse will be indicated. Complications of chronic radial tunnel syndrome include ongoing forearm pain with or without neurogenic pain symptomatology.

Radial Nerve Entrapment at the Humeral Groove

As the radial nerve passes into the upper arm, it winds around the humerus in a groove known as the humeral groove. Here, it has an intimate relationship with the humerus. Distally, the nerve branches into the superficial radial nerve and the posterior interosseous nerve, both described previously. In a motor vehicle accident, a direct blow to the upper arm can injure this nerve. More commonly, injury to the radial nerve in this location occurs with fractures of the humerus. This can lead to severe complications.

The patient with a radial nerve injury will complain of numbness and weakness in the extremity. The weakness will involve all radially innervated muscles (triceps, brachio-radialis, supinator, wrist and finger extensor muscles). Patients will complain of arm pain, paresthesias in a radial nerve distribution, nocturnal paresthesias, and lancinating (electrical shooting) pain.

Physical examination will demonstrate tenderness of the radial nerve as it courses around the humeral groove. There may be a positive Tinel's sign with tapping of the nerve at this site. Motor changes may include weakness involving the triceps, brachioradialis, supinator, wrist extensor, and finger extensor musculature. There will be abnormalities of sensation involving the dorsum of the hand including the thumb and overlying the first web space.

Treatment for a radial nerve laceration after fracture of the humerus will require surgical intervention. If surgery is performed, or if there is significant weakness in the extremity as a result of radial nerve damage, a prolonged course of occupational or physical therapy will be necessary for progressive strengthening including neuromusculature re-education utilizing electrical stimulation.

For milder degrees of entrapment, a TENS unit, medications for pain, muscle spasm, and neurogenic pain, topical creams, and anti-inflammatories may be helpful in conjunction with the physical and occupational therapy. A steroid injection into the region of maximal discomfort may help accelerate recovery. When symptoms persist, surgical intervention is occasionally necessary for neurolytic procedures to relieve pressure around the radial nerve, which may be entrapped in scar tissue. Complications of radial nerve injury include ongoing sensory and motor disturbance in a radial distribution and chronic neurogenic pain, including the development of reflex sympathetic dystrophy.

Thoracic Outlet Syndrome

Frequently, entrapment of the brachial plexus occurs within the thoracic outlet. As noted previously, nerve roots from C4 through T1 coalesce to form a cluster of nerves known as the brachial plexus. The brachial plexus passes through several anatomic structures in the neck and shoulder region before passing into the respective extremity (anterior and middle scalene muscles, clavicle and first rib, pectoralis minor muscle). It courses through the thoracic outlet with the subclavian artery and vein. Therefore, with more advanced thoracic outlet syndrome (TOS) there will be both vascular and neurological abnormalities in the extremity.

Myogenic TOS is fairly common after motor vehicle accidents. It develops in conjunction with muscle spasm and tightness of the scalene or pectoral muscles. Such proximal muscle spasm commonly occurs after whiplash injury. The scalenus anticus syndrome refers to brachial plexus entrapment as a result of chronic scalene muscle tightness. Tightness of the pectoral muscles may also occur with neck or trunk injury. TOS may also occur due to cervical and thoracic malalignment resulting from the whiplash injury. This malalignment may alter the normal anatomic arrangement of the clavicle and first rib which could irritate the adjacent brachial plexus.

Patients with TOS complain of shoulder pain, and arm pain, numbness, paresthesias and weakness. There may be nocturnal paresthesias involving the entire arm, or just in an ulnar distribution. Some patients complain of decreased grip, dropping objects, decreased dexterity, and a heaviness of the arm. There may be associated neck pain, facial pain and headaches. If there is also compression of the subclavian vein or artery (which accompany the brachial plexus through the thoracic outlet), patients may complain of vascular symptoms including color and/or temperature changes in the involved extremity.[22,23] Physical findings that are present in over 90 percent of TOS patients are supraclavicular tenderness and reproduction of symptoms with certain postural maneuvers.

Supraclavicular Tenderness

The anterior scalene muscle is usually extremely tender in the TOS patient. It lies about 3 cm lateral to the trachea and 2 to 3 cm above the clavicle. The supraclavicular space is directly over the brachial plexus. It is located 1 cm posterior to the anterior scalene muscle. The thumb presses over the plexus of each side, holding pressure for 20 to 30 seconds. A positive response is an onset of paresthesias or pain radiating to the arm and hand, similar to the patient's symptoms. Another way of observing the same response is by tapping over the brachial plexus with a finger or reflex hammer to elicit a Tinel's sign.

Postural Maneuvers

Placing the arms in specific positions and noting pulse alterations and/or neurologic symptoms is important in the evaluation of TOS patients, which has been one of the important aspects of physical examination. Common tests include the Adson's maneuver,[24] and the 90 degree abduction external rotation (AER) position.[25]

For many years, the Adson's maneuver was considered to be the principal clinical test in the evaluation of TOS. The test is performed with the patient's hands at the side:

The patient takes a long deep breath, elevates the chin, and turns it to the affected side. A decreased or obliteration of the radial pulse is a pathognomonic sign of scalenus anticus syndrome.[24,26]

The 90 degree AER position will reproduce symptoms in over 90 percent of patients with TOS. Obliteration of the radial pulse is much less consistent, ranging from 24 percent to 51 percent. It is a more reliable maneuver than the Adson's maneuver because positive responses in normal patients are only 5 percent to 10 percent.[27-29]

When performing the 90 degree AER position test, the degree of shoulder flexion (forward) or extension (backward) is critical. The arm position should be straight with the elbows in line with the shoulder, in such a way that if the patient were standing with his/her back against a wall, the abducted, externally rotated arms would lie flat against the wall. If the arms are held too far forward, a negative response can occur. The neck should be extended when performing this maneuver.[30]

Motor examination usually demonstrates mild generalized weakness due to the pain and paresthesias. Sensory abnormalities may involve the whole hand, but usually occur in an ulnar distribution. There may be a Tinel's sign with tapping of the brachial plexus in the supraclavicular space. If there is vascular involvement, the involved extremity may appear pale or bluish in discoloration, with a lower temperature and poor capillary refill as compared to the uninvolved side. Nail changes (thickening and cracking of the nails) suggests chronic arterial insufficiency.

Diagnostic workup includes electrodiagnostic and blood flow studies. Electrodiagnostic studies are usually normal for patients with myogenic TOS. The most common finding is prolongation of the ulnar F-wave when compared to the contralateral ulnar F-wave and the ipsilateral median F-wave. This occurs due to the fact that the most common portion of the brachial plexus involved in TOS is the medial cord (which ultimately makes up the ulnar nerve). Sensory and motor studies are usually normal, but with more advanced TOS may demonstrate decreased amplitudes of CMAPs and SNAPs. Electromyographic examination may demonstrate denervation in hand intrinsic musculature (abductor digiti quinti minimi and/or first dorsal interosseous). However, most of the time, EMG/NCV studies are unrevealing in cases of myogenic TOS.[31]

Blood flow studies may also prove helpful in diagnosing TOS. Venous and arterial Doppler ultrasound may demonstrate the vascular obstruction around the region of the thoracic outlet. The angiogram and venogram are invasive techniques capable of demonstrating obstruction at this level. X-rays may demonstrate an accessory (extra) cervical rib that may be a potential site of entrapment.

Lastly, a scalene anesthetic block can be used as a diagnostic procedure. If the patient's symptomatology diminishes after an anesthetic block of a scalene muscle, this would confirm the diagnosis of myogenic TOS (due to tight scalene musculature).[32]

Treatment for TOS is usually conservative. A physical or occupational therapy program is needed to loosen up, stretch, and recondition structures that make up the thoracic outlet. Modalities (heat, massage), chiropractic manipulation and myofascial release techniques are important adjunctive treatments in the management of thoracic outlet syndrome.

When pain is severe, medications (muscle relaxants, anti-inflammatories, and analgesics) may prove necessary. If there is evidence of nerve damage or nerve irritation, neurogenic medications including the anticonvulsants may be helpful. A TENS unit may help with shoulder discomfort. Trigger point injection therapy in conjunction with physical therapy may further help to loosen up thoracic outlet musculature. Botulinum toxin (Botox) injections can be used to loosen up thoracic outlet musculature on a more long-term basis. To perform Botox injections, diluted botulinum toxin can be injected into the tight scalene or pectoral musculature. A Botox block will provide muscle relaxation that can last anywhere from 6 to 9 months during which time other therapeutic measures can be instituted.[33] As a last resort, surgery may be indicated to treat thoracic outlet syndrome. The most common surgical procedures include scalenectomy and first rib removal.

Complications of TOS include immobilization of the involved shoulder, which over time could lead to adhesive capsulitis (frozen shoulder). There may be chronic upper extremity pain, paresthesias, and weakness. If there is vascular involvement due to poor blood flow, trophic changes involving the skin and nails may occur over time.[34–37]

CERVICAL RADICULOPATHY

Cervical Anatomy

There are eight cervical vertebrae labeled C1 through C8. The first two cervical vertebrae are known as the Atlas (C1) and the Axis (C2). The Atlas articulates with the occipital condyles of the skull. Flexion and extension is the only motion that occurs at this joint. In contrast, only rotation occurs between the C1 and C2 vertebra.

There are no intravertebral discs between the occiput and Atlas and the C1 and C2 vertebras. However, between C2 and C3 and the remaining cervical, thoracic, and lumbar vertebras are fibrocartilaginous intervertebral discs. The cervical intervertebral disc typically has a thick posterior arrangement of annular fibers and its nucleus pulposis tends to be anteriorly located. There are also pseudoarticulations known as the joints of Luschka located posterolateral to each vertebral body, which helps protect against posterolateral disc herniations. Lastly, there is a strong and broad posterior longitudinal ligament in the cervical region. The combination of the anteriorly displaced nucleus pulposis, thick laminated arrangement of posterior annular fibers, broad posterior longitudinal ligament, and the joints of Luschka all combine to help minimize the occurrence of a cervical disc herniation. The facet joints are the posterior articulations between cervical vertebrae from C2 caudally. The facet joints are synovial joints whose articulating bones are lined by cartilage and surrounded by a capsule.

The cervical region has six planes of motion: flexion, extension, rotation to either side, and side bending to either side. Much of the motion occurs between vertebrae C4–5, C5–6, and C6–7, and these are the most likely levels to show degeneration with aging and after trauma.

There are eight cervical nerve roots that emanate from the spinal cord and pass through foramina between each cervical vertebra. They are labeled C1 through C8. The nerves exit above the level of the named vertebra (except for C8 which exits above the T1 vertebra). For example, the C4 nerve root exits from the neuroforamina between vertebrae C3 and C4. Cervical nerve roots C4 through T1 coalesce to form the brachial plexus and peripheral nerves of the respective extremity. Nerve roots C1 through C3 combine to become the greater and lesser occipital nerves, nerves that supply sensation to the scalp. When irritated, they can cause rather significant headaches. Nerve roots C2 through C4 combine to become the phrenic nerve, the motor nerve that controls the diaphragm.

Each cervical nerve root from C5 through T1 supplies a specific sensory distribution in the respective upper extremity known as a dermatome (Figure 5-29). The motor rootlet of each cervical nerve root supplies distinct muscles in the chest, upper back, and upper extremity. A myotome refers to the distribution of muscles supplied by a particular nerve root. The cervical nerve rootlets from C4 through T1 supply muscles listed in Table 5-1.

The upper extremity neurological examination is helpful in determining if nerve root damage is contributing to upper extremity symptomatology. The upper extremity neurological examination includes motor and sensory testing, assessment of reflexes, and several provocative tests that can provide further information on nerve injury.

Motor testing should include:

- hand intrinsic musculature (C8-T1)
- finger flexion and extension (C6, C7)
- wrist flexion and extension (C6, C7)
- elbow extension (C7)
- elbow flexion (C5, C6)
- arm abduction (C4, C5).

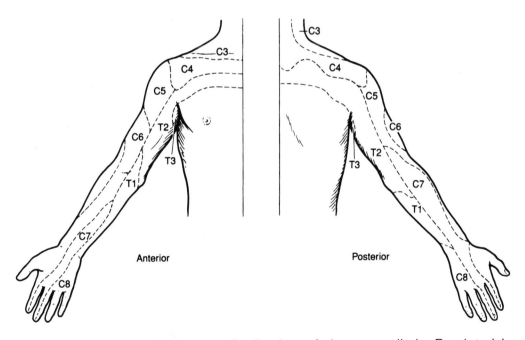

Figure 5-29 Segmental sensory distribution of the upper limb. Reprinted by permission from Unwin A, Jones K (eds). *Emergency Orthopaedics and Trauma*, p 104 (fig 11.5). Oxford, Elsevier Science Ltd, 1995.

Table 5-1 Upper extremity muscles and their nerve root innervation

Muscle	Nerve Root(s)
Rhomboids	C5
Rotator cuff:	C5, C6
-Supraspinatus	
-Infraspinatus	
-Teres minor	
Deltoid	C5, C6
Biceps	C5, C6
Brachioradialis	C5, C6
Wrist extensors	C5, C6
Triceps	C6, C7, C8
Supinator	C6, C7
Finger extensors	C7, C8
Pronator teres	C6, C7
Flexor carpi radialis	C6, C7
Finger flexors:	
-Flexor digitorum sublimes	C7, C8, T1
-Flexor digitorum profundus	C7, C8
Pronator quadratus	C7, C8
Hand intrinsic muscles:	C8, T1
-Adductor pollicis	
-Abductor digiti minimi	
-Opponens digiti minimi	
-Lumbricals	
-Interossei	
-Abductor pollicis brevis	

Sensory testing to pinprick should be assessed for:

- thumb (C6)
- middle finger (C7)
- small finger (C8)
- overlying the deltoid muscle (C5 distribution).

Upper extremity reflex testing should include:

- the biceps (C5, C6)
- triceps (C7)
- brachioradialis (C5, C6) muscles.

The Spurling maneuver is performed by asking the patient to extend and turn their head to one side. Then, gentle compression on the top of the skull will generate radiating pain in the extremity if there is nerve root damage or irritation. This test is then repeated on the other side.[38] The clinical workup to rule out a nerve root lesion includes:

- electrodiagnostic studies
- somatosensory evoked potentials
- MRI scanning
- CT scanning
- myelography
- x-rays including flexion and extension views.

Electrodiagnostic studies include NCV studies and EMG testing of individual muscles. Usually, motor and sensory NCVs will be within normal limits in patients with single root level radiculopathies. If multiple nerve roots are involved, there may be slowing of the motor NCVs, prolongation of F-waves, and decreased amplitude of CMAPs. EMG testing is the more sensitive study when evaluating for actual nerve root damage. The damaged root(s) can be determined based on the patterns of denervation. For example, the triceps muscle is principally supplied by the C7 nerve rootlet. Denervation seen in the triceps muscle is suggestive of an acute C7 radiculopathy. The pronator muscle is principally a C6 innervated muscle, and denervation in this muscle suggests C6 radiculopathy. Along with extremity denervation, denervation potentials are also seen in the paracervical musculature with acute cervical radiculopathy.[39]

MRI imaging of the cervical spine can provide detailed information about nerve root impingement due to a variety of causes including arthritic bone spurs and protruding or herniated discs. Likewise, CT scanning of the cervical region will give information about nerve root impingement particularly due to bony arthritic changes. However, CT scanning is not quite as accurate as MRI imaging in evaluating soft tissue structures such as the intervertebral discs. However, when CT scanning is performed after myelography, it can provide highly detailed information about nerve root impingement due to soft tissue and bony structures. A myelogram is performed by injecting radiopaque dye into the spinal canal following which conventional x-rays are performed. Cervical nerve root impingement may be demonstrated by poor filling of the root sleeve(s) indicating pressure on the nerve by some structure. The post-myelogram CT scan provides further information as to exactly what is causing the obstruction or impingement.

X-rays including AP, lateral, and oblique views are useful in demonstrating bony arthritic changes that may compromise nerve roots as they pass through the neuroforamen. X-rays are excellent for demonstrating degenerative changes, spinal instability (through flexion and extension views), bone spurs, and patency of the neuroforamina through which the nerve roots pass.

Specific Radiculopathy Syndromes

Cervical radiculopathy usually occurs somewhere between the C4–5 vertebrae and the cervical thoracic junction. Therefore, the most common radiculopathy syndromes include C5, C6, C7, and C8. With a C5 radiculopathy, the patient will complain of pain involving the neck, shoulder, and interscapular region. There may be an electrical shooting quality to the pain. Typically, patients do not complain of numbness in their hands as the C5 nerve root dermatome typically overlies the deltoid muscle. There may be complaints of numbness or tingling in that region.

Physical examination may demonstrate a diminished biceps and brachioradialis reflex (both being C5–6 reflexes). Triceps reflex will be normal. Sensory testing may demonstrate decreased pinprick sensation overlying the deltoid muscle. On motor testing, muscles innervated by C5, including the deltoid, biceps, and brachioradialis, may demonstrate weakness.

Patients with C6 radiculopathy will also complain of neck, shoulder, and radiating arm pain. Classically, the radiating pain extends to the patient's thumb. There may be pain and paresthesias involving the patient's thumb and index finger which are both part of the C6 dermatome. There may be an electrical shooting quality to the pain.

Physical examination may demonstrate a diminished biceps and brachioradialis reflex (both being C5–6 innervated muscles). The triceps reflex will be normal. Sensory examination will demonstrate decreased pinprick sensation in the thumb. On motor testing, there will be weakness of C6 innervated muscles (biceps, brachioradialis and pronator).

Symptomatology for a C7 radiculopathy is similar to the C6 radiculopathy except the dermatomal referral pain involves the middle finger. On physical examination there will be a diminished triceps reflex with sparing of the biceps and brachioradialis reflexes. Sensory examination will demonstrate decreased pinprick sensation in the middle finger. On motor testing, there will be weakness of the triceps, wrist flexor, and wrist extensor muscles.

With a C8 radiculopathy, patients typically complain of pain and paresthesias radiating in an ulnar distribution. Therefore, a C8 radiculopathy is also in the differential diagnosis for TOS and ulnar neuropathy at the elbow or wrist. Physical examination will demonstrate normal biceps, brachioradialis and triceps reflexes, decreased sensation of the small finger, and weakness of hand intrinsic musculature.

Treatment

Treatment for cervical radiculopathy ranges from conservative to invasive. Initially, a patient with an acute cervical radiculopathy may require conservative measures such as physical therapy to decrease pain and associated muscle spasm. Modalities such as traction, hot packs, ultrasound, electrical stimulation, and massage may all prove helpful in decreasing symptomatic pain and muscle spasm. In general, cervical immobilization is not indicated in the management of radiculopathy unless the patient is postoperative. Anti-inflammatory agents such as nonsteroidal anti-inflammatory drugs and oral steroids may prove helpful in decreasing the symptoms of acute radiculopathy. Anti-inflammatories in conjunction with the above-mentioned conservative measures may be all that is necessary to help alleviate radicular pain and enable the patient to recuperate without invasive procedures.

However, if the patient fails to improve with conservative treatment, he or she may be a candidate for cervical epidural steroid injection(s). Epidural steroid injections are usually given as a series of three, over several weeks or months. After that, repeat injections can be performed every few months for symptomatic management of chronic radiculopathy.[40]

However, if conservative and epidural steroid injection therapy fails or only provides short-term relief, the patient may require surgical intervention to cure and relieve the effects of the cervical radiculopathy. The most common surgical procedure for treatment of cervical radiculopathy is an anterior approach discectomy of the involved disc followed by interbody fusion utilizing hardware or bone graft. Postoperatively, immobilization is necessary for several weeks. This is usually followed by postoperative rehabilitation.

Patients with chronic radiculopathy may benefit from medications to decrease pain (opioids, anti-inflammatories, and muscle relaxants) and nerve irritation (anticonvulsants, clonidine, Mexitine, or tricyclic antidepressants). Acupuncture is another conservative modality that may help patients with intractable radicular pain. Likewise, a TENS unit may provide some symptomatic relief.

REFERENCES

1. Cailliet R. Nerve control of the hand. In Cailliet R (ed). *Hand Pain and Impairment*, p 93. Philadelphia, F.A. Davis Company, 1986.
2. Cailliet R. Tendons: injuries and diseases. In Cailliet R (ed). *Hand Pain and Impairment*, p 122. Philadelphia, F.A. Davis Company, 1986.
3. Cailliet R. Functional anatomy. In Cailliet R (ed). *Shoulder Pain*, pp 1–37. Philadelphia, F.A. Davis Company, 1987.
4. Moore KL. The upper limb. In Moore KL: *Clinically Oriented Anatomy*, p 686. Baltimore, Williams & Wilkins, 1980.
5. Cailliet R. Traumatic pain. In Cailliet R (ed): *Shoulder Pain*, p 136. Philadelphia, F.A. Davis Company, 1987.
6. Hoppenfeld S. Physical examination of the shoulder. In Hoppenfeld S (ed). *Physical Examination of the Spine and Extremities*, p 33. New York, Appleton-Century-Crofts, 1976.
7. Myers KA. Utility of the clinical examination for carpal tunnel syndrome. *CMAJ* 2000; 163(5): 605.
8. D'Arcy CA, McGee S. Does this patient have carpal tunnel syndrome? *JAMA* 2000; 283(23): 3110.
9. Johnson EW, Kukla RD, Wogsam PE, Piedmont A. Sensory latencies to the ring finger: Normal values and relation to carpal tunnel syndrome. *Arch Phys Med Rehabil* 1981; 62: 206.
10. Cassvan A, Ralescu S, Shapiro E, *et al.* Median and radial sensory latencies to digital 1 as compared with other screening tests in carpal tunnel syndrome. *Am J Phys Med Rehabil* 1988; 67: 221.
11. Jackson DA, Clifford JC. Electrodiagnosis of mild carpal tunnel syndrome. *Arch Phys Med Rehabil* 1989; 70: 199.
12. Dawson D, Hallett M, Millender LH. Carpal tunnel syndrome. In Dawson D, Hallett M, Millender LH (eds). *Entrapment Neuropathies*, pp 25–93. Boston, Little, Brown & Co, 1990.
13. Kimura J. The carpal tunnel syndrome: localization of abnormalities within the distal segment of the median nerve. *Brain* 1979; 102: 619.
14. Kuo MH, Leong CP, Cheng YF, Chang HW. Static wrist position associated with least median nerve compression–sonographic evaluation. *Amer J Phys Med Rehabil* 2001; 80 (4): 256.
15. Dammers JWHH, Veering MM, Vermeulen M. Injection with methylprednisolone proximal to the carpal tunnel: Randomized double blind trial. *BMJ* 1999; 319(2): 884.
16. Katz JN, Losina E, Amick BC, *et al.* Predictors of outcomes of carpal tunnel release. *Arthritis Rheum* 2001; 44(5): 1184.

17. Pecina MM, Krmpotic-Nemanic J, Markiewitz AD: Tunnel syndromes in the upper extremities. In Pecina MM, Krmpotic-Nemanic J, Markiewitz AD (eds). *Tunnel Syndromes*, pp 11–84. Boca Raton, FL, CRC Press, 1991.

18. Dawson D, Hallett M, Millender LH. Median nerve entrapment. In Dawson D, Hallett M, Millender LH (eds). *Entrapment Neuropathies*, pp 93–124. Boston, Little, Brown & Co., 1990.

19. Dawson D, Hallett M, Millender LH. Ulnar nerve entrapment at the wrist. In Dawson D, Hallett M, Millender LH (eds). *Entrapment Neuropathies*, pp 177–198. Boston, Little, Brown & Co., 1990.

20. Dawson D, Hallett M, Millender LH. Ulnar nerve entrapment at the elbow. In Dawson D, Hallett M, Millender LH (eds). *Entrapment Neuropathies*, pp 125–176. Boston, Little, Brown & Co., 1990.

21. Dawson D, Hallett M, Millender LH. Radial nerve entrapment. In Dawson D, Hallett M, Millender LH (eds). *Entrapment Neuropathies*, pp 199–232. Boston, Little, Brown & Co., 1990.

22. Sanders R. Clinical presentation. In Sanders R (ed). *Thoracic Outlet Syndrome, a Common Sequela of Neck Injuries*, pp 71–84. Philadelphia, J.B. Lippincott Co, 1991.

23. Parziale JR, Akelman E, Weiss APC, Green A. Thoracic outlet syndrome. *Amer J Orthop* 2000: 353.

24. Adson AW, Coffey JR. Cervical rib: A method of anterior approach for relief of symptoms by division of the scalenus anticus, *Ann Surg* 1927; 85:839.

25. Eden KC. Complications of cervical rib. Vascular complications of cervical ribs and 1st thoracic rib abnormalities, *Br J Surg* 1939; 27: 111.

26. Adson AW. Surgical treatment for symptoms produced by cervical ribs and the scalenus anticus muscle. *Surg Gynecol Obstet* 1947; 85: 687.

27. Gilroy J, Meyer JS. Compression of the subclavian artery as a cause of ischemic brachial neuropathy. *Brain* 1963; 86:733.

28. Winsor T, Brow R. Costoclavicular syndrome, its diagnosis and treatment. *JAMA* 1966; 196: 109.

29. Telford ED, Mottershead S. The costoclavicular syndrome. *BMJ* 1947; 1: 325.

30. Roos DB, Owens JC. Thoracic outlet syndrome. *Arch Surg* 1966; 93: 71.

31. Dawson D, Hallett M, Millender LH. Thoracic outlet syndrome. In Dawson D, Hallett M, Millender LH (eds). *Entrapment Neuropathies*, pp 233–252. Boston, Little, Brown & Co, 1990.

32. Sanders RJ, Smith R. Diagnostic studies. In Sanders R (ed). *Thoracic Outlet Syndrome, a Common Sequela of Neck Injuries*, pp 85–94. Philadelphia, J.B. Lippincott Co., 1991.

33. Jordan SE, Ahn SS, Freischlag JA, Galabert HA, Machleder HI. Selective botulinum chemodenervation of the scalene muscles for treatment of neurogenic thoracic outlet syndrome. *Ann Vasc Surg* 2000; 14(4): 365.

34. Maxwell-Armstrong CA, Noorpuri BS, Haque SA, *et al.* Long-term results of surgical decompression of thoracic outlet compression syndrome. *J R Coll Surg Edinb* 2001; 46(1): 35.

35. Sharp WJ, Nowak LR, Zamani T, *et al.* Long-term follow-up and patient satisfaction after surgery for thoracic outlet syndrome. *Ann Vasc Surg* 2001; 15(1): 32.

36. Landry GJ, Moneta GL, Taylor LM, *et al.* Long term functional outcome of neurogenic thoracic outlet syndrome in surgically and conservatively treated patients. *J Vasc Surg* 2001; 33(2): 312.

37. Franklin GM, Fulton-Kehoe D, Bradley C, Smith-Weller T. Outcome of surgery for thoracic outlet syndrome in Washington state workers' compensation. *Neurology*, 2000; 54: 1252.

38. Gile LGF, Singer KP. Cervical spine pain. In Gile LGF, Singer KP (eds). *Clinical Anatomy and Management of Cervical Spine Pain*, p118. Boston, Butterworth-Heinemann, 1998.

39. Dillingham TR, Lauder TD, Andary M, *et al.* Identification of cervical radiculopathies: optimizing the electromyographic screen. *Amer J Phys Med Rehab* 2001; 80:(2): 84.

40. Vallee JN, Feydy A, Carlier RY, *et al.* Chronic cervical radiculopathy: lateral-approach periradicular corticosteroid injection. *Radiology* 2001; 218(3): 886.

6

Lower Extremity Pain

Jack L Rook

THE FOOT

Anatomy

Each foot consists of 26 bones including 14 phalanges, 5 metatarsals, and 7 tarsal bones (Figure 6-1). Synovial joint capsules surround bony articulations between the interphalangeal, metatarsal, tarsal, and ankle joints.

The foot has a rich neural innervation. The major nerve supplying motor and sensory function to the foot is the tibial nerve which courses around the medial malleolus where it branches into medial and lateral plantar nerves. The medial and lateral plantar nerves further branch into interdigital nerves which course between the metatarsal and phalangeal bones. The tibial nerve sensory branches provide sensation for the plantar surface of the foot and toes. Other nerves, which cross the ankle are the superficial and deep peroneal nerves and the sural nerve. The medial plantar nerves send cutaneous sensory branches to the plantar surface of the medial three toes and the medial aspect of the fourth toe. Its motor branches supply the abductor hallucis, flexor hallucis brevis, flexor digitorum brevis, and the first two lumbricals.

The lateral plantar nerve passes across the plantar surface of the foot and, after dividing into deep and superficial branches, supplies sensation to the plantar surface of the remaining toes on the lateral aspect of the foot. It supplies the motor innervation to the quadratus plantae, flexor digiti quinti brevis, abductor digiti quinti, and the remaining plantar interosseous and lumbrical muscles.

The superficial peroneal nerve descends the leg in front of the fibula and supplies the evertor muscles of the foot. The sensory area of the superficial peroneal nerve is the lateral aspect of the lower leg and the dorsum of the foot. The deep peroneal nerve proceeds to the interosseous membrane between the tibia and fibula, and descends the leg supplying the dorsiflexors of the foot and ends supplying the extensor digitorum brevis. It supplies a small area of sensation between the first two toes on the dorsum of the foot.[1] The sural nerve courses around the lateral malleolus to supply sensation to the lateral aspect of the foot (Figure 6-2).

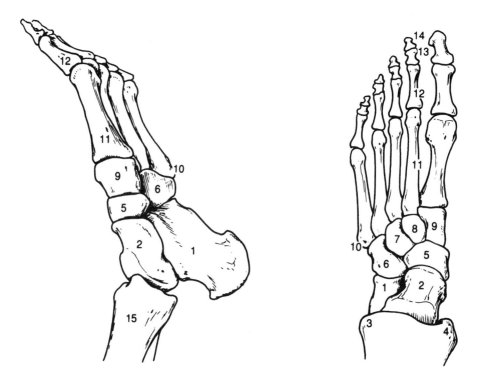

Figure 6-1 AP and lateral views of the foot: 1. Calcaneum; 2. Talus; 3. Medial malleolus; 4. Lateral malleolus; 5. Navicular; 6. Cuboid; 7. Lateral cuneiform; 8. Intermediate cuneiform; 9. Medial cuneiform; 10. Base of fifth metatarsal; 11. Metatarsal shafts; 12. Proximal phalynx; 13. Middle phalynx; 14. Distal phalynx; and 15. Tibia. Reprinted by permission from Unwin A, Jones K (eds). *Emergency Orthopaedics and Trauma*, p 177 (fig 18.4). Oxford, Elsevier Science Ltd, 1995.

On the bottom of the foot is the plantar fascia (aponeurosis), a ligamentous structure that extends between the metatarsal heads and the calcaneous. This fascia helps to maintain the arch of the foot under normal circumstances (Figure 6-3).

Two major arteries provide blood flow to the foot. On the dorsum of the foot is the dorsalis pedis artery, and adjacent to the medial malleolus is the posterior tibial artery. Under normal circumstances, the pulses in these arteries are readily palpable.

Each toe has a nail that emanates from its nail bed. The normal nail should appear smooth, without cracks, striations, or hypertrophy. In addition, color of the nailbed should be pink and capillary refill should be prompt when assessed.

Mechanism of Injury

The foot may be injured in a motor vehicle accident. Most commonly, this occurs due to bracing of one or both feet prior to impact. If the driver or passenger anticipates an impending collision, the natural reaction is to brace the arms, legs, or both against

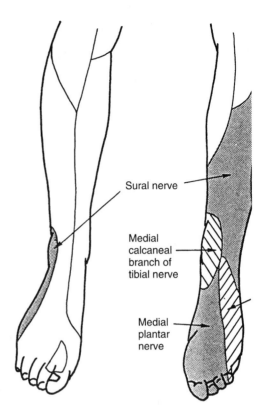

Sural nerve

Medial
calcaneal
branch of
tibial nerve

Medial
plantar
nerve

Figure 6-2 The sural nerve courses around the lateral malleolus to supply sensation to the lateral aspect of the foot. Reprinted by permission from Palastanga N, Field D, Soames R (eds). *Anatomy and Human Movement—Structure and Function*, 3rd ed. p 563 (fig 4.162). Oxford, Elsevier Science Ltd, 1998.

the dash and floorboard. A braced extremity will be subject to injury as the collision forces pass into it. For the driver, the most common reaction is to brace the right leg against the brake and the left leg against the floorboard. A passenger's leg(s) may be braced against the floorboard or back seat. There may also be direct trauma to one or both feet as a result of impact against various structures within the car after impact. Common pathological conditions that can involve the foot after a motor vehicle accident include:

- interdigital neuroma formation
- plantar fasciitis
- fracture(s)
- development of neurogenic pain states.

Interdigital Neuroma

An interdigital neuroma is a damaged interdigital nerve that is surrounded by scar tissue at the site of injury. Each interdigital nerve (a final branch of the tibial nerve) courses between two metatarsal bones to supply sensation to their respective phalanges. In total, there are eight interdigital nerves that can be involved in neuroma formation. A neuroma will form whenever one of these nerves is damaged or torn after an accident. Traumatized

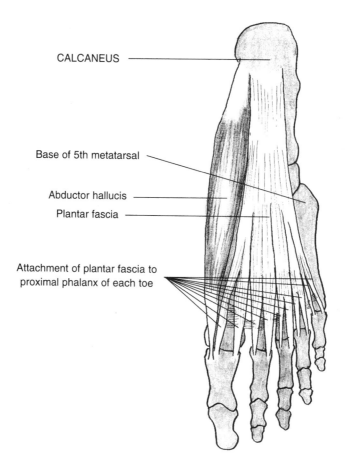

CALCANEUS

Base of 5th metatarsal

Abductor hallucis

Plantar fascia

Attachment of plantar fascia to
proximal phalanx of each toe

Figure 6-3 On the bottom of the foot is the plantar fascia (aponeurosis), a ligamentous structure that extends between the metatarsal heads and the calcaneus. Reprinted by permission from Field D (ed). *Anatomy: Palpation and Surface Markings,* 2nd ed. (fig 3.23-drawing to right). Boston, Butterworth-Heinemann, 1997.

tissues in the region of nerve injury stimulate an inflammatory reaction that promotes the development of scar tissue that may envelope the injured nerve.

Interdigital nerve damage along with the constant irritation caused by surrounding scar tissue can contribute to chronic foot pain that worsens with weightbearing activities. The pain is usually felt on the bottom of the forefoot, often described as being sharp, aching or burning in nature. On physical examination, there will be point tenderness between the metatarsal bones where the involved nerve courses, discomfort with compression of the metatarsal heads, and possibly a decrease in sensation in the respective web space.

The principal diagnostic test to assess for this diagnosis is a selective nerve block into the region of suspected interdigital nerve damage. This can be done with an anesthetic alone or in combination with steroids. If the patient has analgesic relief with a localized injection, this suggests that the diagnosis of interdigital neuroma is likely. Radiographic techniques are not of any assistance in making the diagnosis of interdigital neuroma.

Treatment for an interdigital neuroma would include a series of steroid injections to help decrease any inflammation in the region of the damaged nerve. Orthotics may help relieve pressure on the interdigital nerve during gait. Physical therapeutic modalities that may be helpful include ultrasound, iontophoresis and scar tissue mobilization. For a period of time, it may be helpful for the patient to utilize a cane or crutches to minimize weightbearing to the painful extremity.

Medications that may be helpful for this condition include anti-inflammatories and medications to reduce neurogenic pain (clonidine, mexiletine, and the anticonvulsants Tegretol and Neurontin). Topical creams that may prove helpful include capsaicin cream and anti-inflammatory/lidocaine cream derivatives.

Those patients who fail to improve may be candidates for surgery either to remove the offending neuroma (neurectomy) or to try to release it from its surrounding adhesions (neurolysis). Complications associated with interdigital neuritis include persistent foot pain. This may result in chronic limping with compensatory gait changes that can cause pain in other areas of the leg, in the contralateral leg, or in the trunk or pelvis.

Plantar Fasciitis

The plantar fascia, which extends from the tip of the calcaneous to the metatarsal heads, helps to support the arch of the foot. This ligamentous structure most commonly becomes inflamed at its insertion into the calcaneous. However, inflammation of the plantar fascia can occur anywhere along its length creating pain at the bottom of the foot that worsens with weightbearing activities and is relieved by rest.

On physical examination, there will be discomfort with palpation along the plantar aspect of the foot, including the insertion points at the heel and metatarsal heads. The diagnosis is a clinical one based on history and physical examination. The diagnostic workup is typically unrevealing. With longstanding plantar fasciitis, the patient may develop a heel spur at the insertion site of the plantar fascia into the calcaneous. The presence of a heel spur is suggestive of a chronic inflammatory process at that site.

The treatment for plantar fasciitis includes a trial of orthotics to help maintain the arch of the foot, thereby taking some pressure off of the plantar fascia. Physical therapeutic modalities (i.e., ultrasound) may also prove helpful. Since this is an inflammatory process, the patient may benefit from anti-inflammatory medications. Frequently, steroid injections may prove beneficial. Assistive devices that reduce weightbearing of the involved foot (cane or crutches) may provide the relative rest needed for some of the inflammation to subside. However, if conservative measures (physical therapeutic modalities, NSAIDS, assistive devices, orthotics, and steroid injections) are not beneficial, the patient may require surgical intervention, usually for removal of the heel spur. This may or may not prove beneficial.

Long-term complications of plantar fasciitis include ongoing discomfort that does not subside despite the above interventions. The patient with chronic foot pain may develop an abnormal limp with compensatory body changes which can result in discomfort involving the proximal lower extremity, contralateral extremity, trunk or low back.

Bony Fractures

As a result of motor vehicle accident trauma, the patient may fracture one or more of the bones within their foot. A hairline or "occult" fracture may not become clinically apparent early on in the diagnostic workup. The patient with a fractured foot bone will have sharp, localized foot discomfort that worsens with weightbearing. Physical examination will demonstrate localized tenderness with surrounding soft tissue swelling. Usually initial x-rays will demonstrate the fracture(s). Hairline fractures may not be evident on initial x-rays. A bone scan is more sensitive than x-rays in demonstrating this degree of bone pathology.

Depending on the bone involved, treatment for a fracture may include taping, splinting, or casting the foot. For more complicated fractures, surgery for open reduction and internal fixation will become necessary. After the fracture heals, the patient may be a candidate for a short course of physical therapy to improve range of motion of toe and ankle joints and to improve lower extremity strength (assuming there has been some level of inactivity or immobilization). Medications may be required for the acute pain of the fracture and for any postoperative pain. Assistive devices such as a cane or crutches may be necessary to promote limited weightbearing status after the fracture or surgical intervention.

Complications of a foot fracture include ongoing discomfort even after the bony fracture heals, chronic limping and the development of discomfort in the contralateral leg, low back or torso due to the compensatory gait abnormality. Depending on the need for immobilization, there may be a loss of range of motion at toe, mid-foot, or ankle joint.

Neurogenic Pain/Reflex Sympathetic Dystrophy

As noted earlier, the superficial peroneal, sural, and tibial nerves all have branches to each foot. Damage or trauma to any of these nerves can result in the development of neurogenic foot pain. The patient with neurogenic pain typically has a variety of characteristic symptoms including: numbness (usually in the sensory distribution of the involved nerve), annoying paresthesias (pins and needles/tingling), burning pain, and hypersensitivity to light. Neurogenic pain is usually present both during weightbearing and at rest. It often worsens when the patient lies down at night to go to sleep.

Physical examination may demonstrate abnormal sensation to pinprick and light touch in distribution of the involved nerve. There may be a localized irritation of the nerve characterized by a positive Tinel's sign with tapping of the involved nerve. There may be extreme hypersensitivity with light palpation over the sensory distribution of the nerve, a phenomenon known as allodynia.

Tarsal tunnel syndrome (described later) causes neurogenic foot pain due to entrapment of the tibial nerve as it courses through medial ankle ligaments. These patients complain of ankle pain and foot pain that worsens with weightbearing. Many of the above signs and symptoms of neurogenic pain may be present. Tinel's sign will be positive with tapping of the tibial nerve adjacent to the medial malleolus.

A less common but more serious form of neurogenic pain is due to the development of reflex sympathetic dystrophy syndrome (described in detail in a separate chapter). The patient with reflex sympathetic dystrophy may complain of temperature and color changes of the involved foot. Other signs include excessive sweating (hyperhidrosis), swelling in the foot, poor capillary refill, cracked nails and a diminished hair pattern.

Diagnostic workup for neurogenic pain might include electrodiagnostic studies, thermography, bone scanning, and diagnostic anesthetic blockade. Electrodiagnostic studies will be helpful in identifying an entrapped or damaged nerve. X-rays of the foot are typically unrevealing with neurogenic pain. However, bone scanning may be abnormal if the patient develops a reflex sympathetic dystrophy syndrome and has vasomotor abnormalities (increased or decreased blood flow). Patients with long-term reflex sympathetic dystrophy may develop osteoporosis due to the blood flow abnormalities and disuse over time. This would be appreciated on conventional x-rays. Thermography is also a useful diagnostic tool in the evaluation of reflex sympathetic dystrophy. It employs infrared imaging of bodily structures, which readily demonstrate asymmetric temperature changes between the symptomatic and uninvolved feet.

Lastly, diagnostic blocks with anesthetic may help identify exactly which nerve(s) is/are precipitating the neurogenic pain. Occasionally, these injections can be therapeutic if steroids are also infused with the anesthetic. For the patient with suspected reflex sympathetic dystrophy, lumbar sympathetic ganglion blocks may help prove or disprove this diagnosis. Such injections can be both diagnostic and potentially therapeutic.

The treatment for neurogenic pain includes conservative measures, such as the prescription of orthotics and a trial of physical therapy. Physical therapeutic modalities (ultrasound, iontopheresis) may help reduce inflammation around an involved nerve. The therapist may employ a variety of desensitization techniques. There are a number of medications which may be helpful for the patient with neurogenic pain including clonidine, mexiletine, tricyclic antidepressants, anticonvulsants, and some topical creams (capsaicin and anti-inflammatory/lidocaine derivatives). Steroid injections into localized inflamed nerves may prove efficacious. Occasionally, surgery for release of an entrapped nerve may be necessary. For example, patients with tarsal tunnel syndrome may require release of the entrapped tibial nerve adjacent to the medial malleolus. Complications of neurogenic pain include ongoing persistent discomfort with compensatory gait patterns that may contribute to the development of chronic pain in other areas of the body.

THE ANKLE

Anatomy

The bones of the ankle joint include the talus, tibia and fibula (Figure 6-4). The dome of the talus articulates with the distal portion of the tibia and fibula. This joint is held together by strong ligaments along its medial and lateral aspects. The lateral collateral ligament supports the lateral aspect of the ankle. The medial aspect of the ankle joint is strongly supported by the deltoid ligament, which courses from the medial malleolus to the navicular, the sustentaculum talus, and the posterior aspect of the talus.[1]

Nerves that course around the ankle joint are the sural (adjacent to the lateral malleolus), superficial peroneal (which courses through the anterior tarsal tunnel), and

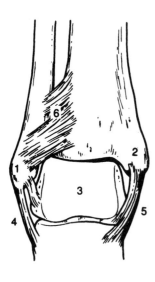

Figure 6-4 The normal ankle: 1. lateral malleolus; 2. medial malleolus; 3. talus; 4. lateral ligament; 5. medial (deltoid) ligament; and 6. inferior tibio-fibular ligament. Reprinted by permission from Unwin A, Jones K (eds). *Emergency Orthopaedics and Trauma*, p 234 (fig 24.1). Oxford, Elsevier Science Ltd, 1995.

tibial (which courses behind the medial malleolus). Major arteries about the ankle include the dorsalis pedis artery anteriorly and the tibial artery adjacent to the medial malleolus. Multiple tendons cross the ankle joint and attach to foot bones. These include tendons that contribute to toe flexion (flexor hallucis brevis, flexor hallucis longus, flexor digitorum brevis, flexor digitorum longus), foot inversion (anterior and posterior tibial), foot eversion (peroneous longus), foot dorsiflexion (anterior tibial and extensor digitorum), and great toe extension (extensor hallucis longus). The major tendon crossing the posterior ankle joint is the Achilles tendon, which emanates from the gastrocnemius and soleus muscles and inserts onto the calcaneous bone. The retrocalcaneal bursa lies between the anterior surface of the Achilles tendon and the posterior superior angle of the calcaneus. The calcaneal bursa lies between the insertion of the Achilles tendon and the overlying skin. These two bursae can become inflamed as a result of either damage to the tendon or excessive pressure upon the area.[2]

The tibial nerve's two terminal branches, the medial and lateral plantar nerves, pass around the medial malleolus through a fibro-osseous tunnel, the tarsal tunnel. The tarsal tunnel has bony walls consisting of a bony sulcus on the medial side of the calcaneus, the posterior talar process, and the medial malleolus. The medial wall of the tunnel is formed by the ligamentum lacinatum and tendonous arch of the abductor hallucis muscle. Tendons overly this fibro-osseous vault.[3] The tarsal tunnel is a potential site of entrapment of the tibial nerve.

Mechanism of Injury

The ankle joint may sustain injury during a motor vehicle accident when the driver or passenger braces their leg(s) prior to impact. The forces generated at the braced foot are transmitted through the foot to all joints of the lower extremity. The ankle may twist causing stretching and/or tearing of the medial or lateral collateral ligaments. There may also be direct trauma to the joint by some structure within the vehicle.

Common ankle injuries include:

- fracture
- sprain
- nerve injury
- bursitis
- tendonitis.

Ankle Fracture

The patient with a fractured ankle will have severe ankle pain and swelling immediately after the accident. With open fractures, bone penetrates through the skin. The patient with a fractured ankle will be unable to bear weight. Physical examination will reveal swelling, ecchymosis and extreme tenderness on palpation. X-rays are diagnostic.

With regards to treatment, if alignment remains good, bracing and/or casting of the ankle for a period of time will be all that is necessary. Malaligned bones and will require closed reduction followed by casting whereas more complex fractures (comminuted, open) will require surgery for open reduction and internal fixation followed by a period of casting and non-weightbearing status. Once the brace or cast comes off, patients will require physical therapy to work on ankle range of motion and lower extremity strengthening. Medications to control pain, including opioids, may be necessary immediately post injury or surgery.

Complications of an ankle fracture include persistent pain, limited ankle range of motion, and the development of a limp which can alter body mechanics, possibly leading to painful disorders involving the ipsilateral extremity, contralateral extremity, pelvis or back. A chronic pain syndrome may ensue.

Ankle Sprain

The sprained ankle is the most common injury that causes pain in the ankle. This condition varies from a simple strain of the ligaments to tearing of the ligaments with or without avulsion of the bones to which they attach. Ankle ligaments are copiously supplied with sensory nerve endings that relay pain impulses into the spinal cord when ligaments are stretched or torn. This will invoke reflex muscle spasm that protects the joint from further motion.

A *strain* is merely an over stretching of a ligament without disruption of the integrity of its fibers or avulsion from its bony attachment. Recovery from a strain typically occurs within a few weeks. If the stress is more severe, the fibers may tear and a severe *sprain* has occurred. A sprain may be defined as a rupture of some or all of the fibers of the ligament. It is considered minor when the number of ruptured fibers does not cause instability of the joint. A major sprain results in joint instability. An ankle ligament rarely tears in its middle, but sustains a tear at its proximal or distal point of attachment. A small fragment of bone may be avulsed with the ligament rather than the ligament itself being torn.

The differentiation of a simple strain from a sprain is suspected clinically and verified by x-ray examination. On examination, an inversion stress when the foot is slightly plantar flexed, results in stretch of the lateral collateral ligaments. In the simple inversion strain, if the foot is passively inverted, the talus remains in its proper position and no gap can be palpated between it and the malleolus. If a tear has occurred, the foot can be inverted to a greater degree than normal and the talus separates from the lateral malleolus. A palpable sulcus may permit insertion of a fingertip between the talus and the lateral malleolus. X-ray films taken with the foot inverted will reveal abnormal tilt of the talus within the mortise.

An injury to the ankle that forcefully everts the ankle will usually cause bony damage rather than straining or tearing of the medial ligament alone as in the inversion type of injury. In an eversion injury the medial ligament is so strong that fracture or avulsion of the tibia will occur before the ligament tears. Although tearing of the medial collateral (deltoid) ligament is infrequent, it must be constantly suspected to prevent the serious consequences of improper treatment (chronic pain and premature degenerative changes involving the ankle joint).[4]

Immediately after the sprain/strain occurs, there will be considerable swelling and inflammation. Anti-inflammatories, wrapping the ankle, compression garments, elevation of the leg, and ice packs during the first few days will help to minimize swelling. An advanced strain may require bracing, casting, and limited weight-bearing status to help promote healing. Some patients require surgical intervention to repair the torn ligaments. Assistive devices (canes, crutches, walker, wheelchair) may be needed to help maintain non- or partial weightbearing status. Patients with more complicated strains (that often require weeks or months to heal) usually need a course of physical therapy for modalities to improve ankle range of motion and for progressive muscle strengthening.

Complications of an ankle strain include persistent pain and ankle instability. This could result in limping with altered body mechanics that may lead to pain in other areas (contralateral leg, pelvis, trunk).

Tarsal Tunnel Syndrome

A tarsal tunnel syndrome may develop after ankle trauma. The tibial nerve courses through the tarsal tunnel (flexor retinaculum) adjacent to the medial malleolus. This is a small caliber area within which pressure can build up if there is local swelling or inflammation (Figure 6-5).

Patients with tarsal tunnel syndrome complain of plantar foot pain that worsens with weightbearing. There may be an electrical shooting quality to the pain, tingling, numbness, or other paresthesias involving the plantar surface of the foot.

Physical examination will demonstrate hypersensitivity of the tibial nerve as it passes through the tarsal tunnel (characterized by a positive Tinel's sign at that site), and there may be decreased sensation on the plantar aspect of the foot. The most important test in the diagnostic workup of tarsal tunnel syndrome is the electrodiagnostic study which will demonstrate slowing of distal motor latencies of the medial and lateral plantar branches of the involved tibial nerve (as compared to normal values and/or the asymptomatic contralateral side). Electromyogram (EMG) may demonstrate denervation potentials in the foot intrinsic musculature supplied by these nerves (the abductor digiti quinti minimi, abductor hallucis).[5]

Treatment for tarsal tunnel syndrome includes orthotics, steroid injections (to reduce local inflammation), and physical therapy modalities. The modalities iontophoresis and

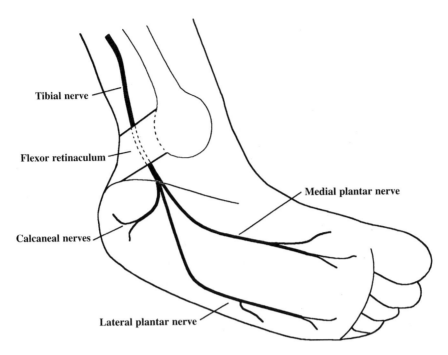

Figure 6-5 The tibial nerve courses through the tarsal tunnel (flexor retinaculum) adjacent to the medial malleolus. Reprinted by permission from Preston DC, Shapiro BE (eds). *Electromyography and Neuromuscular Disorders—Clinical-Electrophysiologic Correlations* (fig 21.1). Boston, Butterworth-Heinemann, 1998.

ultrasound are helpful in decreasing inflammation, while friction massage may help loosen a nerve trapped within scar tissue. A period of non- or partial weightbearing status through the use of assistive devices (cane, crutches, wheelchair) may also be necessary. Anti-inflammatories provide for pharmacologic reduction of inflammation. For patients who have associated neurogenic pain, medications such as clonidine, mexiletine, tricyclic antidepressants, anticonvulsants, and some topical creams (Zostrix, anti-inflammatory/lidocaine derivatives) may be helpful. Some patients require surgery for decompression of the tarsal tunnel. This usually proves to be a curative procedure for the patient with tarsal tunnel syndrome.

Complications of tarsal tunnel syndrome include persistent neurogenic pain and paresthesias. Some patients may develop a localized causalgia and/or reflex sympathetic dystrophy because of the nerve damage. Chronic ankle pain may also cause altered body mechanics with its associated sequela.

Osteoarthritis of the Ankle Joint

Patients who have had fairly significant ankle strains (grade III or IV), ligament tears, and/or fractures will be prone to the development of accelerated degenerative arthritis or osteoarthritis of the ankle joint. As the cartilaginous surfaces of the joint break down, bony surfaces grind against each other contributing to low-grade inflammation and chronic pain. The patient with an arthritic ankle joint will complain of ankle discomfort that worsens with weightbearing, limitations of range of motion, crepitations within the joint, and pain that worsens with changes in weather (barometric changes).

On examination, there will be tenderness about the ankle joint. There may be some degree of deformity and ankle range of motion may be diminished. X-rays will demonstrate the arthritic changes characterized by irregularity and narrowing of the joint space. Osteophytes (bone spurs) may be present. More advanced scanning techniques such as computerized tomography (CT), magenetic resonance imaging (MRI), or bone scanning may demonstrate further details of the arthritic joint. Bone scans can demonstrate active inflammation while CT and MRI may demonstrate intra-articular cartilaginous and ligamentous changes.

The conservative treatment approach to an arthritic ankle joint includes the use of physical therapy modalities to improve range of motion of the joint and to strengthen surrounding musculature. Deep heating (ultrasound) and superficial heating and cooling modalities all may prove helpful. An ankle brace may provide added support for the joint, thereby decreasing pain. Some patients benefit from steroid injection therapy into the ankle joint to reduce inflammation and hopefully minimize discomfort for several months at a time. Patients may require assistive devices to unload the involved ankle joint. Anti-inflammatory medications are appropriate assuming there are no contraindications to their use. A transcutaneous electrical nerve stimulation (TENS) unit and topical creams for arthritis (capsaicin or anti-inflammatory creams) may also prove efficacious. Complications of this diagnosis include persistent arthritic pain, limping, and altered body mechanics with chronic pain sequela.

Achilles Bursitis/Tendonitis

Achilles bursitis refers to inflammation of the bursal tissue beneath the Achilles tendon, whereas Achilles tendonitis is inflammation of the tendon itself. Both of these conditions will produce posterior ankle and heel pain that worsens with weightbearing activities and alleviates with rest. Physical examination will demonstrate localized tenderness involving the Achilles tendon, the bursal tissue beneath it, or both. There may be some boggy inflammation and swelling appreciated. If the Achilles tendon has been torn, there will be weakness of plantar flexion and perhaps a palpable defect appreciated within the tendon. Patients with a complete Achilles tendon rupture will be unable to plantarflex their ankle. This would represent a surgical situation.

Diagnostic x-rays would be unrevealing as soft tissue structures including inflamed tendon or bursal tissue cannot be visualized by this technique. MRI imaging will demonstrate the damaged or inflamed tissue.

After the diagnosis is made, treatment to alleviate pain and inflammation using appropriate analgesics and anti-inflammatories will be necessary. Anti-inflammatories help with both pain and inflammation. Shoe orthotics and heel lifts are helpful in that elevation of the heel takes some stress off the Achilles tendon. Patients with tearing of the Achilles tendon may require bracing or casting for several weeks to allow healing to commence. A steroid injection into the bursa may help with Achilles bursitis. However, steroids should not be injected directly into the Achilles tendon, as intratendonous injections could cause a tendon rupture. The patient may need to alter weightbearing status (partial or non-weightbearing). This will require the use of assistive devices (cane, crutches, wheelchair). Physical therapeutic modalities to reduce inflammation (ultrasound and iontophoresis) may be helpful early on. As the inflammation subsides, stretching and strengthening of the calf musculature will be necessary.

Patients with a significant tear or rupture of the Achilles tendon will require surgical intervention to repair the torn tissue. Such a surgery requires a prolonged recovery period consisting of immobilization followed by appropriate therapy for stretching and progressive strengthening. Complications of Achilles bursitis, tendonitis, or Achilles tendon tear include persistent pain and limitations of ankle range of motion. This may result in a limp with chronic pain sequela due to altered body mechanics.

THE KNEE JOINT

Anatomy

The bones that make up the knee joint include the femur, tibia, and the patella. The distal-most portion of the femur forms two large condyles, rounded structures which articulate intimately with shallow grooves in the tibial plateau, each groove a concave structure that accepts the convex femoral condyle (Figure 6-6). The patella, the largest sesamoid (free floating) bone in the body, guides the knee in flexion and extension as it glides between the groove formed by the femoral condyles (Figure 6-7). The patella is suspended within the knee joint by the quadriceps muscle above, its tendon below, and from the sides by the medial and lateral retinacular ligaments. The patella ligament connects the inferior border of the patella with the tibial tubercle (Figure 6-8).

A capsule of strong ligaments surrounds the knee joint. The medial and lateral collateral ligaments reinforce the capsule medially and laterally, respectively. Within the knee joint are the anterior and posterior cruciate ligaments, ligaments that provide anterior/posterior stability and control flexion and extension by preventing excessive anterior or posterior translation of the knee joint during movement (Figure 6-9). The bony articulating surfaces within the knee joint are all lined by cartilaginous tissue, smooth lubricated tissue that permits low friction gliding of these bony structures against each other.

Embedded within the medial and lateral tibial plateaus are the medial and lateral menisci, respectively. These fibrocartilaginous structures act as cushions or shock absorbers for the femoral condyles as they glide within the recessed portions of the medial and lateral tibial plateau (Figure 6-10). Anteriorly, are the superficial and deep patella bursas. These synovial tissues help promote gliding of the patella tendon during flexion and extension of the knee.

Mechanism of Injury

The knee joint can be injured in a motor vehicle accident. The most common mechanism of injury is direct impact of the individual's knee against the dashboard or back seat. This

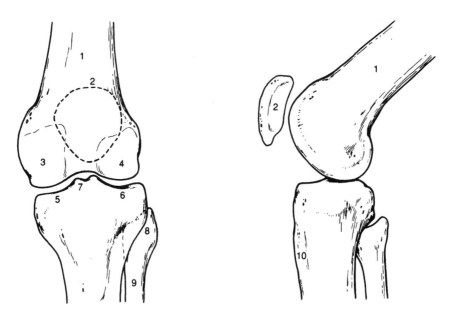

Figure 6-6 AP and lateral views of the knee: 1. Shaft of femur; 2. Patella; 3. Medial femoral condyle; 4. Lateral femoral condyle; 5. Medial tibial plateau; 6. Lateral tibial plateau; 7. Anterior and posterior tibial spines; 8. Head of fibula; 9. Neck of fibula; 10. Tibial tuberosity. Reprinted by permission from Unwin A, Jones K (eds). *Emergency Orthopaedics and Trauma*, p 176 (fig 18.2). Oxford, Elsevier Science Ltd, 1995.

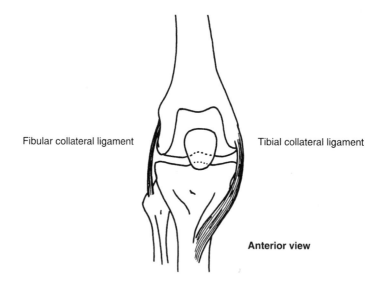

Figure 6-7 The patella guides the knee in flexion and extension as it glides between the groove formed by the femoral condyles. Reprinted by permission from Palastanga N, Field D, Soames R (eds). *Anatomy and Human Movement—Structure and Function*, 3rd ed. p 441 (fig 4.84a). Oxford, Elsevier Science Ltd, 1998.

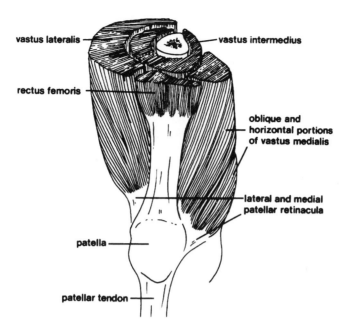

vastus lateralis

vastus intermedius

rectus femoris

oblique and
horizontal portions
of vastus medialis

lateral and medial
patellar retinacula

patella

patellar tendon

Figure 6-8 The patella is suspended within the knee joint by the quadriceps muscle above, its tendon below, and from the sides by the medial and lateral retinacular ligaments. Reprinted by permission from Macnicol MF (ed). *The Problem Knee*, 2nd ed. p 121 (fig 7.12). London, Hodder Arnold, 1995.

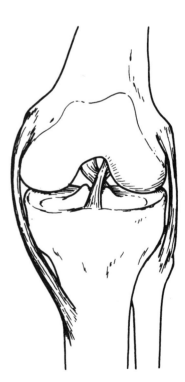

Figure 6-9 The knee joint is reinforced medially and laterally by the medial (left) and lateral (right) collateral ligaments. Within the knee joint are the anterior and posterior cruciate ligaments. Reprinted by permission from Unwin A, Jones K (eds). *Emergency Orthopaedics and Trauma*, p 212 (fig 22.3). Oxford, Elsevier Science Ltd, 1995.

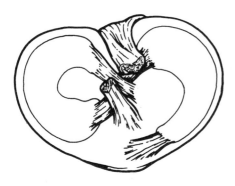

Figure 6-10 Embedded within the medial and lateral tibial plateaus are the medial and lateral menisci, fibro-cartilaginous shock absorbers for the medial and lateral tibial plateaus. Reprinted by permission from Unwin A, Jones K (eds). *Emergency Orthopaedics and Trauma*, p 209 (fig 22.1). Oxford, Elsevier Science Ltd, 1995.

type of injury is commonly known as a "dashboard knee." There is a direct compression injury of the patella against the underlying bony structures of the knee joint. This can result in tearing or laceration of the cartilaginous surface of all bones within the knee. The most common cartilage breakdown occurs on the undersurface of the patella.

The knee may also undergo a direct blow against the door, stick shift, or another passenger as the patient is tossed about after impact. Lastly, the patient may injure one or both knees as a result of leg bracing prior to impact. This will result in transmission of forces throughout the leg after impact. These forces may traumatize the extended knee, possibly injuring cartilaginous structures, ligaments, or the fibrocartilaginous menisci.

Common pathological conditions involving the knee that can be related to motor vehicle accidents include:

- dashboard knee or chondromalacia
- a sprain of a major knee ligament
- development of bursitis or tendonitis
- tearing of a medial or lateral meniscus
- fracture.

Chondromalacia Patella/Dashboard Knee

The patient who develops chondromalacia patella usually has a history of a direct impact of the knee against the dash or back seat. This type of injury compresses the patella against the femoral condyles causing tearing and fissuring of the cartilage tissue. These patients complain of pain within the knee joint or directly under the patella, which worsens with kneeling, going up and down stairs, and/or with ambulation.

Physical examination may or may not demonstrate signs of inflammation. There may be an effusion present early on, but this usually dissipates over time. There may be crepitations appreciated with flexion and extension of the knee. There will be tenderness of the chondral structures including the undersurface of the patella and possibly the cartilage overlying the femoral condyles. The patient will experience increasing pain with downward pressure on the patella, which forces its undersurface to abut the femoral condyles. The discomfort increases if the patient contracts his/her quadriceps while the examiner presses downward. This is known as a positive patella grind test (Figure 6-11).[6]

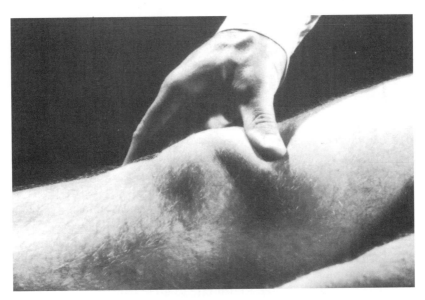

Figure 6-11 The patella grind test. Reprinted by permission from Macnicol MF (ed). *The Problem Knee*, 2nd ed. p 21 (fig 2.7). London, Hodder Arnold, 1995.

X-rays may or may not demonstrate pathology. In general, cartilaginous tissue is radiolucent and any fragmentation of cartilage will not show up on traditional x-rays. Special axial views (sunrise, sunset, or Merchant views) are frequently helpful in determining if patella malalignment is contributing to the underlying condition. Arthrograms are usually not diagnostic. MRI scan of the knee will demonstrate intra-articular pathology including chondromalacia. Joint arthrography may also demonstrate the irregular intra-articular surfaces consistent with chondromalacia. A diagnostic and possibly therapeutic steroid injection may also provide valuable information. If the pain lessens after an anesthetic/steroid injection, this is suggestive of interarticular pathology including chondromalacia.

Early treatment for dashboard knee includes relative rest, immobilization of the joint, gentle compression if swelling is present, and application of ice. A patella tracking brace allows the patella to glide freely without lateral movement, which might aggravate the pain. Anti-inflammatories may be helpful in reducing inflammation and decreasing pain. Some patients need to reduce weightbearing for a period of time, requiring either a cane or crutches. A TENS unit may provide some symptomatic relief of knee discomfort. Topical creams including capsaicin cream and anesthetic/anti-inflammatory creams may provide additional analgesia. A steroid injection may reduce inflammation and help accelerate the recovery to some degree.

Patients in whom discomfort persists, despite these conservative measures, may be candidates for arthroscopic surgery. In such a procedure, the orthopedist arthroscopically inspects the knee, determines what areas have developed cartilage degeneration, and then shaves away the friable cartilage tissue in those areas. This usually provides symptomatic relief to the patient with chondromalacia.[7]

Complications of chondromalacia include chronic knee discomfort and gait abnormalities including limping. Limping will alter body mechanics, predisposing the patient to the development of other limb and trunk pain problems.

Ligament Strain/Sprain

A number of ligaments help maintain structural integrity of the knee including the medial and lateral collateral ligaments (which prevent medial and lateral instability) and the anterior and posterior cruciate ligaments (which prevent anterior and posterior translation of the joint). Trauma to these ligaments can occur after a motor vehicle accident either due to a direct impact or indirectly by forces transmitted through a braced leg.

The patient with a torn (strained) knee ligament post motor vehicle accident will have severe pain, swelling, and limited range of motion of the joint. As the swelling diminishes and weightbearing ensues, these patients continue to complain of knee pain, and they may also complain about instability of the joint (popping and giving way of the joint during ambulation or going up and down stairs). Patients may fall if their knee gives out on them. The patient may be unable to run due to knee pain and instability.

Physical examination may demonstrate swelling and effusion. The patient with a medial or lateral collateral ligament strain or tear will have increasing discomfort when a valgus or varus stress is placed upon the knee joint, respectively. To test the medial collateral ligament, apply valgus stress to open the knee joint on the medial side. To test the lateral need for stability, apply varus stress to open the knee joint on the lateral side (Figure 6-12).[6]

Patients with an anterior or posterior ligament injury, will have increasing pain or frank instability demonstrated with anterior or posterior drawer testing, respectively. To test the integrity of the anterior cruciate ligament, the patient lies supine on the examination table with his knees flexed to 90 degrees and his feet flat on the table. The examiner positions him or herself so as to stabilize the patient's foot and cups his/her hands around the patient's knee. The examiner then draws the tibia toward him or herself. If it slides forward from under the femur (positive anterior draw sign), the anterior cruciate ligament may be torn. The posterior cruciate ligament is tested in a similar manner. The examiner stays in the same position and pushes the tibia posteriorly. If it moves backward on the femur, the posterior cruciate ligament it is probably damaged (positive posterior draw sign) (Figure 6-13).

The anterior draw sign is more common than the posterior sign, since the incidence of damage to the anterior cruciate is much higher than to the posterior cruciate. In fact, an isolated case of a torn posterior cruciate ligament is rare.[6]

With regards to diagnostic workup, standard knee x-rays will not demonstrate torn ligaments. Arthrography may demonstrate intra-articular pathology including torn ligaments. MRI scanning is very accurate in demonstrating torn and ruptured ligaments, as well as inflamed ligaments that have been strained.

Early treatment for a knee ligament strain includes efforts to reduce pain and inflammation through the use of anti-inflammatories, compression, analgesics, immobilization, and alteration of weightbearing status. The patient may require a cane or crutches for a period of time.

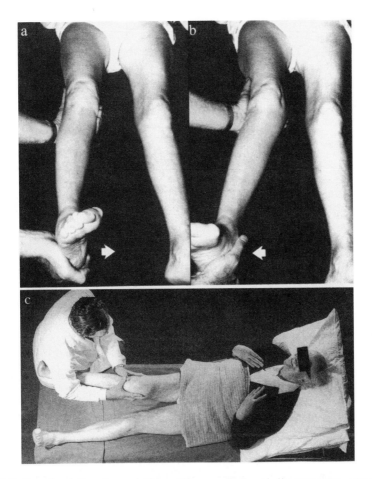

Figure 6-12 Testing for instability: The collateral ligaments can be tested by stressing first the lateral and then the medial side (a, b). If the leg is tucked under the examiner's arm (c), the knee can be steered medially and laterally with greater control. Reprinted by permission from Apley AG, Solomon L (eds). *Concise System of Orthopaedics and Fractures*, 2nd ed. p 197 (fig 20.4 a,b,c). London, Hodder Arnold, 1994.

After the acute pain and inflammation subsides, the patient may benefit from physical therapy for knee strengthening and range of motion. Ultrasound may be helpful in reducing pain and inflammation and improving range of motion. A TENS unit may help decrease acute or chronic discomfort. The patient with knee instability, who chooses not to pursue surgery, will require knee bracing to help stabilize the joint. Many patients pursue surgical treatment to repair torn ligaments. A discussion of surgical techniques is beyond the scope of this text.

Complications of this condition include chronic knee instability and discomfort. The patient with knee instability will be prone to falling. A torn ligament may lead to an altered gait and changes in body mechanics, with resultant contralateral extremity and trunk discomfort.

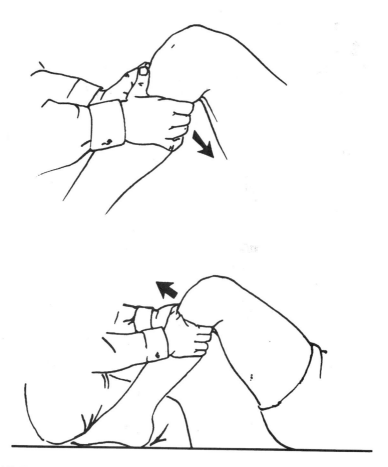

Figure 6-13 The posterior (upper) and anterior (lower) draw tests. Reprinted by permission from Macnicol MF (ed). *The Problem Knee*, 2nd ed. p 25 (fig 2.10). London, Hodder Arnold, 1995.

Bursitis/Tendonitis

The patient with knee trauma may develop a bursitis in one of several bursas that surround the joint. Anterior to the joint are the suprapatellar, prepatellar, deep infrapatellar, and infrapatellar bursas. Inferomedial to the medial knee is the pes anserine bursa under the common tendon of the medial hamstring muscles. All of these bursas may become inflamed as a result of a direct injury post motor vehicle accident.

The major tendon extending across the anterior knee is the patella (quadriceps) tendon. This tendon extends distally from the patella to insert onto the tibial tubercle. The quadriceps tendon may become chronically inflamed. The history for a patient with patella bursitis and/or quadriceps tendonitis includes pain in the region of the patella or infrapatellar space. In the case of pes anserine bursitis, there is discomfort along the inferomedial knee. There may be swelling due to inflammation. The pain of these disorders worsens with kneeling and weightbearing activities.

On physical examination, there will be tenderness of the structure involved in the inflammatory process. In the case of patella tendonitis, there will be tenderness along the course of the tendon itself, as well as its insertion site at the tibial tubercle.

Diagnostic x-rays are not particularly helpful for these soft tissue conditions. MRI scanning is more effective in demonstrating the inflammation seen with tendonitis and bursitis. Selective anesthetic/steroid injections may be both diagnostic and therapeutic. Diagnostically, they help localize the focus of pain. Therapeutically, once the steroids kick in, the patient may have a prolonged analgesic effect or an accelerated recovery. Intratendinous steroid injections should not be performed as they could promote tendon rupture. Therapeutic injections for tendonitis should be performed into tissues adjacent to the tendon following which diffusion of the solution will help promote the desired anti-inflammatory effect.

Conservative treatment measures for bursitis and/or tendonitis includes the use of anti-inflammatories, the application of ice, and relative immobilization or altered weightbearing status for the patient. A cane or crutches may be indicated for a short period of time. Physical therapy including therapeutic modalities to reduce inflammation (ultrasound and iontophoresis), as well as range of motion and strengthening once the inflammation subsides may prove particularly helpful for the patient. Application of topical creams (capsaicin, anesthetic/anti-inflammatory cream) may be helpful. A TENS unit may also provide symptomatic pain relief. The principal complication seen in these cases would be chronic pain and inflammation, which may impair gait.

Torn Meniscus

Trauma to the knee could also result in tearing of the medial or lateral meniscus. These are the fibrocartilaginous shock absorbers, located on the tibial plateaus, that accept the femoral condyles and allow for smooth gliding motion of the knee joint. When traumatized, they may tear and fragment. The patient with a torn meniscus complains of discomfort and intermittent catching, popping, and/or locking of the knee. The symptomatology worsens with weightbearing activities.

Physical examination may demonstrate tenderness along the involved medial or lateral tibial plateau. There may be swelling or an effusion within the knee joint. Special tests to help identify torn menisci include the McMurray test and Apley's compression test. Posterior meniscal tears are difficult to identify. The McMurray test was originally developed to assist in making these difficult diagnoses. The patient lies supine with legs flat in the neutral position. The examiner takes hold of the patient's heel in one hand and flexes his/her leg fully. With the leg externally rotated, the examiner places a valgus stress to on the knee. With the knee in this position, the leg is slowly extended. If this maneuver causes a palpable or audible "click" within the joint, there is a probable tear in the medial meniscus, most likely in its posterior half.

Apley's compression test is another procedure designed to aid in the diagnoses of a torn meniscus. The patient lies prone on the examination table with the involved leg flexed to 90 degrees. The examiner applies downward pressure to the plantar surface of the foot, compressing the medial and lateral meniscus between the tibia and femur. The examiner rotates the tibia internally and externally on the femur while maintaining firm compression. If this maneuver elicits pain, there is probable meniscal damage. Pain on the medial side indicates a damaged medial meniscus; pain on the lateral side suggests a lateral meniscal tear (Figure 6-14).[6]

With regard to diagnostic workup, x-ray evaluation tends to be unrevealing. However, arthrography and MRI scanning usually demonstrates the torn meniscus.[8–10] Sometimes, the pathology is not revealed until arthroscopic evaluation.

Treatment of a meniscus injury includes physical therapy to strengthen muscles about the knee, maintain its range of motion, and for modalities to reduce inflammation. Knee braces can help reduce pain and provide stability for the joint. Steroid injections may be helpful if there is inflammation present. Topical creams and a TENS unit may also provide some symptomatic relief. However, highly symptomatic patients will need to proceed with arthroscopic surgery to remove meniscal fragments that are causing pain and interfering with smooth knee motion.[11,12]

Complications of a torn meniscus include chronic knee discomfort and/or popping, particularly if the patient has not undergone reparative surgery. Even if surgery is performed, the patient now has an underlying degenerative process within the knee that may be prone to further degeneration over time. Chronic knee pain with altered gait and body mechanics may ensue.

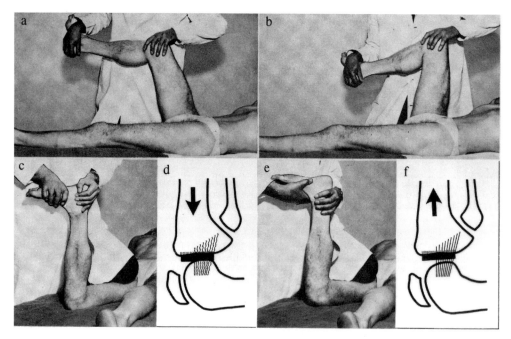

Figure 6-14 Torn medial meniscus—tests: (a, b) McMurray's test is performed at varying angles of flexion. (c, d) Apley's grinding test relaxes the ligaments but compresses the meniscus—it causes pain with meniscus lesions. (e, f) the distraction test release the meniscus but stretches the ligaments and causes pain if these are injured. Reprinted by permission from Apley AG, Solomon L (eds). *Concise System of Orthopaedics and Fractures*, 2nd ed. p 201 (fig 20.10a–f). London, Hodder Arnold, 1994.

Fracture

The tibia, patella, and femur may fracture as a result of motor vehicle accident. The patient with a fractured bone will have severe localized pain, swelling, ecchymoses, and will be unable to bear weight. There may be bleeding within the knee joint (hemarthroses). With more severe fractures, bones may penetrate through the skin.

Examination of the knee will demonstrate tenderness, swelling, ecchymoses, joint effusion and limited/painful range of motion. Routine x-rays will delineate the fractured bone. Occasionally, bone scanning or MRI scanning may be necessary to demonstrate compression deformities of the tibial plateaus or occult fractures that are not picked up by traditional x-rays.

Once a fracture is diagnosed, treatment usually includes closed or open reduction (surgical intervention to reduce the fracture and for internal fixation) followed by bracing or casting. A period of non-weightbearing status with appropriate assistive (crutches, walker or wheelchair) may be necessary early on. Over time, partial weightbearing with crutches or a cane may be necessary until the patient can progress to full weightbearing. Medications to control pain and inflammation are appropriate. A TENS unit may help control some of the discomfort associated with fractures. Once the patient is able to bear weight, he or she should begin physical therapy for knee range of motion, and exercises to strengthen muscles about the joint. Progressive ambulation utilizing a treadmill is often incorporated into the physical therapy program.

Complications of fractures about the knee include persistent knee discomfort and the development of an accelerated arthritic condition within the joint. As with other lower extremity painful conditions, this could result in an altered gait that affects other parts of the body.

THE HIP

Anatomy

The hip articulation is formed by the ball-shaped head of the femur which lies within a socket, the acetabulum. Each acetabulum lies within its respective iliac bone (Figure 6-15). This "ball and socket" articulation is extremely stable. Aside from the inherent stability that occurs with this anatomical arrangement, there is also a strong ligamentous capsule surrounding the hip joint that provides additional stabilization.

A bursa lies between the greater trochanter of the femur and the tensor fascia lata muscle. Its purpose is to allow smooth gliding of the overlying musculature across the greater trochanter, thereby minimizing friction and potential muscle damage. The tensor fascia lata muscle extends from the pelvis to the lateral aspect of the knee. It serves to assist in abduction of the hip joint. The hip flexors (iliopsoas muscle) extend from the lumbar spine to the proximal femur. On the side of the hip is the gluteus medius, the principal abductor of the joint.

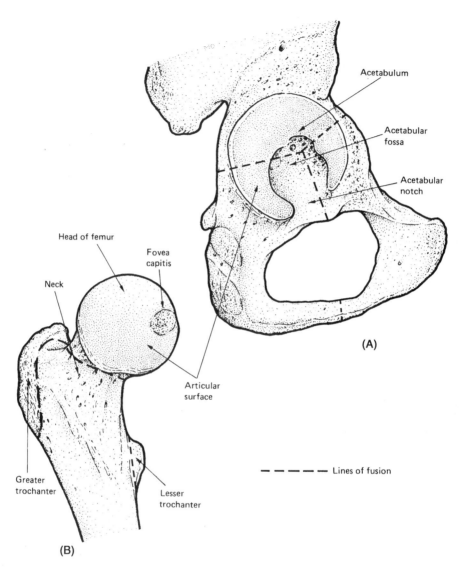

Figure 6-15 The articular surfaces of the hip joint: (A) acetabulum; (B) head of femur. Reprinted by permission from Palastanga N, Field D, Soames R (eds). *Anatomy and Human Movement—Structure and Function*, 3rd ed. p 407 (fig 4.65a,b). Oxford, Elsevier Science Ltd, 1998.

Mechanics of Injury

The patient who braces for impact with legs extended against the floorboard or brake pedal will have the resulting forces of impact spread throughout his/her leg, causing potential trauma to the hip joint. There may also be a direct blow of the hip region against the door, stick shift, seatbelt, or perhaps another passenger. This could result in trauma to the hip, the musculature about the hip, or to the trochanteric bursa.

Common pathological conditions related to the hip joint that can occur after a motor vehicle accident include:

- trochanteric bursitis
- strain of the hip joint
- fracture
- aseptic necrosis of the femoral head
- myofascial pain syndrome involving surrounding musculature.

Trochanteric Bursitis

Trochanteric bursitis can occur after a motor vehicle accident if a hip impacts against the doorframe, stick shift, or another passenger. In addition, when seatbelts catch, they may traumatize tissues adjacent to the hip. The patient with trochanteric bursitis complains of pain along the lateral aspect of the hip and an inability to lie on the involved side without discomfort. Pain may be associated with weightbearing activities.

Physical examination will demonstrate extreme tenderness with palpation of the greater trochanter and the overlying trochanteric bursa. There may be muscle spasm in surrounding musculature particularly involving the gluteus medius and tensor fascia lata. Diagnostic workup is typically unrevealing. X-rays will not demonstrate this soft tissue abnormality. However, MRI scanning may demonstrate the acute inflammation seen with bursitis.

With regards to conservative treatment, changes in weightbearing status may be necessary for a period of time along with the use of anti-inflammatories, analgesics, and application of ice. Physical therapy deep heating modalities (ultrasound) may be helpful in decreasing this deeply seated inflammatory process. Therapy to alleviate surrounding muscle spasm including stretching, massage, ultrasound, and a home exercise program may be necessary. It is particularly important to work on stretching of the tensor fascia latae muscle. When this muscle is tight, it applies direct pressure against the trochanteric bursa, which perpetuates the condition. If the patient fails to improve, they may benefit from one or a series of trochanteric steroid injections to reduce inflammation and accelerate recovery. In the rare instance that bursitis does not improve with these conservative measures, a bursectomy (surgical procedure to remove the bursa) may become necessary.

Complications of trochanteric bursitis include chronic hip pain that could alter gait and lead to more distant pain problems.

Hip Strain

The hip joint capsule may be strained in a motor vehicle accident. The patient with a hip strain complains of hip discomfort that worsens with range of motion of the joint, weightbearing activities, walking, and running. On examination, there will be discomfort associated with range of motion and direct palpation of the joint. There may be a positive Patrick's test (hip pain elicited by flexion, abduction, and external rotation of the involved hip).[13] X-rays are typically are unrevealing unless there is associated arthritis within the joint. However, tearing and inflammation of the joint capsule may be evident on MRI scanning.

Initial treatment for a hip strain includes temporary alteration of weightbearing status as appropriate, anti-inflammatories, and application of ice or heating modalities. Over time, physical therapy may be necessary for deep heating modalities (ultrasound), and for exercises to maintain hip range of motion and strength. A home stretching program is important so that range of motion does not diminish as a result of the pain. A TENS unit may provide some symptomatic relief. Some patients benefit from intra-articular steroid injections to alleviate pain and inflammation associated with the strained capsule.

Complications include chronic hip or pelvic discomfort, chronic spasm of overlying musculature, hip instability, and premature degenerative arthritis of the joint. Chronic hip pain may cause limping and altered body mechanics, which may be associated with distant pain processes.

Hip Fracture

A hip may fracture during a motor vehicle accident. The patient with a hip fracture will have difficulty with any hip movement and will be unable to bear weight. On examination, there will be swelling and ecchymoses about the hip with limited and painful range of motion. Diagnostic x-rays will reveal the fractured bone. Treatment usually includes surgery for open reduction and internal fixation for the fractured bone. Non- or partial-weightbearing status will be necessary for a period of time after surgery.

After surgery, physical therapy will be necessary to improve range of motion of the joint, strengthen surrounding musculature, and for progressive ambulation. Appropriate analgesics will be necessary throughout the course of treatment for a fractured hip. Long-term potential complications include the accelerated development of degenerative arthritis of the joint, chronic hip pain with limping, and the sequela that may occur with alteration of body mechanics.

Aseptic Necrosis

A rare complication of trauma to the hip joint is the development of aseptic necrosis. When this occurs, there is disruption of the blood supply to the femoral head resulting in premature arthritis and degeneration. There is gradual deformation of the femoral head, which limits range of motion. These patients complain of hip pain with weight-bearing activities.

The physical examination of a patient with aseptic necrosis is similar to someone with a strain or arthritis of the hip. They will exhibit discomfort with range of motion of the joint, and a positive Patrick's test (hip pain elicited with flexion, abduction, and external rotation). X-rays of the hip usually demonstrate the degenerative process associated with aseptic necrosis. MRI imaging will be needed to demonstrate mild cases of aseptic necrosis, not seen on conventional radiographs.

Conservative treatment of aseptic necrosis includes measures to maintain range of motion of the hip joint and to maintain strength in the surrounding musculature. Deep heating modalities such as ultrasound may help in diminishing pain and inflammation about the joint. Anti-inflammatories and analgesics may help relieve discomfort. Some patients require assistive devices to alter weightbearing status. A TENS unit may also help reduce hip discomfort. In advanced stages, these patients will require hip arthroplasty to alleviate the symptomatology of aseptic necrosis. If the patient chooses not to pursue surgery, he or she may have chronic hip discomfort which may be associated with a leg length discrepancy, limping, and altered body mechanics.

Myofascial Pain

Myofascial pain involving musculature about the hip joint commonly occurs after a motor vehicle accident. Muscles involved may include the iliopsoas muscle anteriorly, the gluteus medius and the tensor fasciae latae muscles laterally, and the gluteus maximus and piriformis muscles posteriorly. Patients with myofascial pain describe aching discomfort in the hip region while at rest. This pain worsens with weightbearing activities and range of motion of the joint.

Physical examination will demonstrate the tender muscles with associated spasm and trigger points. There will be limitations in hip range of motion. Diagnostic workup is typically unrevealing. Myofascial pain syndrome is a soft tissue condition that will not be revealed on x-rays, CT or bone scanning, or MRI imaging.

The treatment of a myofascial pain syndrome includes physical therapeutic modalities to lengthen the involved muscles (massage, a stretching program, and deep heating modalities such as ultrasound). The patient must ultimately become involved in an aggressive stretching and exercise program for the involved musculature. Anti-inflammatories, analgesics, and TENS may provide symptomatic relief for these patients. Complications include chronic myofascial hip discomfort that may refer distally to the knee and proximally to the low back. The patient with hip pain may develop a limp with the sequela of altered body mechanics.

THE PELVIS

Anatomy

Four bones make up the bony pelvis including the two iliac bones, sacrum and coccyx (Figure 6-16). Both the sacrum and coccyx are made up of fused vertebrae. The anterior portions of the iliac bones are held together by fibrocartilaginous tissue at the pubic symphysis. Posteriorly, the iliac bones articulate with the sacrum at the sacroiliac joints. These are very strong synovial joints between the articular surfaces of the sacrum and the ilium. These articular surfaces have irregular elevations with depressions in the opposing surfaces, producing joints with little movement. The articular capsule is attached close to the articulating surfaces of the sacrum and the ilium. The sacrum is suspended between the iliac bones and the bones are firmly held together by very strong ligaments.

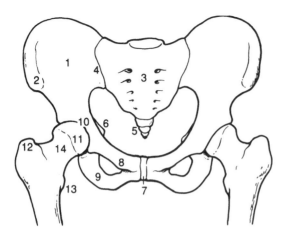

Figure 6-16 AP of the pelvis. 1. Ilium; 2. Anterior superior iliac spine; 3. Sacrum; 4. Sacroiliac joint; 5. Coccyx; 6. Pelvic brim; 7. Pubic symphysis; 8. Superior pubic ramus; 9. Inferior pubic ramus; 10. Acetabulum; 11. Femoral head; 12. Greater trochanter; 13. Lesser trochanter; and 14. Femoral neck. Reprinted by permission from Unwin A, Jones K (eds). *Emergency Orthopaedics and Trauma*, p 175 (fig 18.1). Oxford, Elsevier Science Ltd, 1995.

Little movement occurs at the sacroiliac joints because they are designed primarily for weightbearing. Movement of the sacroiliac joints is limited to a slight gliding and rotary movement.[14] A number of muscles are intimately related to the bony pelvis. The iliopsoas muscle originates from the ventral lumbosacral spinous processes, passes through the pelvis, and inserts on the proximal femur. The iliopsoas muscle is a hip flexor. The hip extensor muscles (gluteus maximus and the hamstrings) have their origins on the posterior bony pelvis. The hip abductor muscles (gluteus medius and the tensor fasciae lata) originate from the lateral pelvis. Posteriorly, under the gluteus maximus is the piriformis muscle, under which the sciatic nerve passes as it exits the pelvis and passes into the respective extremity (Figure 6-17).

Mechanism of Injury

The pelvis may be injured during a motor vehicle accident through a variety of mechanisms. The patient may sustain a hyperflexion/hyperextension injury involving the low back and bony pelvis. The pelvis may sustain a direct blow against the door, stick shift, seatbelt, or another passenger. A pelvic injury may occur as a result of bracing a leg against the floorboard or pedal at time of impact. Resultant forces will spread throughout the extremity, to the pelvis and sacroiliac joint.

Another mechanism of chronic pelvic injury is the gradual cumulative microtrauma that occurs secondary to compensatory gait changes resulting from other injuries to lower extremity structures. Any lower extremity injury that results in limping could, over time, result in pelvic injury. There are a number of pathological conditions that can affect the pelvis after a motor vehicle accident. Some of the more common ones include:

- sacroiliac joint dysfunction
- piriformis syndrome
- pelvic myofascial pain syndrome
- pelvic fracture
- severe pelvic floor strain or tear.

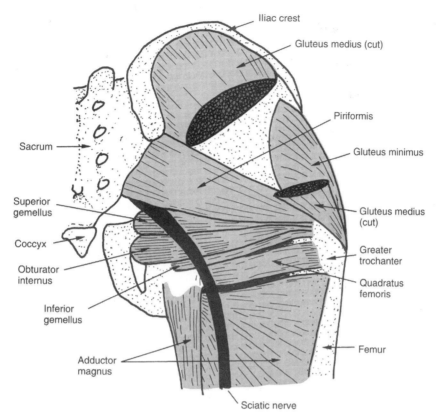

Figure 6-17 Under the piriformis muscle passes the sciatic nerve. Reprinted by permission from Palastanga N, Field D, Soames R (eds). *Anatomy and Human Movement—Structure and Function*, 3rd ed. p 323 (fig 4.20). Oxford, Elsevier Science Ltd, 1998.

Sacroiliac Joint Dysfunction

The sacroiliac (SI) joint(s) may be injured in a motor vehicle accident. With more severe trauma, there may be a subluxation or dislocation of the joint with associated tearing of the sacroiliac joint capsule and surrounding ligaments. More commonly, the joint is strained. The patient with sacroiliac joint dysfunction complains of hip or low back pain on the involved side, and difficulty with weightbearing activities. The sacroiliac joint is critically involved in both weightbearing activities and change of position. These patients may complain of SI joint pain when trying to get out of a chair (they may have to use their arms to push themselves out of the chair), going up and down stairs, and when getting in and out of cars. If there is any instability of the sacroiliac joint, patients complain of popping in the hip region and giving way or buckling of the involved leg.

On physical examination, lower extremity neurological evaluation may be unrevealing. On the other hand, a dislocating sacroiliac joint or tight piriformis muscle may irritate the adjacent sciatic nerve causing sciatica-like signs and symptoms (positive straight leg raising, lower extremity weakness and decreased sensation).

With the patient prone, the involved sacroiliac joint will be tender to palpation. With the patient supine, there are several provocative tests used to delineate SI joint dysfunction. The most common is the Patrick or Faber test. To perform this test, the examiner flexes, abducts, and externally rotates each leg. When the end point of flexion, abduction, and external rotation has been reached, the patient's femur is fixed in relation to the pelvis. To stress the sacroiliac joint, the examiner places one hand on the flexed knee joint and the other hand on the anterior superior iliac spine of the opposite side. The examiner then presses down on these two points. If the patient complains of increased pain, there may be pathology in the sacroiliac joint.[13] Complaints of hip pain may indicate a sacroiliac joint problem. Another commonly used provocative test is the Gaenslen's test. The patient lies supine on the examination table and is asked to draw both legs onto his/ her chest. The patient then shifts to the side of the table so that one buttock extends over the side of the table while the other remains on it. The patient then drops his unsupported leg over the edge, while the other leg remains flexed. Complaints of pain in the area of the sacroiliac joint suggest pathology in that area.[13]

Diagnostic workup of the sacroiliac joint(s) includes x-rays, MRI, CT or bone scanning, the use of diagnostic steroid injections, or the application of a spica body cast. Conventional x-rays may demonstrate arthritic changes involving the sacroiliac joint. The arthritic changes may be further delineated using MRI, CT, or bone scanning techniques. CT scanning is particularly useful in evaluating this joint and it can be used to help guide intra-articular steroid injections. A bone scan performed early on after injury may demonstrate an acute bony or ligamentous sacroiliac joint injury. The radioactive isotope injected during the scan is drawn to any traumatized tissues.

Occasionally, a sacroiliac joint steroid injection can be both diagnostic and therapeutic. A selective steroid injection into the involved sacroiliac joint will help make the diagnosis of sacroiliac joint dysfunction if there is pain relief post injection. Once the steroids take effect, such an injection may provide long-lasting relief of pain. At the very least, the sacroiliac injection is helpful in determining if the joint is a pain generator. Another way of determining if there is a problem with the sacroiliac joint is to put the patient into a spica body cast. If there is chronic pelvic pain due to sacroiliac joint instability, the pain should be alleviated after the patient is placed in the body cast. The patient who benefits from spica body cast application may ultimately be a candidate for sacroiliac joint fusion.

The patient with a sacroiliac joint strain may benefit from conservative treatment including physical therapy and/or chiropractic. The patient with malalignment or subluxation of the sacroiliac joint will need to have mobilization of the joint performed. Deep heating modalities including ultrasound may help to reduce inflammation of the joint. Stretching of pelvic, back, and lower extremity musculature is followed by a series of pelvic stabilization exercises. Strong pelvic muscles will enhance stability of a joint compromised by a torn capsule.

The patient that fails to improve with conservative measures may require a series of steroid injections. The patient may also benefit from a sacroiliac joint belt, which winds around the pelvis providing stabilization of both sacroiliac joints. Analgesic medications (including opioids) may be required. A TENS unit may also prove helpful. If the patient continues to be highly symptomatic, he/she may need to proceed with surgery for a sacroiliac joint fusion.

Complications of chronic sacroiliac joint dysfunction include chronic joint pain, instability, referred lower extremity pain and sciatica like symptomatology. The patient may develop a chronic limp that will alter body mechanics, possibly contributing to more distant pain problems.

Piriformis Syndrome

The piriformis muscle originates from the sacrum and inserts onto the greater trochanter of the femur (see Figure 6-17). Under this muscle passes the sciatic nerve. If this muscle goes into chronic spasm, the patient may develop sciatica-like symptomatology. Pelvic injuries after a motor vehicle accident may contribute to the development of a piriformis syndrome. The patient with piriformis syndrome complains of severe gluteal pain that radiates in a radicular fashion into the involved extremity. There may be paresthesias or numbness in the involved extremity. The pain typically worsens with weightbearing activities and prolonged sitting.

On examination, there will be tenderness with palpation of the piriformis muscle. The supine patient with piriformis syndrome will experience increased pain if the involved leg is externally rotated against resistance or with passive internal rotation (the piriformis muscle is an external rotator of the leg). These maneuvers increase pressure between the two heads of the piriformis muscle, thereby increasing symptomatology. Lower extremity neurological examination is usually normal. However, the patient may have a subjective decrease in pinprick sensation, often in a nonanatomic stocking-like distribution.

Since the piriformis muscle is a soft tissue structure, diagnostic imaging workup tends to be unrevealing. However, a steroid/anesthetic injection into the involved piriformis muscle may provide diagnostic information. If the patient obtains relief with the injection, it suggests that the piriformis muscle is a focus of pain. The injection may also have some therapeutic value.

Conservative treatment of piriformis syndrome includes physical therapy to loosen up the tight piriformis muscle. This may require massage and deep heating modalities such as ultrasound. The patient should be given a piriformis-stretching program to be performed both at the clinic and at home. If the patient fails to improve, they may benefit from one or a series of piriformis injections utilizing anesthetic and steroids. Analgesics may be necessary if the pain is severe. A TENS unit may also be helpful. Complications of piriformis syndrome include ongoing chronic hip and lower extremity discomfort that could alter body mechanics, causing distant pain problems.

Myofascial Pain Syndrome

The patient who strains their low back and pelvis may develop a localized myofascial pain syndrome (MPS). Pelvic muscles that may be involved include the gluteus medius and maximus, piriformis, tensa fasciae latae, and the iliopsoas. The patient with pelvic MPS will complain of pelvic and/or low back discomfort, which increases with change of position, bending, range of motion, and walking.

On physical examination, the involved musculature will be tender to palpation. There may be associated spasm and trigger points identified. The tight muscles will produce limitations in range of motion of the low back and hip joint(s). Involvement of the gluteal and piriformis muscles cause posterior pelvic pain whereas psoas spasm will result in groin and anterior thigh pain. Spasm of the tensa fascia lata typically causes discomfort along the side of the leg. Diagnostic imaging workup (x-rays, MRI, CT and bone scanning) tends to be unrevealing for this soft tissue condition.

Treatment for the myofascial pain syndrome includes physical therapy for massage, modalities, and initiation of a stretching and strengthening program for the involved musculature. The patient should be instructed on a home exercise program, which needs to be performed regularly. Some patients benefit from one or a series of trigger point injections into the involved musculature. Formal massage therapy, trial of a TENS unit, and medications (muscle relaxants, analgesics, and anti-inflammatories) may also help promote recovery.

Complications of pelvic MPS include chronic muscular discomfort with functional limitations. There may be an alteration of normal body mechanics that can affect regions distant from the pelvis.

Pelvic Floor Strain

The female patient with a severe strain of pelvic floor musculature may develop problems with maintaining urinary continence. The pelvic floor muscles form a sling that extends across the bottom of the bony pelvis (Figure 6-18). Through it passes the anal canal and the urethra. A loss of strength or integrity of these muscles can result in varying degrees of stress urinary incontinence. The history will suggest the development of stress incontinence (urinary leakage with exertion) occurring within a reasonable time frame after a motor vehicle accident. A history of having had a traumatic or multiple vaginal deliveries may predispose the individual to develop this problem.

The typical musculoskeletal and neurological examination performed by most clinicians after a motor vehicle accident is inadequate to determine the cause of a patient's incontinence. Usually, the patient needs to be referred to a urologist for a more complete physical and urodynamic workup. The urodynamic workup may include urine flow studies, cystometrogram, and video urodynamics. These studies will demonstrate whether the incontinence is due to weakness of pelvic floor musculature.

Treatment for pelvic floor weakness associated with incontinence includes physical therapeutic modalities. Pelvic muscle strengthening exercise programs are available. The most commonly known exercises are known as Kegel exercises whereby the female patient actively attempts to contract pelvic floor and vaginal musculature in an effort to strengthen those muscles. There are also electrical stimulation and biofeedback techniques available to strengthen the weakened muscles. This type of therapy usually requires the assistance of a therapist or nurse who is specially trained in this area.

If the patient fails to improve with conservative treatment measures, they may benefit from medications (alpha adrenergic agents) that strengthen contraction of the urinary

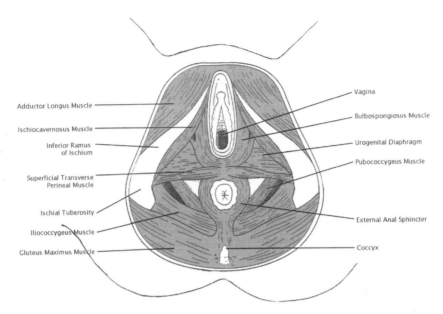

Figure 6-18 The pelvic floor muscles (pelvic diaphragm) extend from the anterior to the posterior aspects of the bony pelvis, forming a sling that supports the pelvic contents. The urethra, vagina, and anal canal perforate the pelvic diaphragm. Reprinted by permission from Rook JL. Anatomy of the urinary system. In Rook JL, Weiss LD, Hagler DD (eds). *Skin Care Triad—Continence Management, Wound Care, and Therapeutic Positioning*, p 25 (fig 1.20). Oxford, Elsevier Science Ltd, 2000.

sphincter muscles. As a last resort, there are a variety of urological surgical procedures available to strengthen the sphincter mechanism. A description of these procedures is beyond the scope of this text. Complications of weakened pelvic floor musculature include chronic incontinence, which predisposes the patient to develop urinary tract infections and/or skin breakdown.

LUMBAR RADICULOPATHY

Lower extremity pain may occur as a consequence of lumbar pathology, which causes nerve irritation or damage. Lumbosacral nerve roots can be adversely affected by degenerative processes involving vertebrae or intervertebral discs.

Lumbar Anatomy

Five lumbar vertebrae seat themselves upon the sacrum. Each lumbar vertebra has an anterior solid portion known as the vertebral body and a posterior bony vertebral arch. The posterior arrangement helps to protect the spinal cord and its nerve roots. The vertebral body serves as a weightbearing structure.

Two adjacent vertebrae in the lumbar region form a "functional unit" characterized by a three-joint complex.[15] The first joint, the intervertebral disc, exhibits minimal motion. In contrast, the two posterior facet joints are articulating synovial joints connecting facets of the superior and inferior vertebrae of the functional unit. Movement occurs at the lumbar facet joints in four planes, flexion, extension, and side bending to the left and right.

There are a number of ligaments that add stability to the lumbar spine including the anterior and posterior longitudinal ligaments, ligamentum flavum, and the interspinous ligaments. The anterior longitudinal ligament resides anterior to the vertebral bodies and the intervertebral discs. The posterior longitudinal ligament extends along the posterior surface of the vertebral bodies and their discs. The ligamentum flavum lines the posterior vertebral arch, and the interspinous ligaments connect adjacent spinous processes. All of these ligaments provide stability to the lumbar spine. Stability is also maintained due to the orientation of facet joints, their joint capsules, and the strength of both abdominal and lumbar paraspinal musculature.

The spinal cord terminates at approximately the T12 vertebral level. Caudal to this point are the lumbar and sacral nerve roots which course for a distance before exiting from their respective neuroforamina. This region of the spinal cord is known as the "cauda equina," a Greek phrase for "horse's tail." In the lumbar region, the nerve roots exit the neuroforamen above the level of the vertebra for which it is named. For example, the S1 nerve root exits from the neuroforamina formed by the L5 and S1 vertebra. This is in contrast to the cervical nerve roots that exit below the vertebra for which they are named.

The lumbar-sacral nerve roots coalesce in the pelvis to form the pelvic plexus, which rearranges itself to form the sciatic, femoral, and obturator nerves (Figure 6-19). The sciatic nerve branches into the peroneal and tibial nerves. The spinal nerve roots that make up the sciatic nerve run from L4 through S3. The upper lumbar nerve roots (L2–L4) coalesce to form the femoral and obturator nerves.

Each lumbar spinal nerve supplies distinct muscles, although several different nerve roots may supply a single muscle (Table 6-1). For example, the quadriceps, a rather large muscle, receives its innervation from the L2, L3, and L4 lumbar nerve roots. The tibialis anterior receives its innervation from L4 and L5, although it is principally an L4 innervated muscle. The extensor hallucis longus is innervated by L5 and S1, although it is principally innervated by L5. The motor supply of a nerve root is known as a myotome. Likewise, there are sensory dermatomes in each lower extremity (Figure 6-20). These represent a particular region of skin supplied by the sensory portion of a lumbosacral nerve root. Knowing the dermatomes and myotomes will help the clinician distinguish which lumbosacral nerve is being compromised in a lumbosacral radiculopathy.

The clinical presentation of the patient with lower extremity pain due to a lumbar radiculopathy may vary. Classically, the lower extremity discomfort is described as a lancinating, electrical or shooting-type pain. The patient may complain of numbness in a particular dermatome distribution (corresponding to the nerve root involved with the radiculopathy). There may be weakness of lower extremity musculature characterized by dragging of the foot or buckling of the knee. With a severe impingement involving the L4 or L5 nerve root, the patient may develop a frank foot drop due to weakness or paralysis of the foot dorsiflexor muscles. There may also be bowel or bladder dysfunction as the autonomic nerve supply to these structures travel through the lumbosacral nerve roots.

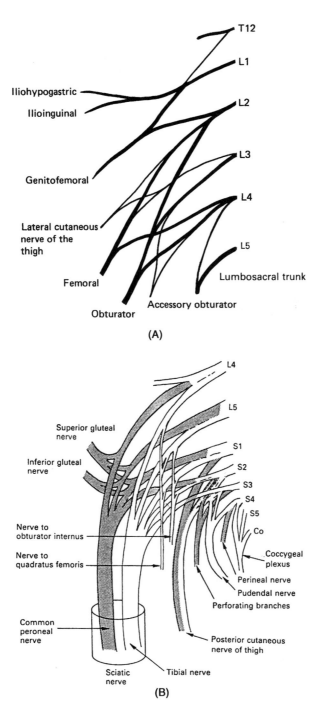

(A)

(B)

Figure 6-19 Diagram to show the formation of (A) the lumbar plexus and (B) the lumbosacral plexus. Reprinted by permission from Palastanga N, Field D, Soames R (eds). *Anatomy and Human Movement—Structure and Function*, 3rd ed. p 555 (fig 4.158). Oxford, Elsevier Science Ltd, 1998.

Table 6-1 Lower extremity muscles and their nerve root innervation

Muscle	Nerve Root(s)
Iliopsoas	L2, L3, L4
Quadriceps:	L2 ,L3, L4
Rectus femoris	
Vastus lateralis	
Vastus medialis	
Gluteus medius	L4, L5, S1
Gluteus maximus	L5, S1, S2
Hamstrings:	L5, S1, S2
Biceps femoris (short head)	
Semitendinosus	
Semimembranosus	
Tibialis anterior	L4, L5
Extensor hallucis longus	L5, S1
Peroneus longus	L5, S1
Peroneus brevis	L5, S1
Gastrocnemius	S1, S2
Soleus	S1, S2
Foot Intrinsics	S1, S2

The development of muscle paralysis or bowel or bladder dysfunction represents a neurosurgical emergency necessitating urgent decompression of the involved nerve root(s).

The patient with lower extremity pain due to a suspected radiculopathy must undergo an appropriate neurological examination including testing of lower extremity motor strength, sensation and reflexes. The straight leg raising test is commonly used to delineate nerve root impingement and is designed to reproduce back and leg pain so that its cause can be determined. The test is performed with the patient lying supine on the examination table. The examiner lifts the patient's leg upward while supporting his foot around the calcaneus. The patient's knee should remain straight. Hamstring pain involves only the posterior thigh, whereas sciatic pain can extend all the way down the leg.[13]

Manual motor testing should be performed on all major lower extremity muscle groups including dorsi and plantar flexors of the foot, the knee flexor and extensor muscles, and the hip flexion, extension, abduction, and adduction muscles. Various nerve roots in the lumbosacral region supply all of these muscles. Sensation is assessed for pinprick and light touch in all sensory dermatomes in both lower extremities.

Reflex testing includes assessment of the knee jerks (L2, L3, L4), ankle jerks (S1), and the tibialis posterior reflexes (L5). The bulbocavernous reflex or "anal wink" reflex test is reserved for those patients suspected of having a sacral nerve root lesion (S1 through S3). These patients typically have pelvic floor weakness and may have bowel or bladder incontinence. To perform the bulbocavernous reflex, a gloved index finger is inserted into the patient's anal canal while the other hand taps or compresses the glans penis in the

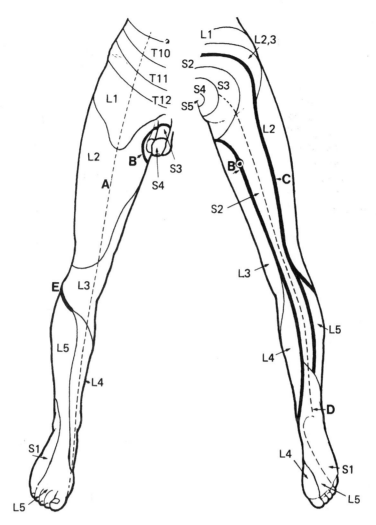

Figure 6-20 Dermatomes of the lower limb. A = Preaxial border; B = Ventral axial line; C = Dorsal axial line; D = Postaxial border; E = Extension from dorsal axial line. Reprinted by permission from Palastanga N, Field D, Soames R (eds). *Anatomy and Human Movement—Structure and Function*, 3rd ed. p 567 (fig 4.164). Oxford, Elsevier Science Ltd, 1998.

male or the clitoris in the female. Normally, there will be a reflexive contraction of the anal sphincter (anal wink) around the examiner's index finger. Absence of this reflex suggests a sacral nerve root lesion.

The straight leg-raising test can be performed with the patient supine or sitting. For the sitting straight leg raising, the examiner lifts the patient's respective extremity from a flexed knee to a knee extension position. This brings the leg close to a 90 degree angle to the body. If the patient feels shooting pain down the lifted extremity this would constitute a positive straight leg raising test, possibly consistent with a lumbar-sacral radiculopathy.

The procedure is repeated on the contralateral side. This test can also be performed with the patient lying supine by lifting one leg at a time. Some patients complain simply of back pain or hamstring tightness while performing the straight leg raising. This may be an indication of a mechanical back problem or tight hamstring musculature as opposed to an acute lumbosacral radiculopathy.

As noted above, bowel and/or bladder dysfunction may occur as a result of a lumbosacral radiculopathy. The nerve supply to the bladder emanates from spinal cord segments T10 through L2 and S1 through S3. Aside from the motor and sensory fibers, nerve roots in the cauda equina carry autonomic nerve fibers of both the sympathetic and parasympathetic nervous system to innervate the bladder, colon and pelvic floor (Figure 6-21). Lumbar pathology that compresses nerve rootlets, particularly sacral nerve rootlets, may cause damage to the neural supply to these structures. This could result in incontinence.

The workup for lumbar radiculopathy includes imaging techniques, electrophysiologic studies, urodynamic studies (for suspected bladder dysfunction), and selective nerve root blocks. Electrodiagnostic studies include nerve conduction studies (NCVs), electromyography, and somatosensory evoked potentials. With significant nerve root damage, there may be abnormalities both on nerve conduction testing and needle electromyography corresponding to the damaged root(s). For example, EMG of an L5 radiculopathy, may demonstrate denervation potentials involving the tibialis anterior, tibialis posterior, and extensor hallucis longus muscles. With an S1 radiculopathy, there may be abnormalities seen in the posterior calf musculature. However, occasionally, motor nerve roots are spared by the radiculopathy as the patient has irritation or damage principally to sensory nerve rootlet(s). In such cases, somatosensory evoked potentials (SSEPs) may prove useful as they principally measure conduction of electrical impulses along sensory nerve pathways.

For patients with bladder dysfunction, there are a number of urodynamic studies available that can be used to determine if neurological damage is contributing to the dysfunction. These studies include urine flow studies, cystometry, the urethral pressure profile, and video fluoroscopic evaluation of the lower urinary tract.

Conventional x-rays may demonstrate bony abnormalities that are causing nerve root impingement. For example, neuroforaminal narrowing or posterior vertebral body osteophytes (bone spurs) may indicate a source of impingement. Flexion and extension x-rays can be obtained to demonstrate whether or not instability in the low back is contributing to spinal canal or lateral recess stenosis and radiculopathy. A myelogram is performed by injecting dye into the spinal canal and allowing it to travel throughout the lumbar region. The dye is radiopaque and will appear as bright white on x-rays. Any disc material or abnormal bone formation impinging upon a nerve root will be outlined as a lucent area within the radiopaque background. The myelogram procedure is more physiologic than MRI or CT scanning in that it can be performed with the patient upright, rather than while the patient is supine (a position often not associated with radicular symptoms).[16]

More sensitive spinal imaging studies include MRI and CT scanning. With these techniques, cross sectional images are taken through each lumbar disc demonstrating soft tissue abnormalities, which cannot be demonstrated on conventional x-rays. These imaging studies will demonstrate herniated discs, swollen nerve roots, distorted thecal sacs, and compressed nerve rootlets (Figure 6-22).

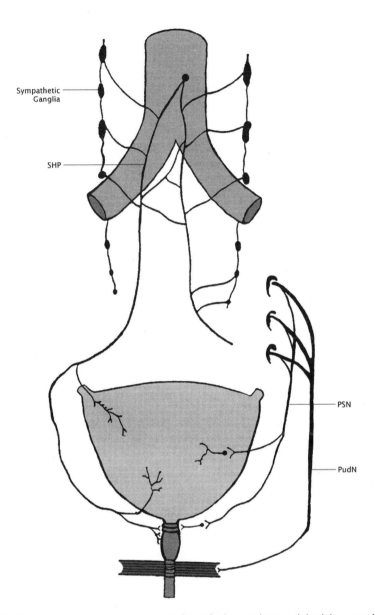

Figure 6-21 The afferent nerve supply of the urinary bladder and sphincter includes the sympathetic and parasympathetic outflow, and the somatic fibers. The sympathetic fibers travel along the superior hypogastric plexus (SHP) to the bladder and bladder outlet. The parasympathetic fibers travel through the pelvic splachnic nerve (PSN) to the same structures. The preganglionic parasympathetic fibers synapse with short postganglionic fibers located near the innervated structure. The somatic lower motor neuron fibers originate in the sacral spinal cord and travel via the pudendal nerve (PudN) to the external sphincter and pelvic floor. Reprinted by permission from Rook JL. Anatomy of the urinary system. In Rook JL, Weiss LD, Hagler DD (eds). *Skin Care Triad—Continence Management, Wound Care, and Therapeutic Positioning* p 38 (fig 2.8). Oxford, Elsevier Science Ltd, 2000.

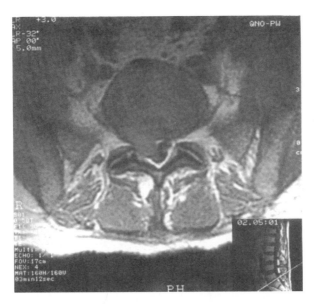

Figure 6-22 MRI scan through the level of the disc between L5 and S1 showing a large protrusion, compressing the nerve root on the right. Reprinted by permission from Osselton JW, Binnie CD, Cooper R, *et al* (eds). *Clinical Neurophysiology—Electromyography, Nerve Conduction and Evoked Potentials* (fig 2.6.26). Boston: Butterworth-Heinemann, 1995.

Lastly, important information concerning potential nerve compression can be obtained from selective nerve blocks or epidural steroid injections. Selective nerve blocks are performed by trained personal and require fluoroscopic guidance. The suspected injured nerve rootlet is identified fluoroscopically following which an anesthetic is infiltrated into the region. If the patient gets excellent pain relief after the injection, it suggests that the injected nerve rootlet is damaged or inflamed. This then becomes a diagnostic procedure. If steroids are also infused along with the anesthetic, and if the patient obtains long-term relief, then the injection becomes therapeutic. With a lumbar epidural steroid injection, the patient with radiculitis and/or radiculopathy may experience an overall decrease in pain as the steroids reduce inflammation about the damaged or irritated nerve root(s). This is also indicative of a nerve root problem, but it is a less sensitive diagnostic procedure than selective nerve root blocks.

Treatment for lumbosacral radiculopathy includes conservative measures, semi-invasive measures, and surgical procedures. Physical therapy should include abdominal and back strengthening exercises. Lumbar traction may relieve pressure on an impinged nerve root. Modalities (massage, ultrasound, hot packs, cold packs, electrical stimulation) can be used to treat reactive muscle spasm associated with the radicular process. In conjunction with the therapy, some form of anti-inflammatory should be utilized. Oral anti-inflammatories can be tried but may be associated with GI side effects. A short course of oral steroids such as a Medrol Dosepak may help reduce inflammation associated with a suspected radiculopathy. Steroids are potent anti-inflammatories and a short course of low dose treatment is usually well tolerated.

Chiropractic treatment may also prove helpful for the patient with lumbar radiculo-pathy. A home exercise program including lower extremity and back stretches, and abdominal strengthening exercises should be continued for a period of time after symptoms resolve or diminish.

If the patient fails to improve, and if there is no frank neurological damage evident, a trial of lumbar epidural steroid injection(s) are usually the next step. The steroids are injected into the epidural space where they exert a potent localized anti-inflammatory effect. Occasionally, a series of two or three injections is necessary before patients achieve optimal improvement in radicular symptomatology. Intermittent blocks may subsequently be required. Other medications may be necessary during the acute phase of a radiculopathy including opioid analgesics and medications to diminish neurogenic pain (mexiletine, anticonvulsants, clonidine and tricyclic antidepressants). Trial of a TENS unit may prove helpful.

The patient who has chronic bladder dysfunction may require medications to improve the integrity of the pelvic floor and sphincter, or to improve contraction of bladder musculature. Such medications are available and are usually prescribed by a urologist.

If the patient fails to improve with conservative and semi-invasive measures, then he or she may be a candidate for surgery. The most commonly performed procedure is the lumbar laminectomy with discectomy. More extensive procedures (such as spinal fusion) may be necessary depending on the degree of disc derangement. Most patients have good outcomes from laminectomy procedures. Occasionally, a patient will develop chronic radicular symptoms with ongoing lower extremity discomfort that has a neurogenic quality (burning pain, paresthesias, hypersensitivity). These patients may require ongoing analgesics or medications to decrease neurogenic pain.

REFERENCES

1. Cailliet R. Structural anatomy. In Cailliet R (ed). *Foot and Ankle Pain*. Philadelphia, F.A. Davis Company, 1985.
2. Hoppenfeld S. Physical examination of the foot and ankle. In Hoppenfeld S (ed). *Physical Examination of the Spine and Extremities*. Norwalk, CT, Appleton-Century-Crofts, 1976.
3. Pecina MM, Krmpotic-Nemanic J, Markiewitz AD. Tarsal tunnel syndrome. In Pecina MM, Krmpotic-Nemanic J, Markiewitz AD (eds). *Tunnel Syndromes*. Boca Raton, CRC Press, 1991.
4. Cailliet R. Injuries to the ankle. In Cailliet R (ed). *Foot and Ankle Pain*. Philadelphia, F.A. Davis Company, 1985.
5. Dawson DM, Hallett M, Millender LH. Tarsal tunnel syndromes. In Dawson DM, Hallett M, Millender LH (eds). *Entrapment Neuropathies*. Boston, Little, Brown & Company, 1990.
6. Hoppenfeld S. Physical examination of the knee. In Hoppenfeld S (ed). *Physical Examination of the Spine and Extremities*. Norwalk, CT, Appleton-Century-Crofts, 1976.
7. Kruger T, Wohlrab D, Birke A, Hein W. Results of arthroscopic joint debridement in different stages of chondromalacia of the knee joint. *Arch Orthop Trauma Surg* 2000; 120(5–6): 338.
8. Lecas LK, Helms CA, Kosarek FJ, Garret WE. Inferiorly displaced flap tears of the medial meniscus: MR appearance and clinical significance. *AJR Am J Roentgenology*; 174: 161.
9. Van de Berg BC, Lecouvet FE, Duchateau F, *et al.* Lesions of the menisci of the knee: value of MR imaging criteria for recognition of unstable lesions. *AJR Am J Roentgenology* March 2001; 176: 771-776.

10. Van de Berg BC, Lecouvet FE, Poilvache P, *et al.* Dual-detector spiral CT arthrography of the knee: accuracy for detection of meniscal abnormalities and unstable meniscal tears. *Radiology* 2000; 216(3): 851.

11. Koski JA, Ibarra C, Rodeo SA, Warren RF. Meniscal injury and repair: clinical status. *Orthop Clin North Am* 2000; 31:(3). 419.

12. Macnicol MF. Thomas NP. The knee after meniscectomy. *J Bone Joint Surg Br* 2000; 82-B(2):157.

13. Hoppenfeld S. Physical examination of the lumbar spine. In Hoppenfeld S (ed). *Physical Examination of the Spine and Extremities*, pp 237-264. Norwalk, CT, Appleton-Century-Crofts, 1976.

14. Moore KL. The perineum and pelvis. In Moore KL (ed). *Clinically Oriented Anatomy*. Baltimore, Williams & Wilkins, 1988.

15. Cailliet R. Low back pain. In Cailliet R (ed). *Soft Tissue Pain and Disability*, p 49. Philadelphia, F.A. Davis Company, 1988.

16. Botwin KP, Skene G, Torres-Ramos FM, *et al.* Role of weightbearing and flexion and extension myelography in evaluating the intervertebral disc. *Am J Physical Med Rehabil* 2001; 80(4): 289.

7

Spine Pain

Jack L Rook

ANATOMY

The human spine has five distinct segments including the cervical, thoracic, lumbar, sacral, and coccygeal regions. The cervical spine consists of eight vertebrae normally aligned in a lordotic curvature. The thoracic vertebrae, 12 in number, articulate with ribs, have limited motion, and with normal posture have a kyphotic curvature. There are five lumbar vertebrae, larger in size than the cervical and thoracic, as they have a major weight-bearing function. The normal lumbar spine has a lordotic curvature (Figure 7-1).

The lowest or most caudal spinal segments are fused vertebrae known as the sacrum and coccyx. The sacrum is a major weight-bearing bone and a principal component of the pelvis. Nerve roots pass through foremena within the sacrum. Although the human coccyx does not serve any function, it can be a source of significant discomfort if fractured or when its sacrococcygeal ligaments are strained. (See Figure 6-16.)

Range of motion is achieved at all non-fused vertebral levels (cervical, thoracic and lumbar). The greatest motion occurs in the cervical region when the vertebrae are oriented in such a way as to achieve six planes of motion (flexion, extension, right and left rotation and right and left lateral flexion). In contrast to the cervical region, thoracic vertebrae have the least movement, principally due to rib attachments, which limit vertebral motion. The principal motions of the thoracic region are flexion and rotation. Lumbar vertebrae permit four ranges including flexion, extension, and lateral bending from side to side. There is no movement within the sacrum or coccyx.

The Vertebrae

Each vertebra from C3 through the sacrum has a characteristic shape which includes an anterior weightbearing portion and a posterior arch that is designed to protect the spinal cord. As we move from the base of the skull to the pelvis, each vertebral body enlarges in size, as it is required to bear more weight.

The anterior vertebral body is designed for weightbearing. It is an oval shaped bone with flattened superior and inferior surfaces. To these flat sides attach fibers of

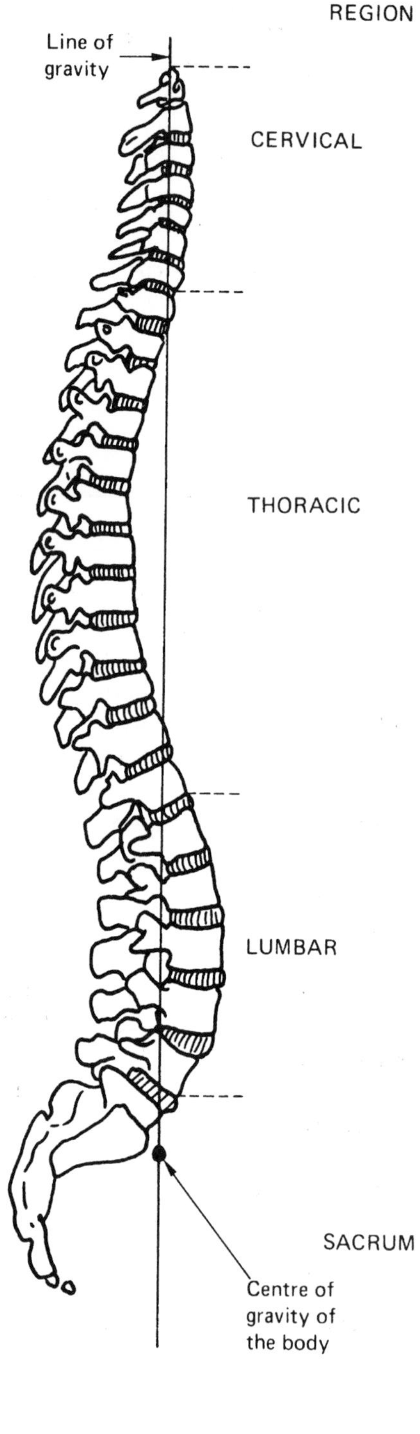

REGION

Figure 7-1 Adult vertebral column, lateral view. Reprinted by permission from Palastanga N, Field D, Soames R (eds). *Anatomy and Human Movement—Structure and Function*, 3rd ed. p 585 (fig 5.3). Oxford, Elsevier Science Ltd, 1998.

the intervertebral discs. The bone of the vertebral body is quite dense particularly along its sides and endplates adjacent to the intervertebral discs. It is richly innervated by blood vessels and nerves, and therefore, can be a source of pain when traumatized or fractured.

The vertebral arch extends posteriorly from the vertebral body. Components of vertebral arches include pedicles, lamina, spinous processes, neural foramen, the pars interarticularis, and the facet joints. The pedicles extend posteriorly from the vertebral body. Superior and inferior to the pedicles pass spinal nerves. The pedicles branch out to form the transverse spinous processes and further extend posteriorly as the lamina of the vertebral arch. Another spinous process extends dorsally, and in thin individuals can be seen and readily palpated (Figure 7-2). The pars interarticularis refers to the bony region between the superior and inferior facet joints. It is a potential site of fracture, known as a spondylolysis.

The Intervertebral Disc

Between each vertebra is an intervertebral disc (IVD). It functions as a shock absorber for the vertebral bones above and below it. The IVD has two principal components, an outer fibrous layer and a jelly-like central portion (nucleus pulposus). The outer portion is known as the annulus fibrosis. It is composed of numerous thin collagen layers arranged concentrically, each layer composed of tightly bound collagen fibers oriented in a particular direction. The collagen fibers attach from the periphery of one vertebral body and pass obliquely at a 30 degree angle connecting to the endplate of the adjacent vertebral body.[1] The next annular sheet has its fibers running at a 30 degree angle in the opposite direction (Figure 7-3). There are numerous concentric layers (lamellae) composing each annulus fibrosis that surround the inner nucleus pulposus. The nucleus pulposus is a centrally located, well hydrated mass of reticular and collagenous fibers embedded in mucoid material. In young adults the water content of the nucleus pulposus is about 88 percent and their fullness, or turgor, is great.[2] The nucleus pulposus is normally well contained within the annular envelope and between adjacent vertebral endplates (Figure 7-4).

The disc functions in a "hydrodynamic" fashion. Downward pressure against the nucleus pulposus (due to weightbearing) causes it to exert outward forces against the annulus fibrosis. However, the nucleus maintains its shape because of the inward pressure exerted by an intact annulus fibrosis. This phenomenon contributes to the shock absorber function of the intervertebral disc.

The oblique arrangement of collagen fibers within layers of the annulus fibrosis provides for a limited degree of flexibility for the intervertebral disc. This movement allows some distortion of the nucleus pulposus so that it can better serve as a shock absorber between the respective vertebral bodies.[1]

If an external stressor causes excessive movement between two adjacent vertebrae, beyond what its annular fibers are capable of handling, there will be a tearing of annular fibers, loss of integrity of the intervertebral disc, and the loss of its ability to function as a shock absorber. Two adjacent vertebrae and the intervening IVD are referred to as the "functional unit."[1]

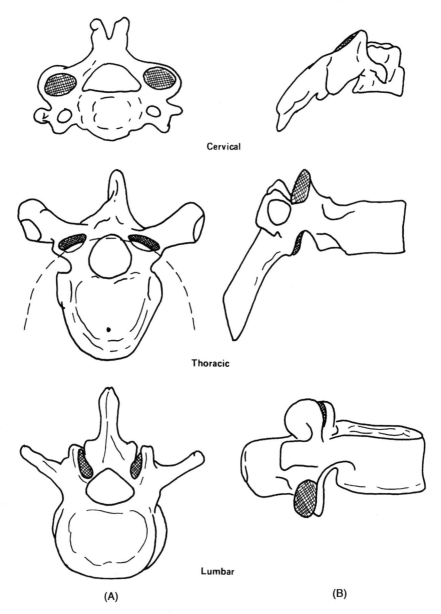

Cervical

Thoracic

Lumbar

(A)   (B)

Figure 7-2 Cervical, thoracic and lumbar vertebral bodies: (A) from above; (B) lateral view. Reprinted by permission from Palastanga N, Field D, Soames R (eds). *Anatomy and Human Movement—Structure and Function*, 3rd ed. p 647 (fig 5.35). Oxford, Elsevier Science Ltd, 1998.

There are notable differences between the cervical and lumbar intervertebral discs and vertebrae (Figure 7-5). In the cervical region the nucleus pulposus is anteriorly displaced and the annular fibers are more prominent posteriorly. The posterior longitudinal ligament is broad. Lastly, there are two bony protuberances on the superior endplate of each

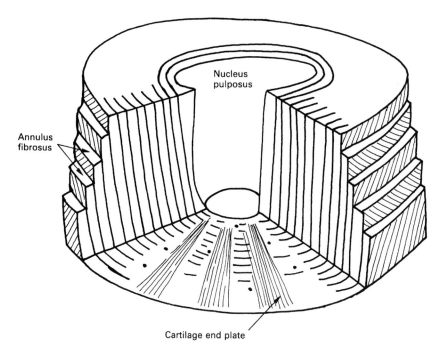

Figure 7-3 The intervertebral disc has two principal components, an outer fibrous layer and a jelly-like central portion (nucleus pulposus). The outer portion is known as the annulus fibrosis. It is composed of numerous thin collagen layers arranged concentrically. The collagen fibers attached from the periphery of one vertebral body. The next annular sheet has its fibers running at a 30 degree angle connecting to the end plate of the adjacent vertebral body. The next annular sheet has its fibers running at a 30 degree angle in the opposite direction. Reprinted by permission from Palastanga N, Field D, Soames R (eds). *Anatomy and Human Movement—Structure and Function*, 3rd ed. p 637 (fig 5.29a). Oxford, Elsevier Science Ltd, 1998.

cervical vertebra known as uncovertebral joints. This anatomical arrangement is designed to protect the cervical region from posterior and posterolateral disc herniation.

In contrast, the nucleus pulposus in the lumbar region has a more central location and the annular fibers are organized more evenly in a circular fashion. There's no additional bone such as the uncovertebral joints to protect the lumbosacral spinal cord. Lastly, the posterior longitudinal ligament, which is broad in the cervical region (for additional posterior protection) tapers in the lumbar region. Disc herniation with neurological impairment is more likely to occur in the lumbar region because of these differences.[3] (See Figure 7-5)

Spinal Ligaments

A number of spinal ligaments help maintain the integrity and normal orientation of the vertebrae. Alignment of the spinal canal is maintained by the intervertebral disc, anterior and posterior longitudinal ligaments, the interspinous ligaments, and the ligamentum

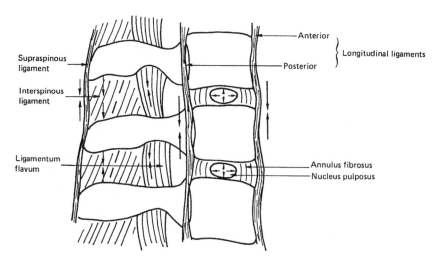

Figure 7-4 The nucleus pulposus is normally well contained within the annular envelope and between adjacent vertebral endplates. Reprinted by permission from Palastanga N, Field D, Soames R (eds). *Anatomy and Human Movement— Structure and Function*, 3rd ed. p 661 (fig 5.43b). Oxford, Elsevier Science Ltd, 1998.

flavum. Anterior to spinal vertebrae is the broad anterior longitudinal ligament. This ligament covers the anterior surface of the vertebral bodies and its fibers fuse with the anterior outer layer of each annulus fibrosis. It has limited flexibility. Thus, the anterior longitudinal ligament limits anterior translation of the spinal vertebrae and reinforces the anterior annulus of the disc.

The posterior longitudinal ligament covers the posterior aspect of all vertebral bodies and joins with the outer posterior layer of the intervertebral disc. It is broad in the cervical region and tapers in the lumbar spine, providing less protection and support at that level.

The ligamentum flavum is an elastic tissue that lines the posterior vertebral arch. Because of its elasticity, it does not contribute any significant stability to the spinal column. Lastly, ligaments that extend between the posterior spinous processes of the spine are known as the interspinous ligaments. They provide further stability to the respective spinal segments.

The Facet Joints

The functional unit of the spine includes two adjacent vertebrae and the interposed IVD. The spinal functional unit is a three-joint complex with the intervertebral disc representing one of the joints. This type of joint is known as a *synarthrosis*. Very little movement occurs within a synarthrosis. However, the two posterior joints, known as the facet joints, are synovial joints that have a good deal of motion. A synovial joint is characterized by two articulating surfaces that are lined by cartilage and connected to each other by ligaments or a capsule. Synovial joints are lubricated by synovial fluid that is produced by synovial tissues within the joint.

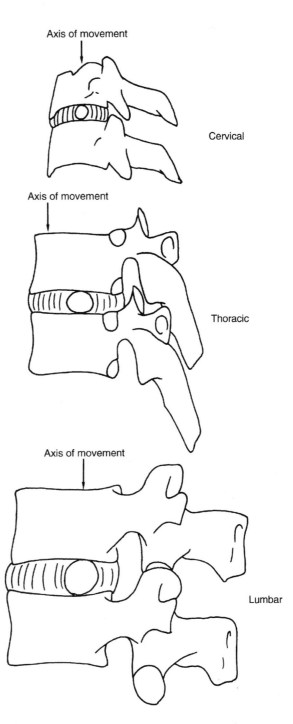

Axis of movement

Cervical

Axis of movement

Thoracic

Axis of movement

Lumbar

Figure 7-5 There are notable differences between the cervical, thoracic and lumbar intervertebral discs and vertebrae. In the cervical region the annular fibers are more prominent posteriorly. The posterior longitudinal ligament is broad. There are bony protuberances on the superior endplate of each cervical vertebra (uncovertebral joints). Each thoracic vertebra is a five-joint complex (two facet joints, the intervertebral disc, and two articulating ribs). In contrast, in the lumbar region the annular fibers are thin posteriorly, there is no additional bone to protect the lumbosacral spinal cord, and the posterior longitudinal ligament tapers. Reprinted by permission from Palastanga N, Field D, Soames R (eds). *Anatomy and Human Movement—Structure and Function*, 3rd ed. p 639 (fig 5.30). Oxford, Elsevier Science Ltd, 1998.

Posterior facet joints are located throughout the spine. They are formed by superior and inferior extensions of adjacent vertebral arches. The facet joints normally bear little or no weight. The orientations of the facet joints help define the planes of motion characteristic of each spinal region. In the lumbar region, the facet joints have a vertical alignment. This joint orientation permits principally flexion and extension with limitation of lateral bending. In contrast, cervical facet joints have a more horizontal orientation, which allows for movement in six different planes (flexion, extension, side bending and rotation to either side).

The facet joints are reinforced by a capsule that surrounds the joint and affords it a certain degree of stability. With extreme motion of the spine due to trauma, there can be stretching and tearing of capsular fibers with loss of integrity of the joint, and the development of instability or premature arthritis.

BIOMECHANICS OF SPINAL INJURY

Normally, there is no appreciable horizontal movement occurring between the superior and inferior vertebral bodies of the functional unit. This is due to the arrangement of fibers in an intact annulus fibrosis, further reinforced by the anterior and posterior longitudinal ligaments, the interspinous ligaments and the surrounding paravertebral musculature. There is a certain amount of spinal flexibility achieved despite this spinal arrangement due to the orientation of the facet joints in each spinal region. However, excessive forces, such as those generated in a motor vehicle accident, can stress and tear ligamentous fibers contributing to spinal pain and instability.

The flexibility of the annulus fibrosis is permitted by the angulation of the fibers forming each annular sheet. As noted above, the individual fibers that make up each circumferential sheet of the annulus have a specific orientation, 30 degrees from the vertical. Each successive row of the annulus has its fibrils oriented at a 30 degree angle either to the right or to the left.[1] This arrangement allows for controlled movement within the disc including flexion, extension, and shear/torque movements.

The fibrils of each annulus extend from the inferior endplate of the cephalad vertebral body to the superior endplate of the vertebra below. Ligamentous fibers have a parallel organization that adds to their strength. Therefore, ligaments throughout the body are organized in such a way as to resist pulling. However, if the pulling forces to these structures become excessive, the individual fibers that make up the ligament can tear.

With excessive motion of annular collaginous fibers, there can be tearing of individual fibrils leading to loss of integrity of the intervertebral disc. With extreme flexion and/or extension of a functional unit there is stress placed on all layers of the annulus. With shear or torque (rotational) forces there is stretching of those fibrils oriented in the direction of shear, whereas the fibrils in adjacent lamina shorten.[1] Ultimately, the disc may bulge and the nucleus pulposus may protrude through tears created within the annular fibers. In addition, as the disc loses its shock absorber function, the adjacent vertebrae come into closer opposition, leading to other problems, which are discussed later.

Excessive flexion also causes opposition of the anterior portions of the superior and inferior vertebral bodies of the functional unit. This can lead to chip fractures or compression fractures of the respective vertebrae. Therefore, an excessive flexion injury may not only cause tearing of posterior annular fibers, but also can damage the vertebral body. In contrast, hyperextension may disrupt anterior annular fibers and will result in compression of the opposing facet joints causing cartilage damage or facet fractures.

THE CERVICAL SPINE

Cervical vertebral movement is more complicated then movement in the lumbar region. The first cervical vertebra (Atlas) articulates with the occiput of the skull (Figure 7-6). It has a distinct shape, as does the C2 vertebra (axis) (Figure 7-7). The remaining cervical vertebrae (C3 through C8) are similar in structure and function.

At the occipital-atlas articulation only flexion and extension can occur with 10 degrees of flexion and 25 degrees of extension from a neutral position. Between the atlas and axis (C1–C2), only rotation occurs. Approximately 45 degrees of rotation to either side, a total of 90 degrees, occurs just at this articulation. Therefore, the two uppermost cervical vertebrae account for 35 degrees of flexion-extension and 90 degrees of rotation.[3] No intervertebral discs exist at the occipital-atlas or the atlas-axis articulations. The remainder of the cervical vertebrae has the characteristic anatomy described above including the anterior vertebral body, the intervertebral disc, the bony posterior arch, and the facet joints.

The horizontal orientation of the C3 through C8 facet joints allows for six planes of cervical motion (flexion, extension, rotation, and side bending to either side). Anatomical variations found in the cervical region, which help protect the spinal cord, include the

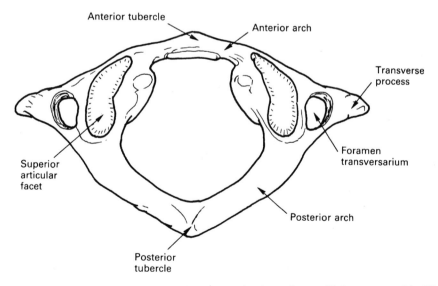

Figure 7-6 The Atlas. Reprinted by permission from Palastanga N, Field D, Soames R (eds). *Anatomy and Human Movement—Structure and Function*, 3rd ed. p 595 (fig 5.11). Oxford, Elsevier Science Ltd, 1998.

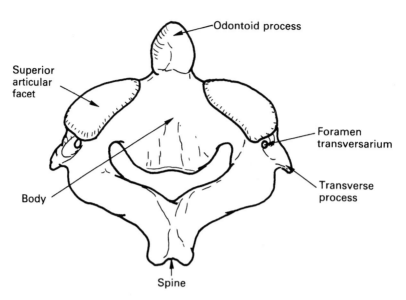

Figure 7-7 The Axis posterior view. Reprinted by permission from Palastanga N, Field D, Soames R (eds). *Anatomy and Human Movement—Structure and Function*, 3rd ed. p 595 (fig 5.10), Oxford, Elsevier Science Ltd, 1998.

anteriorly located nucleus pulposus, the thicker arrangement of posterior annular fibers, the presence of the uncovertebral joints and the broad posterior longitudinal ligament. The posterior spinal arch protects and houses the spinal cord.

THE SPINAL CORD AND NERVE ROOTS

The brain and spinal cord make up the central nervous system (CNS). Within the CNS originate nerve fibers that control both voluntary and involuntary activities of the body. Voluntary activities include planned motion. Involuntary activities include bowel and bladder functioning, modulation of heart rate and blood pressure, gastrointestinal activity, glandular activity, sweating, sexual functioning, and pupillary constriction (meiosis). The spinal cord component of the CNS is a critical structure, which is why it is carefully protected by the vertebral bodies anteriorly and by the vertebral arch laterally and posteriorly. The spinal cord begins at the base of the brain and passes into the spine through a large opening in the skull, the foramen magnum. It is approximately 30 cm in length and it terminates at the T12–L1 vertebral bodies. At that level, the spinal cord tapers to a point known as the conus medullaris. From that point on, the remainder of the cord consists of elongated nerve roots, collectively termed the cauda equina (Greek for "horse's tail") (Figure 7-8).

The nerve roots exit the spinal cord at different levels that correspond to the cervical, thoracic, and lumbar vertebrae. In the cervical region, the C1 nerve root passes between the base of the skull and the atlas (C1). The C2 nerve root passes between the atlas (C1) and axis (C2) vertebrae. Therefore, in the cervical region, the cervical nerve roots

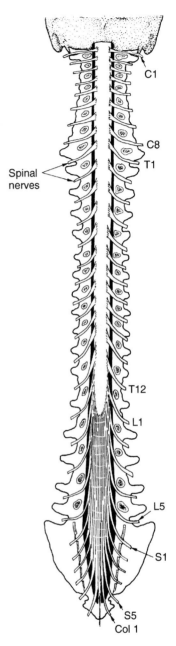

Figure 7-8 The spinal cord begins at the base of the brain. It is approximately 30 cm in length and it terminates at the T12–L1 vertebral bodies. At that level, the spinal cord tapers to a point known as the conus medullaris. From that point on, the remainder of the cord consists of elongated nerve roots, collectively termed the cauda equina. Reprinted by permission from Palastanga N, Field D, Soames R (eds). *Anatomy and Human Movement—Structure and Function*, 3rd ed. p 817 (fig 8.20a). Oxford, Elsevier Science Ltd, 1998.

are numbered based on the vertebrae immediately *below* it, except for the C8 nerve root, which exits immediately above the T1 vertebrae. This is because there are eight cervical nerve roots and seven cervical vertebrae. From C8–T1 caudally, the thoracic, lumbar, and sacral nerve roots are named based on the vertebrae immediately *above* them. For example, a nerve root that passes through the foramen at the L5–S1

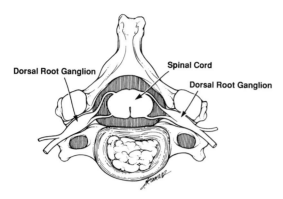

Figure 7-9 Cervical region, transverse section, showing the relationship of the spinal cord, spinal roots, and the dorsal root ganglia to the surrounding bone structures. The dorsal root ganglia are within the intervertebral foramina. Reprinted by permission from Brown WF, Bolton CF (eds). *Clinical Electromyography*, 2nd ed. (fig 7.10). Boston, Butterworth-Heinemann, 1993.

level would be the L5 nerve root. Understanding this arrangement is important when considering what nerve roots might be affected by disc pathology in the various spinal regions.

Each nerve root exits through a space known as the neural foramen. Between each functional unit, there are two neural foramina through which pass the right and left nerve roots corresponding to their respective level. The neural foramen is a space bounded superiorly and inferiorly by the pedicles of the functional unit, posteriorly by a facet joint, and anteriorly by the annulus fibrosis (Figure 7-9). Each nerve root passes a neuroforamen, and in the cervical and lumbar region, eventually coalesce to form the brachial and lumbosacral plexus, respectively. The brachial plexus is a cluster of nerve fibers formed from ipsilateral C3 through T1 spinal cord rootlets. These nerves further divide into individual nerves that enter the respective upper extremity. The lumbosacral plexus fibers separate to form the sciatic and femoral nerves that supply motor and sensory functions to the lower extremities.

Each sensory nerve that enters the dorsal horn of a spinal cord segment is composed of an anterior primary division (carrying sensory information from the ipsilateral extremity) and a posterior primary division (carrying sensory information from the bony spinal canal and posterior soft tissues). Collectively, the posterior primary divisions form a sensory nerve known as the recurrent nerve of Luschka. This nerve innervates pain sensitive structures in the spinal region.[1]

The tissue sites of the functional unit, which when injured, irritated, or inflamed are capable of transmitting nociceptive stimuli, include the anterior and posterior longitudinal ligaments, outer layers of the annulus fibrosis, dura of nerve roots, capsule of the facets, interspinous ligaments, and the posterior spinal erector muscles. The vertebral bodies have also been shown to be sites of pain in fractures and malignant invasion. Structures that are not considered to be pain sensitive include the inner portions of the intervertebral disc and the ligamentum flavum. The yellow ligamentum flavum is totally without nerve supply and is, therefore, insensitive.[1] The nucleus pulposus has no nerve supply and thus is essentially insensitive. Sensory end organs and unmyelinated nerve fibers have never been anatomically traced to the annular fibers either. Studies have suggested that sensory end organs have been located in the outer annular fibers, possibly representing an invasion of sensory end organs from the anterior and posterior longitudinal ligaments. The presence of these nerves in the periphery of the annulus is the basis for "disc pain."[1]

The anterior and posterior longitudinal ligaments are copiously supplied with end organs of unmyelinated and myelinated nerve fibers from the recurrent nerve of Luschka. Clinically, these long ligaments have been shown to be sites of low back pain when irritated chemically or mechanically.[1] The sheaths of nerve roots (dura) within the foramena are also amply supplied by branches of the recurrent nerve of Luschka and have clinically been confirmed as sites of back and referred leg pain.[1]

The interspinous ligaments are well innervated by nerve fibers capable of transmitting nociceptive stimuli. The posterior facet joints are also well innervated by branches of the posterior primary division nerve roots and, like any synovial joint, are sites of pain when injured or inflamed.[1]

The deep muscles of the spine have been confirmed as sites of pain. With reflex contraction known as "protective spasm," these muscles can enhance pain already coming from underlying sites and may ultimately become the major pain generator.

In conclusion, sensory pain receptors are present in the outer layers of the annulus fibrosis, both the anterior and posterior longitudinal ligaments, the vertebral bones, the facet joints and their surrounding capsules, the interspinous ligaments, and the posterior paraspinal musculature.

SITES OF SPINAL PAIN AFTER MOTOR VEHICLE ACCIDENT

With knowledge of pain sensitive spinal structures, one can understand which tissues produce pain (nociception) after traumatic motor vehicle accidents that involve hyperflexion, hyperextension or torquing injuries. The tissues that can become sites of nociception include the vertebral body, anterior longitudinal ligament, the annulus fibrosis, the posterior longitudinal ligament, nerve rootlet(s) and their surrounding dura, the facet joint(s) and their capsules, the paraspinal musculature, and the interspinous ligaments.

With extreme flexion, spinal structures experience the following:

- excessive pressure against the anterior longitudinal ligament
- excessive stretch of the posterior fibers of the annulus fibrosis, possibly leading to tearing of fibers and associated pain
- stretching and/or tearing of posterior longitudinal ligament fibers
- anterior translation of the superior facet joint possibly impinging the exiting nerve root as it passes through the foramina
- stretching of the facet capsule as the superior facet slides anteriorly
- stretching and possible tearing of interspinous ligaments and/or surrounding paraspinal musculature.

All of these sites can be potential foci of pain after traumatic hyperflexion.

With a hyperextension injury, traction forces will stress the anterior annular fibers and the anterior longitudinal ligament, while compression of the facet joints could cause joint/bony injury. Hyperextension will cause spinal facets to come into opposition, grind against each other, and cause pain. Additionally, with hyperextension, there is narrowing of the neural foramina that can cause impingement of the exiting nerve root, dural irritation, nerve root damage, and associated pain. Intervertebral disc bulging and arthritic changes such as posterior vertebral osteophytes will further compromise the neural foramina, contributing to potential nerve root damage with a hyperextension injury.

In summary, tissues that can be stretched and/or damaged as a result of hyperflexion injuries include the posterior longitudinal ligament, posterior annular fibers of the intervertebral disc, the facet joint capsule, the interspinous ligaments, and the posterior spinal muscles. With hyperextension injury, there can be damage to the anterior longitudinal ligament and anterior annular fibers, impingement upon nerve roots due to decrease in size of neural foramen, and damage to the articulating surfaces of the facet joint(s).

SPINAL PAIN

Spinal pain complaints may emanate from:

- the vertebral body
- facet joints and intervertebral disc, due to nerve or spinal cord impingement
- the sacral iliac joints.

Vertebral Body Fracture

Pain can emanate from a fractured/compressed vertebral body (Figure 7-10). Such a fracture is known as a compression fracture. Radiographs will demonstrate loss of vertebral body height as compared to its normal appearance. Compression fractures occur as a consequence of extreme trunk hyperflexion. Compression fractures are graded as 1 through 4, with each grade indicating a progressive increase in the degree of compression as characterized by loss of vertebral height on radiographs. A grade 1 compression fracture involves 0 to 25 percent loss of vertebral height; grade 2, 25 to50 percent; grade 3, 50 to 75 percent; and grade 4, 75 to 100 percent (Figure 7-11a,b).

Spinal compression fractures can cause severe, potentially incapacitating spinal pain, which worsens with any trunk movement. Treatment for spinal compression fractures includes immobilization and pain control. Immobilization can be accomplished through the use of a variety of thoraco lumbosacral orthoses (TLSO), which maintain the back in a slight degree of hyperextension. Progressive collapse can be prevented by internal fixation (Figure 7-11c,d). Appropriate pain management is an essential part of the treatment of compression fractures. Anti-inflammatories may help, but frequently the pain is of such severity that patients require opioid analgesics. Over time, physical therapy can be instituted for gentle stretching (with the avoidance of excessive flexion), progressive back strengthening, and modalities such as electrical stimulation and ultrasound. Massage therapy and muscle relaxants are frequently indicated to treat reactive muscle spasm in the region of the bony fracture.

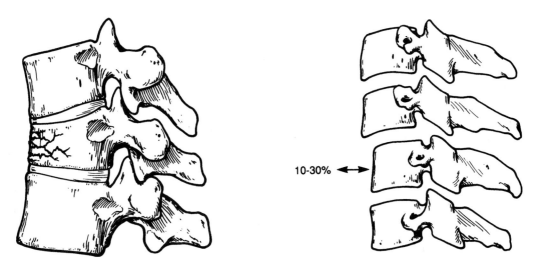

Figure 7-10 Compression fracture. Reprinted by permission from Unwin A, Jones K (eds). *Emergency Orthopaedics and Trauma*, p 36 (fig 9.16). Oxford, Elsevier Science Ltd, 1995.

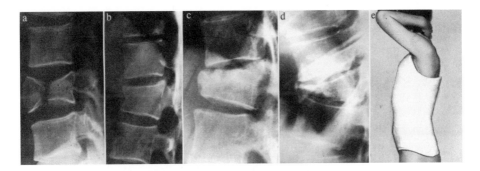

Figure 7-11 Wedge compression: (a) Grade 1, with 20 percent loss of height, and (b) grade 3 with greater than a 50 percent loss of height; (c) both of these could be treated in a plaster jacket; (d) progressive collapse can be prevented by internal fixation. Reprinted by permission from Apley AG, Solomon L (eds). *Concise System of Orthopaedics and Fractures*, 2nd ed. p 306 (fig 29.10). London, Hodder Arnold, 1994.

With a severe spinal compression fracture, there may be retropulsion of bone into the spinal canal. This can lead to damage of neural structures (nerve roots or spinal cord) with the development of radiculopathy or spinal cord injury after a motor vehicle accident.

Intervertebral Disc Degeneration

Intervertebral disc degeneration is a common phenomenon, occurring as a consequence of aging. Often times, mild degenerative changes can be present in an individual who is without symptomatology, other than perhaps a subtle unrecognized decrease in range of motion in the cervical or lumbar region. However, an asymptomatic individual with disc degeneration may be predisposed to developing a spinal pain syndrome after a motor vehicle accident.

The intact intervertebral disc serves as a shock absorber. It functions hydrodynamically as intact annular fibers help prevent deformation of the jelly-like nucleus pulposus it surrounds. Slight bulging or deformation of the disc may occur as pressure within it increases. However, when the stress is removed, the intact disc returns to its normal shape and height. With an intact disc, the vertebral bodies are separated by 1 to 2 cm. At this distance, there is maximal space within the spinal canal (for the spinal cord) and intervertebral foramina (for the nerve roots), and the facet joints are separated by a joint space (Figure 7-12).

A number of things happen as a consequence of disc degeneration.

- The vertebral bodies come closer together.
- This causes a bulging of the outer layers of the annular fibers.
- As these fibers bulge, they tug on the superior and inferior vertebral endplates. This tugging action causes localized microtrauma with tearing of the ligaments as they insert into the vertebral endplate bone.
- Blood flows into these tears.

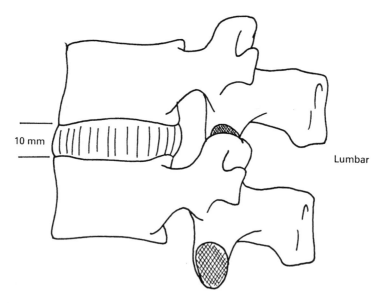

Figure 7-12 With an intact disc, the lumbar vertebral bodies are separated by 1 to 2 cm. At this distance, there is maximal space within the spinal canal (for the spinal cord) and intervertebral foramina (for the nerve roots), and the facet joints are separated by a joint space. Reprinted by permission from Palastanga N, Field D, Soames R (eds). *Anatomy and Human Movement—Structure and Function*, 3rd ed. p 635 (fig 5.28-bottom right). Oxford, Elsevier Science Ltd, 1998.

- Calcification ensues causing the development of "osteophytes". Osteophytes are small bone spurs that make their appearance at the bony vertebral end plates.
- As the vertebral bodies come closer together, the facet joints come into closer opposition, grind against each other, and can degenerate over time. The term facet arthropathy refers to degenerative changes occurring within the facet joints. Facet arthropathy is a consequence of disc degeneration.
- Osteophytes or bone spurs may grow off the facet joints impinging upon the neural foramina and possibly injuring the exiting nerve roots.

Disc degeneration will contribute to neural foraminal narrowing due to the superior and inferior pedicles coming closer together (narrowing the superior-inferior dimensions of the neural foramen), the intervertebral disc bulging into the anterior neural foramen, and facet osteophytes projecting from posteriorly. All of these factors lead to narrowing of the involved neural foramen increasing the potential for nerve impingement (Figure 7-13).

In addition to neuro foraminal stenosis with impingement (also known as lateral recess stenosis), central canal stenosis will also occur with this degenerative process, due to bulging of the intervertebral disc anteriorly and kinking of the ligamentum flavum posteriorly. Pain can occur as a consequence of the disc degeneration itself. As mentioned above, a number of spinal structures are heavily supplied by sensory pain and mechanoreceptors.

Three different types of pain can result as a consequence of disc degeneration including neurological or radicular pain, discogenic pain, and pain due to facet arthropathy. Each

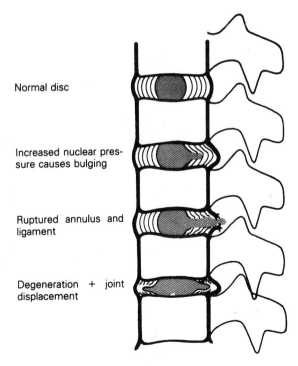

Normal disc

Increased nuclear pressure causes bulging

Ruptured annulus and ligament

Degeneration + joint displacement

Figure 7-13 Disc degeneration will contribute to neural foraminal narrowing due to the superior and inferior pedicles coming closer together and the intervertebral disc bulging into the anterior neural foramen. Reprinted by permission from Apley AG, Solomon L (eds). *Concise System of Orthopaedics and Fractures*, 2nd ed. p 167 (fig 18.12). London, Hodder Arnold, 1994.

type has a characteristic presentation. However, often the patient will have more than one type of discomfort occurring as a consequence of the disc degeneration.

Facet arthropathy can produce pain as the involved facet bones grind against each other, and due to stretching and distortion of the synovial capsule (which is heavily innervated by pain receptors). Facet arthropathy pain principally occurs in the low back. Such patients complain of discomfort with spinal extension, a movement that causes the irritated facet joints to generate discomfort as they grind against each other.

Disc degeneration associated with lateral recess stenosis may cause irritation of nerve(s) and their surrounding dura. This can lead to a neurogenic type of pain known as radiculopathy. A radiculopathy in the cervical or lumbar region classically results in extremity pain with associated paresthesias (numbness, tingling).

Advanced degenerative changes in the cervical and lumbar region could lead to central spinal stenosis, which, if severe, may cause spinal cord compression. In the cervical region, spinal cord compression could lead to pain, spasticity, bowel and bladder dysfunction, and varying degrees of motor and sensory loss. In the lumbar spine, central spinal stenosis causes entrapment of multiple nerve roots as the cauda equina passes through the lumbar vertebral canal. This can produce "neurogenic claudication" whereby the patient experiences lower extremity pain and paresthesias with standing and walking, and resolution of symptoms with sitting or flexion of the trunk.

With loss of integrity of the annulus, the patient may develop instability whereby the superior and inferior vertebrae of the functional unit start moving pathologically one upon the other. This type of movement can be very painful, and in conjunction with the torn annulus can contribute to back pain. In contrast to radicular pain, discogenic low back pain causes principally back discomfort that radiates into the hips and pelvis. Such patients may complain of intermittent painful movement of their unstable vertebrae.

The Herniated Disc and Radiculopathy

Occasionally, the terms "herniated disc" and "disc bulge" are used interchangeably. The difference between the terms "disc bulge" and "herniated disc" is really a matter of semantics. It is impossible say exactly when a disc bulge becomes a herniation. Some radiologists refer to a herniated disc as representing a more severe bulging of annular fibers or extrusion of the nucleus pulposus through the passageway created by torn annular fibers. As the herniated disc (HNP) extrudes into the spinal canal, it can impinge against neural structures. In its most severe form, an HNP fragment breaks loose and migrates caudally or cephalad causing nerve irritation and/or frank radiculopathy.

The term "radiculitis" refers to irritation of a nerve root without actual damage to the root itself. In contrast, a "radiculopathy" refers to sensory, motor, and reflex changes that occur in response to nerve damage. Nerve impingement can result from spinal degenerative changes or an intervertebral disc herniation.

Cervical disc herniations occur less frequently than in the lumbar region. The cervical HNP tends to be central in location due to the presence of the uncovertebral joints, which protect the lateral recesses. In contrast, in the lumbar region, posterolateral disc herniations are common due to the fact that the posterior longitudinal ligament tapers as it proceeds caudally (Figure 7-14).

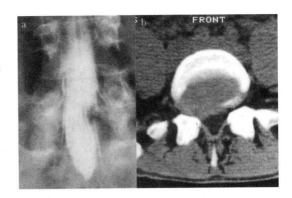

Figure 7-14 Lumbar disc–imaging: (a) myelogram in which absence of the contrast medium shows where a disc has protruded; (b) CAT scan showing how disc protrusion can obstruct the intervertebral foramen. Reprinted by permission from Apley AG, Solomon L (eds). *Concise System of Orthopaedics and Fractures*, 2nd ed. p 169 (fig 18.15). London, Hodder Arnold, 1994.

Patients who have already had spinal surgery may develop scar tissue formation as a consequence of the surgical intervention. The scar tissue may entrap or irritate nerve rootlets in that region. The term arachnoiditis refers to excessive scar tissue in the lumbar spinal canal that entraps and irritates lumbosacral nerve rootlets producing post operative back and lower extremity pain.

Characteristic symptoms of radiculopathy include an electrical radiating-type pain into the respective extremity, neck or back pain, paresthesias (numbness, tingling, or burning pain) and/or weakness of the involved extremity. Lower extremity weakness may manifest as knee buckling, foot dragging, foot drop, or falls. Upper extremity motor loss may be characterized by complaints of decreased grip or dropping objects. Physical examination of the patient with a frank radiculopathy will reveal characteristic motor, sensory, and reflex changes depending upon the cervical and/or lumbar level(s) involved by the radicular process. For further elaboration on the signs, symptoms, and physical examination findings for both cervical and lumbar radiculopathy, please refer to the cervical and lumbar radiculopathy sections of this text.

Soft Tissue and Bony Pain

Spinal soft tissue structures may be the focus of pain after a motor vehicle accident. Soft tissue structures supplied by pain fiber sensory nerve endings include the outer layers of the annulus fibrosis, the anterior and posterior longitudinal ligaments, the nerve rootlets and their surrounding dura, the facet joint capsules, the interspinous ligaments, and the paraspinal musculature.

Disc bulging results in increased pressure on the outer annular fibers as well as the anterior and posterior longitudinal ligaments. Disc bulging can contribute to spinal discomfort in the region of the disc. Annular tears also contribute to discogenic pain especially if they are so severe that movement results between the respective vertebral bodies. With facet arthropathy, the facet capsules can become an inflamed soft tissue focus of pain. The patient may develop pain emanating from torn interspinous ligaments, injured with an extreme hyperflexion injury. Lastly, the patient may have pain emanating from paraspinal musculature, that is either strained or in reactive muscle spasm. Reactive muscle spasm occurs as a consequence of pain generated from underlying vertebrae, facet joints, or irritated nerves. These primary nociceptive foci send pain impulses into the spinal cord triggering reflex spasm in the paraspinal musculature. This then becomes a secondary focus of discomfort.

Spondylosis, Spondylolysis, and Spondylolisthesis

Several terms that are often confused are spondylosis, spondylolysis, and spondylolisthesis. The term "spondylo", common to all three, is Greek terminology for the spine.

- *Spondylosis* refers to degenerative changes within the spine.
- *Spondylolysis* refers to a fracture of the pars interarticularis that lies in the posterior vertebral arch between the facet joints.
- *Spondylolisthesis* is derived from the Greek term "olisthesis" which means to slide. The term spondylolisthesis refers to movement of two adjacent vertebrae upon each other.

Movement of the superior vertebra in an anterior direction is known as a spondylolisthesis or anterolisthesis. Backward movement of the superior vertebra is referred to as retrolisthesis.

A spondylolysis refers to a fracture in the region of the posterior vertebral arch known as the pars interarticularis (Figure 7-15). This fracture site can be a source of discomfort with spinal movement, particularly with hyperextension. Figure 7-16 demonstrates the characteristic x-ray findings for spondylolysis in the lumbar region. Oblique x-rays will show the "broken neck of the Scottish terrier." The "broken neck" is the fracture of the pars interarticularis.

A spondylolisthesis can occur as a consequence of spondylolysis or spinal degenerative changes. The spondylolisthesis is graded using Roman numerals I through V. Grade I spondylolisthesis refers to movement of 0 to 25 percent of the superior vertebral body against the one below it. Grade II spondylolisthesis refers to 25 to 50 percent, grade III 50 to 75 percent, and grade IV 76 to 100 percent movement (Figure 7-17). Grade V spondylolisthesis represents a slippage of greater than 100 percent.[4]

The vertebral movement of spondylolisthesis may cause pain as a result of the instability itself, traction upon annular or spinal ligaments, impingement of the superior and inferior facet joints, strain of the adjacent interspinous ligaments or paraspinal musculature, and traction of adjacent nerve roots with development of radiculitis and/or radiculopathy.

The most common sight of a spondylolisthesis is at the L5–S1 level. This is in part to due to the effect of gravity on the lumbosacral angle. The lumbosacral angle refers to the downward tilt of the L5 vertebra as compared to the horizontal, normally about 30 degrees. Because of this downward angle and the effect of gravity, there is a tendency of the L5 vertebra to want to slide forward (Figure 7-18). Therefore, the L5–S1 level is the most common location for an anterior spondylolisthesis. In contrast, after traumatic events such as a motor vehicle accident, spondylolisthesis may occur at more superior levels. Spondylolisthesis due to degenerative changes most frequently occurs at the L45 level.

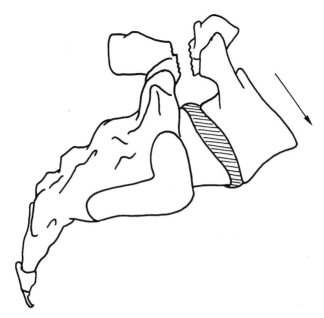

Figure 7-15 A spondylolysis refers to a fracture in the region of the posterior vertebral arch known as the pars interarticularis. Reprinted by permission from Palastanga N, Field D, Soames R (eds). *Anatomy and Human Movement— Structure and Function*, 3rd ed. p 671 (fig 5.49b). Oxford, Elsevier Science Ltd, 1998.

Sacroiliac Joint Dysfunction

The sacroiliac joints are often responsible for low back discomfort after a motor vehicle accident. These joints lie between the sacrum and the iliac bones of the pelvis. (See Figure 6-16.) The joint that forms between these bones has a movable synovial and an immobile fibrous portion. An extensive series of ligaments about this joint provide stability, which is further enhanced by surrounding intra and extra pelvic musculature. Therefore, the sacroiliac joint has both great stability and controlled movement.

The sacroiliac joint is a critical joint because of its location at the transition between the trunk and lower extremities. It is a major weight-bearing joint that plays a role in both walking and change of position. For example, getting in and out of a car or a chair, bending, lifting, and going up and down stairs all involve some movement of the sacroiliac joints. In addition, the sacroiliac joints have close proximity to the sciatic nerve and the lumbosacral plexus within the pelvis. Outside of the pelvis, the sacroiliac joint is adjacent to the piriformis muscle, through which the sciatic nerve passes. Therefore, trauma and pathology involving this joint can lead to both low back pain and lower extremity symptomatology (because of its relationship with adjacent nerves).

After trauma, the fibers of this joint can be torn or strained. When tearing is significant, the sacroiliac joint may actually sublux intermittently resulting in the symptoms of hip popping, lower extremity pain, and weakness and nerve irritation with sciatica symptoms. Therefore, symptoms of sacroiliac joint dysfunction include low back pain, hip pain or

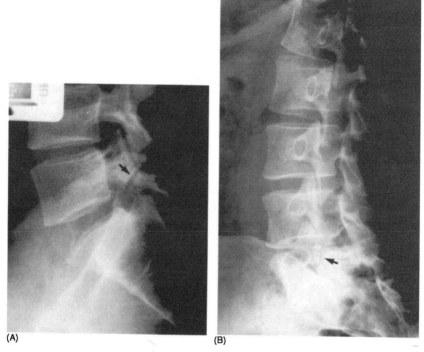

(A)   (B)

Figure 7-16 Spondylolysis and spondylolisthesis. (A) lateral and (B) oblique plain films demonstrate the presence of a pars defect (arrows). Note the classic appearance of the collar (or broken neck) of the Scottie dog on the oblique view. Reprinted by permission from Rucker KS, Cole AJ, Weinstein SM. *Low Back Pain: a Symptom-based Approach to Dagnosis and Treatment* (fig 5.13 a,b). Boston, Butterworth-Heinemann, 2001.

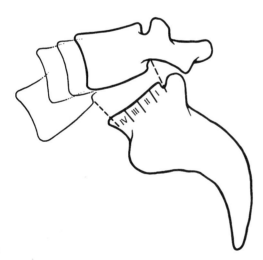

Figure 7-17 Grade I-IV spondylolisthesis.

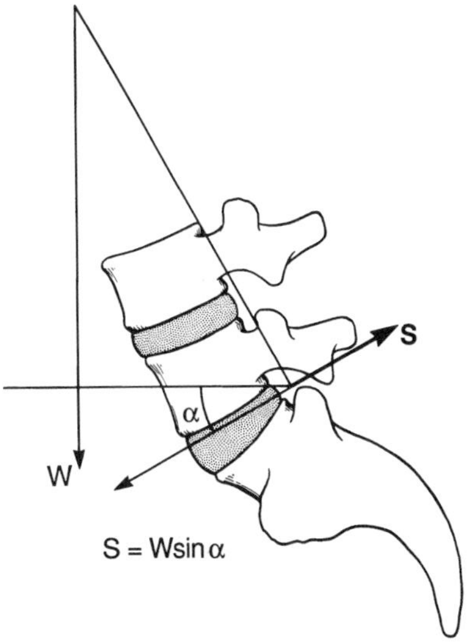

Figure 7-18 The most common sight of a spondylolisthesis is at the L5–S1 level. This is in part to due to the effect of gravity on the lumbosacral angle (α). The lumbosacral angle refers to the downward tilt of the L5 vertebra as compared to the horizontal, normally about 30 degrees. Because of this downward angle and the effect of gravity, there is a tendency of the L5 vertebral to want to slide forward.

$$S = W \sin \alpha$$

popping, lower extremity pain and/or paresthesias, altered gait, trouble getting out of a seat or a car, trouble ascending or descending stairs, and trouble walking.

The physical examination of sacroiliac joint dysfunction will demonstrate direct tenderness of the joint and a positive provocation test. The two most common tests used to define SI joint pathology are the FABER and Gaenslen tests. To evaluate for Gaenslen's sign, the patient lies supine on the examination table and is asked to draw both legs onto his/her chest. The patient is then shifted to the side of the table so than one buttock extends over the edge of the table while the other remains on it. The unsupported leg is allowed to drop over the edge, while the opposite leg remains flexed. Complaints of pain in the area of the sacroiliac joint indicate pathology in that area.

The Patrick test or FABER test can also be used to detect pathology in the hip and/or sacroiliac joint(s). The supine patient places the foot of his/her involved side on the opposite knee. The hip joint is then flexed, abducted, and externally rotated. In this position, inguinal pain is a general indication that there is pathology in hip joint or the surrounding muscles. When the end point of flexion, abduction, and external rotation has been reached, the femur is fixed in relation to the pelvis. To stress the sacroiliac joint, the examiner extends the range of motion by placing one hand on the patient's flexed knee joint and the other hand on the anterior superior iliac spine of the opposite side. Pain associated with pressure on each of these points may indicate pathology within the sacroiliac joint. The term "FABER" is an acronym for flexion (F), abduction (A B), and external rotation (E R). The patient with sacroiliac joint dysfunction may or may not have x-ray abnormalities. Pelvic A–P x-rays and CT scans may demonstrate sclerosis on opposing sides of the sacroiliac joint indicating the degenerative process.

The treatment for sacroiliac joint dysfunction includes physical therapy for modalities and initiation of a pelvic stabilization exercise program. Such exercises help strengthen the pelvic musculature surrounding the joint, hopefully providing for further stability. Some patients have a dislocation of the sacroiliac joint, and they may respond favorably to manipulation of the joint to obtain better alignment. A pelvic stabilization program should follow this. The patient might also benefit from a sacroiliac joint elastic belt, which generates compression of the sacroiliac joints and affords some degree of stabilization. If the patient fails to improve with conservative measures, he or she may benefit from a sacroiliac joint injection with steroids, which can be done with CT guidance. As a last resort, surgery to fuse the unstable joint may be the only option to achieve stability.

REFERENCES

1. Cailliet R. Low back pain. In Cailliet R (ed). *Soft Tissue Pain and Disability*, p 53. Philadelphia, F.A. Davis Co, 1988.
2. Moore KL. The back. In Moore KL (ed). *Clinically Oriented Anatomy*, p 627. Baltimore, Williams and Wilkins, 1980.
3. Cailliet R. Functional anatomy. In Cailliet R (ed). *Neck and Arm Pain*, p 5. Philadelphia, F.A. Davis Co, 1987.
4. Turek SL. The back. In Turek SL (ed). *Orthopedics–Principles and Their Applications* 4th ed, pp 1524–1551. Philadelphia, J.B. Lippincott, 1984.

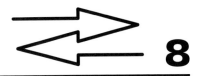

Headaches

Jack L Rook

Headaches are a common symptom following a motor vehicle accident, occurring as a result of a variety of pathophysiological mechanisms: a direct blow to the head may cause pain to emanate from cranial structures that have been traumatized; as a result of a whiplash injury, the patient may develop myofascial pain and spasm in the suboccipital cervical muscles. This can result in tension (muscle contraction) headaches, or headaches due to irritation of one of the four occipital nerves which course posteriorly along the scalp (occipital neuralgia); those patients who sustain head trauma may develop migraine/vascular headaches due to a traumatic brain injury; individuals with a pre-existing history of migraines may develop more intense vascular headaches, precipitated by nociceptive input from cervical and craniofacial structures (paracervical muscles or temporomandibular joints); lastly, those patients with temporomandibular joint dysfunction may have associated headaches as a result of referred pain from the involved joint(s).

This chapter reviews the pathophysiology, diagnosis, and treatment of the most common types of headaches associated with motor vehicle accidents. Included will be a discussion of tension headaches/occipital neuralgia, headaches that develop secondary temporomandibular joint dysfunction, and vascular headaches. More than one type of headache can coexist, in which case treatment will be more challenging.

TENSION-TYPE HEADACHE/OCCIPITAL NEURALGIA

Chronic cervical muscle contraction can result in entrapment or irritation of the occipital nerves (Figure 8-1). The C1 through C3 nerve roots coalesce to form these nerves, which supply sensation to the scalp. Entrapment of any of these nerves within tight musculature could lead to chronic tension-type headaches (TTH).[1-5] Muscle spasm and irritated occipital nerves are the primary contributing factors to TTH. The term TTH is often used in place of muscle contraction headache and/or occipital neuralgia.

The onset of pain in the tension-type headache (TTH) is generally more gradual than with migraine, and the pain sensation described by TTH patients includes fullness, tightness, or pressure, on which waves of aching pain are superimposed. Psychogenic factors (e.g., stress, anxiety, depression) may trigger or aggravate attacks.[6]

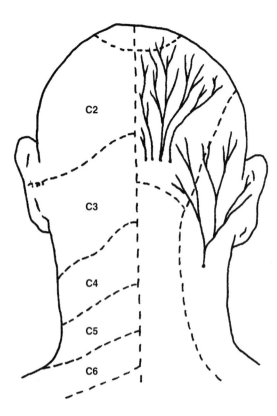

Figure 8-1 Chronic cervical muscle contraction can result in entrapment or irritation of the occipital nerves C2–C6, which may lead to chronic tension headaches. Reprinted by permission from Cassvan A, Weiss LD, Weiss JM, Rook JL, Mullens SU (eds). *Cumulative Trauma Disorders*. Newton, MA, Butterworth-Heinemann, 1997.

For patients who suffer from TTH, muscle-contraction headaches or occipital neuralgia, treatment modalities that promote relaxation of head and neck musculature will help reduce headaches by relieving spasm and associated pressure on the involved occipital nerves. Modalities available include physical therapy, massage therapy, and psychotherapy (biofeedback and behavioral/cognitive therapies). Among headache sufferers are some with clear evidence of psychiatric, stress-induced, and behavioral disturbances that contribute to, or occur as a response to, the headaches or chronic pain. Biofeedback, stress management, and behavioral and cognitive therapies can constitute primary, effective intervention in many patients with headache, even those without psychological problems or evident distress. These therapies also serve as adjunctive interventions in patients who suffer frequent headaches for which medications are required. Use of these therapies, which should be administered by expert professionals, well versed in headache disorders, is recommended whenever appropriate.

HEADACHES SECONDARY TO TEMPOROMANDIBULAR JOINT DYSFUNCTION

Temporomandibular joint syndrome (TMJ) may occur after a MVA either due to direct trauma with damage to the joint(s), or as a consequence of reactive spasm in the periarticular muscles. Cervical myofascial pain syndrome (MPS) can refer pain to facial (pterygoid and masseter) muscles, thereby activating latent trigger points (Figure 8-2). Over time, MPS may develop in these muscles, and chronic muscle contraction may cause slight alteration of the TMJ. Slight malalignment of the jaw could cause chronic tension of the temporalis muscle tendon, which attaches to the coronoid process of the mandible (Figure 8-3). This chronic strain could lead to muscle-contraction headaches.

Travell and Simons have pointed out that pterygoid muscle trigger points may develop as satellites in response to trigger-point activity of the neck muscles.[7] Furthermore, the

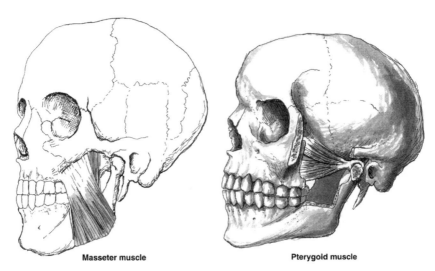

Masseter muscle   Pterygoid muscle

Figure 8-2 Masseter and pterygoid muscle trigger points may be activated by referred pain from cervical myofascial pain syndrome. Reprinted by permission from Cassvan A, Weiss LD, Weiss JM, Rook JL, Mullens SU (eds). *Cumulative Trauma Disorders*. Newton, MA, Butterworth-Heinemann, 1997.

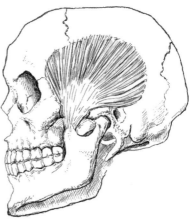

Figure 8-3 Slight malalignment of the jaw could cause chronic tension of the temporal muscle tendon, which attaches to the coronoid process of the mandible. Reprinted by permission from Cassvan A, Weiss LD, Weiss JM, Rook JL, Mullens SU (eds). *Cumulative Trauma Disorders*. Newton, MA, Butterworth-Heinemann, 1997.

masseter muscles often remain contracted for abnormally long periods in patients who develop the temporomandibular pain and dysfunction syndrome.[8,9]

Patients who suffer headaches associated with TMJ dysfunction must undergo a dental evaluation. Treatment might include trigger-point injections and massage therapy for head, neck, and facial (pterygoid and masseter) musculature. Often, such treatment in combination with dental splinting is sufficient to alleviate headaches associated with TMJ dysfunction.

VASCULAR HEADACHES

Vascular or migraine headaches may occur as a result of traumatic injury after a motor vehicle accident. Migraine headaches commonly occur as a symptom of a closed head injury. The head trauma leads to pathophysiological and chemical changes within the brainstem that produce the vascular changes associated with migraine. Similar pathophysiological changes may occur without a closed head injury, as a result of nociceptive input coming from painful head and neck structures.

Nociceptive impulses from head and neck structures are relayed to the nucleus caudalis. The nucleus caudalis is analogous to the spinal cord dorsal horn. It occupies a similar location in the brainstem and actually extends caudally into the upper cervical cord. In fact, in view of its association with nociceptive transmission and its structural and functional similarities to the spinal cord dorsal horn, the nucleus caudalis has been termed the *medullary dorsal horn* (Figure 8-4).[10–13]

The exact pathophysiology of vascular headaches has never been elucidated completely. However, extensive research since 1983 seems to implicate an ascending serotonergic neural system from midbrain raphe nuclei, which when activated leads to the release of substance P and calcitonin gene-related polypeptide (CGRP) from trigeminal nerve peripheral nociceptor terminals that innervate cerebral blood vessels.[14,15]

The first step in the development of vascular headaches is the convergence of nociceptive information from head and neck structures onto second-order pain transmission cells in the nucleus caudalis. In the neck, nociceptive information from cervical MPS or irritated occipital nerves (C1–C3) travels via C and A-delta fibers into the upper spinal cord portion of the nucleus caudalis. Likewise, nociceptive impulses from cranial structures (masseter, pterygoid, and temporalis muscles and the TMJ) are transmitted via C and A-delta fibers of cranial nerve V to the medullary nucleus caudalis.

Animal experiments have indeed demonstrated extensive convergence of neural input from neck and jaw musculature onto second-order pain transmission cells in the nucleus caudalis. Sessle *et al.* showed that stimulation of high-threshold (nociceptive) afferents from cat jaw, tongue, and neck muscles caused excitation of Wide Dynamic Range Neurons (WDRNs) and Nociceptor Specific Pain Transmissions Cells (NSPTCs) in the nucleus caudalis.[10]

In addition to this nociceptive input, neurons in the nucleus caudalis of the trigeminal nuclear complex also may integrate both excitatory and inhibitory supraspinal impulses. Supraspinal impulses generated by tension, stress, anxiety and depression

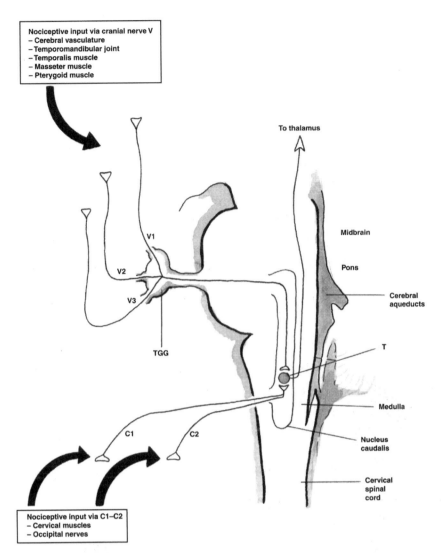

Nociceptive input via cranial nerve V
– Cerebral vasculature
– Temporomandibular joint
– Temporalis muscle
– Masseter muscle
– Pterygoid muscle

To thalamus

V1

V2

V3

Midbrain

Pons

Cerebral
aqueducts

TGG

T

Medulla

C1

C2

Nucleus
caudalis

Cervical
spinal
cord

Nociceptive input via C1–C2
– Cervical muscles
– Occipital nerves

Figure 8-4 Pathophysiology of vascular headaches. Nociceptive impulses from head (via cranial nerve V) and neck (via C1–C2 nerve roots) structures are relayed to second-order pain transmission cells (T) in the nucleus caudalis (medullary dorsal horn). Transmission cells relay the information to thalamic nuclei. (V1, V2, V3 = three divisions of trigeminal nerve; TGG = trigeminal ganglion.) Reprinted by permission from Cassvan A, Weiss LD, Weiss JM, Rook JL, Mullens SU (eds). *Cumulative Trauma Disorders.* Newton, MA, Butterworth-Heinemann, 1997.

probably have an excitatory effect on the trigeminal nucleus caudalis projection neuron (Figure 8-5). Over time, the convergence of noxious and supraspinal impulses may sensitize second-order pain transmission cells within the nucleus caudalis.[16] Activity in these second-order cells activates the ascending pain pathway, which travels towards the thalamus via the STT. However, before this pathway reaches the thalamus, neural

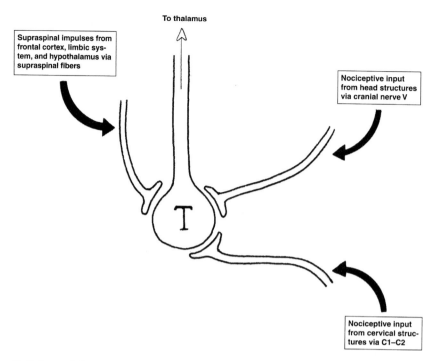

Figure 8-5 In addition to nociceptive input from head and neck structures, transmission neurons (T) in the nucleus caudalis also may integrate both excitatory and inhibitory supraspinal impulses. Reprinted by permission from Cassvan A, Weiss LD, Weiss JM, Rook JL, Mullens SU (eds): *Cumulative Trauma Disorders.* Newton, MA, Butterworth-Heinemann, 1997.

connections at midbrain raphe nuclei stimulate an ascending serotonergic system that travels toward cerebral blood vessels, ultimately releasing serotonin at the blood vessel level. It is the release of serotonin that may underlie the vascular abnormalities seen in migraine headaches (Figure 8-6). Therefore, some discussion of serotonin receptors is warranted.

There are at least four classes of serotonin (5-hydroxytryptamine, or 5-HT) receptors—5-HT_1 through 5-HT_4—and subtypes of these classes. The 5-HT_1 receptors are inhibitory, whereas the other types are excitatory. In humans, there are at least three 5-HT_1 receptors subtypes: 5-HT_{1A}, 5-HT_{1C}, and 5-HT_{1D}. The 5-HT_{1D} receptor is the most widespread serotonin receptor in the brain and functions as an autoreceptor modulating neurotransmitter release. Presynaptic 5-HT_{1D} receptor activation *inhibits* the release of 5-HT, norepinephrine, acetylcholine, CGRP, and substance P. Moreover, postsynaptic 5-HT_{1D} receptors are found on cerebral blood vessels. Agonist action of these receptors appears to produce vasoconstriction.[17,18]

The serotonin released from the ascending system, binds to 5-HT receptors on nerve terminals of C and A delta fibers surrounding the cerebral blood vessels (the trigeminal vascular system). The binding of serotonin to these nociceptive nerve terminals causes release of various neurotransmitters, including substance P, CGRP, and other

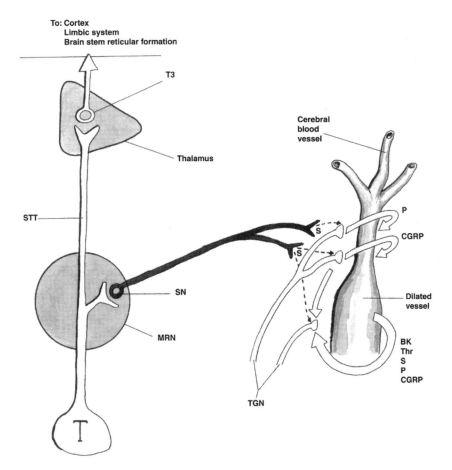

To: Cortex
Limbic system
Brain stem reticular formation

T3

Thalamus

Cerebral
blood
vessel

STT

SN

MRN

S

S

P

CGRP

Dilated
vessel

BK
Thr
S
P
CGRP

TGN

T

Figure 8-6 Activity in second-order pain transmission cells (T) activates the ascending pain pathway, which travels toward the thalamus via the spinothalamic tract (STT). Before this pathway reaches the thalamus, neural connections at midbrain raphe nuclei (MRN) stimulate an ascending serotoninergic system that travels toward cerebral blood vessels, ultimately releasing serotonin (S) at the blood vessel level. It is the release of serotonin that may underlie the vascular abnormalities seen in migraine headaches. Refer to the text for details. (T3 = third-order pain transmission cell; SN = serotoninergic neuron; BK = bradykinins; Thr = thromboxanes; TGN = trigeminal nerve fibers; P = substance P; CGRP = calcitonin gene-related polypeptide.) Reprinted by permission from Cassvan A, Weiss LD, Weiss JM, Rook JL, Mullens SU (eds). *Cumulative Trauma Disorders*. Newton, MA, Butterworth-Heinemann, 1997.

neuropeptides. The released neuropeptides interact with the blood vessel wall, producing dilatation, plasma extravasation, and sterile inflammation. Released substance P is postulated to increase vascular permeability and dilate cerebral blood vessels. Substance P has been shown to activate macrophages to synthesize thromboxanes, to activate lymphocytes, and, at high concentrations, to degranulate mast cells, with local release of histamine. Local inflammation ensues. The presence of pain-producing substances causes orthodromic conduction of nociceptive impulses along trigeminal nerve fibers, toward the second-order pain transmission cells in the nucleus caudalis, thereby perpetuating this cycle.[14,15]

Many of the drugs effective in treating migraines are believed to work in one of two ways. Some of the medications—including ergot, amitriptyline, propanolol (Inderal), dihydroergotamine (D.H.E.), and verapamil—possess serotonin receptor-blocking properties and are useful in both the prophylaxis and short-term treatment of migraine. Calcium ions are essential for neurotransmitter release, and calcium channel blockers therefore may owe some of their effectiveness to this action on perivascular sensory nerve fibers.[14,19,20] D.H.E. 45 and the triptan derivatives (see below) interact at 5-HT_{1A} and 5-HT_{1D} receptors, which, as mentioned previously, are inhibitory. They prevent the release of vasoactive neuropeptides from the nociceptive nerve terminals by having an inhibitory rather than a stimulatory (serotonergic) effect on these receptors.[16]

Understanding the foregoing pathophysiologic model will be helpful in formulating a plan for treatment of vascular headaches. Efforts to decrease nociceptive input to the nucleus caudalis should be made. Physical modalities and medications aimed at decreasing such noxious input from the TMJ, cervical muscles, occipital nerves, and facial structures might prove helpful. In addition, it would be beneficial to decrease supraspinal influences that may be up-regulating the nucleus caudalis projection neurons. To diminish such influences will require psychotherapeutic techniques and medications aimed at treating depression, tension, and anxiety. Finally, medications that prevent the release of serotonin at the cerebral blood vessel level (triptan derivatives, D.H.E. 45, verapamil), as well as medications that block the effect of serotonin (tricyclic antidepressants, ergotamines, Inderal), also have proven efficacious in the treatment of vascular headaches.

TREATMENT OF VASCULAR HEADACHES

As noted above, a vascular or migraine headache syndrome may develop as a response to the chronic nociceptive input from head and neck structures. The vascular component of the headache syndrome will vary from case to case. Some patients will have mild, chronic daily vascular headaches, whereas others will experience intermittent classic migraine attacks interspersed among chronic daily musculoskeletal headaches. Identification of mild, chronic, daily vascular headaches is difficult; these often are not diagnosed until patients respond to symptomatic or prophylactic migraine medications. Treatment of vascular headaches includes pharmacological and nonpharmacologic interventions. Medications usually are described as being either symptomatic or preventative.[21]

Pharmacologic Treatment

Symptomatic Therapy

The symptomatic treatment of head pain involves the use of agents that reverse, abort, or reduce pain once it has begun or is anticipated. Symptomatic treatment should be considered when attacks are infrequent (two or fewer per week). Many symptomatic headache medications are combinations of vasoconstrictive agents and muscle relaxants, aspirin, acetaminophen, narcotics, tranquilizers, or caffeine. Caffeine produces vasoconstriction, enhances analgesia, and increases gastrointestinal absorption. Whereas modest caffeine intake might have no adverse effect on headache patients and might even help some, excessive caffeine intake can aggravate or induce headaches. High daily intake greater than 500 mg per day can produce dependency, leading to withdrawal headaches 8–16 hours after the last dose. The total daily caffeine intake of headache patients should be calculated or at least carefully estimated (Table 8-1), as caffeine overuse can be an important contributing factor in some cases.[22–24]

Symptomatic headache treatment medications include traditional analgesics, combination analgesics, opioids, antiemetics, ergotamine derivatives, steroids, and the oral, injectable or inhalation migraine medications (Table 8-2). Opioids may be necessary for symptomatic relief of intermittent migraine headaches. Most patients respond to oral opioids of mild to moderate strength. Parenteral opioids (meperidine [Demerol], morphine, butorphanol [Stadol]) are occasionally required for severe intractable migraines in the emergency-room setting. Prochlorperazine (Compazine), promethazine (Phenergan), and metoclopramide (Reglan) may aid in the treatment of nausea and vomiting that frequently occurs with severe vascular headaches.

Ergotamine derivatives are occasionally-used drugs for moderate to severe migraine headaches. Cafergot and dihydroergotamine (D.H.E. 45) are commonly used agents. Proposed mechanisms for the ergotamines include agonist action on 5-HT_{1A} and 5-HT_{1D} receptors (inhibiting release of substance P and calcitonin gene-related polypeptides from trigeminal nerve endings), agonist action at alpha-adrenergic receptors (directly promoting vasoconstriction), and re-uptake inhibition of norepinephrine at sympathetic nerve endings (also producing vasoconstriction of involved cerebral vessels). Recommended use of ergotamine derivatives include moderate to severe migraine, intractable migraine, and intractable chronic daily headache. Cafergot is appropriate for initial treatment of acute attacks of migraine. D.H.E. 45 (inhalation, intravenously, intramuscularly, or subcutaneously) is appropriate for more severe attacks or prolonged intractable attacks.[21,22,25–29]

Steroids are occasionally useful adjuncts in the treatment of severe vascular headaches, helping to reduce inflammation within the involved cerebral vessels.[22] Sumatriptan succinate (Imitrex), a selective 5-HT_1 agonist agent, is considered useful for symptomatic treatment of acute migraine headache. This drug produces vasoconstriction and reverses neurogenic inflammation. It is available orally, or via inhalation or injection delivery system.[30] Other selective 5-HT_1 agonist agents now available for migraine sufferers include naratriptan hydrochloride (Amerge), rizatriptan benzoate (Maxalt), zolmitriptan (Zomig) and dihydroergotamine mesylate (Migranol).

Preventive Therapy

For those patients who suffer frequent attacks of migraine, a combination of preventive and symptomatic treatment is often necessary. Preventive (prophylactic) treatment is

Table 8-1 Caffeine content of foods, beverages, and drugs

	Serving Size or Dose	Caffeine (mg)
Beverages		
Coffee, drip	5 oz	110–150
Coffee, perked	5 oz	60–125
Coffee, instant	5 oz	40–105
Coffee, decaffeinated	5 oz	2–5
Tea, 5-min steep	5 oz	40–100
Tea, 3-min steep	5 oz	20–50
Tea, 1-min steep	5 oz	9–33
Hot cocoa	5 oz	2–10
Coca-Cola	12 oz	45
Canned iced tea	12 oz	22–36
7-Up/Diet 7-Up	12 oz	0
Diet Pepsi	12 oz	34
Dr. Pepper	12 oz	38
Fresca	12 oz	0
Ginger ale	12 oz	0
Mountain Dew	12 oz	52
Pepsi-Cola	12 oz	37
Tab	12 oz	44
Foods		
Milk chocolate	1 oz	1–15
Bittersweet chocolate	1 oz	5–35
Chocolate cake	1 slice	20–30
Baking chocolate	1 oz	35
Chocolate candy bar	1 oz	25
Over-the-Counter Drugs		
Anacin, Empirin, or Midol (analgesics)	2 tablets	64
Excedrin (analgesic)	2 tablets	130
NoDoz (stimulant)	2 tablets	200
Aqua-Ban (diuretic)	2 tablets	200
Dexatrim (weight-control aid)	1 tablet	200
Vanquish (analgesic)	1 tablet	33
Vivarin tablets (stimulant)	1 tablet	200
Prescription Drugs		
Darvon (propoxyphene)	1 tablet	32.4
Esgic (butalbital, acetaminophen, caffeine)	1 tablet	40
Fioricet (butalbital, acetaminophen, caffeine)	1 tablet	40
Fiorinal (butalbital, aspirin, caffeine)	1 tablet	40
Norgesic (orphenadrine, aspirin, caffeine)	1 tablet	30
Norgesic Forte (orphenadrine, aspirin, caffeine)	1 tablet	60
Synalgos-DC (dihydrocodeine, aspirin, caffeine)	1 tablet	30

Reprinted by permission from Cassvan A, Weiss LD, Weiss JM, Rook JL, Mullens SU (eds). *Cumulative Trauma Disorders*. Newton MA, Butterworth-Heinemann, 1997.

Table 8-2 Symptomatic medications in the treatment of migraine

Trade Name	Generic Name
Traditional Analgesics	
Tylenol	Acetaminophen
Bufferin, Ecotrin, etc.	Acetylsalicylic acid
Anaprox, Naprosyn, Ibuprofen, Motrin, etc.	Nonsteroidal anti-inflammatory drugs
Combination Analgesics	
Esgic	Butalbital 50 mg + acetaminophen 325 mg + caffeine 40 mg
Esgic with codeine	Butalbital 50 mg + acetaminophen 325 mg + caffeine 40 mg + codeine 30 mg
Fioricet	Butalbital 50 mg + acetaminophen 325 mg + caffeine 40 mg
Fiorinal	Butalbital 50 mg + aspirin 325 mg + caffeine 40 mg
Fiorinal with codeine #3	Butalbital 50 mg + aspirin 325 mg + caffeine 40 mg + codeine 30 mg
Midrin	Isometheptene mucate 65 mg + dichloralphenazone 100 mg + acetaminophen 325 mg
Phrenilin	Butalbital 50 mg + acetaminophen 325 mg
Phrenilin Forte	Butalbital 50 mg + acetaminophen 650 mg
Phrenilin with codeine #3	Butalbital 50 mg + acetaminophen 325 mg + codeine phosphate 30 mg
Opioids	
Bancap HC	Hydrocodone bitartrate 5 mg + acetaminophen 500 mg
Darvocet-N 100	Propoxyphene napsylate 100 mg + acetaminophen 650 mg
Darvocet-N 50	Propoxyphene napsylate 50 mg + acetaminophen 325 mg
Darvon Compound	Propoxyphene HCl 32 mg + aspirin 389 mg + caffeine 32.4 mg
Darvon Compound-65	Propoxyphene HCl 65 mg + aspirin 389 mg + caffeine 32.4 mg
Darvon with ASA	Propoxyphene HCl 65 mg + aspirin 325 mg
Darvon-N	Propoxyphene napsylate
Darvon-N with ASA	Propoxyphene napsylate 100 mg + aspirin 325 mg
Demerol (tablets or injectable)	Meperidine HCl
Dilaudid	Hydromorphone
DHC Plus	Dihydrocodeine bitartrate 16 mg + acetaminophen 350 mg + caffeine 30 mg
Dolophine HCl (tablets)	Methadone HCl
Empirin with codeine #2	Codeine 15 mg + aspirin 325 mg
Empirin with codeine #3	Codeine 30 mg + aspirin 325 mg
Empirin with codeine #4	Codeine 60 mg + aspirin 325 mg
Levo-Dromoran	Levorphanol tartrate
Lorcet	Hydrocodone bitartrate (5, 7.5, 10 mg) + acetaminophen (500 or 650 mg)
Lortab	Hydrocodone bitartrate (2.5, 5, 7.5 mg) + aspirin 500 mg
Mepergan	Meperidine HCl + promethazine HCl
MS Contin (tablets)	Morphine sulphate

(continued)

Table 8-2 (Continued)

Trade Name	Generic Name
Opioids (continued)	
MSIR (tablets or oral solution)	Morphine sulphate
Percocet	Oxycodone 5 mg + acetaminophen 325 mg
Percodan	Oxycodone HCl 4.5 mg + oxycodone terephthalate 0.38 mg + aspirin 325 mg
Stadol (injectable or nasal spray)	Butorphanol tartrate
Synalgos-DC	Dihydrocodeine bitartrate 16 mg + aspirin 356.4 mg + caffeine 30 mg
Talacen	Pentazocine HCl 25 mg + acetaminophen 650 mg
Talwin compound	Pentazocine HCl 12.5 mg + aspirin 325 mg
Talwin NX	Pentazocine HCl 50 mg + naloxone HCl 0.5 mg
Tylenol #2	Acetaminophen 300 mg + codeine 15 mg
Tylenol #3	Acetaminophen 300 mg + codeine 30 mg
Tylenol #4	Acetaminophen 300 mg + codeine 60 mg
Tylox	Oxycodone 5 mg + acetaminophen 500 mg
Vicodin	Hydrocodone bitartrate 5 mg + acetaminophen 500 mg
Steroids	
Decadron (tablets and suspension)	Dexamethasone
Deltasone (tablets)	Prednisone
Medrol (tablets)	Methylprednisolone
Medrol Dosepak	Methylprednisolone
Solu-Medrol (parenteral)	Methylprednisolone
Antiemetics	
Antivert	Meclizine
Compazine	Prochlorperazine
Phenergan	Promethazine HCl
Reglan	Metoclopramide HCl
Tigan	Trimethobenzamide HCl
Ergotamine Derivatives	
Cafergot (suppositories)	Ergotamine tartrate 2 mg + caffeine 100 mg
Cafergot (tablets)	Ergotamine tartrate 1 mg + caffeine 100 mg
Ergomar (sublingual tablets)	Ergotamine tartrate 2 mg
Ergostat (sublingual tablets)	Ergotamine tartrate 2 mg
Wigraine (suppositories)	Ergotamine tartrate 2 mg + caffeine 100 mg + tartaric acid 21.5 mg
Wigraine (tablets)	Ergotamine tartrate 1 mg + caffeine 100 mg
Injectable Migraine Medications	
Imitrex	Sumatriptan
DHE 45	Dihydroergotamine mesylate
Inhalant Migraine Medications	
Imitrex Nasal Spray	Sumatriptan
Migranol	Dihydroergotamine mesylate

Table 8-2 (Continued)

Trade Name	Generic Name
Oral Triptan Derivatives	
Imitrex	Sumatriptan
Amerge	Naratriptan hydrochloride
Maxalt	Rizatriptan benzoate
Zomig	Zolmitriptan

Modified with permission from Cassvan A, Weiss LD, Weiss JM, Rook JL, Mullens SU (eds). *Cumulative trauma disorders*. Newton MA, Butterworth-Heinemann, 1997.

Table 8-3 Medications used for headache prophylaxis

Drug	Recommended Dose
Tricyclic Antidepressants	
Nortriptyline hydrochloride	10–125 mg/day
Amitriptyline hydrochloride	10–300 mg/day
Doxepin hydrochloride	10–50 mg/day
Antidepressants	
Fluoxetine hydrochloride	20–80 mg/day
Calcium Channel Blockers	
Verapamil hydrochloride	240–720 mg/day
Nifedipine	30–180 mg/day
Nimodipine	60 mg four times daily
Diltiazem hydrochloride	120–360 mg/day
Beta Blockers	
Propranolol hydrochloride	40–320 mg/day
Atenolol	50–150 mg/day
Nadolol	40–240 mg/day
Timolol maleate	10–30 mg/day
Anticonvulsants	
Valproate	250–750 mg/day
Phenytoin sodium	200–400 mg/day

Reprinted by permission from Cassvan A, Weiss LD, Weiss JM, Rook JL, Mullens SU (eds). *Cumulative Trauma Disorders*. Newton MA: Butterworth-Heinemann, 1997.

used to reduce the frequency and severity of headache events.[21,25] It is appropriate when attacks of acute pain occur more than two times per week, when the severity or duration of infrequent attacks justifies the use of preventive treatment, when symptomatic medications are ineffective for infrequent attacks, and to enhance the efficacy of symptomatic medications. Preventive medications include beta-blockers, calcium channel blockers, antidepressants, and anticonvulsants (Table 8-3).

Beta blockers are the group of prophylactic agents most widely used for migraine and related headaches. In 60 to 80 percent of cases, they are effective in reducing frequency of headache by at least 50 percent. They should be administered initially in small, divided doses, titrating upward to tolerance. Two-, three-, or four-times-daily dosing is superior to once-daily dosing. Selected major untoward reactions to beta blockers include fatigue, depression, memory disturbances, impotence, hypotension, bradycardia, weight gain, peripheral vasoconstriction, bronchospasm, and adverse influence on cholesterol and lipid metabolism. Contraindications to beta-blocker use include congestive heart failure (CHF), asthma, significant diabetes or hypoglycemia, bradycardia, hypotension, and moderate to severe hyperlipidemia. Beta-blocker therapy must be individualized. Underdosing is a major cause of therapeutic failure. When discontinuing beta blockers after extended usage, a gradual reduction program is necessary.

Verapamil is the calcium channel blocker most widely used for the treatment of vascular headache. It is an appropriate alternative to beta blockers. As with beta blockers, a small, divided dose should be used initially and then titrated upward to tolerance. High-dose verapamil (160 mg three to four times per day) may be necessary for beneficial effects in some patients. Selected major untoward reactions to verapamil include constipation, atrioventricular block, CHF, hypotension, and reflex tachycardia. Contraindications include CHF, heart block, moderate to severe bradycardia, hypotension, sick sinus syndrome, atrial flutter or fibrillation, and severe constipation.[22,28]

Tricyclic antidepressants (TCAs) are potentially valuable prophylactic agents in patients who suffer chronic daily headache or intermittent migraines, with or without depression. TCAs are sedating, and so patients with associated sleep disturbances may benefit from one of these agents. Generally, TCAs should be administered as a single dose at bedtime. The major TCAs for headache include amitriptyline, nortriptyline, doxepin, desipramine, and protriptyline. Untoward reactions of TCAs include weight gain, dizziness, subtle cognitive impairment, and anticholinergic symptoms (drowsiness, dry mouth, constipation, urinary retention, blurry vision, and tachycardia). Contraindications to TCA use include significant cardiac arrhythmia, glaucoma, and urinary retention.[31–34] Recent studies have advocated the use of tizanidine hydrochloride (Zanaflex) as effective and safe for the prophylactic treatment of chronic daily headaches and/or TTH.[35,36]

Anticonvulsants such as phenytoin (Dilantin), carbamazepine (Tegretol), gabapentin (Neurontin), and valproate (Depakote) occasionally benefit migraine sufferers. They also might help patients who suffer chronic daily headache and occipital neuralgic syndromes. The membrane-stabilizing effects of these drugs might be useful in occipital neuralgia, a condition characterized by entrapment or irritation of the occipital nerves in tight paracervical musculature. Anticonvulsants must be administered carefully, beginning with small, divided doses.

Dilantin is administered in dosages of 100 to 400 mg per day. Tegretol should be given in dosages beginning at 100 to 200 mg two to three times per day, with gradual increase to tolerance or efficacy. Maximum recommended dosage is 1200mg/day. Depakote should be started at a dose of 125 to 250 mg three to four times per day. Doses should be increased gradually to a maximum dose of 1 to 2 g per day.[21,37–39] Neurontin dosages

Box 8-1 Foods that should be avoided by the headache patient

1. Salt on an empty stomach (e.g., snacks of potato chips, popcorn, peanuts)
2. All cheeses except American, cottage, and Velveeta
3. Real sour cream (imitation sour cream acceptable)
4. Live yogurt cultures
5. Fresh breads, raised coffee cakes, raised donuts
6. Beans of any sort—navy, lima, pinto, and so on, and pea pods
7. All nuts, including peanut butter
8. All preserved meats, including sausage, hot dogs, ham, bacon; all deli meats, including chicken and turkey
9. Oranges, orange juice, and other citrus foods, bananas, pineapple
10. Anything pickled, fermented, or marinated
11. Chocolate
12. Monosodium glutamate in any form
13. Excessive caffeine intake
14. Alcoholic beverages

Reprinted by permission from Cassvan A, Weiss LD, Weiss JM, Rook JL, Mullens SU (eds). *Cumulative Trauma Disorders.* Newton MA, Butterworth-Heinemann, 1997.

range from 100 to 3600 milligrams per day. Blood level monitoring is advisable in all patients taking anticonvulsants. Also, periodic evaluation of hematologic and liver function is recommended, per standard protocol.

Nonpharmacologic Treatment

Nonpharmacologic interventions for headache sufferers include applying ice; resting in a cool, quiet, dark environment; practicing biofeedback and relaxation techniques; discontinuing smoking; and exercising regularly. Furthermore, the patient will benefit from keeping activities the same from day to day, insofar as this is possible, and from avoiding foods (Box 8-1) and stressful circumstances that might provoke headache.[22]

REFERENCES

1. Bovim G, Fredriksen TA, Stolt-Neelsen A, *et al.* Neurolysis of the greater occipital nerve in cervicogenic headache. *Headache* 1992; 32: 175.
2. Bogduk N. The anatomy of occipital neuralgia. *Clin Exp Neurol* 1981; 17: 167.
3. Edmeads J. Headaches and head pains associated with diseases of the cervical spine. *Med Clin North Am* 1978; 62: 533.
4. Hammond SR, Danta G. Occipital neuralgia. *Clin Exp Neurol* 1978; 15: 258.
5. Hunter CR, Mayfield FH. Role of the upper cervical roots in the production of pain in the head. *Am J Surg* 1949; 78: 743.
6. Clinch CR. Evaluation of acute headaches in adults. *Am Fam Physician* 2001; 63(4): 685.
7. Travell JG, Simons DG. TMJ dysfunction. In Travell JG, Simons DG (eds). *Myofascial Pain and Dysfunction: The Trigger Point Manual*, p 260. Baltimore, Williams and Wilkins, 1983.

8. Wolff HG. *Wolff's Headache and other Head Pain* 3rd ed, p 550. Oxford: Oxford University Press, 1972.

9. Yemm K. Temporomandibular dysfunction and masseter muscle response to experimental stress. *Br Dent J* 1969; 127: 508.

10. Sessle BJ, Hu JW, Amano N, *et al.* Convergence of cutaneous, tooth pulp, visceral, neck and muscle afferents onto nociceptive and non-nociceptive neurons in trigeminal subnucleus caudalis (medullary dorsal horn) and its implications for referred pain. *Pain* 1986; 27: 219.

11. Gobel S, Hockfield S, Ruda MA. Anatomical similarities between medullary and spinal dorsal horns. In Kawamura Y, Dubner R (eds). *Oral-Facial Sensory and Motor Functions*, p 211. Tokyo, Quintessence, 1981.

12. Hoffman DS, Dubner R, Hayes RL, *et al.* Neuronal activity in medullary dorsal horn of awake monkeys trained in a thermal discrimination task: I. Responses to innocuous and noxious thermal stimuli. *J Neurophysiol* 1981; 46: 409.

13. Hu JW, Dostrovsky JO, Sessle BJ. Functional properties of neurons in cat trigeminal subnucleus caudalis (medullary dorsal horn). I. Response to oral-facial noxious and non-noxious stimuli and projections to thalamus and subnucleus oralis. *J Neurophysiol* 1981; 45: 173.

14. Moskowitz MA. The neurobiology of vascular head pain. *Ann Neurol* 1984; 16: 157.

15. Silberstein SD. Advances in understanding the pathophysiology of headache. *Neurology* 1992; 42(suppl 2): 6.

16. Olesen J. Clinical and pathophysiological observations in migraine and tension-type headache explained by integration of vascular, supraspinal, and myofascial inputs. *Pain* 1991; 46: 125.

17. Saper JR, Silberstein S, Gordon CD, *et al.* Mechanisms and theories of head pain. In Pine JW (ed): *Handbook of Headache Management*, p 16. Baltimore, Williams and Wilkins, 1993.

18. Raskin NH. Serotonin receptors and headache. *N Engl J Med* 1991; 325: 353.

19. Amery WK. Flunarizine, a calcium channel blocker: a new prophylactic drug in migraine. *Headache* 1983; 23: 70.

20. Diamond S, Schenbaum H. Flunarizine, a calcium channel blocker, in the prophylactic treatment of migraine. *Headache* 1983; 23: 39.

21. Shulman EA, Silberstein SD. Symptomatic and prophylactic treatment of migraine and tension-type headache. *Neurology* 1992; 42(suppl 2): 16.

22. Saper JR, Silberstein S, Gordon CD, *et al.* Mechanisms and theories of head pain. In Pine JW (ed). *Handbook of Headache Management*, p 16. Baltimore, Williams and Wilkins, 1993.

23. Matthew RJ, Wilson WH. Caffeine-induced changes in cerebral circulation. *Stroke* 1985; 16: 814.

24. Ward N, Whitney C, Avery D, *et al.* The analgesic effects of caffeine in headache. *Pain* 1991; 44: 151.

25. Ward TN. Providing relief from a headache pain—current options for acute and prophylactic therapy. *Postgrad Med J* 2000; 108(3): 121.

26. Callaham MM, Raskin NH. A controlled study of dihydroergotamine in the treatment of acute migraine headache. *Headache* 1986; 26: 168.

27. Goldstein J. Ergot pharmacology in alternative delivery systems for ergotamine derivatives. *Neurology* 1992; 42(suppl 2): 45.

28. Peroutka SJ. The pharmacology of current antimigraine drugs. *Headache* 1990; 30(suppl 1): 5.

29. Silberstein SD, Shulman EA, Hopkins MM. Repetitive intravenous DHE in the treatment of refractory headache. *Headache* 1990; 30: 334.

30. Subcutaneous Sumatriptan International Study Group. Treatment of migraine attacks with sumatriptan. *N Engl J Med* 1991; 5: 316.

31. Couch JR, Hassanein RS. Amitriptyline in migraine prophylaxis. *Arch Neurol* 1979; 21: 263.

32. Gomersall JD, Stuart A. Amitriptyline in migraine prophylaxis. *J Neurol Neurosurg Psychiatry* 1973; 36: 684.

33. Diamond S, Baltes BJ. Chronic tension headache treated with amitriptyline—a double blind study. *Headache* 1971; 11: 110.

34. Lance JW, Curran DA. Treatment of chronic tension headache. *Lancet* 1964; 1: 1236.

35. Saper JR, Winner PK, Lake AE. An open-label dose-titration study of the efficacy and tolerability of tizanidine hydrochloride tablets in the prophylaxis of chronic daily headaches. *Headache* 2001; 41: 357.

36. Shimomura T, Awaki E, Kowa H, Takahasho K. Treatment of tension-type headache with tizanidine hydrochloride: Its efficacy and relationship to the plasma MHPG concentration. *Headache* 1991; 31(9): 601.

37. Herring R, Kuritzky A. Sodium valproate in the prophylactic treatment of migraine: a double-blind study vs. placebo. *Cephalgia* 1992; 12: 81.

38. Mathew NT, Ali S. Valproate in the treatment of persistent chronic daily headache. An open-label study. *Headache* 1991; 31: 71.

39. Sorensen KV. Valproate: a new drug in migraine prophylaxis. *Acta Neurol Scand* 1988; 78: 346.

9

The Chronic Pain Patient

Jack L Rook

The patient who develops a chronic pain syndrome after a motor vehicle accident represents a worse case scenario with regards to the individual's pain and suffering, the multitude of symptoms that challenge the treating physician, and the significant cost for third party payers. The patient with a chronic pain syndrome typically presents with a constellation of symptoms including:

- ongoing pain which can occur either intermittently (with certain activities) or continuously with fluctuations depending on activities;
- complaints of discomfort and suffering that often do not correlate with objective pathology;
- functional limitations that vary from mild to extreme. For example, some patients may be able to do all prior activities of daily living, but not without discomfort. Other patients become unable to participate in activities that require prolonged weightbearing or sitting, bending, twisting, repetitive or forceful upper extremity use, or presence in environmental extremes;
- depression due to the ongoing discomfort with associated functional limitations;
- sleep disturbance due to the chronic discomfort interfering with the individual attaining deep levels of sleep;
- vocational and avocational losses. A chronic pain patient may lose his/her job because of stringent restrictions that preclude them from performing their occupation. Avocational activities such as engaging in sports, housecleaning and yard work, hobbies, or gardening may also be precluded by the chronic pain and restrictions. Inability to work or to participate in pleasurable avocational activities further aggravates the patient's depression;
- family discord. The chronic pain patient interactions with his or her spouse and/ or family are usually adversely affected by the chronicity of the pain, complaints of suffering, ongoing depression, functional limitations, and vocational losses. The financial ramifications associated with job loss will further stress family relationships;
- decreased libido occurs due to the pain itself (which may cause discomfort during sexual activity), depression, and possibly due to side effects from medications used to treat chronic pain;

- a perception that they have become victims. They were initially victimized by the person who caused the accident, and subsequently by family members or treatment providers whom they perceive as not taking their complaints seriously. Lastly, they become victimized by third party payers who they may feel are not covering their bills adequately;
- a loss of quality of life. This occurs due to all the above-mentioned reasons including the ongoing discomfort, vocational, avocational, and functional limitations, poor sleep, damage to family relationships, and associated depression;
- some patients who initially present with a fairly localized pain process may, over time, develop a migrating pain syndrome. For example, the patient with proximal myofascial discomfort (involving the cervical, upper back, and upper chest region) may develop headaches or upper extremity symptomatology (pain, numbness, and paresthesias).

THE TOTAL COST OF PAIN

According to the NIH Institute of Neurological Disorders, chronic pain is the most expensive health problem in the United States today at $50 billion annually.[1] The average chronic pain patient has suffered seven years, has undergone three major surgeries, and has current medical bills in the range of $50,000 to $100,000. Co-morbid conditions that occur with chronic pain (depression, anxiety and chronic fatigue) increase the overall cost of treatment for these patients substantially.

Inappropriate assessment and management of chronic pain patients takes its toll on all aspects of the medical and business community. It has been estimated that patients lose 515 million workdays per year as a result of inadequate pain management.

According to the Department of Health and Human Services, Acute Pain Management Guidelines, "the ethical obligation to manage pain and relieve the patient's suffering is at the core of a health care professional's commitment." The Joint Commission for the Accreditation of Hospital Organizations (JCAHO) has new mandates for the treatment of chronic pain, which became effective in the year 2000. It has been stated that such treatment should not increase expense per patient, but may in fact lessen the burden on a per case basis.[2]

DISABILITY DUE TO CHRONIC PAIN

Disability is a societal problem. A number of studies have been performed over the years in an effort to define its prevalence in the United States population. A recent study included a self-report through personal interviews of 36,700 households, representing civilian, non-institutionalized population, greater than 15 years of age.[3] For the population in the age range of 18 to 64 years, 16.5 percent reported a disability and 10.5 percent reported limitations at work. The disabling conditions included arthritis (17.5 percent) spine problems (16.5 percent) and mental/emotional problems (3.7 percent).

Disability was also studied in a large banking company.[4] The productivity of workers and time lost from work was studied in a population of 364 telephone customer service agents. Of note, musculoskeletal disorders accounted for the second highest loss of time from work (after digestive disorders).

DISABILITY MANAGEMENT

A quick return to activity is better for patients than rest, to prevent long-term disability. Multiple studies have shown that prolonged absence from work can lead to long-term disability. Early activation for patients with first-time musculoskeletal conditions can significantly decrease the risk of developing chronic pain.[5] However, motivating a patient to return to activity may be more complex. Some patients place all responsibility on the physician to take care of them. These patients are said to have an *external focus of control*. Other patients wish to control the outcome themselves. Those patients are considered to have an *internal focus of control*, and are likely to be active participants in their recovery. Those with an external focus of control tend to be more passive, and depend on others to fix their problem.[6]

The patient should be encouraged to have an internal focus of control. Such patients are likely to respond more readily to their physician's suggestions as compared to those patients with an external focus of control. Those patients with an external focus may require further encouragement to participate in the therapeutic plan. Patients with musculoskeletal pain will need to take an active role in their own recovery. Physicians can encourage this by promoting the benefits of activity and other self-management techniques.

The first step in managing a patient with chronic pain is for the physician to show respect for the patient. The physician should respond to the patient's complaints of pain and concerns or fears regarding their current situation.

The feeling of being understood by another person is intrinsically therapeutic; it bridges the isolation of illness and helps to restore connectedness that patients need to feel whole. A growing body of research suggests an association between clinicians caring, and the appropriateness, effectiveness and satisfaction with care.[7]

Once a good doctor/patient relationship has been established, the clinician should educate the patient with regards to his or her diagnoses, likely time for recovery, and need for any diagnostic tests and treatment. Patient education is advocated as a fundamental treatment.[8] The AMA considers patient education an essential portion of medical care. Patient education on activity recommendations, diagnoses and mechanisms of self-management of care are indispensable to prevent short and long-term disability. The patient should always be motivated to increase their activity. The focus should always be on increasing activity levels: personal, family and work.

THE PATIENT WITH DELAYED RECOVERY

Those patients who demonstrate delayed recovery should have a psychosocial evaluation within 6 to 12 weeks of identification of the delayed recovery. Depressed patients show poorer overall functioning than those with major chronic medical conditions.[9] The cost of screening for depression is low in primary care.[10] In general health care studies, patients with psychological problems which are left untreated cost the system more money, whereas patients who received treatment did not increase the overall cost of their general health care.[11] Mental illness is a major cause of lack of productivity at work as well as time lost from work.[9] Multiple papers support the concept that psychosocial problems are predictors of low back disability and musculoskeletal disability.[12–14]

In conclusion, disability is a societal problem. The physician can improve the functional outcome for their patient by respecting the patient, educating the patient, activating the patient for functional goals, and supporting self-sufficiency. Psychosocial issues should be evaluated and treated early in an effort to prevent long-term disability.[15]

MYOFASCIAL PAIN SYNDROME

Most, if not all patients with chronic pain have some sort of muscular component. These patients are said to have chronic myofascial pain or the myofascial pain syndrome (MPS). Myofascial pain can be localized (e.g., a neck and shoulder MPS), or it can be quite diffuse (e.g., the fibromyalgia syndrome).

Clinical features of the MP syndrome include:

- continuous, dull, deep aching pain
- pain produced by pressure on tender spots or bands (trigger points) in muscles
- pain relieved by inactivation of trigger points
- restricted range of motion in the affected muscle
- local muscle twitch produced by trigger-point stimulation
- patient startle or jump sign with trigger-point pressure.[16–20]

Trigger points have another characteristic, referral pain patterns when pressed or irritated. Specifically, pressure on a trigger point will cause it to refer pain to other locations in the general proximity. That could result in the activation of latent trigger points in distant muscles, which can ultimately contribute to migration of the chronic myofascial condition.

The myofascial pain syndrome is often a self-sustaining process unless some intervention occurs to break the cycle. Muscle contraction will produce a more severe and sustained secondary pain if the contracting muscle contains a latent trigger point. Travell and Simons believe that MPS occurs when the latent trigger points are activated.[19] Trigger points have particularly sensitive muscle nociceptors. The nociceptor input from trigger points feeds back to the spinal cord to cause further muscle contraction and sustain the pain.[21]

Migration of myofascial pain occurs as the irritated trigger points refer pain to various locations activating latent trigger points in other muscles, with gradual migration of the myofascial pain.[17,19] In addition, spread of impulses in the spinal cord may occur in a cephalad-caudal direction as well as segmentally. Such impulse propagation could lead to activation of the alpha motor neurons at adjacent spinal segments, causing spread of myofascial pain due to activity within the central nervous system. The myofascial pain may continue indefinitely. MPS must be addressed to decrease overall pain levels and to prevent its migration over time.

Physical and occupational therapy play an important role in the management of MPS. Therapeutic modalities (hot packs, cold packs, ultrasound, massage, and electrical stimulation), daily stretching, and therapeutic exercise can be applied to loosen up tight painful muscles, break myofascial adhesions, and improve blood flow to tissues. A goal of treatment is to decrease afferent nociceptive input from these tissues, thereby lessening or breaking the vicious cycle of pain and reactive spasm that perpetuates the condition.

Other treatments available for the management of chronic MPS include trigger-point injection therapy, transcutaneous electrical nerve stimulation (TENS), and medications such as nonsteroid anti-inflammatory drugs and muscle relaxants. Nonsteroidal anti-inflammatory drugs may or may not be effective analgesics for patients with MPS or fibromyalgia. However, a component of low-grade inflammation may be present that might respond favorably to this class of medication.[22,23] In summary, myofascial pain is a self-perpetuating condition that can migrate over time producing a more severe chronic pain syndrome.

DEPRESSION

Depression in the chronic pain patient may occur secondary to functional losses, the chronic unrelenting pain, inability to engage in vocational or avocational pursuits, financial worries, and family stressors. When depression is mild, psychological counseling, perhaps in conjunction with a low-dose antidepressant, may be all that is needed. However, when major depression occurs, consultation with a psychiatrist is strongly recommended for medical management. A major depressive episode implies a prominent and relatively persistent depressed and dysphoric mood that usually interferes with daily functioning (nearly every day for at least 2 weeks). At least four of the following eight symptoms should be demonstrated:

- change in appetite
- change in sleep
- psychomotor agitation or retardation
- loss of interest in usual activities or decrease in sexual drive
- increased fatigue
- feelings of guilt or worthlessness
- slowed thinking or impaired concentration
- a suicide attempt or suicidal ideation.[24]

Psychological counseling for depressed patients with chronic pain often requires special emphasis on and instruction in pain management strategies, pacing, relaxation techniques including biofeedback, and stress management. Involvement of other family members often is helpful.

With regard to pathophysiology, depressed patients have been found to have alterations of neurotransmitters within the brain. The neurotransmitters most frequently implicated include serotonin and norepinephrine whose absolute levels seem to decrease in depressed patients. Anxiety and depression both have an adverse effect on the perception of chronic pain. Typically, the depressed patient perceives their pain as being more severe than an individual who has pain but is not depressed.

Treatment of depression includes conservative modalities and pharmacologic agents. Management of depression in the chronic pain patient should start by actually addressing the underlying cause of the depression, the chronic unrelenting pain with impaired sleep. Appropriate analgesic therapy and physical therapeutic modalities will be necessary to manage the pain, and hypnotics are often necessary for the associated sleep disturbance. Once that is optimally addressed, traditional pharmacologic antidepressant agents and psychologic counseling/behavior modification are available for the depressed individual. The pharmacologic treatment of depression includes the use of old generation antidepressants (tricyclic antidepressants), as well as an expanding array of newer agents, which include the SSRIs, Effexor, Serzone, Wellbutrin, and Remeron.

SLEEP DISTURBANCE

Sleep disturbance is another problem commonly associated with chronic pain syndromes. It is characterized by: difficulty falling asleep; restlessness (nocturnal myoclonus), to the extent that the patient may kick his/her covers off the bed while sleeping; inability to find a comfortable position; frequent awakening with discomfort; inability to enter deeper stages of sleep; daytime fatigue, ranging from bothersome tiredness to overwhelming exhaustion.

Restlessness at night causes increased pain and discomfort during the day. Pain in conjunction with chronic fatigue can lead to impaired cognitive processes. Therefore, sleep disturbance in this context needs to be addressed. Conservative treatment might include behavioral and cognitive techniques such as relaxation training or listening to relaxation cassette tapes, which should be attempted at bedtime by patients who have difficulty falling asleep. However, pharmacologic management of sleep disturbances is often necessary. Such management includes the use of TCAs, conventional hypnotics, muscle relaxants, and the drug clonazepam (Klonopin).

Important concerns when choosing sedatives and hypnotics should include effectiveness of the drug, cost, side effects (including daytime fatigue and hangover effect), and presence or absence of nocturnal myoclonus or muscle spasm. Occasionally, combinations of different classes of medications prove most helpful (e.g., a low dose TCA with Klonopin).

Tricyclic Antidepressants (TCAs)

TCAs play an important role in the treatment of patients with chronic pain.[25–38] These agents offer the chronic pain patient three potentially useful effects: analgesia, sedation, and an antidepressant action. TCAs relieve pain and help promote sleep at lower dosages, at lower plasma levels, and in a shorter period of time than normally are required for treatment of depression. For example, chronic pain sufferers often benefit from low-dose

Table 9-1 Commonly used tricyclic antidepressant drugs

Drug (Trade Name)	Usual Daily Dose (mg)
Amitriptyline HCl (Elavil)	75–150
Desipramine HCl (Norpramin)	75–200
Doxepin HCl (Adapin, Sinequan)	75–150
Imipramine HCl (Tofranil)	50–200
Nortriptyline HCl (Pamelor)	75–100
Trazodone HCl (Desyrel)	150–200

Reprinted by permission from Rook JL. Symptom management. In Cassvan A, Weiss DL, Weiss JM, Rook JL, Mullens SU (eds). *Cumulative Trauma Disorders*. Boston, Butterworth-Heinemann, 1997.

amitriptyline (Elavil, 10 to 75 mg), the drug's positive analgesic and hypnotic effects being seen within days. On the other hand, the severely depressed patient will require higher doses (100 to 150 mg), and several weeks usually will go by before a therapeutic effect is realized.[39] Of the TCAs (Table 9-1), amitriptyline and imipramine are the most sedating. Trazodone also is quite sedating, although structurally it is not a true TCA.

Hypnotics

Conventional hypnotics are also available for patients with sleep disturbances. Among these are over-the-counter medications, benzodiazepines (temazepam [Restoril], flurazepam [dalmane], triazolam [halcion], clonazepam [Klonopin]), or non-benzodiazepine hypnotics (zolpidem tartrate [Ambien], Zalepon [Sonata]). Klonopin (0.5 to 2.0 mg at bedtime) is useful in decreasing night-time restlessness (nocturnal myoclonus); patients tend to feel more rested during the day if this phenomenon is lessened. Cyclobenzaprine HCl (Flexeril), which is structurally similar to the TCAs, may be helpful in promoting sleep in patients whose muscle spasms contribute to their chronic pain syndrome. The administration of hypnotic medications must be individualized.

Traditional hypnotics alone may be insufficient to induce sleep in the patient with unrelenting discomfort. In such cases, the patient should be provided with an appropriate analgesic medication at time of sleep so that the traditional hypnotic or tricyclic antidepressant will be able to exert their sedative side effects appropriately.

THE CHRONIC PAIN CLINIC

Occasionally patients fail to improve with conservative or invasive treatment measures. Some of these people may be appropriate for a chronic pain clinic. The typical chronic pain clinic lasts anywhere between three to six weeks. It is run by a multidisciplinary collection of professionals including a physician, psychologist, physical therapist, occupational therapist, social worker, and a nurse.

There are a number of skills that can be achieved by the patient during their pain clinic course. Patients need to be taught pain management skills, the importance of appropriate pacing of activities, and relaxation techniques. A good amount of time is devoted to exercise and generalized reconditioning. Most commonly, these patients have already had extensive courses of therapy, but nevertheless, are relatively inactive. The physical and occupational therapist works on increasing overall physical activity of the patient and assuring that they have an adequate home exercise program of stretches and exercises.

Many patients are referred to chronic pain clinics for alterations of their pharmacologic regimen, which might include detoxification. There is a medical school of thought that suggests that function is actually impaired by medications. Certainly, there are cases when patients are overmedicated with regards to analgesics and benzodiazepines (tranquilizers and hypnotics). In certain cases, it is definitely appropriate to decrease or terminate such medications. This process is usually done by providing the patient with what is known as a "pain cocktail" in which the patient receives an unknown medication (usually a liquid) whose various constituents are gradually altered by the physician running the clinic.

On the other hand, it may be more appropriate to simply modify the patient's pharmacologic regimen, to add appropriate analgesics, discontinue inappropriate medications, and perhaps to add other medications that might help with pain, sleep, depression, and neurogenic discomfort. Vocational counseling is an important component of the pain clinic. Often times, the patient with chronic pain has strict limitations that may preclude previous vocational pursuits. The vocational counselor discusses potential options given the patient's interests and restrictions.

Many patients enter the pain clinic chronically depressed as a result of the discomfort and the functional limitations. Treatment of depression is an important part of the pain clinic program. This would include individual counseling with a psychologist, perhaps on a daily basis, as well as manipulation of psychotropic medications in an effort to optimally stabilize the patient's mood during the several weeks that the patient participates in the clinic.

The chronic pain clinic also provides an environment for some degree of socialization for the patient. Often times, patients with chronic pain tend to avoid group activities and socialization that previously may have been a large part of their lives. This is due to the discomfort and functional limitations, as well as depression and irritability associated with chronic discomfort.

Lastly, a very important purpose of these clinics is to work on case closure from a legal and medical standpoint. The goal for many third party payers who fund these programs is to have the patient achieve some status of medical stability (also known as maximum medical improvement). Usually, at this stage, there can be some degree of administrative and/or legal closure of a case. When a patient is at maximum medical improvement, he or she can be provided with restrictions and an impairment rating. With the restrictions, determination can be made as to whether or not the patient can return to competitive employment. With the impairment rating, there can be legal closure to many cases. The physician of the team also needs to determine whether or not the patient will require maintenance care. Maintenance care refers to ongoing medical treatment without which the patient's condition will deteriorate.

Not all patients are appropriate for chronic pain clinics. For example, patients with borderline intellectual capabilities may not be appropriate as this type of clinic relies heavily on lectures and education concerning self-management of the chronic discomfort (relaxation strategies, pacing techniques, etc.). Patients with borderline intellectual capabilities are often unable to comprehend these strategies and they get very little out of this expensive environment. There are other patients who are physically unable to handle the rigors of going through a three- to six-week program. This type of program usually includes five very full days per week. Patients must have a critical level of endurance or else they will be unable to fully participate in this clinic. In some instances, the clinic program can be modified with shorter days. However, if patients cannot sit for more than a few minutes at a time and if they need to lie down frequently during the day, they may not be appropriate even for this modified program.

Patients who are profoundly depressed may not be able to actively participate in this type of social environment. They may require some treatment of their depression prior to their attempting entrance into this program. Usually, this is accomplished through pharmacologic manipulation, aggressive counseling, and psychiatric treatment for a period of time prior to their admittance into the pain clinic.

Treatment provided during the three- to six-week pain clinic includes the following:

- daily lectures concerning pacing strategies, pain management techniques, and relaxation strategies
- psychological counseling including both group sessions and one-on-one treatments with a psychologist
- pharmacologic manipulation by the physician running the clinic. As described above, this may include addition of psychotropic medications, hypnotics, and/or analgesics vs. detoxification from habituating medications
- physical therapy and occupational therapy on a daily basis
- instruction on home exercises to use upon completion of the clinic
- many pain clinics have a pool so that patients can participate in hydrotherapy
- vocational counseling
- towards the end of the program, patients may undergo a functional capacity assessment (FCA) or functional capacity evaluation (FCE), a rather extensive physical test performed by the patient in an effort to determine appropriate restrictions. Specific restrictions regarding ability to sit, stand, walk, change positions (bend, twist, kneel, crouch), use of the upper or lower extremities repetitively, and determination of the maximum weight that the patient should lift can be determined by this test. This determination will help label the patient as being in one of several physical demand levels including sedentary, light, medium, heavy, and very heavy
- at the end of the functional capacity evaluation, range of motion assessment is performed so that the patient can be provided with an impairment rating
- towards the end of the clinic, the staff meets to discuss issues of maximum medical improvement, impairment rating, and maintenance care
- it is important for the staff to determine necessary maintenance care so that the patient's condition does not deteriorate. This might include the ongoing need for medications and/or therapeutic modalities (physical or occupational therapy, chiropractic, massage therapy, psychological counseling).

PHARMACOLOGIC MANAGEMENT OF CHRONIC PAIN

Over the past ten years there has been a revolutionary movement in medicine, that of the more aggressive pharmacologic management of chronic pain. Over the past few years, legislation has been enacted in many states making it easier for physicians to prescribe opioid medications without the fear of sanctions against their licensure.

The Analgesic Ladder

If pharmacologic management of chronic pain is to be entertained, then the physician should follow a stepwise approach to medication management. The World Health Organization has described this approach to pain management as "the analgesic dosing ladder."[40] At the bottom of the ladder, are the weakest oral analgesics with the fewest side effects, and, at the top of the ladder, are the most potent opioid analgesics. In between are combinations of stronger, shorter-acting analgesics in conjunction with adjuvant medications (medications that enhance the potency of traditional analgesics, but do not necessarily have analgesic qualities by themselves).

At the bottom of the ladder are Tylenol, aspirin, or the nonsteroidal anti-inflammatory drugs (NSAIDs). Tylenol works as an analgesic and an antipyretic through its action in the central nervous system. This is in contrast to aspirin and the NSAIDs, which have a more peripheral action, inhibiting inflammation at the site of the injured tissue.

Physicians prefer to use Tylenol to the NSAIDs due to its lower toxicity profile. However, it is not completely benign. The maximum recommended dosage for Tylenol (acetaminophen) is 4 gm per day. Keeping in mind that a regular-strength Tylenol has 325 mg of acetaminophen, and an extra-strength Tylenol has 500 mg of acetaminophen, one must understand that a physician should not prescribe more than 12 or 8 of these pills per day, respectively. Physicians must also be aware that many scheduled medications include Tylenol in conjunction with the scheduled portion of the medication. For example, hydrocodone is available with combinations of acetaminophen ranging from 325 mg to 750 mg. This information must be kept in mind by the prescribing physician, who must advise the patient not to take more than 4 gm of Tylenol either alone or through a combination of these medications.

NSAIDs and aspirin are useful for pain associated with inflammation. There are many different NSAIDs available, each with a slightly different mechanism of action. The two newest NSAIDs, celecoxib (Celebrex) and rofecoxib (Vioxx), have minimal gastrointestinal side effects. The principal side effect of all anti-inflammatories is stomach irritation. Other potential side effects include liver and kidney damage, elevation of blood pressure, and impairment of bone healing.

Adjuvant Medications

There are a variety of medications that are known as adjuvants. These medications can be combined with traditional analgesics at any level in the analgesic dosing ladder. By themselves, these medications may not have analgesic potency. However, when combined with traditional analgesics, they tend to enhance the potency of those medications. Some examples would include caffeine, antihistamines, tricyclic antidepressants, and anticonvulsants.

Caffeine is frequently added to traditional analgesics to enhance potency. It is also helpful when added to headache medications as caffeine is a vasoconstrictor that helps with migraines (headaches characterized by vasodilatation of cerebral blood vessels). Caffeine is also added to several opioid medications, both to enhance potency and to prevent sedation caused by these medications. Antihistamines also can be added to traditional analgesic regimens to enhance potency of the analgesics. Additionally, antihistamines are somewhat sedating, and, when given at night, may help the chronic pain patient to sleep better.

It is well known that tricyclic antidepressant medications are helpful both as primary analgesics and as adjuvant medications. The tricyclic antidepressants have been around for more than 50 years. They have become well known in the field of chronic pain due to their analgesic and adjuvant qualities. They also help with sleep disturbance and depression, two symptoms common with chronic pain patients. The most commonly used tricyclic antidepressant is amitriptyline. Dosage can range anywhere between 10 to 150 mg, usually prescribed at night. Some patients suffer from a hangover effect during the day, which may preclude use of this class of medication. Therefore, tricyclic antidepressants are helpful for different types of chronic pain problems. They enhance traditional analgesics. When given at night, they may help with pain and sleep. The dosage for pain is usually lower than the dosage for depression. When used at higher dosages, it may be effective for depression.

Muscle relaxants are frequently helpful for chronic pain associated with increased muscle tone and spasm. The problem with most muscle relaxants is that they are sedating which may preclude daytime usage. However, when used at night, they may help promote better quality sleep. There are many different muscle relaxants available (Table 9-2). Flexeril can be used in the management of the fibromyalgia syndrome with dosages ranging between 10 to 40 mg per day. One muscle relaxant that is prone to abuse is Soma, which breaks down into a potentially habituating component, meprobamate.[41-44] However, it is generally a well tolerated and very effective muscle relaxant.

Several muscle relaxants exert their effect at the spinal cord level. The most well known is baclofen which is used principally for severe spasticity associated with spinal cord injuries or multiple sclerosis. However, it is also an effective muscle relaxant in patients with varying types of chronic myofascial pain and it is generally well tolerated. Other muscle relaxants similar to baclofen include methocarbamol (Robaxin) and metaxalone (Skelaxin). The mechanism of action of these medications has not been established, but may be due to general central nervous system depression. It has no direct action on the contractile mechanism of striated muscle, the motor endplate or the nerve fiber.[45]

The patient with severe, acute muscle spasm may benefit from Valium. However, Valium is very sedating, and of all the muscle relaxants, has the greatest risk of addiction. Nevertheless, in select instances, it is an extremely effective muscle relaxant.

Table 9-2 Common muscle relaxants

Trade Name	Generic Name
Flexeril	Cyclobenzaprine
Lioresal	Baclofen
Norflex	Orphenadrine citrate
Norgesic	Orphenadrine citrate 25 mg + aspirin 385 mg + caffeine 30 mg
Norgesic Forte	Orphenadrine citrate 50 mg + aspirin 770 mg + caffeine 60 mg
Parafon Forte DSC	Chlorzoxazone
Robaxin	Methocarbamol
Robaxin-750	Methocarbamol
Skelaxin	Metaxalone
Soma	Carisoprodol 350 mg
Soma Compound	Carisoprodol 200 mg + aspirin 325 mg
Valium	Diazepam

Reprinted by permission from Rook JL. Symptom management. In Cassvan A, Weiss DL, Weiss JM, Rook JL, Mullens SU (eds). *Cumulative Trauma Disorders*. Boston, Butterworth-Heinemann, 1997.

Pharmacologic Management of Neurogenic Pain

There are a number of medications that are effective for pain generated by the peripheral or central nervous system, also known as neurogenic pain. Several medications that have been advocated for use in patients with neurogenic pain include clonidine, mexiletine, anticonvulsants, tricyclic antidepressants, and various topical preparations.

Clonidine

Clonidine is a blood pressure medication that has analgesic qualities. It works by acting on alpha-receptors within the central nervous system. This interaction decreases the patient's perception of pain. It is also somewhat sedating, and when used at night, it may help promote better quality sleep. Another important quality of this medication is that it decreases the intensity of withdrawal symptomatology that might occur with the detoxification from a habituating medication. It is frequently advocated for use in chronic pain states of neurogenic etiology. It is available in oral tablets (0.1 mg, 0.2 mg, and 0.4 mg), and as a transdermal patch that gives continuous levels of medication with the convenience of only needing to be changed on a weekly basis. The principal side effect to this medication is sedation and orthostatic hypotension (as the medication is an antihypertensive). The patches may also cause a localized skin irritation secondary to the adhesive. Therefore, clonidine is an antihypertensive agent that has several potential uses in chronic pain patients including analgesia, sedation, adjuvant qualities, and its ability to minimize withdrawal side effects from habituating medications.[46–52]

Mexiletine

Mexiletine is the oral version of lidocaine. We are most familiar with the use of lidocaine as an injectable anesthetic agent. In this context it works by inhibiting nerve conduction across nerve segments that have been infiltrated by this medication. The principal purpose for the drug mexiletine is as an antiarrhythmic agent. Frequently, patients who are hospitalized with heart attacks and arrhythmias are given intravenous lidocaine to prevent ectopic cardiac activity that could lead to ventricular fibrillation and death. However, it was noted that the intravenous lidocaine also had analgesic properties. An oral lidocaine derivative (Mexiletine or Mexitil) was fabricated for use in ambulatory patients with arrhythmias. This medication is now also being used for treatment of various types of neurogenic pain. It has a more systemic effect than injected lidocaine, which acts only locally. This medication calms down hyperactive nervous system tissue by interfering with the conduction of pain impulses. The principal side effect of mexiletine is gastrointestinal irritation and nausea. It is recommended that mexiletine be taken with food to prevent these side effects. Therefore, mexiletine is an oral derivative of the anesthetic lidocaine. It is useful for pain states associated with nerve injury. Initial dosage can range between 150 to 300 mg. The total daily dosage should not exceed 1200 mg/day. This medication will need to be titrated. Its principal side effects are gastrointestinal.[53–59]

Anticonvulsants

Anticonvulsant drugs traditionally are used for patients who have a seizure disorder. They work by calming down irritated foci of brain tissue, which initiate the seizures. It has been found that these medications also decrease irritated nervous tissue that contributes to various neurogenic pain states. For example, patients who have peripheral nerve entrapments have localized nervous tissue irritation at the site of entrapment. The anticonvulsants work by decreasing the painful discharges emanating from those sites.[39,60–62] This class of medications has been found useful in treating neurogenic pain due to peripheral nerve entrapment, radiculopathy, nerve damage within the central nervous system, reflex sympathetic dystrophy, and diabetic peripheral neuropathy. There are a number of anticonvulsants that can be used for this purpose. Some of the more common ones include Tegretol, Dilantin, Depakote, Neurontin, and Klonopin.

Tegretol, when used in the seizure disorder patient requires dosages up to 1600 mg per day. The dosage for neurogenic pain is typically lower. Pain patients can start at a very low dosage (100 mg to 200 mg per day) and the medication can be titrated upwards slowly until it becomes efficacious or until there are unacceptable side effects. This medication can cause liver toxicity and frequent monitoring of the Tegretol level, blood counts, and liver functions are required when managing neurogenic pain with this class of medication. If Tegretol is not helpful, trials can be attempted with other anticonvulsants such as Depakote (250 to 1000 mg per day), Neurontin (300 to 3600 mg per day), Dilantin (100 to 400 mg per day), or Klonopin (0.5 to 6 mg per day). All anticonvulsants have associated side effects that vary from individual to individual. Depakote, Neurontin, Tegretol, and Dilantin all can potentially damage the liver, and, as noted above, frequent liver function studies are necessary. Klonopin tends to be very sedating and when used during the day can cause drowsiness and subtle cognitive impairment. However, these medications as a group may be efficacious in decreasing various types of neurogenic pain experienced by some patients.[63–72]

Tricyclic Antidepressants

Tricyclic antidepressants are occasionally helpful in treating neurogenic pain. The most common TCA is Elavil. It can be started at a low dosage of 10 mg and titrated up to a maximum dosage of 150 mg per day. Other TCAs are listed in Table 9-1.

PHARMACOLOGIC MANAGEMENT OF DEPRESSION

Depression, a common symptom amongst chronic pain patients, can occasionally be managed through conservative measures (psychological counseling, pain management). However, pharmacologic management is usually necessary to help minimize the depressive episode. It is certainly reasonable for the primary care physician or the pain specialist to attempt early trials of pharmacologic management of the depression. However, if the patient fails to improve, it would be wise to refer him or her to a psychiatrist for more precise adjustment and titration of psychotropic medications.

There are many different antidepressants currently available for treatment. In the past, older antidepressant classes included the TCAs, trazodone, and the Monoamine Oxidase (MAO) Inhibitors. Since the introduction of Prozac in the 1980s there has been an explosion in research and production of a number of new families of antidepressants.

Tricyclic Antidepressants

TCAs have several qualities that are useful for chronic pain patients. Higher dosages often are required to achieve the antidepressant effects then are necessary for analgesia and sleep. Occasionally, TCA use is limited by anticholinergic side effects (dry mouth, constipation, and urinary retention), daytime sedation, disturbed concentration, cardiac arrhythmias (heart block, tachycardia, and palpitations), and weight gain (particularly with Elavil).

TCAs inhibit the membrane pump mechanisms responsible for reuptake of norepinephrine and serotonin in adrenergic and serotoninergic neurons. The increased synaptic availability of these neurotransmitters is believed to underlie the antidepressant activity of the TCAs. Likewise, increased availability of norepinephrine and serotonin in the noradrenergic and serotoninergic descending pain pathways may explain the analgesic abilities of this antidepressant class.[25–34]

Selective Serotonin-reuptake Inhibitor Antidepressants

Over the past decade, a new family of antidepressants has evolved that works by selectively inhibiting reuptake of the neurotransmitter serotonin. In general, this class of medication is better tolerated than the TCAs with fewer side effects and sedative qualities. The medications available include fluoxetine hydrochloride (Prozac), sertraline hydrochloride (Zoloft), paroxetine hydrochloride (Paxil), nefazodone hydrochloride (Serzone), and citalopram hydrobromide (Celexa). These drugs all are orally administered antidepressants chemically unrelated to TCAs or other available antidepressants. Their mechanism of action is believed to be via selective inhibition of normal serotonin reuptake. As opposed to the TCAs, the selective serotonin-reuptake inhibitor antidepressants (SSRIs) have little affinity for muscarinic, histaminergic, and adrenergic receptors; stimulation of such receptors has been hypothesized to be associated with the various anticholinergic, sedative, and cardiovascular effects seen with the TCAs.

The SSRIs are metabolized in the liver and excreted in the kidneys. Consequently, dosages must be adjusted appropriately in patients with liver and kidney disease. A serious and possibly fatal reaction can occur if SSRIs are used in conjunction with monoamine oxidase inhibitors (MAOIs). Therefore, SSRIs should not be used in combination with, or within 14 days of discontinuation of, an MAOI. The most commonly observed adverse reactions to SSRIs are listed in Box 9-1. The usual dose ranges are 20 to 80 mg per day for Prozac, 50 to 200 mg per day for Zoloft, 20 to 60 mg per day for Paxil, and 20 to 40 mg for Celexa. As with other antidepressants, the full antidepressant effect of SSRIs may be delayed until 4 weeks or more after treatment begins.[73–79]

Venlafaxine Hydrochloride

Venlafaxine hydrochloride (Effexor) is chemically unrelated to the TCAs or SSRIs. The antidepressant action of Effexor is believed to be due to potent inhibition of norepinephrine and serotonin neuronal reuptake.[80] However, as opposed to the TCAs

Box 9-1 Commonly observed adverse reactions for the selective serotonin-reuptake inhibitors

Nervous system
  Anxiety
  Nervousness
  Insomnia
  Somnolence
  Tremor
  Dizziness
Gastrointestinal system
  Nausea
  Diarrhea
  Dyspepsia
  Anorexia
  Dry mouth
Other reactions
  Increased sweating
  Male sexual dysfunction (ejaculatory delay)

Reprinted by permission from Rook JL: Symptom management. In Cassvan A, Weiss DL, Weiss JM, Rook JL, Mullens SU (eds). *Cumulative Trauma Disorders.* Boston, Butterworth-Heinemann, 1997.

(which also inhibit norepinephrine and serotonin), Effexor has no significant affinity for muscarinic, histaminergic, and adrenergic receptors, thereby avoiding the anticholinergic, sedative, and cardiovascular effects of TCAs.[80–82] Effexor is metabolized extensively in the liver and excreted in the kidney. Like SSRIs, it should not be administered to patients on MAOIs or for two weeks after discontinuation of these drugs, and there is a similar side effect profile. Dosage can range from 75 to 225 mg per day for mild to moderate depression and up to 350 mg per day for severely depressed patients.

Bupropion Hydrochloride

Bupropion hydrochloride (Wellbutrin) is chemically unrelated to TCAs, SSRIs, and Effexor. The neuro chemical mechanism of its antidepressant effect is not known, but it appears to be a stimulant for the central nervous system. There is a fourfold increased incidence of seizure activity in patients on Wellbutrin as compared with other marketed antidepressants. Therefore, Wellbutrin is contraindicated in patients with a seizure disorder and in patients with anorexia and bulimia, because of a higher incidence of seizures in such patients. Common side effects of this drug include agitation, dry mouth, insomnia, headaches, nausea, vomiting, constipation, and tremor. The usual adult dose is 300 mg per day in divided doses.[83,84]

Mirtazapine

Mirtazapine (Remeron) is an antidepressant for oral administration. It has a chemical structure unrelated to SSRIs, tricyclics or MAO inhibitors. The mechanism of action of Remeron is unknown. Clinical studies suggest that Remeron enhances central noradrenergic and serotinergic activity. Remeron is a potent antagonist of histamine receptors, a property that may explain its prominent sedative effects. Commonly observed adverse effects associated with the use of this drug include somnolence, increased appetite, weight gain and dizziness. The recommended starting dose for Remeron is 15 mg/day, administered as a single dose, preferably prior to sleep. The effective dose range is between 15 and 45 mg/day.[45]

REFERENCES

1. Johnson S. Disciplinary actions and pain relief: analysis of the Pain Relief Act. *J Law Med Ethics* 1996; 24(4): 319.
2. Arnst C, Licking E, *et al.* Conquering pain. *Business Week* Mar 1 1999.
3. Centers for Disease Control. Prevalence of disabilities and associated health conditions among adults—United States. 1999. *Morb Mortal Wkly Rep CDC Surveill Summ* 2001; 50(7): 120.
4. Burton WN, Conti DJ, Chen CY, *et al.* The role of health risk factors and disease on worker productivity. *J Occup Environ Med* 1999; 41(10): 863.
5. Linton SJ, Hellsing AL, Andersen D. A controlled study of the effects of an early intervention on acute musculoskeletal pain problems. *Pain* (Netherlands) 1993; 54(3): 353.
6. Lohman WH. Resources for disability prevention. Occupational medicine update: selected topics in occupational medicine. St. Paul, MN, p 72.

7. Suchman AL, Markakis K, Bechman HB, *et al.* A model of empathic communication in the medical interview. *JAMA*, Feb 26 1997; 277(8): 678.
8. The Robert Wood Johnson Foundation Staff Planning Committee. *Patient education and consumer activation in chronic disease.* Princeton, NJ, The Robert Wood Johnson Foundation meeting proceedings, July 6–7 2000.
9. Wells KB, Stewart A, Hays RD, *et al.* The functioning and well-being of depressed patients—results from the medical outcomes study. *JAMA* 1989, 262(7): 914.
10. Valenstein M, Vijan S, Zeber JE, *et al.* The cost-utility of screening for depression in primary care. *Ann Intern Med* 2001; 134(5): 345.
11. Kesterson CM, Tierney WM. Association of symptoms of depression and diagnostic test charges among older adults. *Ann Intern Med* 1997; 126(6): 426.
12. Gatchel RJ. The dominant role of psychosocial risk factors in the development of chronic low back pain disability. *Spine* 1995; 20(24): 2702.
13. Burton AK. Psychosocial predictors of outcome in acute and subchronic low back trouble. *Spine* 1995; 20(6): 722.
14. Crook J, Moldofsky H, Shannon H. Determinants of disability after a work related musculoskeletal injury. *J Rheumatol* 1998; 25(8): 1570.
15. The Colorado Department of Labor and Employment, Division of Workers Compensation. *Disability management.* Workers compensation level II re-accreditation course, August 2001.
16. Gutstein M. Diagnosis and treatment of muscular rheumatism. *BMJ* 1938; 1: 302.
17. Kellgren JH. A preliminary account of referred pains arising from muscle. *BMJ* 1938; 1: 325.
18. Simons DG, Travell JG. Myofascial origins of low back pain. *Postgrad Med* 1983; 73: 66.
19. Travell JG, Simons DG. *Myofascial Pain and Dysfunction. The Trigger Point Manual.* Baltimore, Williams and Wilkins, 1983.
20. Harden RN, Bruehl SP, Gass S, *et al.* Signs and symptoms of the myofascial pain syndrome. A national survey of pain management providers. *Clin J Pain* 2000; 16(1): 64.
21. Fields HL. Evaluation of patients with persistent pain. In Fields HL (ed). *Pain*, p 205. New York, McGraw-Hill, 1987.
22. Esenyel M, Caglar N, Aldemir T. Treatment of myofascial pain. *Am J Phys Med Rehabil* 2000; 79(1): 48.
23. Hanten WP, Olson SL, Butts NL, *et al.* Effectiveness of a home program of ischemic pressure followed by sustained stretch for treatment of myofascial trigger points. *Phys Ther* 2000; 80(10): 997.
24. American Psychiatric Association. *Diagnostic and Statistical Manual of Mental Disorders.* DSM-IV, 4th ed. Washington, DC, American Psychiatric Association, 1994.
25. Couch JR, Hassanein RS. Amitriptyline in migraine prophylaxis. *Arch Neurol* 1979; 21: 263.
26. Gomersall JD, Stuart A. Amitriptyline in migraine prophylaxis. Changes in pattern of attacks during a controlled clinical trial. *J Neurol Neurosurg Psychiatry* 1973; 36(4): 684.
27. Diamond S, Baltes BJ. Chronic tension headache treated with amitriptyline–a double blind study. *Headache* 1971; 11(3): 110.
28. Lance JW, Curran DA. Treatment of chronic tension headache. *Lancet* 1964; 1: 1236.
29. Watson CP, Evans RJ, Reed K, *et al.* Amitriptyline versus placebo in postherpetic neuralgia. *Neurology* 1982; 32: 671.
30. Gomez-Perez FJ, Rull JA, Dies H, *et al.* Nortriptyline and fluphenazine in the symptomatic treatment of diabetic neuropathy. A double-blind cross-over study. *Pain* (Netherlands) 1985; 23(4): 395.
31. Kvinesdal B, Molin J, Froland A, *et al.* Imipramine treatment of painful diabetic neuropathy. *JAMA* 1984; 251(13): 1727.
32. Turkington RW. Depression masquerading as diabetic neuropathy. *JAMA* 1980; 243: 1147.
33. Gringas M. A clinical trial of Tofranil in rheumatic pain in general practice. *J Int Med Res* 1976; 4: 41.
34. Scott WAM. The relief of pain with an antidepressant in arthritis. *Practitioner* 1969; 202: 802.
35. Descombes S, Brefel-Courbon C, Thalamas C, *et al.* Amitriptyline treatment in chronic drug-induced headache. a double blind comparative pilot study. *Headache* 2001; 41(2): 178.

36. Plesh O, Curtis D, Levine J, McCall WD. Amitriptyline treatment of chronic pain in patients with temporomandibular disorders. *J Oral Rehabil* 2000; 27(10): 834.
37. Lynch ME. Antidepressants as analgesics. a review of randomized controlled trials. *J Psychiatry Neurosci* 2001; 26(1): 30.
38. Sindrup SH, Jensen TS. Effectiveness of pharmacological treatments of neuropathic pain. An update and the effect related to mechanism of drug action. *Pain* 1999; 83(3): 389.
39. Fields HL. Anticonvulsants, psychotropics, and anti-histamine drugs in pain management. In Fields HL (ed). *Pain*. New York, McGraw-Hill, 1987.
40. World Health Organization. *Cancer Pain Relief*. Geneva, World Health Organization, 1986.
41. Bennett RM, Gatter RA, Campbell SM, *et al*. A comparison of cyclobenzaprine and placebo in the management of fibrositis. A double-blind controlled study. *Arthritis Rheum* 1988; 31(12): 1535.
42. Hamaty D, Valentine JL, Howard R, *et al*. The plasma endorphin, prostaglandin and catecholamine profile of patients with fibrositis treated with cyclobenzaprine and placebo: a 5-month study. *J Rheumatol* 1989; 19(suppl): 164.
43. Reynolds W, Moldofsky H. The effects of cyclobenzaprine on sleep physiology and symptoms in FMS. *J Rheumatol* 1991; 18: 452.
44. Littrell RA, Hayes LR, Stillner V. Carisoprodol (Soma). A new and cautious perspective on an old agent. *South Med J* 1993; 86: 753.
45. *Physicians' Desk Reference*, 52nd ed, pp 830, 1957, 2428. Montvale, NJ, Medical Economics, 1998.
46. Fleetwood-Walker S, Mitchell R, Hope PJ, *et al*. An alpha 2 receptor mediates the selective inhibition by noradrenaline of nociceptive responses of identified dorsal horn neurones. *Brain Res* (Netherlands), 1985; 334(2): 243.
47. Yaksh TL, Reddy SVR. Studies in the primate on the analgesic effects associated with intrathecal actions of opiates, adrenergic agonists and baclofen. *Anesthesiology* 1981; 54: 451.
48. Wong KC, Franz DN, Tseng J. Clinical pharmacology of alpha 2-agonist and beta-adrenergic blocker. *Anaesth Sinica* 1989; 27: 357.
49. Spaulding TC, Fielding S, Venafro JJ, *et al*. Anti-nociceptive activity of clonidine and its potentiation of morphine analgesia. *Eur J Pharmacol* 1979; 58: 19.
50. Zemlan FP, Corrigan SA, Pfaff DW. Noradrenergic and serotonergic mediation of spinal analgesia mechanisms. *Eur J Pharmacol* 1980; 61: 111.
51. Reddy SVR, Maderdrut JL, Yaksh TL. Spinal cord pharmacology of adrenergic agonist-mediated antinociception. *J Pharmacol Exp Ther* 1980; 213: 525.
52. Fielding S, Spaulding T, Lal H. Antinociceptive action of clonidine. In Fielding S, Spaulding T, Lal H (eds). *Psychopharmacology of Clonidine*, p 225. New York, Alan R Liss, 1981.
53. Davis RW. Phantom sensation, phantom pain, and stump pain. *Arch Phys Med Rehabil* 1993; 74: 79.
54. Chabal C, Russell LC, Burchiel KJ. The effect of intra-venous lidocaine, tocainide, and mexiletine on spontaneously active fibers originating in rat sciatic neuromas. *Pain* 1989; 38: 333.
55. Dejgaard A, Petersen P, Kastrup J. Mexiletine for the treatment of chronic painful diabetic neuropathy. *Lancet* 1988; 29: 9.
56. *Physicians' Desk Reference*, 48th ed, p 616. Montvale, NJ. Medical Economics, 1994.
57. Sloan P, Basta M, Storey P, von Gunten C. Mexilitine as an analgesic for the management of neuropathic cancer pain. *Anesth Analg* 1999; 89(3): 760.
58. Mao J, Chen LL. Systemic lidocaine for neuropathic pain relief. *Pain* 2000; 87(1): 7.
59. Wallace MS, Magnuson S, Ridgeway B. Efficacy of oral mexilitine for neuropathic pain with allodynia. a double-blind, placebo-controlled, crossover study. *Reg Anesth Pain Med* 2000; 25(5): 459.
60. Wall PD. Changes in damaged nerve and their sensory consequences. In Bonica JJ, Liebeskind JC, Albe-Fessard D (eds). *Proceedings of the Second World Congress on Pain*, p 39. New York, Raven, 1979.
61. Yaari Y, Devor M. Phenytoin suppresses spontaneous ectopic discharge in rat sciatic nerve neuromas. *Neurosci Lett* 1985; 58: 117.

62. Burchiel KJ. Carbamazepine inhibits spontaneous activity in experimental neuromas. *Exp Neurol* 1988; 102: 249.

63. Blom S. Tic douloureux treatment with new anticonvulsant. *Arch Neurol* 1963; 9: 285.

64. Maciewicz R, Bouckoms A, Martin JB. Drug therapy of neuropathic pain. *Clin J Pain* 1985; 1: 39.

65. Dunsker SB, Mayfield FH. Carbamazepine in the treatment of the flashing pain syndrome. *J Neurosurg* 1976; 45: 49.

66. Espir MLE, Millac P. Treatment of paroxysmal disorders in multiple sclerosis with carbamazepine (Tegretol): *J Neurol Neurosurg Psychiatry* 1970; 33: 528.

67. Fields HL, Raskin NH. Anticonvulsants and pain. In Klawans HL (ed). *Clinical Neuropharmacology*, p 173. New York, Raven, 1976.

68. Shibasaki H, Kuroiwa Y. Painful tonic seizure in multiple sclerosis. *Arch Neurol* 1975; 30: 47.

69. Rull JA, Quibrera R, Gonzalez-Millan H, *et al*. Symptomatic treatment of peripheral diabetic neuropathy with carbamazepine (Tegretol). double blind crossover trial. *Diabetologia* 1969; 5: 215.

70. Laird MA, Gidal BE. Use of Gabapentin in the treatment of neuropathic pain. *Ann Pharmacother* 2000; 34(6): 802.

71. Wiffen P, Collins S, McQuay H, *et al*. Anticonvulsant drugs for acute and chronic pain. *Cochrane Database Syst Rev* 2000; (3).CD 001133.

72. Tremont-Lukats IW, Megeff C, Backonja MM. Anticonvulsants for neuropathic pain syndromes. mechanisms of action and place in therapy. *Drugs* 2000; 60(5): 1029.

73. Stokes PE. Fluoxetine. a five-year review. *Clin Ther* 1993; 15: 216.

74. Potter WZ, Rudorfer MV, Manji H. The pharmacologic treatment of depression. *N Engl J Med* 1991; 325: 633.

75. Tollefson GD. Antidepressant treatment and side effect consideration. *J Clin Psychiatry* 1991; 52(suppl 6): 4.

76. Thomas DR, Nelson DR, Johnson AM. Biochemical effects of the antidepressant paroxetine, a specific 5-hydroxytryptamine uptake inhibitor. *Psychopharmacology* 1987; 93: 193.

77. Bergstrom RF, Lemberger L, Farid NA, *et al*. Clinical pharmacology and pharmacokinetics of fluoxetine. a review. *Br J Psychiatry* 1988; 153(suppl 3): 47.

78. *Physicians' Desk Reference*, 47th ed, p 2058. Montvale, NJ, Medical Economics, 1993.

79. Cooper GL. The safety of fluoxetine–an update. *Br J Psychiatry* 1988; 153(suppl 3): 77.

80. *Effexor (venlafaxine HCl) prescribing information*. Philadelphia, Wyeth-Ayerst Laboratories.

81. Richelson E. Synaptic pharmacology of antidepressants. An update. *McLean Hosp J* 1988; 13: 67.

82. Preskorn SH, Burke M. Somatic therapy for major depressive disorder. selection of an antidepressant. *J Clin Psychiatry* 1992; 53(suppl 9): 5.

83. Feinberg M. Bupropion. new therapy for depression. *Am Fam Physician* 1990; 41: 1787.

84. Bupropion for depression. *Med Lett* 1989; 31(804): 97.

10

Neurogenic Pain

Jack L Rook

ANATOMY AND PATHOPHYSIOLOGY

An in-depth discussion of the anatomy of ascending and descending pain pathways can be found in Chapter 2. In review, the nervous system is broken down into central and peripheral components. The central nervous system consists of the brain and spinal cord and the peripheral nervous system is all of the nerves that emanate from the brainstem and the spinal cord (12 cranial, 8 cervical, 12 thoracic, and 5 sacral nerves).

The cervical spinal nerve roots coalesce in the shoulder region as the brachial plexus, which further organizes to form distinct peripheral nerves which supply each upper extremity. The major peripheral nerves in the upper extremities are the median, ulnar, radial, musculocutaneous, and axillary nerves. The thoracic nerve roots become the intercostal nerves, supplying intercostal and abdominal musculature and thoraco-abdominal sensory dermatomes. The lumbosacral nerve roots coalesce as the lumbar plexus within the pelvis. The lumbar plexus further organizes into two major peripheral nerves, the femoral and sciatic. The femoral nerve branches to form the saphenous nerve, and the sciatic nerve branches into the tibial and peroneal nerves.

Each peripheral nerve analyzed microscopically will demonstrate a variety of different sized fibers within the nerve trunk. Some of the nerve fibers are surrounding by a waxy covering known as myelin. These nerve fibers, known as A-alpha, are the largest and they have been found to conduct electrical impulses at velocities in the range of 50 to 70 m/sec. Other nerve fibers contain little or no myelin at all. These fibers of smaller diameter are known as the C (unmyelinated) and A-delta (small myelinated) fibers. It is these smaller fibers that transmit impulses concerned with nociception (pain).

The nociceptive C and A-delta fibers transmit their impulses into the dorsal horn of the spinal cord where there are connections (synapses) with second order pain transmission cells. These second order cells send their fibers across the spinal cord, where they then ascend towards the brain in a "tract" of fibers known as the spinothalamic tract (STT). Once the spinothalamic tract reaches the brain, the second order pain fibers within it separate out into two distinct pathways known as the neospinothalamic tract (NSTT) and the paleospinothalamic tract (PSTT).[1]

The neospinothalamic tract transmits information that helps to localize the origin of the pain impulses. These fibers, which have a lateral course through the brainstem, travel to the somatosensory cortex to relay information about location of pain. The more medial pathway is the paleospinothalamic tract (PSTT). It travels through the thalamus to a number of areas in the brain that control the emotional responses to chronic pain (depression, anxiety). PSTT connections with the brainstem modulate the sleep disturbances associated with chronic pain.[1] (See Figures 2-2 and 2-3.) This summarizes the ascending pain pathways.

There is a descending pain modulatory system that travels from the brain to the spinal cord. This system helps an individual to modulate their pain. The major nuclei centers in the descending modulatory pain system can be found in the pons (dorsal lateral pons), the medulla (rostroventral medulla), and the outer layers (dorsal horn) of the spinal cord.[2–15]

Impulses from cortical centers have connections with the pontine center. The nuclei in the dorsal lateral pons have connections with nuclei in the rostroventral medulla. Synaptic connections with cells in the rostroventral medulla involve endorphins (opioid like substances made by the body to help control pain) as the neurotransmitters. The endorphins stimulate descending nerve fibers that travel to the dorsal horn of the spinal cord where they liberate the neurotransmitters serotonin and/or norepinephrine. These chemicals directly inhibit the first and second order pain transmission cells with which they synapse, or they stimulate small interneurons that then release endorphins, which can inhibit the second order cells.[16–21] (See Figure 2-4.)

SYMPTOMS OF NEUROGENIC PAIN

The patient with neurogenic pain usually complains of severe pain that seems to be out of proportion to the physical examination. The pain may be deep or aching, may have a burning quality, or there may be an electrical shooting sensation known as lancinating pain. Some patients complain of being excessively sensitive to stimuli that normally would not be painful. For example, a patient with reflex sympathetic dystrophy may hold his or her hand in a protective fashion because of its hypersensitivity to seemingly harmless stimuli such as a gentle breeze. Some patients complain of temperature or color changes in their extremities.

SIGNS/PHYSICAL EXAMINATION

Whenever there is nerve damage, there will be characteristic signs seen on physical examination. The signs that are seen depend on the degree of damage and whether or not there is a predilection for damage to large vs. small peripheral nerve fibers. The large fibers are concerned with non-noxious sensation (light touch or vibration) and muscle control. Therefore, if there is significant damage to large fibers within a peripheral nerve, the patient will have principally motor and sensory abnormalities.

The clinician must become familiar with the motor distributions of upper and lower extremity peripheral nerves in order to determine the site of injury. Spinal nerve root or peripheral nerve damage will produce specific patterns of weakness in the extremity. For example, damage to the C5 nerve root may result in weakness of shoulder abduction and elbow flexion (the deltoid and biceps are innervated by nerve roots C5 and C6), a median nerve lesion at the level of the wrist will result in weakness of thumb movement (the median nerve controls the thenar muscle known as the abductor pollicis brevis), and a radial nerve lesion at the mid humerus, will result in weakness of wrist and finger extension. Along with motor weakness, with nerve injury there will be muscle atrophy seen on physical examination.

Sensory abnormalities may also be detected. The sensory examination can give important information to help localize the site of injury. The clinician must become familiar with sensory dermatomes corresponding to spinal nerve roots (see Figure 6-20), as well as the sensory distributions of peripheral nerves (Figure 10-1).

At the site of nerve injury, the clinician may detect a positive Tinel's sign. This sign indicates nerve damage with associated hypersensitivity at a particular location. The test is performed by tapping along the course of a nerve. At the site of nerve damage or entrapment a shooting pain or paresthesia may be generated.

- A positive Tinel's sign at the wrist is indicative of carpal tunnel syndrome (entrapment of the median nerve at the level of the transverse carpal ligament)
- A positive Tinel's sign just above the clavicle may be an indication of thoracic outlet syndrome
- A positive Tinel's sign in the lower extremity adjacent to the medial malleolus may be an indication of tarsal tunnel syndrome.

The patient with carpal tunnel syndrome may also have a positive Phalen's maneuver. To perform this test, the patient flexes their wrist(s). (See Figure 5-23B.) If a hand "falls asleep," it suggests median nerve compression through the carpal tunnel.

The hyperabduction test (or 90 degree abduction external rotation [AER]) is used to assess for thoracic outlet syndrome. To perform this test, the patient raises both arms over his or her head. The development of upper extremity paresthesias (particularly in an ulnar distribution) is highly suggestive of thoracic outlet syndrome. This and other tests for thoracic outlet syndrome are elaborated upon in the chapter on upper extremity pain syndromes.

A physical finding consistent with small fiber (nociceptive) nerve damage is the phenomenon of allodynia. The patient with allodynia describes a noxious sensation from non-noxious stimuli. For example, light stroking of the hand may be described as being extremely painful. This hypersensitivity is allodynia.

Color and temperature changes in an extremity suggest an abnormality of the sympathetic nervous system, a system also modulated by small unmyelinated fibers. The sympathetic nervous system is hyperactive in the chronic painful condition known as reflex sympathetic dystrophy. This hyperactivity causes decreased blood flow in the involved extremity. Chronic decreased blood flow results in trophic changes in the extremity (dry skin, brittle nails, muscle atrophy, and/or contractures).

There may be changes in normal reflexes of the respective extremity. Reflexes that are commonly assessed include the biceps, triceps, and brachioradialis in the upper extremities, and the knee jerk, ankle jerk, and tibialis posterior reflexes in the lower extremities. Reflex abnormalities may indicate a lesion of a particular nerve root or a peripheral nerve. In conjunction with the remainder of the physical examination, reflex assessment will help to localize the nerve lesion.

A provocative test used to determine cervical nerve root injury is known as Spurling's maneuver. To perform this test, the examiner asks the patient to hyperextend his or her head and then move it laterally. If the patient experiences paresthesias or an electrical radiation of the pain into the respective extremity when the examiner applies downward pressure to the patient's head, this suggests a cervical nerve root injury.[22] The straight leg

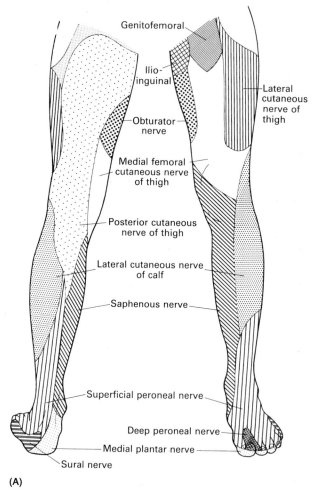

(A)

Figure 10-1 (A) Cutaneous innervation of the left lower limb. (B) Cutaneous innervation of the left arm. Reprinted by permission from Osselton JW, Binnie CD, Cooper R, et al. (eds): *Clinical Neurophysiology—Electromyography, Nerve Conduction and Evoked Potentials*, pp 127, 114. Boston, Butterworth-Heinemann, 1995.

raising test is a provocative maneuver used to assess for lumbar-sacral nerve root injury. It can be performed with the patient sitting or lying supine. The examiner raises the patient's leg, and, if the patient experiences paresthesias or pain into the respective extremity, then the straight leg raising test is positive. This suggests a pinched nerve at the lumbosacral level.

NEUROGENIC PROBLEMS RELATED TO MOTOR VEHICLE ACCIDENTS

Upper Extremity Nerve Entrapments

A variety of neurological problems can occur after a motor vehicle accident. Nerve damage in the upper extremities can involve one or more of the major peripheral nerves in the extremity (median, radial, and ulnar). The major sites of entrapment of the median nerve are

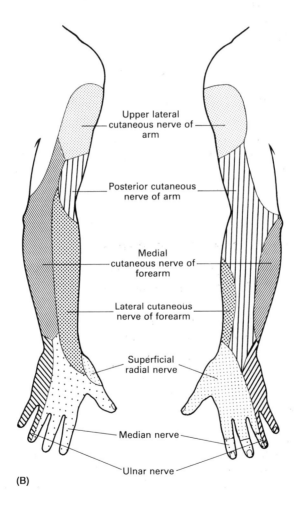

(B)

at the wrist (carpal tunnel syndrome), and in the forearm (pronator syndrome). The ulnar nerve may be entrapped at the level of the wrist (Guyon's canal syndrome), or as it courses around the elbow (cubital tunnel syndrome). The radial nerve may be entrapped just above the wrist on the radial aspect of the forearm (superficial radial nerve entrapment), as it courses through the supinator muscle (radial tunnel syndrome or supinator syndrome), or more proximally as it courses along the radial groove of the humerus. Entrapment of the brachial plexus can occur at the level of the clavicle and surrounding musculature. This is referred to as a brachial plexopathy or thoracic outlet syndrome.

Upper extremity nerve entrapments may complicate motor vehicle accidents for a variety of reasons. Often, patients brace themselves prior to impact, grasping the steering wheel tightly, or bracing against the dashboard or back seat. Hyperextension wrist injuries could result in a nerve entrapment syndrome anywhere throughout the involved extremity. The accident victim who bangs his/her arm against the door could develop cubital tunnel, radial tunnel, or pronator syndrome as a result of the elbow trauma. Patients who sustain whiplash or shoulder injuries may ultimately develop thoracic outlet syndrome due to spasm of surrounding thoracic outlet musculature (pectoral or scalene muscles) which causes irritation of the underlying brachial plexus.

An interesting phenomenon that occurs with brachial plexus irritation is the development of hypersensitivity in all *distal* peripheral nerves. When this occurs, a previously asymptomatic peripheral nerve compression may become symptomatic. For example, some patients develop symptoms of carpal tunnel syndrome after a motor vehicle accident with whiplash injury and proximal muscle spasm. On electrical testing, the patient is found to have abnormalities consistent with carpal tunnel syndrome. These electrical abnormalities may have pre-existed the motor vehicle accident, but the syndrome was asymptomatic until the brachial plexus became irritated in tight thoracic outlet musculature. Therefore, proximal nerve injury will make distal extremity nerves become hypersensitive, a common neurological phenomenon often described as a "double crush syndrome."

Lower Extremity Nerve Entrapments

Lower extremity nerve entrapments may also occur after a motor vehicle accident, possibly due to bracing the leg against the brake or floorboard prior to impact. Common lower extremity nerve entrapments include tarsal tunnel syndrome (entrapment of the tibial nerve as it courses along the medial ankle), or anterior tarsal tunnel syndrome (entrapment of the superificial peroneal nerve as it courses over the anterior ankle). A less common entrapment may involve the common peroneal nerve as it courses around the fibular head. This region may be affected by direct trauma with bruising to the lateral foreleg.

Nerve Root Irritation

The patient may develop nerve root irritation as a result of a motor vehicle accident. In the cervical region, a hyperflexion hyperextension injury may traumatize nerve roots. For example, during hyperextension, the neural foramina (the passageway through which the nerve roots exit the spinal canal), decrease in caliber to a point where there may actually be bony entrapment of its nerve root. This sudden pinching may irritate and/or damage the nerve resulting in a radiculitis or radiculopathy. Disruption of intervertebral discs in the cervical and lumbar region may cause their herniation. A herniated disc may directly impinge against a nerve root. Pre-existing degenerative changes may further reduce the caliber of the spinal canal and neuroforamina predisposing to peripheral nerve or spinal cord compression as the neck or trunk moves through flexion and extension during the whiplash.

Radiculopathy

A cervical and/or lumbar radiculopathy may result from a motor vehicle accident. These patients complain of extremity pain and paresthesias and physical examination will reveal motor and sensory abnormalities.

Headaches

Patients with whiplash injuries frequently complain of headaches that may be a result of mechanical irritation of the occipital nerves. These nerves emanate from spinal nerve roots C1, C2, and C3 that coalesce to form two greater and two lesser occipital nerves. These nerves supply sensation to the head and scalp. One or more of the four occipital nerves may become entrapped in tight paracervical musculature. (See Figure 10-1.)

In contrast, vascular or migraine headaches may occur after a motor vehicle accident. Some individuals who have a pre-existing history of well controlled migraines may note that their headaches have become markedly accentuated in intensity and frequency after an accident. This may require modulation of a prior medical regimen or initiation of new medications for management of this worsened condition. The pathophysiology of this condition is described in the chapter on headaches.

Neuroma

Nerve damage may occur along any upper or lower extremity peripheral nerve. Wherever there is nerve damage, a patient may develop a neuroma, a cluster of damaged nerve fibers surrounded by scar tissue. The scar tissue entraps the nervous tissue, causing chronic pain. A common site of neuroma formation is between the metatarsal bones of the foot. These are known as interdigital neuromas and they can cause chronic foot pain that worsens with weightbearing.

Each of the above-mentioned neurogenic problems are discussed in separate chapters within this text.

WORKUP FOR NEUROGENIC PAIN

The workup of neurally mediated pain begins with the history and physical examination. Ancillary testing which may demonstrate peripheral or central nervous system damage includes electrodiagnostic studies, thermography, diagnostic nerve blocks, and somato-sensory evoked potentials.

Electromyography (EMG/NCV)

Electrodiagnostic studies are used to evaluate for nerve injury involving the peripheral nervous system (nerve roots, brachial and lumbar plexus, and peripheral nerves of the upper and lower extremities). The electrodiagnostic evaluation consists of nerve conduction velocity studies (NCVs) and the electromyographic examination (EMG). Nerve conduction studies are performed by stimulating a peripheral nerve at two different sites in the respective extremity. These stimulations result in a motor or sensory response that can be reported on an oscilloscope. By knowing the amount of time it takes to produce these responses and the distance between the two stimulation sites, the examiner is able to determine how well the nerve conducts electricity.

When performing NCVs, nerve damage is indicated by a slowing of velocity or a decrease in amplitude of the sensory or motor response. All nerves have characteristic velocities with normal usually being in the range of 50 to 70 m/sec in the upper extremities, and 40 to 50 m/sec in the lower extremities. The results of the NCV studies can be compared with normal values, or the asymptomatic extremity can be used as a control.

The EMG portion of the electrodiagnostic study is performed using needles that are inserted into various muscles in the involved extremity, and neck or back muscles. Each muscle is supplied by a distinct nerve root and peripheral nerve distribution. By recording electrical potentials in specific muscles, the examiner can determine very precisely the location of a neurological lesion. The electrodiagnostic examination can provide valuable physiologic adjunctive information to complement the physical examination and imaging studies.

Somatosensory Evoked Potential (SSEP)

Another type of electrodiagnostic study is the somatosensory evoked potential (SSEP). This study is performed by stimulating skin in a distal extremity with a repetitive electrical discharge and recording how long those impulses take to reach active electrodes overlying the spinal cord and sensory cortex of the brain. The amount of time it takes for the sensory impulses to reach active electrodes along the neck, back, or head is compared to normals. This test may be useful in detecting both peripheral and central nervous system injury.

Thermography

Thermography is a test used to assess for abnormal temperature changes in an extremity. The machinery includes a special camera that, instead of taking formal pictures, maps out temperature distributions throughout the body. Different temperature gradients are seen as different colors on the thermography images. This test is particularly useful in helping to diagnose the neurological disorder reflex sympathetic dystrophy. Patients with reflex sympathetic dystrophy typically have vasomotor abnormalities that cause abnormal changes in blood flow. These blood flow changes produce temperature changes in the respective extremity and these temperature changes can be picked up on thermographic images. Thermography is much more sensitive in detecting subtle temperature differences than the physical examination. In addition, special stress testing can be performed to precipitate abnormal vasomotor responses in potential RSD patients.

Selective Nerve Blocks

Selective nerve blocks can be performed by trained personal to determine if a particular nerve or nerve root has been damaged or traumatized. For example, if a clinician suspects a herniated disc at the L4 level with radiculopathy due to an L4 nerve lesion, a nerve block selectively anesthetizing the suspected L4 nerve root will help determine if indeed, that nerve root is involved in the neurological pain process (if sciatica is relieved by the injection, the nerve root is involved). This type of blocking procedure can also be performed on peripheral nerves in the extremities and on the occipital nerves in a patient who has post traumatic headaches. Once again, nerve blocks help to localize those nerves that contribute to the nociceptive process.

Sympathetic Blockade

Lastly, sympathetic blocks are performed to help evaluate whether or not the patient has reflex sympathetic dystrophy syndrome. These blocks must be performed by trained personnel (usually an anesthesiologist) who have resuscitative equipment available should the patient develop a complication to one of the blocks. After blocking the sympathetic nervous system, a significant decrease in pain in conjunction with improved blood flow is usually consistent with an abnormality of the sympathetic nervous system. Sympathetic blocks are not only diagnostic, but they may be therapeutic for these individuals.

TREATMENT OF NEUROGENIC PAIN

Treatment modalities for patients with neurogenic pain include:

- physical and occupational therapy
- medications
- electrical stimulation devices (ranging in complexity from the transcutaneous electrical nerve stimulation [TENS] unit to a spinal cord stimulator)
- surgical procedures
- nerve blocking procedures.

Physical and Occupational Therapy

Physical and occupational therapy techniques that may be helpful for the patient with neurogenic pain include a variety of desensitization techniques for the involved extremity.

Use of a symptomatic extremity is encouraged to help prevent muscle atrophy. Additionally, movement of an extremity can help to modulate the pain itself. Activation of movement receptors (proprioceptive nerve fibers) has an inhibitory effect at the dorsal horn (pain center) of the spinal cord. Therefore, use of the involved extremity should be encouraged as part of both the therapy and daily life of these patients. The patient may also require splinting, and modalities such as ultrasound and iontophoresis, which can be helpful in reducing inflammation and/or scar tissue about an entrapped nerve.

Medication

There are a whole host of medications that may be helpful for patients with neurogenic pain. The most commonly used "neurogenic" medications include anticonvulsants, tricyclic antidepressants, mexiletine, clonidine, opioid analgesics, and topical creams.

The most common *anticonvulsants* utilized for neurogenic pain are Tegretol and Neurontin. These medications are particularly useful for patients who complain of lancinating (electrical shooting) pain.[23-25]

Mexiletine is an oral medication analogous to lidocaine, the anesthetic given to numb nerves (e.g., at the dentist's office). Lidocaine works by decreasing or eliminating neural transmission in the area where it has been injected. Oral lidocaine works in a similar fashion, decreasing the hypersensitivity of irritated or damaged nervous tissue.[26-28]

Clonidine is an antihypertensive agent that has analgesic properties. It can be administered both orally and via transdermal patches. It is now also used intrathecally, administered via an implanted infusion pump system.

Tricyclic antidepressants are frequently used in the treatment of a variety of pain states including neurogenic pain. They also help promote better quality sleep and in treating depression (a common problem in patients suffering from chronic pain).[29-32]

Capsaicin cream is an over-the-counter preparation that may help certain types of neurogenic pain. It is a derivative of the chili pepper and it works by inactivating Substance P, a chemical liberated by small fiber pain cells. Other topical creams can be individually compounded, using combinations of anti-inflammatories and anesthetics (e.g., Indocin-lidocaine cream). Such creams are frequently helpful for patients with neurogenic pain and skin hypersensitivity.

Electrical Stimulation Devices

A TENS unit is always worth trying in a patient with neurogenic pain. The theory behind TENS unit efficacy is the "gait control hypothesis" of Melzack and Wall. They proposed that stimulation of the fast-conducting, large, myelinated fibers with gentle electrical stimulation will help to modulate and decrease nociceptive information traveling on the slower A-delta and C-fibers by blocking those impulses at the dorsal horn/spinal cord level.[33,34] TENS units are frequently effective for the patient with chronic neurogenic pain, and certainly an attempt of this conservative modality is worthwhile. However, proper equipment and proper instruction on its use is essential.

Spinal cord stimulation refers to a high technology surgical treatment technique whereby a pacemaker-like device is implanted under the skin with electrodes inserted adjacent to the spinal cord. When it works, the spinal cord stimulator will produce a non-noxious paresthetic sensation (i.e., tingling) in place of the former region of neurogenic pain. When successful, spinal cord stimulation can provide pain relief, improved function, and decrease an individual's reliance on medications and other modalities offered by the health care system.

Surgical Procedures

There are a number of surgical procedures that may be indicated for patients with intractable neurogenic pain. In those cases where a nerve is entrapped under a ligament, within scar tissue, or underneath a muscle that is chronically in spasm, a *neurolysis* of the nerve is indicated. This refers to a surgical procedure whereby the nerve fibers are released from the entrapping ligament, scar tissue, or tight musculature respectively.

Rarely, a *neurectomy* is the procedure of choice. For example, when there has been significant nerve damage to a small peripheral sensory nerve, and there is a considerable amount of surrounding scar tissue constantly irritating that small sensory nerve, transection of the nerve (neurectomy) may be helpful. For example, neurectomy may be required when an interdigital nerve in the foot or the superficial radial nerve of the upper extremity is entangled within scar tissue. A neurectomy is a neuroablative procedure in that it results in the destruction of nervous tissue. It should never be performed on a major mixed (motor and sensory) nerve.

Other neuroablative procedures that are occasionally indicated include *rhizotomies* (transection of sensory spinal nerves that innervate painful facet joints), and *sympathectomy* (a procedure to eliminate sympathetic nervous tissue that lies alongside the spinal cord in an effort to decrease the symptoms of reflex sympathetic dystrophy). In general, the results of neuroablative procedures are unpredictable. Occasionally, they are helpful, but usually with a self-limited positive response. On other occasions, the neurogenic pain actually worsens after such procedures.

Nerve Blocking Technique

Lastly, there are a variety of *nerve-blocking techniques* that are frequently helpful for individuals with neurogenic pain. Steroid injections may be helpful in treating entrapped peripheral nerves. For example, the patient with carpal tunnel syndrome may benefit from a steroid injection underneath the transverse carpal ligament. This may reduce inflammation sufficiently so that the patient can accelerate recovery and perhaps avoid a surgical procedure. Other upper extremity peripheral nerves that can be injected include the ulnar nerve at the cubital tunnel or at Guyon's canal, the radial nerve at the supinator mass, and the superficial radial nerve in the distal radial forearm. In the lower extremities, steroid injections may be performed to help alleviate tarsal tunnel (tibial nerve) and/or anterior tarsal tunnel (superficial peroneal nerve) syndrome. Such steroid injections may help accelerate recovery.

More proximal steroid blocks, into the spinal canal, may be indicated if the patient has a nerve root entrapment with radiculopathy. These blocks must be administered by specially trained personnel, usually an anesthesiologist, who have resuscitative equipment available should complications occur. In the cervical region, the injection technique is known as a cervical epidural steroid injection, and in the lumbar region it is known as a lumbar epidural steroid injection. These injections may help accelerate recovery in patients with cervical or lumbar radiculitis respectively. Usually, a series of such injections are indicated.

Sympathetic blockade is useful for patients with neurogenic pain due to the reflex sympathetic dystrophy syndrome. For a more complete discussion on sympathetic nerve blocks, see Chapter 11, Reflex Sympathetic Dystrophy Syndrome.

REFERENCES

1. Fields HL. Pain pathways in the central nervous system. In Fields HL (ed). *Pain*. New York, McGraw-Hill, 1987.
2. Baskin DS, Mehler WR, Hosobuchi Y, *et al.* Autopsy analysis of the safety, efficiency, and cartography of electrical stimulation of the central gray in humans. *Brain Res* 1986; 371: 231.
3. Hosobuchi Y, Adams JE, Linchitz R. Pain relief by electrical stimulation of the central gray matter in humans and its reversal by naloxone. *Science* 1977; 197: 183.
4. Richardson DE, Akil H. Pain reduction by electrical brain stimulation in man. *J Neurophysiol* 1977; 47: 178.
5. Abols IA, Basbaum AI. Afferent connections of the rostral medulla of the cat. A neural substrate for midbrainmedullary interactions in the modulation of pain. *J Comp Neurol* 1981; 201: 285.
6. Beitz AJ. The organization of afferent projections to the midbrain periaqueductal gray of the rat. *Neuroscience* 1982; 7: 133.
7. Mantyh PW. The ascending input to the midbrain periaqueductal gray of the primate. *J Comp Neurol* 1982; 211: 50.
8. Zorman G, Hentall ID, Adams JE, *et al.* Naloxone-reversible analgesia produced by microstimulation in the rat medulla. *Brain Res* 1981; 219: 137.
9. Fields HL, Heinricher MM. Anatomy and physiology of a nociceptive modulatory system. *Philos Trans R Soc Lond B Biol Sci* 1985; 308: 361.
10. Bowker R, Westlund KN, Coulter JD. Origins of serotonergic projections of the spinal cord in rat: an immunocytochemical retrograde transport study. *Brain Res* 1981; 226: 187.
11. Fields HL, Basbaum AI, Clanton CH, *et al.* Nucleus raphe magnus inhibition of spinal cord dorsal horn neurons. *Brain Res* 1977; 126: 441.
12. Willis WD. *Control of Nociceptive Transmission in the Spinal Cord*. New York, Springer, 1982.
13. Westlund KN, Bowker RM, Ziegler MG, *et al.* Descending noradrenergic projections and their spinal terminations. *Prog Brain Res* 1982; 57: 219.
14. Westlund KN, Bowker RM, Ziegler MG, *et al.* Origins and terminations of descending noradrenergic projections into the spinal cord of the monkey. *Brain Res* 1984; 292: 1.
15. Reddy SVR, Yakah TL. Spinal noradrenergic terminal system mediates antinociception. *Brain Res* 1980; 189: 391.
16. Fields HL. Central nervous system mechanisms for control of pain transmission. In Fields HL (ed), *Pain*, p 99. New York, McGraw-Hill, 1987.
17. Glazer EJ, Basbaum AI. Axons which take up [^{3}H] serotonin are presynaptic to enkephalin immunoreactive neurons in cat dorsal horn. *Brain Res* 1984; 298: 389.
18. Ruda MA. Opiates and pain pathways: demonstration of enkephalin synapses on dorsal horn projection neurons. *Science* 1982; 215: 1523.
19. Fields HL, Emson PC, Leigh BK, *et al.* Multiple opiate receptor sites on primary afferent fibers. *Nature* 1980; 284: 351.

20. Hiller JM, Simon EJ, Crain SM, *et al.* Opiate receptors in culture of fetal mouse dorsal root ganglia (DRG) and spinal cord. predominance in DRG neurites. *Brain Res* 1978; 145: 396.
21. Mudge AW, Leeman SE, Fischbach GD. Enkephalin inhibits release of substance P from sensory neurons in culture and decreases action potential duration. *Proc Natl Acad Sci USA* 1979; 76: 526.
22. Calliet R. Medical management of neck pain of mechanical origin. In Giles LGF, Singer KP (eds). *Cervical Spine Pain*, p 118. Boston, Butterworth Heinemann, 1998.
23. Laird MA, Gidal BE. Use of Gabapentin in the treatment of neuropathic pain. *Ann Pharmacother Jun* 2000; 34(6): 802.
24. Wiffen P, Collins S, McQuay H, *et al.* Anticonvulsant drugs for acute and chronic pain. *Cochrane Database Syst Rev* 2000; (3): CD 001133.
25. Tremont-Lukats IW, Megeff C, Backonja MM. Anticonvulsants for neuropathic pain syndromes. mechanisms of action and place in therapy. *Drugs* 2000; 60(5): 1029.
26. Sloan P, Basta M, Storey P, *et al.* Mexilitine as an analgesic for the management of neuropathic cancer pain. *Anesth Analg* 1999; 89(3): 760.
27. Mao J, Chen LL. Systemic lidocaine for neuropathic pain relief. *Pain* Jul 2000; 87(1): 7.
28. Wallace MS, Magnuson S, Ridgeway B. Efficacy of oral mexilitine for neuropathic pain with allodynia: a double-blind, placebo-controlled, crossover study. *Reg Anesth Pain Med* 2000; 25(5): 459.
29. Descombes S, Brefel-Courbon C, Thalamas C, *et al.* Amitriptyline treatment in chronic drug-induced headache: a double-blind comparative pilot study. *Headache* 2001; 41(2): 178.
30. Plesh O, Curtis, Levine J, McCall WD. Amitriptyline treatment of chronic pain in patients with temporomandibular disorders. *J Oral Rehabil* 2000; 27(10): 834.
31. Lynch ME. Antidepressants as analgesics: a review of randomized controlled trials. *J Psychiatry Neurosci* 2001; 26(1): 30.
32. Sindrup SH, Jensen TS. Effectiveness of pharmacological treatments of neuropathic pain. An update and the effect related to mechanism of drug action. *Pain* 1999; 83(3): 389.
33. Melzack R, Wall PD. Pain mechanisms. a new theory. *Science* 1965; 150: 971.
34. Melzack R, Wall PD. *The Challenge of Pain*. New York, Basic Books, 1982.

11

Reflex Sympathetic Dystrophy Syndrome

Jack L Rook

The human body normally recovers from injury in a manner that is thoroughly predictable and consistent with the type and severity of trauma. This statement holds true for the vast majority of traumatic injuries where patients receive appropriate treatment for their condition. Occasionally, instead of improving, a patient's condition worsens; the patient develops a degree of pain and disability that is disproportionate to the original injury and persists long after the injury has healed.[1,2] This may be attributable to development of the reflex sympathetic dystrophy syndrome (RSDS), a constellation of signs and symptoms first described in 1864 by Weir Mitchell, a Civil War surgeon.[3] Mitchell used the terms *causalgia* (Greek for "burning pain") and *erythromelalgia* (redness and pain) to describe this new syndrome seen in soldiers who had major nerve injuries due to gunshot wounds.

Since Mitchell's time, numerous names have been applied to RSDS (Table 11-1).[3–18] Most recently, the umbrella term *complex regional pain syndrome* (CRPS) has been adopted.[10] Two types of CRPS have been recognized: type I corresponds to RSDS that occurs without a definable nerve lesion, whereas type II, formerly called *causalgia*, refers to cases in which a definable nerve lesion is present.

TERMINOLOGY

The original terms *erythromelalgia* and causalgia were coined by Mitchell in the 1860s.[3,4] At the turn of the twentieth century, Sudeck[11] described bony changes seen with this disorder and, in 1937, DeTakats[12] described reflex dystrophy of the extremities. In the 1940s, causalgia was further subdivided into minor and major causalgia and, in 1947, Evans first used the term *reflex sympathetic dystrophy syndrome*.[16] Even since that time, additional terms for this entity have evolved, including *reflex algodystrophy, mimocausalgia*, and *sympathetically maintained pain*.[5–7,9,15–20]

Causalgia refers to RSDS that occurs after nerve injury, minor causalgia being caused by minor injury to a sensory nerve and major causalgia being caused by injury to a major mixed nerve (e.g., median nerve, brachial plexus). The pain of minor causalgia tends to be less severe and fairly localized initially, but it may spread rapidly.[2,21]

Table 11-1 Alternative terms for the reflex sympathetic dystrophy syndrome

Year	Term	Describer
1864	Erythromelalgia	Mitchell[3,4]
1867	Causalgia	Mitchell[3,4]
1900	Sudeck's atrophy of bone	Sudeck[11]
1929	Peripheral acute trophoneurosis	Zur Verth[5,6]
1931	Traumatic angiospasm	Morton and Scott[5]
1933	Post-traumatic osteoporosis	Fontaine and Herrmann[5]
1934	Traumatic vasospasm	Lehman[18]
1937	Reflex dystrophy of the extremities	DeTakats[12]
1940	Minor causalgia	Homans[13]
1947	Reflex neurovascular dystrophy	Steinbrocker[15]
1947	Reflex sympathetic dystrophy syndrome	Evans[16]
1967	Reflex algodystrophy	Serre[17]
1973	Mimocausalgia	Patman[14]
1973	Algoneurodystrophy	Glick[7]
1986	Sympathetically maintained pain	Roberts[9]
1995	Complex regional pain syndrome	Stanton-Hicks et al[10]

Reprinted by permission from Rook JL. Reflex sympathetic dystrophy syndrome. In Cassvan A, Weiss LD, Weiss JM, Rook JL, Mullens SU (eds). *Cumulative Trauma Disorders*, p 156. Boston, Butterworth-Heinemann, 1997.

Shoulder-hand syndrome refers to RSDS that begins in the shoulder and spreads distally, causing swelling and burning pain in the hand. The shoulder-hand syndrome is most frequently associated with hemiparetic stroke syndromes, but it has also been described after shoulder injury and in association with referred shoulder pain due to cervical radiculopathy.[2]

The term *Sudeck's atrophy of bone* refers to osteoporotic bony changes that may occur in association with RSDS. Current common terminology for this condition includes *reflex sympathetic dystrophy* (RSD), *reflex sympathetic dystrophy syndrome* (RSDS), *sympathetically maintained pain* (SMP), and *complex regional pain syndrome*. In this chapter, RSDS is used to refer to this entity. Later in this chapter, SMP is discussed briefly as a variant of RSDS.

EPIDEMIOLOGIC FEATURES

RSDS occasionally complicates injuries sustained in a motor vehicle accident. It may complicate an upper or lower extremity injury, particularly if there is some sort of nerve damage involved. The injury that precipitates the development of an RSDS, can be major, minor, or even trivial. It may result from injury to bone, muscle, or ligament. However, the most likely etiology of this neurogenic pain phenomenon involves some sort of damage to a peripheral nerve.

In the upper extremity, nerve damage can occur as a result of essentially any trauma. The peripheral nerves of the upper extremity emanate from the anterior rami of cervical nerve roots C5 through T1. These nerves coalesce at the level of the neck and shoulder into the collection of nerves known as the brachial plexus. Distal to this point, the brachial plexus divides into distinct peripheral nerves including the median, ulnar, radial, and musculocutaneous nerves. These nerves further branch in the forearm and hands to supply sensation to the digits, hand, and forearm. Small branches of the peripheral nerves are scattered throughout the hand and forearm region. Many of these nerves are subcutaneous and can easily be injured with the type of trauma experienced in a motor vehicle accident.

For example, a hyperextension wrist injury (as may occur with grasping the steering wheel or bracing oneself at time of impact) may traumatize the median and ulnar nerves where they cross the wrist. Nerve injury in this fashion could underlie a subsequent RSDS.

Any traumatic event, including a direct blow to the extremity at time of impact, could ultimately precipitate an RSDS. Localized swelling will increase pressure against an adjacent subcutaneous nerve. For example, elbow trauma with localized swelling could affect the ulnar nerve as it courses through the ulnar groove of the medial elbow. Whenever a nerve is damaged, it could set into motion the pathophysiological changes that contribute to the development of RSDS.

Patients who develop proximal myofascial discomfort and spasm after whiplash injury, may develop entrapment of the brachial plexus through the thoracic outlet, particularly as the nerves pass through the scalene and pectoral muscles. Nerve irritation or damage due to thoracic outlet syndrome could precipitate the development of an RSDS.

Occasionally, RSDS may complicate a fracture. This may result from actual nerve irritation or damage by the fractured bony segment, or it may result as a complication of prolonged immobilization via casting.

Lower extremity RSDS may also complicate a traumatic motor vehicle accident. A significant ankle strain could traumatize peripheral nerves that cross the ankle joint (superficial peroneal, tibial, and sural nerves). Fractured bones may precipitate the development of an RSDS, either due to the fracture itself, associated damage to an adjacent nerve, or as a result of prolonged immobilization. The knee, a heavily innervated joint, may sustain a neurologic injury after striking against the dashboard. This may precipitate the development of RSDS.

A patient may develop RSDS after surgical treatment for an injury sustained in a motor vehicle accident. For example, RSDS has developed after first rib resection for the treatment of a thoracic outlet syndrome,[22] and after carpal tunnel surgery. Such procedures require manipulation of underlying nerves. Other potential iatrogenic problems including tight-fitting casts applied after fractures, and long-term casting of nonfracture diagnoses (e.g., epicondylitis, severe strain, ulnar neuritis, ankle strain) may initiate an RSDS.[23] The long-term casting prevents joint movement which causes a loss of proprioceptive afferent input (which can down-regulate the sympathetic nervous system) into the spinal cord dorsal horn. These events may precipitate the development of RSDS (Box 11-1).

Box 11-1 Common causes of reflex sympathetic dystrophy syndrome after motor vehicle accident

Soft Tissue Injury
Tendonitis
Bursitis

Operative Procedures
Brachial plexopathy
Scalenus anticus syndrome
Cervical radiculopathy
Cervical cord injury

Immobilization with Cast or Splint
Dashboard knee
Ankle sprain
Wrist hyperextension injury

Reprinted by permission from Rook JL. Reflex sympathetic dystrophy syndrome. In Cassvan A, Weiss LD, Weiss JM, Rook JL, Mullens SU (eds). *Cumulative Trauma Disorders*, p 157. Boston, Butterworth-Heinemann, 1997.

THREE STAGES OF REFLEX SYMPATHETIC DYSTROPHY SYNDROME

The symptoms of RSDS might begin gradually, days or weeks after injury, or they may manifest within a few hours. The patient suffers greatly and protects the affected area. Classical literature discussing this disorder describes how it typically progresses in stages:

1. The first, *acute* stage, can last up to three months. It is characterized by signs and symptoms of sympathetic underactivity. RSDS is normally considered to be a process characterized by excessive activity of the sympathetic nervous system (SNS), with vasoconstriction and decreased blood flow. However, in the acute stage, blood flow actually increases, and there is redness, warmth, and soft swelling of the extremity. Increased blood flow to hair follicles and nail beds leads to increased hair and nail growth. Patients find that pain worsens with heat application and that generalized stiffness can occur owing to soft swelling. Lastly, osteoporosis may commence after approximately three weeks due to a combination of intraosseous hyperemia and disuse of the extremity.[1,2,21,24-34]

2. The second stage, the *dystrophic* stage, usually occurs between the third and ninth months. In this stage, pain progressively worsens, and the patient begins to develop characteristic psychological and behavioral changes. The swelling spreads and becomes firm and fixed over time (brawny edema). In the dystrophic stage, we begin to see sympathetic overactivity, with decreased blood flow (cyanotic, pale, cool skin), increased sweating (hyperhidrosis), and decreased hair growth. Cold will worsen pain in this stage. The osteoporosis that began in stage 1 becomes marked and diffuse. Owing to a localized lack of nutrition, nails becomes brittle, skin begins

to atrophy, fibrosis of joints commences and patients develop increasing stiffness in their affected extremity.[1,2,12,21,24,25,27,31,32,34,35]

3. The third stage, the *atrophic* stage, usually occurs after nine months. The patient's pain reaches a plateau, swelling decreases, and skin appears pale, cool, and dry. The skin begins to atrophy, tightening around the fingers, and patients may develop "pencil-pointing" of the fingertips (extreme tapering of the digits). Osteoporosis, contractures, and muscle wasting now involve most of the extremity. In general, patients with stage 3 RSDS are left with a nonfunctional contracted extremity.[2,12,13,21,24,25,27,32,35,36]

These characterize the classical textbook description of the stages of RSDS. In actuality, a patient may skip a stage and/or may find themselves permanently within a particular stage. If there is identification of this neurological phenomenon, and if patients receive appropriate treatment, many of the signs that will occur with later-stage disease would be absent. For example, the patient who tries to utilize their extremity and does the exercises outlined by their therapist, may avoid development of atrophic phenomena characteristic of stage 3 RSDS. In addition, those patients who receive sympathetic blockade, or sympatholytic medications will not necessarily demonstrate the characteristic findings seen in stage 2 of this disorder (with decreased blood flow, brittle nails, decreased hair growth, and cold extremities).

SIGNS AND SYMPTOMS

Pain

Pain is the most prominent symptom, distinguished by its intensity. It seems disproportionate to the injury, constant, and burning, and tends to spread in a nonanatomic distribution, proximally through the extremity, to the contralateral extremity, or even throughout the body.[37–39] The symptoms' disproportionate pain that spreads in a nonanatomic distribution represent two positive Waddell signs. Therefore, the use of Waddell signs to guide management of affected individuals could prove harmful, as necessary care might be delayed in these patients.

The pain is increased by motion of the involved extremity and by anything that increases sympathetic tone (excessive exercise; being startled; and anxious emotional states).[2,37–40] Heat or cold will aggravate the pain, depending on the stage of the disorder: heat aggravates the involved extremity in the first stage and cold in the later stages. *Allodynia* refers to pain that worsens with non-noxious stimuli (e.g., gentle pressure, clothing, or a breeze). Because of this phenomenon, the RSDS patient tends to hold the involved extremity close to the body in a protective fashion.[41]

Other Clinical Signs and Symptoms

Edema, localized at first, may spread proximally through the extremity. Early in the process, the edema is soft but, over time becomes firm and fixed (i.e., brawny edema) as the proteinaceous edema fluid organizes, resulting in fibrosis and contractures.

Vasomotor instability results in color and temperature changes throughout the extremity. Redness and warmth are characteristic early in the process. Over time, the extremity may appear blotchy, cyanotic, pale, and cool. Sudomotor changes (abnormalities of sweating) include hyperhidrosis (stage 2) and excessive dryness of the extremity (stages 1 and 3). Osteoporosis may begin by the third week after onset of the disorder. Initially, it is spotty and periarticular but, over time, it can become homogeneous and diffuse.

Trophic changes occur owing to lack of nutrition to the extremity. The skin becomes shiny, thin, and tight, causing a loss of skin creases. There is atrophy of subcutaneous fat, muscle wasting and, occasionally, pencil-pointing of the fingertips. Over time, fibrosis and contractures will develop if mobility of the extremity is not maintained through physical therapy and independent exercise.[2,21] Some RSDS patients experience involuntary movements, such as jerking, twisting, writhing motions, or muscle spasm. The presence of such activity suggests involvement of the central nervous system.[39,42,43]

Psychological and Behavioral Characteristics

A number of psychological and behavioral characteristics might become evident in RSDS patients over time, leading some researchers to describe these patients as having a "causalgic personality," characterized by withdrawn, fearful, and suspicious behavior, a low pain threshold, and preoccupation with protection of the painful extremity.[1] Such patients present as chronic complainers who are depressed and emotionally unstable.[2,24,44] Eighty percent of patients in one series scored high on the hysteria, hypochondriasis, and depression scales of the Minnesota Multiphasic Personality Inventory, a report that has incited debate as to whether RSDS occurs because patients have a predisposing diathesis.[45]

Although injuries are very common, only a very small fraction of injured patients go on to develop RSDS. Of patients with nerve injuries, only approximately 2 to 5 percent develop causalgia,[21] and of patients with all kinds of trauma, the incidence of RSDS has been estimated at between 5 percent and 15 percent.[45] It has been suggested that those individuals who do develop the disease have a predisposing diathesis which may be either physiological or psychological.[1,2]

The *physiologic diathesis* refers to an underlying autonomic imbalance (history of cold hands or feet, pre-existing Raynaud's phenomenon, excessive sweating, fainting, migraine headaches, or blushing) before the onset of RSDS.[2] *Personality diathesis* refers to a psychological predisposition to development of RSDS. The theoretic model for this suggests that the premorbid presence of depression, anxiety, and life stress may result in sympathetic hyperarousal, which can contribute to the development or maintenance of RSDS. The RSDS personality diathesis is a controversial issue, as many researchers believe that the personality changes are secondary to the chronic, unrelenting pain.[40] However, the disparity between the often minor trauma believed to have initiated the RSDS and the extreme pain experienced by the patient can cause health professionals to conclude that the RSDS patient is malingering, neurotic, or emotionally unstable. Certainly, further investigation is needed in this area.[46–51]

DIAGNOSIS

Diagnosis is based on clinical criteria, x-rays, techniques that measure skin temperature, bone scans, blood tests, electrodiagnostic studies, and response to sympathetic interruption. A thorough history and physical examination might reveal the characteristic signs and symptoms consistent with a diagnosis of RSDS (Box 11-2). Patients typically

Box 11-2 Characteristic signs and symptoms of the reflex sympathetic dystrophy syndrome

Signs
Allodynia
Edema
Vasomotor changes
  Increased sweating (stage 2)
  Decreased sweating (stages 1, 3)
Osteoporosis
Trophic changes
  Shiny, thin skin
  Loss of skin creases
  Atrophy of subcutaneous fat
  Muscle wasting
  Pencil-pointing of digits
Contractures
Increased hair and nail growth (stage 1)
Decreased hair and nail growth (stages 2, 3)
Nail fragility
Involuntary movements
Muscle spasm

Symptoms
Pain
  Out of proportion to injury
  Burning
  Unrelenting
  Spreads in nonanatomic distribution
  Worsens with anxiety or stress
  Worsens with heat (stage 1)
  Worsens with cold (stages 2, 3)
Skin hypersensitivity
Psychological manifestations
  Depression
  Anxiety
Sleep disturbance

Reprinted by permission from Rook JL. Reflex sympathetic dystrophy syndrome. In Cassvan A, Weiss LD, Weiss JM, Rook JL, Mullens SU (eds). *Cumulative Trauma Disorders*, p 159. Boston, Butterworth-Heinemann, 1997.

complain of pain that is out of proportion to what would be expected, given the degree of injury. Physical examination may demonstrate swelling, stiffness, vasomotor and sudomotor changes, and in late-stage disease, trophic changes, which make the diagnosis more obvious.

Radiographic Studies

X-rays of both involved and uninvolved extremities should be obtained. These may demonstrate peri-articular osteoporosis within a few weeks of injury. The radiological hallmark of RSDS of the limb is unilateral osteoporosis (Sudeck's atrophy). However, osteoporosis can be absent in as many as 33 percent of cases, particularly during the early course of the disease process. The radiologic appearance of RSDS osteoporosis has been characterized as spotty or patchy. Osteoporosis is manifested by the thinning of the cortices, loss of fine trabeculae, and tunneling of the cortex due to widening of intracortical Haversian canals.[2,24,38,44–45,52,53] Although RSDS can exist in the absence of osteoporosis, the diagnosis of RSDS cannot be made on the basis of radiographic appearance of the osteoporosis alone.

Thermography

Thermography, an infrared imaging technique that can measure very subtle temperature differences between involved and uninvolved regions, might provide objective documentation of autonomic dysfunction. Serial thermograms can be used to help determine the effectiveness of treatment over time.[24] Thermography is most useful in identifying early cases of RSDS and, for this purpose, is actually better than triple-phase bone scanning, the sensitivity of which is in the range of 50 to 75 percent. Infrared stress studies significantly improve the sensitivity and the specificity of standard thermographic procedures by challenging the integrity of the autonomic nervous system.

The cold-water stress test is performed as follows.

- A baseline quantitative thermal emission of the symptomatic extremity is obtained.
- After baseline imaging, the contralateral or asymptomatic extremity is immersed for five minutes in a cold-water bath filled with 10 to 15°C water.
- At the end of the five-minute session, a quantitative thermal image of the symptomatic extremity is obtained.
- The quantitative pre vs. post-test image changes in temperature are calculated. Post-test cooling of the non-immersed extremity is the expected result. Paroxysmal warming is strongly suggestive of vasomotor instability.

The warm-water stress test is performed in a similar fashion but with opposite results expected. Physiologic thermovascular challenges may demonstrate decreased autonomic function in suspected cases of sympathetically mediated pain. An asymmetric "thermo-vascular" rate of change in involved extremities has been deemed clinically useful in the study of RSDS.[54–61]

Triple-Phase Bone Scans

Triple-phase bone scans also will demonstrate blood flow abnormalities, providing further supporting objective documentation of the diagnosis, though such scans may be negative in up to 40 percent of patients in whom RSDS is clinically diagnosed.[8,62] Many different types of conditions can produce osteoporosis, and a triple-phase bone scan does not distinguish between the causes of bone demineralization. In general, then, triple-phase bone scanning may be considered a highly sensitive but not very specific tool. Though it will help to support the diagnosis, clinical acumen and correlation ultimately are required to diagnose RSDS.

Clinical information can be derived from each of the three phases of the triple-phase bone scan after injection of the radiopharmaceutical agent. First is the *angiogram phase*, as the compound remains intravascular for one to two minutes immediately following the injection. Serial images are recorded rapidly. Over the next five to ten minutes, the radiopharmaceutical compound diffuses into the extracellular fluid spaces of the body. This period reflects the soft tissue distribution of the compound and is referred to as the *blood pool phase* (phase 2). After two or three hours, the tracer is maximally bound to bone and will increase in areas where there is stimulus of bone turnover. It is during this time (phase 3) that images of the skeleton or bone are obtained.

In early (stage 1) RSDS, uptake of the tracer during phase 1 is increased. However, in disease stages 2 and 3, uptake during phase 1 is decreased. Likewise, in phase 2, which reflects the soft-tissue vascularity, an increased diffuse uptake may be appreciated during the early course of RSDS. During phase 3, one will see diffuse bony uptake in the involved limb, reflecting bone turnover secondary to osteoporosis.[44,45,63–71]

Blood Tests

Blood tests that should be obtained include a complete blood cell count, erythrocyte sedimentation rate, muscle enzyme studies, and rheumatoid factor. In RSDS, these are usually normal, but they do help to differentiate RSDS from other disorders that might present with a similar clinical picture.[44,45,69]

Electrodiagnostic Studies

Electrodiagnostic studies, including electromyography and nerve conduction velocities, generally are not very helpful. Occasionally, severe nerve entrapment or radiculopathy may be causing the RSDS and, in such cases, electromyography and nerve conduction velocities would assist in identifying the underlying lesion.[1]

Sympathetic Blockade

Many authorities consider the diagnosis of RSDS to be confirmed *only* if the patient improves after sympathetic blockade (i.e., stellate ganglion block, Bier block, phentolamine test).[2,8,21,72] Such improvement would imply an abnormality of the SNS, thus helping to confirm the diagnosis of RSDS or a sympathetically maintained pain state. It is recommended that three diagnostic stellate ganglion blocks or Bier blocks should be done. At least 50 percent relief should be experienced for the duration of the local anesthetic. Placebo effects should be checked by injection of sodium chloride solution or by using local anesthetics possessing different durations of action (i.e., procaine, lidocaine, bupivacaine). However, it should be noted that with RSDS, it is not unusual for the relief to last longer than the duration of the local anesthetic. After the administration of a diagnostic block (or blocks), the patient should not be physically stressed or sent to physical therapy in order to assess accurately the results of the procedure.

The phentolamine test is another diagnostic tool for RSDS based upon the principle of sympathetic interruption. Phentolamine is an alpha-adrenoceptor antagonist (alpha$_1$, alpha$_2$). Up to 30 mg phentolamine and 100 ml saline are infused intravenously over about 20 minutes, or 5 to 15 mg are infused over 5 to 10 minutes. Pain is measured using a visual analog scale. If pain is reduced, the SNS is likely to be involved in the generation of pain.[73–75]

PATHOPHYSIOLOGIC FEATURES

RSDS is characterized by dysfunction of the autonomic nervous system. Pupillary changes, heart rate, blood pressure, gastrointestinal peristalsis, and bowel and bladder function all represent involuntary reactions controlled by the autonomic nervous system, which has two divisions, sympathetic and parasympathetic.

The parasympathetic division is concerned with conservation of energy. For example, with activity of the parasympathetic nervous system (PNS), there will be a decrease in heart rate and blood pressure, bronchiolar and pupillary constriction, and stimulation of the gastrointestinal tract so that reabsorption of nutrients can occur during this resting phase.

The energy stored during activity of the PNS can be used on activation of the SNS, which is concerned with energy expenditure. With increased sympathetic activity, there is an elevation of heart rate and blood pressure, bronchiolar dilatation (to provide muscles with greater oxygenation), and pupillary dilation (to enhance peripheral vision). Most importantly, there is a redistribution of blood flow *away* from the skin and gastrointestinal tract and towards muscles.

During stress, sympathetic activity increases, preparing the organism for the so-called fight-or-flight response. In contrast, injury to an arm, leg, hand, or foot may evoke a sympathetic reflex with vasoconstriction only in the injured extremity. This type of sympathetic reflex is designed to help minimize blood loss and swelling. However, the sympathetic reflex will need to diminish over time so that healing can commence.[1,2]

The sympathetic neurotransmitter norepinephrine (NE) causes vasoconstriction of blood vessels and the secretion of sweat from sweat glands. The SNS originates from the intermediolateral gray area of the spinal cord. Myelinated nerve fibers from cell bodies in this region travel out to the sympathetic ganglion, where there is a synaptic connection with an unmyelinated sympathetic nerve that travels outward toward the periphery. The target tissues for adrenergic peripheral neurons have two types of catecholamine receptors, alpha and beta. The alpha-receptor mediates vasoconstriction and the beta-receptor mediates vasodilatation.

Target tissues of particular interest in the RSDS patient include arterioles, systemic veins, and skin (pilomotor muscles and sweats glands). Alpha-receptor stimulation leads to vasoconstriction of arterioles and veins, whereas beta-receptor stimulation causes dilatation. Alpha-receptor stimulation of pilomotor muscles and sweat glands causes piloerection and sweat secretion, respectively.[76]

RSDS results from an abnormality of sympathetic activity. Over the years, many different pathophysiologic theories have been proposed to explain the various clinical signs and symptoms seen in the typical RSDS patient. An optimal pathophysiological model would be able to explain autonomic changes, allodynia, spread of the disease, and psychological manifestations. The following theories explain many of these manifestations.

Activation of the Nociceptive Afferent System

One model suggests that peripheral trauma causes activation of nociceptive afferent (C and A-delta) fibers. The nociceptive impulses enter the dorsal horn, where there is activation of second-order pain transmission cells in layers I (nociceptor-specific pain transmission cells [NSPTCs]) and V (wide dynamic-range neurons [WDRNs]). Increased dorsal horn activity is relayed to the nearby intermediolateral gray region, the origin of the SNS. Increased sympathetic efferent activity causes sensitization of peripheral sensory receptors. The sensitized peripheral nociceptors and mechanoreceptors bombard the dorsal horn with nociceptive input that causes sensitization of NSPTCs and WDRNs. The sensitized WDRN, which responds to a wide range of stimuli, produces the phenomenon of allodynia (Figure 11-1).[9,77–80]

Injury to the Sympathetic Efferent System

Another hypothesis suggests that the initial injury is to the sympathetic efferents and not to the nociceptive afferent system. Such an injury results in decreased sympathetic outflow and the classic description of stage 1 RSDS (hot, red, dry limb with increased nail growth). This hyposympathetic phase causes subsequent upregulation of receptors in the peripheral tissues that could then result in a pathologic response to circulating catecholamines or to NE released from both surviving and re-innervated sympathetic efferents. This hypersensitivity phase would produce the clinical picture of stage 2 RSDS, representing not increased efferent sympathetic activity, but rather an exaggerated response to normal levels of circulating catecholamines or residual sympathetic outflow. The intense nociception could be explained by either upregulation of existing, normally quiescent adrenergic receptors or the development of new pathologic receptors on the nociceptive afferents. This ongoing intense nociceptive barrage might cause altered central processing, with sensitization of the second-order pain transmission cells, including the WDRN, resulting in allodynia.[80]

Activation of Ascending Pain Pathways

Impulses spread cephalad via axons from sensitized second-order pain transmission cells traveling in the spinothalamic tract (STT).[81] The STT is believed to exhibit somatotopic organization, fibers from the WDRN being medially located and fibers from the nociceptor-specific cells occupying a more lateral position as they ascend toward the brain. Two

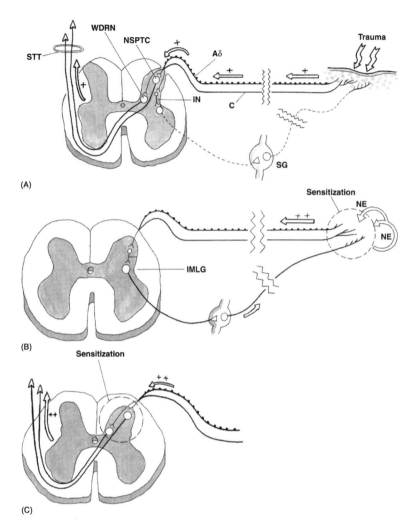

Figure 11-1 Pathophysiologic model for the development of reflex sympathetic dystrophy syndrome. (A) Peripheral trauma causes activation of nociceptive afferent (C and A delta) fibers. The nociceptive impulses enter the dorsal horn, where there is activation of second-order pain transmission cells in layers I (NSPTC) and V (WDRN). (A, C = A delta and C nociceptive fibers; WDRN = wide dynamic-range neuron; NSPTC = nociceptor-specific pain transmission cell; STT = spinothalamic tract; IN = interneuron; SG = sympathetic ganglion; + = nociceptive transmission; + + = sensitized nociceptive transmission.) (B) Increased dorsal horn activity is relayed to the nearby IMLG, the origin of the sympathetic nervous system. Increased sympathetic efferent activity causes sensitization of peripheral sensory receptors. (C) The sensitized peripheral nociceptors and mechanorecep-tors bombard the dorsal horn with nociceptive input, causing sensitization of second-order pain transmission cells. The sensitized WDRN produces the phenomenon of allodynia. (IMLG = inter-mediolateral gray area; NE = norepineph-rine; + + = sensitized nociceptive transmission.) Reprinted by permission from Rook JL. Reflex sympathetic dystrophy syndrome. In Cassvan A, Weiss LD, Weiss JM, Rook JL, Mullens SU (eds). *Cumulative Trauma Disorders*, p 163. Boston, Butterworth-Heinemann, 1997.

distinct pathways have been identified anatomically once the STT enters the brain: the medial paleospinothalamic tract (PSTT), extending to the frontal lobes and limbic system, and the lateral neospinothalamic tract (NSTT), traveling to the somatosensory cortex. It is believed that the medial system modulated by the WDRN is more active in RSDS, the result of which is poorly localized, diffuse, noxious pain with emotional features. The STT, PSTT, and NSTT characterize the ascending system.[79,81,82]

The pain of RSDS is diffuse, burning, intolerable, and unpleasant. Other findings that remain fairly consistent from case to case include strong emotional reactions, a sense of emotional alarm, chronic anxiety, chronic insomnia, depression, and other chronic pain behaviors. Increased activity in the PSTT pathway might account for such behaviors on a physiologic, rather than on a purely psychological, basis.

Activation of Anterior Horn Cells

Nociceptive impulses stimulate the SNS (see Figure 11-1). Likewise, pain impulses via C and A delta fibers have, through interneurons, a stimulating effect on anterior horn cells, possibly resulting in reactive muscle spasm. Muscle spasm is a painful process, and pain fibers originating in the muscle further propagate nociceptive impulses back to the spinal cord, thereby perpetuating the cycle of muscle spasm (Figure 11-2).[77,78]

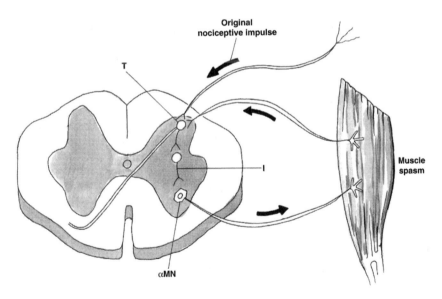

Figure 11-2 Livingston's vicious circle. Increased dorsal horn activity spreads to alpha motor neurons (MNs) in the ventral horn via interneurons (I). The activation of alpha motor neurons results in muscle spasm. The painful muscle's own nociceptive fibers feed back to the spinal cord to sustain the spasm. (T = second-order pain transmission cell.) Reprinted by permission from Fields HL. *Pain*, p 153. New York, McGraw-Hill, 1987.

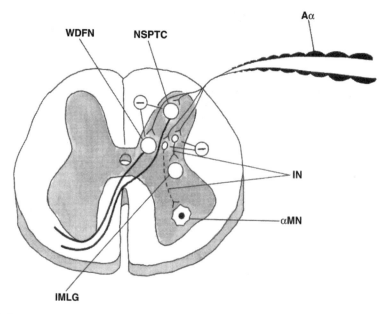

Figure 11-3 Down-regulation by large A-alpha proprioceptive fibers. Increased movement in an extremity relays proprioceptive information to the spinal cord, which down-regulates second-order pain transmission cells, intermedio-lateral gray cells (sympathetic nervous system), and alpha motor neurons. (A = A-alpha myelinated nociceptive fiber; NSPTC = nociceptor-specific pain transmission cell; WDRN = wide dynamic-range neuron; IN = interneuron; MN = alpha motor neuron; − = inhibitory impulse; IMLG = intermediolateral gray area.) Reprinted by permission from Rook JL. Reflex sympathetic dystrophy syndrome. In Cassvan A, Weiss LD, Weiss JM, Rook JL, Mullens SU (eds). *Cumulative Trauma Disorders*, p 164. Boston, Butterworth-Heinemann, 1997.

A-alpha Proprioceptive Fiber Pain Modulation

There is, however, a counterbalancing effect from A-alpha proprioceptive fibers. Increased movement in an extremity relays proprioceptive information into the spinal cord, which down regulates second order pain transmission cells, intermediolateral cells (SNS), and alpha motor neurons (Figure 11-3). Therefore, increased proprioceptive input in an RSDS patient can decrease pain, sympathetic outflow, and muscle spasm.[79] Unfortunately, patients with RSDS tend to avoid use of the involved extremity. With decreased proprioceptive input, the pain impulses become uninhibited, and there is no modulation of the SNS. For this reason, among others, physical therapy (to keep the extremity moving) is of great importance in management of RSDS.

SYMPATHETICALLY MAINTAINED PAIN

The term *sympathetically maintained pain* (SMP) refers to the effect of NE on nerve terminals in the periphery. The three major physiologic changes in SMP include (1) increased activity of the SNS which causes (2) sensitization of peripheral nociceptors and mechanoreceptors and (3) subsequent sensitization of the WDRN.

Increased activity of the SNS results in the release of NE in the periphery. It is believed that NE may increase the baseline tonic firing rate of nociceptors in the periphery to the point at which they begin firing spontaneously, even in the absence of noxious or non-noxious stimuli. The WDRN becomes sensitized by this increased firing rate. The sensitized WDRN perceives this increased firing rate as representing a painful stimulus. At this point, the patient is experiencing pain even in the absence of any cutaneous stimulation: this is SMP.[9]

TREATMENT

RSDS patients will require treatment to relieve pain and prevent disability. Untreated, the pain mechanisms may become "centralized" or irreversibly implanted within the central nervous system. The sooner treatment is begun, the better the prognosis. Of course, implicit in this is the fact that the patient's physician must be capable of making a quick and appropriate diagnosis.

Basic treatment principles include elimination of precipitating factors, relief of pain, and establishment of an active physical therapy program.[1] The hallmark of treatment is to shut down the SNS. Sympathetic interruption can be accomplished either in the periphery through sympatholytic medications or Bier blocks, or centrally via sympathetic ganglion blockade or invasive surgical procedures such as sympathectomy. The goal of such treatment is to desensitize the peripheral sensory receptors and WDRNs.

Some patients will suffer indefinitely from unrelenting neurogenic pain that has become unresponsive to traditional sympatholytic techniques and conservative interventions. These patients may be candidates for pain management via oral opioids, opioid pump implantation, or spinal cord stimulation (Box 11-3).

Sympatholytic Medications

Peripheral interruption of the SNS is accomplished via blockade of sympathetic receptors. The sympathetic neurotransmitter NE binds to alpha receptors on blood vessels, producing vasoconstriction. However, stage 1 RSDS is characterized by vasodilatation, soft edema, and erythema due to underactivity of the SNS. Whereas alpha receptors mediate constriction of blood vessels, beta receptors mediate vasodilatation. Hence, in stage 1 disease, a beta blocker is the drug of choice (Table 11-2).[24,27,72,83]

In contrast, disease stages 2 and 3 are characterized by decreased blood flow due to excessive noradrenergic stimulation of alpha receptors. In late-stage disease, alpha-blocking agents might improve blood flow and minimize trophic changes (Table 11-3).[2,6,24,76,84] Calcium channel blockers such as verapamil or nifedipine also might prove useful in increasing blood flow and decreasing the pain associated with ischemia in late-stage disease.[85]

Box 11-3 Summary of currently available treatment modalities for managing the reflex sympathetic dystrophy syndrome

Sympatholytic Medications
Alpha blockers
Beta blockers
Calcium channel blockers
Sympathetic blockade
Stellate ganglion block
Bier block

Physical Therapy Modalities
Massage
Splinting
Range-of-motion
Functional activities
Stress loading
Contrast baths
Cold packs
Hot packs
Thermoelastic gloves
Transcutaneous electrical nerve stimulation
Acupuncture

Psychotherapy
Treatment of depression
Relaxation training
Biofeedback
Hypnosis

Nonsympatholytic Medications
Nonsteroidal anti-inflammatory drugs
Corticosteroids
Tricyclic antidepressants
Baclofen
Mexiletine
Capsaicin cream

Sympathectomy
Opioid analgesics
Opioid pump implantation
Spinal cord stimulation

Reprinted by permission from Rook JL. Reflex sympathetic dystrophy syndrome. In Cassvan A, Weiss LD, Weiss JM, Rook JL, Mullens SU (eds). *Cumulative Trauma Disorders*, p 165. Boston, Butterworth-Heinemann, 1997.

Bier Blocks

Bier blocks are performed using medications that work either by interfering with NE storage (reserpine, guanethidine) or by preventing NE release from sympathetic nerve endings (guanethidine, bretylium).[76]

Table 11-2 Common beta-blockers

Generic Name	Trade Names
Labetalol	Normodyne, Trandate[a,b]
Nadolol	Corgard[a]
Pindolol	Visken[a]
Propranolol	Inderal[a]
Timolol	Blocadren[a]

[a] Nonselective beta$_1$- and beta$_2$-adrenergic antagonist.
[b] Labetalol is also a potent alpha$_1$-adrenergic antagonist.
Note: Beta$_2$ receptors mediate vasodilatation and, in stage 1 disease, a beta-blocker is the drug of choice.
Reprinted by permission from Rook JL. Reflex sympathetic dystrophy syndrome. In Cassvan A, Weiss LD, Weiss JM, Rook JL, Mullens SU (eds). *Cumulative Trauma Disorders*, p 165. Boston, Butterworth-Heinemann, 1997.

Table 11-3 Alpha-blockers

Generic	Trade Name	Mode of Action
Doxazosin mesylate	Cardura	Selective alpha$_1$-receptor blockers
Phenoxybenzamine HCl	Dibenzyline	Alpha$_1$-, alpha$_2$-receptor blocker
Guanethidine monosulfate	Esimil, Ismelin	Interferes with release of the sympathetic neurotransmitter norepinephrine
Prazosin HCl	Minipress	Alpha$_1$-, alpha$_2$-receptor blocker
Clonidine HCl	Catapres	Central nervous system alpha$_2$ agonist that decreases sympathetic outflow

Reprinted by permission from Rook JL. Reflex sympathetic dystrophy syndrome. In Cassvan A, Weiss LD, Weiss JM, Rook JL, Mullens SU (eds). *Cumulative Trauma Disorders*, p 166. Boston, Butterworth-Heinemann, 1997.

In the Bier procedure, a tourniquet is placed proximally on the involved extremity, and a distal intravenous line is used to infuse the respective medication (guanethidine, reserpine, or bretylium, with anesthetics or steroids). After 15 to 20 minutes, the tourniquet is released. By that time, most of the medication has been absorbed by the tissues, and very little enters the general circulation to exert systemic effects. Patients may experience significant pain relief that can last from one to several days or even months at a time. During the period of pain relief, physical therapy should be instituted.[24,34,72,86–98]

Sympathetic Ganglion Blocks

General Considerations

A ganglion block is frequently successful in the management of RSDS.[99–107] A *ganglion* is a group of nerve cells located outside the central nervous system. The sympathetic ganglia are paired chains of nervous tissue lying on either side of the spinal cord, extending from the neck to the pelvis (Figure 11-4).[1,2]

With each sympathetic ganglion block, the SNS shuts down for the duration of the anesthetic agent's effective period, there is inhibition of NE release in the periphery, and sensitized mechanoreceptors and nociceptors are able to desensitize. In the *ideal* situation, aggressive shutdown of the SNS for a prolonged period (perhaps through a series of sympathetic blocks) will enable the central pathophysiologic abnormalities to return to their baseline (i.e., normal) level.

Basic Principles of Stellate Ganglion Blockade

Infiltration of the appropriate ganglion with local anesthetic interrupts transmission of sympathetic impulses to the painful area. For upper-extremity RSDS, it is necessary to infiltrate the stellate ganglion. The stellate ganglion is the relay station for sympathetic nerves traveling to the head, neck, and upper extremity. If performed early in the course of disease, a single block may produce long-lasting relief. However, usually five to seven and perhaps even more are necessary.[1,2,21,72]

Stellate ganglion blockade is usually performed by anesthesiologists specially trained in invasive pain management techniques. It is necessary to retract the carotid sheath so that the needle can be cleanly inserted down to the stellate ganglion, which overlies a cervical transverse process. There are a number of critical structures adjacent to the stellate ganglion, including the common carotid artery, internal jugular vein, vagus nerve (housed within the carotid sheath), and recurrent laryngeal nerve (which controls the larynx and vocal cords) (Figure 11-5).

The carotid sheath must be retracted before needle insertion (Figure 11-6). The anesthetic can then be injected, most likely without the threat of hemorrhage or vascular collapse.[108] After successful stellate ganglion block, a painful, cold, pale extremity will become pink and warm, and there will be a marked decrease in pain.[2,21,24] The patient will also develop a Horner's syndrome, characterized by ptosis (drooping of the eyelid), miosis (constriction of the pupil), anhidrosis (lack of sweating on the blocked side of the face and arm), eye redness and nasal congestion.[2,24]

It might take several sympathetic blocks to relieve a patient's symptoms for a prolonged period. The absence of pain relief with a block indicates that the diagnosis is in error or that the RSDS has become centralized.[2,39]

Complications of Stellate Ganglion Blockade

There are a host of possible complications of stellate ganglion blockade, including injection of anesthetic directly into an artery (carotid or vertebral), causing seizure activity; infiltration of the recurrent laryngeal nerve, resulting in transient hoarseness and increased risk for aspiration; perforation of the lung apex, causing pneumothorax that could necessitate hospitalization for chest tube placement; and bradycardia. If the anesthetic trickles into the spinal canal, a high spinal cord block can occur, which might necessitate rapid intubation and short-term hospitalization until the anesthetic wears off. Other possible complications are hypotension and allergic or toxic reaction to the anesthetic.[1,24]

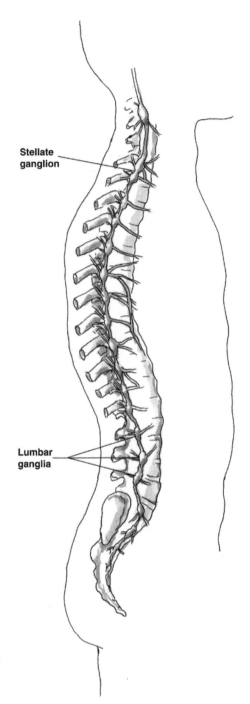

Stellate ganglion

Lumbar ganglia

Figure 11-4 The sympathetic ganglia are paired chains of nervous tissue lying on either side of the spinal cord, extending from the neck to the pelvis. Reprinted by permission from Rook JL. Reflex sympathetic dystrophy syndrome. In Cassvan A, Weiss LD, Weiss JM, Rook JL, Mullens SU (eds). *Cumulative Trauma Disorders*, p 167. Boston, Butterworth-Heinemann, 1997.

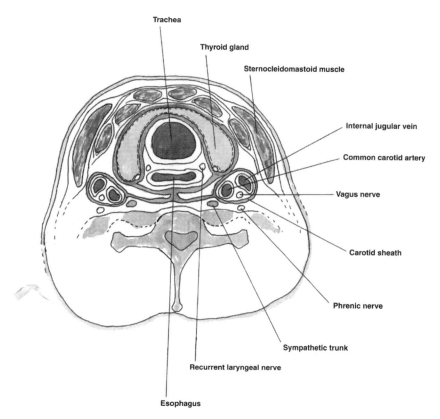

Trachea

Thyroid gland

Sternocleidomastoid muscle

Internal jugular vein

Common carotid artery

Vagus nerve

Carotid sheath

Phrenic nerve

Sympathetic trunk

Recurrent laryngeal nerve

Esophagus

Figure 11-5 Critical structures adjacent to the stellate ganglion. Reprinted by permission from Rook JL. Reflex sympathetic dystrophy syndrome. In Cassvan A, Weiss LD, Weiss JM, Rook JL, Mullens SU (eds). *Cumulative Trauma Disorders*, p 168. Boston, Butterworth-Heinemann, 1997.

Protocol for Stellate Ganglion Blockade

Early in the treatment program, blocks should be done frequently (daily, every other day, or two times per day, depending on the patient's response). During the first 6 to 12 blocks, the patient should be making notable progress in his or her rehabilitation program and achieving an increasingly longer duration of relief between blocks. If appropriate outcomes are not achieved within this treatment period, changes should be made in the treatment regimen. Often, continued blocks are needed, but the duration between the blocks should increase if they are being used as maintenance therapy.

Maintenance blocks are considered appropriate if they provide relief or decreased pain for 6 to 12 weeks at a time. An effective maintenance therapeutic regimen should involve only four to eight blocks during the course of a year. Maintenance blocks are usually combined with and enhanced by appropriate analgesic and neuropharmacologic medications and other care (e.g., self-directed home exercise program, transcutaneous electrical nerve stimulation [TENS], relaxation techniques). It is anticipated that the

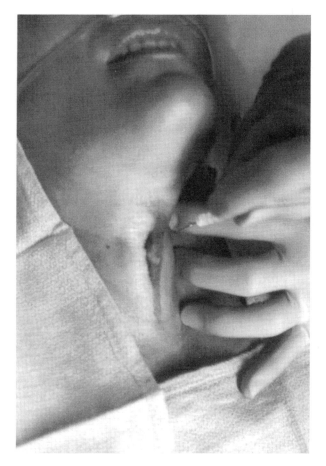

Figure 11-6 The stellate ganglion block. The carotid sheath must be retracted prior to needle insertion. Reprinted by permission from Rook JL. Reflex sympathetic dystrophy syndrome. In Cassvan A, Weiss LD, Weiss JM, Rook JL, Mullens SU (eds). *Cumulative Trauma Disorders*, p 169. Boston, Butterworth-Heinemann, 1997.

frequency of maintenance blocks may need to be increased in cold winter months and decreased in the warmer summer months.

For best results, sympathetic interruption needs to be done as early as possible in the course of RSDS. None-the-less, long-standing disease does not preclude attempts at sympathetic interruption; yet if irreversible fibrosis has already occurred, the patient will experience some permanent disability.

Sympathectomy

If sympathetic ganglion blocks produce good but only temporary relief, surgical or chemical sympathectomy may be indicated, although this is controversial.[2,14,24,72,100,109–119] Much of the research on the effectiveness of sympathectomy is based on short-term postoperative data.[119] Long-term experience suggests only temporary relief with this neuroablative procedure.[32,79] Destruction of part of the SNS should be considered only rarely and very carefully, as long-term success with this treatment is poor.[28,120]

Chemical or surgical sympathectomy can be considered if a patient demonstrates single extremity RSDS and distal pain only. This procedure should *not* be done if the proximal part of the extremity is involved. In addition, destructive sympathectomy should be considered only if the local anesthetic consistently gives excellent (75 to 100 percent) but temporary relief each time a technically good block is performed.

Physical Therapy

Physical therapy is an essential part of RSDS treatment protocol and needs to be instituted early. However, in severe cases, physical therapy should be done under sympathetic interruption (via medications or blocking procedures). The concept of "no pain, no gain" does not hold for patients in whom RSDS has been diagnosed. The disease will worsen and spread faster if excessive exercise is performed without appropriate sympathetic interruption.

The basic principles of physical therapy for RSDS patients include gentle, repetitive, active motion and massage, and weight-bearing activities. Passive motion is not recommended. Between exercising, splinting occasionally is needed to prevent contractures. Exercise will improve mobility, prevent contractures, and reduce pain. Once some degree of active range of motion has been restored, functional activities can be introduced, practicing simple tasks initially and progressing gradually to more complex activities.[1,2,69,110,121–123]

Stress-loading exercise,[124,125] paraffin baths, and contrast baths may be helpful tools in the RSDS therapy protocol, both in supervised treatment and as part of an independent self-treatment regimen. Stress loading consists of active traction (carrying activities) and compression exercises (scrubbing) that provide stressful stimuli to the extremity without joint motion. Contrast baths are done by alternating immersion of extremities in media (generally water) at contrasting (hot and cold) temperatures. Such baths may be useful in decreasing edema, improving peripheral circulation, and decreasing joint pain and stiffness.

Other Treatment Modalities

Other adjunctive treatments that might help the RSDS patient include cold, heat, thermoelastic gloves, TENS, acupuncture, psychotherapy, nonsympatholytic medications, opioid analgesics, spinal cord stimulation, and opioid pump implantation. Cold packs are useful in stage 1 disease, whereas warm moist packs are more helpful in stages 2 and 3, when there is an overall decrease in blood flow. Hot packs decrease muscle spasm and improve blood flow.[126,127] Thermoelastic gloves provide compression, warmth, and protection.[1,2] TENS and acupuncture appear to help some individuals with RSDS.[2,21,24,72,128–135]

Psychotherapy is an extremely important modality for RSDS patients. Depression, anxiety, financial concerns, and fears about the future are common problems encountered in this population. RSDS patients frequently need aggressive treatment of depression through therapy and medications. Biofeedback and hypnosis are occasionally helpful in promoting relaxation, decreasing muscle spasm, and improving circulation through reduction of sympathetic tone.[126,136,137] Relaxation training is important, as a chronically anxious state with high levels of circulating NE from the adrenal glands (which respond in this manner to chronic anxiety) certainly will worsen the pain of RSDS.

Nonsympatholytic medications that might provide analgesic relief for these individuals include nonsteroidal anti-inflammatory drugs, corticosteroids, tricyclic antidepressants, anticonvulsants, baclofen, mexiletine, capsaicin and anesthetic creams, and opioid analgesics.

The primary usefulness of nonsteroidal anti-inflammatory drugs is to deal with the myofascial discomfort associated with physical and occupational therapy.[24,44] Gastrointestinal side effects should be monitored. The use of corticosteroids has been advocated in the literature particularly if there are any contraindications to sympathetic blocks or if the latter are not helpful. Various protocols have been recommended (e.g., 30 mg/day for 12 weeks or 100 to 200 mg/day for 2 to 3 weeks).[7,21,24,72,138–143]

Tricyclic antidepressants (amitriptyline, imipramine, and nortriptyline) are frequently helpful in promoting better-quality sleep, in decreasing neurogenic pain, and in treating depression.[144–150] Anticonvulsants (e.g., phenytoin, carbamazepine, gabapentin, valproic acid) are often helpful in decreasing neurogenic pain, including the pain of RSDS.[21,151,152] Biannual serum studies for anticonvulsant level, liver function, and blood counts should be used to monitor patients maintained on anticonvulsant therapy.

Baclofen (40 to 80 mg/day in divided doses) is useful for sympathetically related abnormalities of tone, especially reactive muscle spasm, dyskinesia or dystonia.[42] Mexiletine (oral lidocaine) is increasingly being used for various types of neurogenic pain, including the pain of RSDS.[153–155] Capsaicin cream depletes nerve terminals of substance P, feels quite warm, and may be soothing for patients with later-stage disease.

The use of oral opioid analgesics, opioid pump implantation, and spinal cord stimulation should be considered if traditional modalities have failed to relieve pain and improve function and quality of life for the suffering RSDS patient. Opioid analgesia, opioid pump implantation, and spinal cord stimulation are discussed in separate chapters.[156–159] Finally, patients should be instructed to stop smoking, as nicotine, a potent vasoconstrictor, often worsens the symptoms of RSDS.[25,44]

THE COST OF TREATING RSDS

Making the diagnosis and subsequently treating RSDS will produce staggering health care costs. There will be a prolonged need for physical or occupational therapy for desensitization, maintenance of movement, strengthening, and as part of the sympathetic blockade protocol. There may very well be a lifelong need for medications, including sympatholytic medications, analgesics, neurogenic medications, hypnotics for those patients with sleep disturbances, and antidepressants as depression is a common lifelong accompaniment of the severe pain and disability associated with this disorder.

The cost of the various sympathetic blockade procedures is significant. Each Bier block and/or sympathetic block carries a price tag between $600 and $1500. These blocks need to be performed by a specialist with training in invasive injection techniques. Frequently, hospital settings with appropriate monitoring are required. Some patients may require hospitalization for several days for continuous epidural analgesia techniques. The cost for such hospitalizations could range between $5000 and $10,000 and perhaps more.

Surgical procedures are often necessitated. We have already discussed the technique of sympathectomy, and a separate chapter is devoted to the discussion of morphine pump implantation and spinal cord stimulator implantation. The cost for the high-technology surgical procedures could range anywhere from $20,000 to $70,000. Sympathectomy frequently needs to be repeated and the cost for that can be significant also. RSDS is a lifelong ailment and the costs of treatment usually continue on a lifelong basis for each patient.

CONCLUSION

RSDS is a neuropathic condition that must be identified and treated early in the course of disease. The disorder, which is difficult to diagnose and to treat, can prove to be frustrating for the physician, and third-party payers (owing to the staggering health care costs associated with diagnosis and treatment). Ultimately, however, it is the patient and his or her family who must deal with a number of unfortunate realities including extreme lifelong pain, prolonged family disruption, disability and unemployment, misdiagnosis by and disbelief of inexperienced physicians, improper treatment, multiple operations, unsuccessful surgery, diminished quality of life, and increased health care costs.

REFERENCES

1. Mausner PA. Reflex sympathetic dystrophy. *Trial Talk* 1987; 36: 92.
2. Lankford LL. Reflex sympathetic dystrophy. In Evarts CM (ed). *Surgery of the Musculoskeletal System*, p 145. New York, Churchill Livingstone, 1983.
3. Mitchell SW, Morehouse GR, Keen WW. *Gunshot Wounds and Other Injuries of Nerves.* New York. Lippincott, 1989.
4. Mitchell SW. *Injuries of Nerves and their Consequences.* New York, Lippincott, 1988.
5. Shelton RM, Lewis CW. Reflex sympathetic dystrophy: a review. *J Am Acad Dermatol* 1990; 22: 513.
6. Escobar PL. Reflex sympathetic dystrophy. *Orthop Rev* 1986; 15: 646.
7. Glick EN. Reflex dystrophy (algoneurodystrophy): results of treatment by corticosteroids. *Rheumatol Rehabil* 1973; 12: 84.
8. Schwartzman RJ, McLellan TL. Reflex sympathetic dystrophy—a review. *Arch Neurol* 1987; 44: 555.
9. Roberts WJ. A hypothesis on the physiological basis for causalgia and related pains. *Pain* 1986; 24: 297.
10. Stanton-Hicks M, Janig W, Hassenbusch S, *et al.* Reflex sympathetic dystrophy: changing concepts and taxonomy. *Pain* 1995; 63: 127.
11. Sudeck P. Dietrophische extremitantensgroung durch periphere (infetoise and traumatische) *Reize Dtsch Z Chir* 1931; 234: 596.

12. DeTakats G. Reflex dystrophy of the extremities. *Arch Surg* 1937; 34: 939.

13. Homans J. Minor causalgia: a hyperesthetic neurovascular syndrome. *N Engl J Med* 1940; 222: 870.

14. Patman RD, Thompson JE, Persson AV. Management of post-traumatic pain syndromes:. a report of 113 cases. *Ann Surg* 1973; 177: 780.

15. Steinbrocker O. The shoulder-hand syndrome. *Am J Med* 1947; 3: 402.

16. Evans JA. Reflex sympathetic dystrophy. *Surg Clin North Am* 1946; 26: 780.

17. Serre H, Simon L, Claustie J. Sympathetic dystrophy of the foot. *Rev Rheum* 1967; 34: 722.

18. Lehman EP. Traumatic vasospasm: a study of four cases of vasospasm in the upper extremity. *Arch Surg* 1934; 29: 92.

19. International Association for the Study of Pain (IASP). *Classification of Chronic Pain: Descriptions of Chronic Pain Syndromes and Definitions of Pain Terms*, 2nd ed. Seattle, IASP Press, 1994.

20. Steinbrocker O, Argyros TG. The shoulder-hand syndrome: present status as a diagnostic and therapeutic entity. *Med Clin North Am* 1958; 42: 1533.

21. Warfield CA. The sympathetic dystrophies. *Hosp Pract* 1984; 19(5): 52C.

22. Horowitz SH. Brachial plexus injuries with causalgia resulting from transaxillary rib resection. *Arch Surg* 1985; 20: 1189.

23. Goldner JD. Causes and prevention of reflex sympathetic dystrophy. *J Hand Surg* 1980; 5: 295.

24. Rowlingson JC. The sympathetic dystrophies. *Int Anesthesiol Clin* 1983; 21(4): 117.

25. Lankford LL, Thompson JE. Reflex sympathetic dystrophy: upper and lower extremity: diagnosis and management. In *The American Academy of Orthopaedic Surgeons Instructional Course Lectures*, vol 26, p 63. St. Louis, Mosby, 1977.

26. Kleinert HE, Cole NM, Wayne L, *et al.* Post-traumatic sympathetic dystrophy. *Orthop Clin North Am* 1973; 4: 917.

27. Hodges DL, McGuire TJ. Burning and pain after injury. Is it causalgia or reflex sympathetic dystrophy? *J Postgrad Med* 1988; 83: 185.

28. Richards RL. Causalgia. *Arch Neurol* 1967; 16: 339.

29. Mayfield FH. *Causalgia*, p 3. Springfield, IL, Thomas, 1951.

30. DeTakats G. Causalgic states in peace and war. *JAMA* 1945; 128: 669.

31. Sylvest J, Jensen EM, Siggaard-Andersen J, *et al.* Reflex dystrophy. *Scand J Rehabil Med* 1977; 9: 25.

32. Bonica JJ. Causalgia and other reflex sympathetic dystrophies. *J Postgrad Med* 1973; 53: 143.

33. Richards RL. Vasomotor and nutritional disturbances after injuries to peripheral nerves. *Med Res Council Spec Rep Ser* 1954; 282: 25.

34. Jaeger SH, Singer DI, Whitenack SH. Nerve injury complications. Management of neurogenic pain syndromes. *Hand Clin* 1986; 2: 217.

35. DeTakats G. Nature of painful vasodilatation in causal-gic states. *Arch Neurol Psychiatry* 1943; 50: 318.

36. Doupe J, Cullen CH, Chance GQ. Post-traumatic pain and the causalgic syndrome. *J Neurol Neurosurg Psychiatry* 1944; 7: 33.

37. Seddon H. *Surgical Disorders of the Peripheral Nerves*, p 239. New York, Churchill Livingstone, 1972.

38. Turek SL. *Orthopaedics Principles and their Application*, p 796. Philadelphia, Lippincott, 1984.

39. Schott GD. Mechanisms of causalgia and related clinical conditions: the role of the central and of the sympathetic nervous systems. *Brain* 1986; 109: 717.

40. Mayfield FH, Devine JW. Causalgia. *Surg Gynecol Obstet* 1945; 80: 631.

41. Meyer RA, Campbell JN, Raja S. Peripheral neural mechanisms of cutaneous hyperalgesia. *Adv Pain Res Ther* 1985; 9: 53.

42. Schwartzman RJ, Kerrigan J. The movement disorder of reflex sympathetic dystrophy. *Neurology* 1990; 40: 57.

43. Geiderman JM. Sympathetic dystrophy. *Ann Emerg Med* 2001; 37: 412.

44. Tietjen R. Reflex sympathetic dystrophy of the knee. *Clin Orthop* 1986; 209: 234.

45. Markoff M, Farole A. Reflex sympathetic dystrophy syndrome: case report with a review of the literature. *Oral Surg Oral Med Oral Pathol* 1986; 61: 23.

46. Weiss WU. Psychophysiologic aspects of reflex sympathetic dystrophy syndrome. *Am J Pain Manage* 1994; 4: 67.

47. Lynch ME. Psychologic aspects of reflex sympathetic dystrophy. a review of the adult and paediatric literature. *Pain* 1992; 49: 337.

48. Van Houdenhove B, Vasquez G, Onghena P, *et al.* Etiopathogenesis of reflex sympathetic dystrophy: a review and biopsychosocial hypothesis. *Clin J Pain* 1992; 8: 300.

49. Bruehl S, Carlson CR. Predisposing psychological factors in the development of reflex sympathetic dystrophy—a review of the empirical evidence. *Clin J Pain* 1992; 8: 287.

50. Egle UT, Hoffman SO. Psychosomatic aspects of reflex sympathetic dystrophy. In Stanton-Hicks M, Janig W, Boas RA (eds). *Reflex Sympathetic Dystrophy*. Boston, Kluwer Academic, 1990.

51. Van Houdenhove B. Neuroalgodystrophy: a psychiatrist's view. *Clin Rheumatol* 1986; 5: 399.

52. Bickerstaff DR, Charlesworth D, Kanis JA. Changes in cortical and trabecular bone in algodystrophy. *Br J Rheumatol* 1993; 32: 46.

53. Kozin F, Genant HK, Bekerman C, *et al.* The reflex sympathetic dystrophy syndrome: 2. Roentgenographic and scintigraphic evidence of bilaterality and of periarticular accentuation. *Am J Med* 1976; 60: 332.

54. Hobbins WB. Differential diagnosis of painful conditions and thermography. In Parris WCV (ed). *Contemporary Issues in Chronic Pain Management*, p 251. Boston, Kluwer Academic, 1991.

55. Hobbins WB. Pain management in thermography. In Raj PP (ed). *Practical Management of Pain*, 2nd ed, p 181. St. Louis, Mosby, 1992.

56. Green J. A preliminary note: dynamic thermography may offer a key to the early recognition of reflex sympathetic dystrophy. *J Acad Neuromusc Thermogr* 1989; 8: 104.

57. Green J. The pathophysiology of reflex sympathetic dystrophy as demonstrated by dynamic thermography. *J Acad Neuromusc Thermogr* 1989; 8: 121.

58. Green J. Tutorial 12:. thermography medical infrared imaging. *Pain Dig* 1993; 3: 268.

59. Uematsu S, Jankel WR. Skin temperature response of the foot to cold stress of the hand: a test to evaluate somatosympathetic response. *Thermology* 1988; 3: 41.

60. Feldman F. Thermography of the hand and wrist: practical applications. *Hand Clin* 1991; 7: 99.

61. Karstetter KW, Sherman RA. Use of thermography for initial detection of early reflex sympathetic dystrophy. *J Am Podiatr Med Assoc* 1991; 81: 198.

62. Kozin F, Soin JS, Ryan LM, *et al.* Bone scintigraphy in the reflex sympathetic dystrophy syndrome. *Radiology* 1981; 138: 437.

63. Weiss L, Alfano A, Bardfeld P, *et al.* Prognostic value of triple phase bone scanning for reflex sympathetic dystrophy in hemiplegia. *Arch Phys Med Rehabil* 1993; 74: 716.

64. Davidoff G, Werner R, Cremer S, *et al.* Predictive value of the three-phase technetium bone scan in diagnosis of reflex sympathetic dystrophy syndrome. *Arch Phys Med Rehabil* 1989; 70: 135.

65. Intenzo C, Kim S, Millin J, *et al.* Scintigraphic patterns of the reflex sympathetic dystrophy syndrome of the lower extremities. *Clin Nucl Med* 1989; 14: 657.

66. Constantinesco A, Brunot B, Demangeat J, *et al.* Three-phase bone scanning as an aid to early diagnosis in reflex sympathetic dystrophy of the hand: a study of 89 cases. *Ann Chir Main Memb Super* 1986; 5: 93.

67. Greyson N, Tepperman P. Three-phase bone studies in hemiplegia with reflex sympathetic dystrophy and the effect of disuse. *J Nucl Med* 1984; 25: 423.

68. Demangeat J, Constantinesco A, Brunot B, *et al.* Three-phase bone scanning in reflex sympathetic dystrophy of the hand. *J Nucl Med* 1988; 29: 26.

69. Berstein BH, Singsen BH, Kent JT, *et al.* Reflex neurovascular dystrophy in childhood. *J Pediatr* 1978; 93: 211.

70. Laxer RM, Malleson PN, Morrison RT. Technetium 99m–methylene diphosphonate bone scans in children with reflex neurovascular dystrophy. *J Pediatr* 1985; 106: 437.

71. Holder LE, Mackinnon SE. Reflex sympathetic dystrophy in the hands: clinical and scintigraphic criteria. *Radiology* 1984; 152: 517.

72. Schutzer SF, Gossling HR. The treatment of reflex sympathetic dystrophy syndrome. *J Bone Joint Surg Am* 1984; 66: 625.

73. Arner S. Intravenous phentolamine test: diagnostic and prognostic use in reflex sympathetic dystrophy. *Pain* 1991; 46: 17.

74. Raja SN, Treede RD, Davis KD, *et al*. Systemic alpha-adrenergic blockade with phentolamine: a diagnostic test for sympathetically maintained pain. *Anesthesiology* 1991; 74: 691.

75. Campbell JN, Meyer RA, Raja SN. Is nociceptor activation by alpha-1 adrenoreceptors the culprit in sympathetically maintained pain? *Am Pain Soc J* 1992; 1: 3.

76. deGroot J. The autonomic nervous system. In de Groot J (ed). *Correlative Neuroanatomy*, p 193. East Norwalk, CT, Appleton & Lange, 1991.

77. Fields HL. Painful dysfunction of the nervous system. In Fields HL (ed). *Pain*, p 133. New York, McGraw-Hill, 1987.

78. Livingston WK. *Pain mechanisms*. New York, Macmillan, 1943.

79. Hooshmand H. *Chronic Pain: Reflex Sympathetic Dystrophy Prevention and Management*. Boca Raton, CRC Press, 1993.

80. Harden RN, Duc TA, Williams TR, *et al*. Norepinephrine and epinephrine levels in affected versus unaffected limbs in sympathetically maintained pain. *Clin J Pain* 1994; 10: 324.

81. Fields HL. Pain pathways in the central nervous system. In Fields HL (ed). *Pain*, p 41. New York, McGraw-Hill, 1987.

82. Melzack R, Casey KL. Sensory, motivational, and central control determinants of pain: a new conceptual model. In Kenshalo D (ed). *The Skin Senses*, p 423. Springfield, IL, Thomas, 1968.

83. Visitsunthorn U, Prete P. Reflex sympathetic dystrophy of the lower extremity: a complication of herpes zoster with dramatic response to propranolol. *West J Med* 1981; 135: 62.

84. Ghostine SY, Comair YG, Turner DM, *et al*. Phenoxybenzamine in the treatment of causalgia: report of 40 cases. *J Neurosurg* 1984; 60: 1263.

85. Prough DS, McLeskey CH, Poehling GG, *et al*. Efficiency of oral nifedipine in the treatment of reflex sympathetic dystrophy. *Anesthesiology* 1985; 62: 796.

86. Pak TJ, Martin GM, Magness JL, *et al*. Reflex sympathetic dystrophy. *Minn Med* 1970; 53: 507.

87. Tabira T, Shibasaki H, Kuroiwa Y. Reflex sympathetic dystrophy (causalgia). Treatment with guanethidine. *Arch Neurol* 1983; 40: 430.

88. Hannington-Kiff JG. Intravenous regional sympathetic block with guanethidine. *Lancet* 1974; 1: 1019.

89. Hannington-Kiff JG. Relief of Sudeck's atrophy by regional intravenous guanethidine. *Lancet* 1977; 1: 1132.

90. Hannington-Kiff JG. Relief of causalgia in limbs by regional intravenous guanethidine. *BMJ* 1979; 2: 367.

91. Hannington-Kiff JG. Hyperadrenergic-affected limb causalgia: relief by IV pharmacologic norepinephrine blockade. *Am Heart J* 1982; 103: 152.

92. Glynn CJ, Basedow RW, Walsh JA. Pain relief following postganglionic sympathetic blockade with IV guanethidine. *Br J Anaesth* 1981; 53: 1297.

93. Loh L, Nathan PW, Schott GD, *et al*. Effects of guanethidine infusion in certain painful states. *J Neurol Neurosurg Psychiatry* 1980; 43: 446.

94. Bonnelli S, Conoscente F, Movilia PG, *et al*. Regional intravenous guanethidine vs. stellate ganglion block in reflex sympathetic dystrophies. A randomized trial. *Pain* 1983; 16: 297.

95. Holland AJC, Davies KH, Wallace DH. Sympathetic blockade of isolated limbs by intravenous guanethidine. *Can Anaesth Soc J* 1977; 24: 597.

96. Chuinard RG, Dabezies FJ, Gould JS, *et al*. Intravenous reserpine for treatment of reflex sympathetic dystrophy. *South Med J* 1981; 74: 1481.

97. Benzon HT, Chomka CM, Brunner EA. Treatment of reflex sympathetic dystrophy with regional intravenous reserpine. *Anesth Analg* 1980; 59: 500.

98. Poplawski ZJ, Wiley AM, Murray JF. Post-traumatic dystrophy of the extremities. *J Bone Joint Surg Am* 1983; 65: 642.

99. DeTakats G. The nature of painful vasodilatation in causalgic states. *Arch Neurol* 1943; 50: 318.

100. Wettrell G, Hallbook T, Hultquist C. Reflex sympathetic dystrophy in two young females. *Acta Paediatr Scand* 1979; 68: 923.

101. Carron H, McCue F. Reflex sympathetic dystrophy in a 10-year-old. *South Med J* 1972; 65: 631.

102. Guntheroth WG, Chakmakjian S, Brena SC, *et al.* Post-traumatic sympathetic dystrophy: dissociation of pain and vasomotor changes. *Am J Dis Children* 1971; 121: 511.

103. Loh L, Nathan PW. Painful peripheral states and sympathetic blocks. *J Neurol Neurosurg Psychiatry* 1978; 41: 661.

104. Loh L, Nathan PW, Schott GD. Pain due to lesions of central nervous system removed by sympathetic block. *BMJ* 1981; 2: 1026.

105. Steinbrocker O. The shoulder-hand syndrome. Present perspective. *Arch Phys Med Rehabil* 1968; 49: 388.

106. Steinbrocker O, Neustadt D, Lapin L. Shoulder-hand syndrome. Sympathetic block compared with corticotropin and cortisone therapy. *JAMA* 1946; 153: 788.

107. Subbarao J, Stillwell GK. Reflex sympathetic dystrophy syndrome of the upper extremity: analysis of total outcome of management of 125 cases. *Arch Phys Med Rehabil* 1981; 62: 549.

108. Ferrante FM. Techniques for blockade of the sympathetic nervous system. *Curr Rev Clin Anesth* 1991; 12: 1.

109. Wirth FP, Rutherford RB. A civilian experience with causalgia. *Arch Surg* 1970; 100: 633.

110. Shumacker HB, Abramson DI. Post-traumatic vasomotor disorders: with particular reference to late manifestations and treatment. *Surg Gynecol Obstet* 1949; 88: 417.

111. Holden WD. Sympathetic dystrophy. *Arch Surg* 1948; 57: 373.

112. Echlin F, Owens FM, Wells WL. Observations on 'major' and 'minor' causalgia. *Arch Neurol* 1945; 62: 183.

113. Szeinfeld M, Palleres VS. Considerations in the treatment of causalgia. *Anesthesiology* 1983; 58: 294.

114. Rasmussen TB, Freedman H. Treatment of causalgia: an analysis of 100 cases. *J Neurosurg* 1946; 3: 165.

115. Spurling RG. Causalgia of the upper extremity: treatment by dorsal sympathetic ganglionectomy. *Arch Neurol* 1930; 23: 784.

116. Barnes R. The role of sympathectomy in the treatment of causalgia. *J Bone Joint Surg Br* 1953; 35: 172.

117. Evans JA. Sympathectomy for reflex sympathetic dystrophy: report of 29 cases. *JAMA* 1946; 132: 620.

118. Hardy WG, Posch JL, Webster JE, *et al.* The problem of major and minor causalgia. *Am J Surg* 1958; 95: 545.

119. Olcott C, Eltherington LG, Wilcosky BR, *et al.* Reflex sympathetic dystrophy—the surgeon's role in management. *J Vasc Surg* 1991; 14: 488.

120. Bingham JA. Some problems of causalgic pain. A clinical and experimental study. *BMJ* 1948; 2: 334.

121. Ruggeri SB, Athreya BH, Doughty R, *et al.* Reflex sympathetic dystrophy in children. *Clin Orthop* 1982; 163: 225.

122. Goodman CR. Treatment of shoulder-hand syndrome. *NY State J Med* 1971; 71: 559.

123. Johnson EW, Pannozzo AN. Management of shoulder-hand syndrome. *JAMA* 1966; 195: 152.

124. Watson HK, Carlson LK. Stress loading treatment for reflex sympathetic dystrophy. *Complications Orthop* 1990; 2: 19.

125. Watson HK, Carlson L. Treatment of reflex sympathetic dystrophy of the hand with an active "stress loading" program. *J Hand Surg [Am]* 1987; 12: 779.

126. Blanchard EB. The use of temperature biofeedback in the treatment of chronic pain due to causalgia. *Biofeed-back Self Regul* 1979; 4: 183.

127. Fermaglich DR. Reflex sympathetic dystrophy in children. *Pediatrics* 1977; 60: 881.

128. Richlin DM, Carron H, Rowlingson JC, *et al.* Reflex sympathetic dystrophy: successful treatment by trans-cutaneous nerve stimulation. *J Pediatr* 1978; 95: 84.

129. Owens S, Atkinson ER, Lees DE. Thermographic evidence of reduced sympathetic tone with transcutaneous nerve stimulation. *Anesthesiology* 1979; 50: 62.

130. Ebersold MJ, Laws ER, Albers JW. Measurements of autonomic function before, during, and after transcutaneous stimulation in patients with chronic pain and control subjects. *Mayo Clin Proc* 1977; 52: 228.

131. Meyer GA, Fields HL. Causalgia treated by selective large fibre stimulation of peripheral nerve. *Brain* 1972; 95: 163.

132. Chan CS, Chow SP. Electroacupuncture in the treatment of post-traumatic sympathetic dystrophy (Sudeck's atrophy). *Br J Anaesth* 1981; 53: 899.

133. Leo KC. Use of electrical stimulation at acupuncture points for the treatment of reflex sympathetic dystrophy in a child. *Phys Ther* 1983; 63: 957.

134. Fialka V, Resch KL, Ritter-Dietrich D, *et al.* Acupuncture for reflex sympathetic dystrophy. *Arch Intern Med* 1993; 153: 661.

135. Hill SD, Sheng LM, Chandler PJ. Reflex sympathetic dystrophy and electroacupuncture. *Tex Med J* 1991; 87: 76.

136. Lauer JW. Hypnosis in the relief of pain. *Med Clin North Am* 1968; 52: 217.

137. Gainer MJ. Hypnotherapy for reflex sympathetic dystrophy. *Am J Clin Hypn* 1992; 34: 227.

138. Kozin F, McCarty DJ, Sims J, *et al.* The reflex sympathetic dystrophy syndrome. I. Clinical and histologic studies. Evidence for bilaterality, response to corticosteroids and articular involvement. *Am J Med* 1976; 60: 321.

139. Ingram GJ, Scher RK, Lally EV. Reflex sympathetic dystrophy following nail biopsy. *J Am Acad Dermatol* 1987; 16: 253.

140. Kozin F, Ryan L, Carerra G, *et al.* The reflex sympathetic dystrophy syndrome (RSDS). III. Scintigraphic studies, further evidence for the therapeutic efficacy of systemic corticosteroids and proposed diagnostic criteria. *Am J Med* 1981; 70: 23.

141. DeTakats G. Sympathetic reflex dystrophy. *Med Clin North Am* 1965; 49: 117.

142. Mowat AG. Treatment of the shoulder-hand syndrome with corticosteroids. *Ann Rheum Dis* 1974; 33: 120.

143. Christensen K, Jensen EM, Noer I. The reflex sympathetic dystrophy syndrome. Response to treatment with systemic corticosteroids. *Acta Chir Scand* 1982; 148: 653.

144. Watson CP, Evans RJ, Reed K, *et al.* Amitriptyline versus placebo in postherapeutic neuralgia. *Neurology* 1982; 32: 671.

145. Gomez-Perez FJ, Rull JA, Dies H, Guillermo J. Nortriptyline and fluphenazine in the symptomatic treatment of diabetic neuropathy. A double-blind crossover study. *Pain* 1985; 23: 395.

146. Kvinesdal B, Molin J, Froland A, Gram LF. Imipramine treatment of painful diabetic neuropathy. *JAMA* 1984; 251: 1727.

147. Turkington RW. Depression masquerading as diabetic neuropathy. *JAMA* 1980; 243: 1147.

148. Gringras M. A clinical trial of Tofranil in rheumatic pain in general practice. *J Int Med Res* 1976; 4: 41.

149. Scott WAM. The relief of pain with an antidepressant in arthritis. *Practitioner* 1969; 202: 802.

150. Kehoe WA. Antidepressants for chronic pain: selection and dosing considerations. *Am J Pain Manage* 1993; 3: 161.

151. Chaturvedi SK. Phenytoin in reflex sympathetic dystrophy. *Pain* 1989; 36: 379.

152. Mellick GA, Mellicy LB, Mellick LB. Gabapentin in the management of reflex sympathetic dystrophy. *J Pain Symptom Manage* 1995; 10: 265.

153. Davis RW. Phantom sensation, phantom pain, and stump pain. *Arch Phys Med Rehabil* 1993; 74: 79.

154. Chabal C, Russell LC, Burchiel KJ. The effect of intra-venous lidocaine, tocainide, and mexiletine on spontaneously active fibers originating in rat sciatic neuromas. *Pain* 1989; 38: 333.

155. Dejgaard A, Petersen P, Kastrup J. Mexiletine for the treatment of chronic painful diabetic neuropathy. *Lancet* 1988; 29: 9.

156. Schwartzman RJ. New treatments for reflex sympathetic dystrophy. *N Eng J Med* 31 2000; 343(9): 654.

157. Claeys LGY. Correspondence: reflex sympathetic dystrophy. *N Eng J Med* 2000; 343(24): 1811.

158. Kemler MA, Barendse GAM, Van Kleef M, *et al.* Spinal cord stimulation in patient with chronic reflex sympathetic dystrophy. *N Eng J Med* 2000; 343(9): 618.

159. Kemler MA, Barendse GAM, Van Kleef M, *et al.* Pain relief in complex regional pain syndrome due to spinal cord stimulation does not depend upon vasodilation. *Anesthesiologist* 2000; 92: 1653.

12

Neuropsychological Evaluation and Treatment of Patients with Whiplash-Induced Mild Traumatic Brain Injury

Dennis A Helffenstein, Robert Sokol

INCIDENCE [1]

If an individual is involved in an accident severe enough to result in soft tissue and skeletal injury, then in some instances those same forces can be significant enough to result in injury to the brain. In the course of a medical practice, the physician may identify a subset of the whiplash patient population that begin to complain of symptoms other than those typically associated with a cervical or soft tissue injury. In those instances, the accurate and timely diagnosis and intervention related to Post-Concussive Syndrome/Mild Traumatic Brain Injury (PCS/MTBI) will be an integral part of the physician's overall treatment of a patient. Uzzell recently entitled a book chapter concerning the topic of MTBI "Mild Head Injury: Much Ado About Something" and states "we owe it to those who truly suffer from MHI to raise this syndrome out of the mire of devisiveness and scientific illegitimacy, and to drop the polemics." This chapter will provide an overview of the evaluation and treatment of individuals with whiplash-induced PCS/MTBI. Previously, the notion has been held that MTBI will occur only in high-speed accidents. More recent studies and clinical experience support the notion that this is not the case. As Parker aptly notes, "whiplash is a grossly underestimated source of neurobehavioral trauma."[2]

Low Impact Forces Can Result in Brain Injury

Some clinicians, including many neuropsychologists, continue to question if symptoms following mild head or whiplash injury truly have an anatomical or physiological basis. They continue to question if the group of individuals who demonstrate persistent PCS symptoms are merely malingerers motivated by secondary gain, neurotics with a psychological predisposition to wallow in the patient role, or individuals whose symptoms are merely the result of a variety of co-morbid factors (e.g., pain, depression, fatigue, or medication effects). For some time, there has been clear and substantial evidence to support the theory that acceleration/deceleration forces to the head and the resulting head movement create a variety of pressure gradients, leading to shear and compression strains within the brain and skull, which can result in injury to the brain.[3] It is important not just to take into account the change in velocity, but also the change in velocity over time (Average Acceleration = Change in Velocity/Change in Time).[4] As a result, significant forces can be generated if a relatively low change in velocity occurs over a very short period of time.

Varney and Varney[5] performed an analysis of the acceleration/deceleration forces resulting in brain injury of 15 individuals who sustained MTBI's in motor vehicle accidents. One of the case studies presented provides rather compelling evidence that brain injury can occur even at low speed impacts. One case study describes an incident in which a woman driving an unloaded, small, pickup truck was traveling at approximately five miles per hour when a sedan backed into her vehicle at ten miles per hour. She was wearing a seatbelt at the time of impact. The woman experienced no external evidence of a head injury and she experienced no alteration of her memories surrounding the accident. An analysis of the biomechanics involved revealed that she experienced an acceleration force to her head of 34g. She was alert and oriented when the police arrived at the scene. Later medical evaluation was positive for cervical strain and she was treated for whiplash injuries. The individual was serving as an officer in the military at the time of the accident. She had an engineering degree and performed highly technical work for the United States Army. Six months after the accident, she was demoted and, 3 months later, was discharged with a 20 percent service-connected disability. Neuropsychological testing revealed a variety of cognitive deficits, inconsistencies, or relative weaknesses that clearly explained her vocational deterioration despite a long history of academic and military/vocational success. Her full scale IQ was measured at 97, which was determined to be well below expectations for an honor graduate of a demanding engineering program. Her short-term memory scores ranged from the 22nd to the 47th percentiles (borderline range to average). Again, these scores were below expectation given her prior academic performance. Arithmetic skills were in the borderline range at the 18th percentile. Performance on four separate tests of executive functioning was consistently impaired, suggesting frontal involvement. In addition, during testing, she demonstrated two clear episodes of loss of mental focus (i.e., cognitive set loss). Her persisting cognitive problems were corroborated by her work associates and friends.

In this paper, Varney and Varney also discuss the similarities of "shaken baby syndrome" to the mechanism of injury in motor vehicle accidents involving acceleration/deceleration forces to the head and brain. They also point out that all of the cases reviewed resulted in cervical injury and, therefore, the forces involved were not trivial. In addition, they suggest that the presence of a cervical injury should be viewed as a clue for the clinician that brain injury may have occurred in the accident. Their ultimate conclusion was that acceleration/deceleration forces greater than 20g are potentially dangerous to the human brain.[5]

A number of studies have been performed utilizing rhesus monkeys to establish that even relatively low acceleration/deceleration forces can result in documented neurological injury. Ommaya, *et al.* simulated rear-impact accidents utilizing rhesus monkeys.[6] They determined that, if a vehicle was hit from behind causing it to move at a speed of

10.8 miles per hour within 0.1 seconds, a 5g horizontal acceleration force would result. Their study revealed that 50 percent of the rhesus monkeys exposed to such a force demonstrated cerebral contusions. They suggested that rotational displacement and acceleration forces exerted on the head accounted for the observed anatomic lesions. Because humans have larger brains, the angular acceleration required to produce cerebral concussion and brain injury will be much lower than that required to produce a similar injury in monkeys.[6] The cerebral contusions were demonstrated on the orbitofrontal and temporal surfaces of the brain. It is crucially important that clinicians investigate and manage the problems associated with whiplash injury not only with regards to the musculoskeletal and peripheral nervous systems, but also with greater attention to the finer details of behavioral and neurological deficits.[6]

Incidence of MTBI in the General Population

The incidence of MTBI varies widely in the studies from 131 per 100,000 to 519 per 100,000.[7] The 519 per 100,000 figure was derived from a national sample conducted through the US Census Bureau. This estimate involved only loss of consciousness and it is noted that this represents a conservative estimate because MTBI may occur without loss of consciousness. Given the national population of 250 million, this would result in an estimate of 1.3 million mild brain injuries per year. Forty percent to 80 percent of the individuals who sustain a mild head injury each year develop PCS.[8] Persistent post-concussive symptoms following mild head injury can occur in 20 to 40 percent of cases.[7] With regard to permanent impairment, Malec states "studies that provide estimates of the number of cases with residual symptoms typically indicate that 20 to 25 percent of individuals who sustain a MTBI will have residual symptoms or disability."[7] Therefore, it is evident that the incidence of a mild head injury resulting in permanent symptoms is quite high and presents a significant health concern.

Underdiagnoses and Misdiagnoses

Those clinicians who do not believe that persistent post-concussive symptoms have a true physiologic or neuro-anatomic basis will often espouse that MTBI is significantly over-diagnosed. However, those clinicians who believe that the symptoms do relate directly to some physical injury to the brain believe that MTBI is often under- or misdiagnosed. In their 1998 Consensus Statement on the rehabilitation of persons with traumatic brain injury, the National Institutes of Health agreed with the second group of clinicians. They noted, "mild TBI is significantly under-diagnosed and early intervention is often neglected."[9] The consensus statement further points out that, even though a MTBI can immediately result in a variety of impairments, the symptoms may be "masked" by more urgent medical problems. The symptoms may be missed or dismissed for a variety of reasons. If a patient is complaining of more prominent or pressing problems, such as pain or other physical symptoms, that is what the patient and physician will focus on. As a result, the patient may not spontaneously report symptoms of a concussion. The physician may not be inclined to ask specifically about concussive symptoms, particularly if there was no blow to the head, no loss of consciousness, or the Glasgow Coma Scale (GCS) was within normal limits. The importance of asking specific questions about PCS or utilizing a post-concussive symptom checklist cannot be over-emphasized. Early and complete documentation of these symptoms in the medical record is also important. Because denial and/or lack of insight may also be a component of an individual's MTBI, it may be also helpful for the physician to obtain collateral data from family members.

Early and proper diagnosis as well as education and appropriate multi-disciplinary intervention will maximize the MTBI patient's potential for recovery. It will also minimize the potential for persistent post-concussive symptoms developing.[1,7]

The importance of early diagnosis and intervention is also emphasized by Jay.[10] He notes that, when patients do discuss symptoms of a concussion with their physician, the physician will often perform a neurological examination, which is within normal limits. The patient is then informed that there is no organic reason for their problems, they should wait longer for recovery, learn to live with their problems, or seek psychiatric help. Jay states, "these iatrogenically induced problems (cause and effect) most likely lengthen the patient's symptomatic period as they begin to feel ever increasing loss of control, fear of the unknown, and concern that they must be going crazy."[10] In the course of our clinical practice, we are often told by our patients after receiving the diagnosis of PCS/ MTBI that they are relieved that there is an explanation for their problems and that indeed they are "not going crazy." There is therapeutic value in validating the patient's symptoms, in normalizing those symptoms, and also in providing the clear message that there are multiple interventions that can assist in recovery.

DEFINITIONS OF MTBI

The issue of rehabilitation of PCS/MTBI must begin with a proper identification of the clinical signs and symptoms associated with the condition. One of the major difficulties complicating the research into the nature and outcome of MTBI has been the lack of consensus regarding the definition of the disorder. The four professional disciplines frequently involved in the treatment of these patients (i.e., rehabilitation medicine, neurology, psychiatry, and neuropsychology) have each offered their own ideas regarding criteria to identify the MTBI patient.

American Congress of Rehabilitation Medicine

The first national attempt to establish diagnostic criteria for PCS/MTBI originated with the American Congress of Rehabilitation Medicine (ACRM). In 1993, the Brain Injury Interdisciplinary Special Interest Group—Mild Traumatic Brain Injury Committee of the American Congress published their definition of PCS/MTBI.[11] The definition states:

A patient with Mild Traumatic Brain Injury is a person who has had a traumatically induced physiological disruption of brain function, as manifested by at least one of the following:

1. Any period of loss of consciousness;
2. Any loss of memory for events immediately before or after the accident;
3. Any alteration in mental state at the time of the accident (e.g., feeling dazed, disoriented, or confused); and

4. Focal neurological deficit(s) that may or may not be transient; but where the severity of the injury does not exceed the following:

- Loss of consciousness of approximately 30 minutes or less;
- After 30 minutes, an initial GCS of 13–15; and
- Posttraumatic amnesia (PTA) not greater than 24 hours.

One important aspect of this definition was the inclusion of whiplash without external trauma to the head as a potential causative factor in the development of a traumatic brain injury. In this regard, the definition clearly indicated the possibility of brain injury without head injury.

The definition also specifies physical symptoms, cognitive deficits, and behavioral changes that can occur alone or in combination with each other. It asserts that such symptoms and deficits can produce a functional disability. The committee noted that such symptoms might persist, for varying lengths of time after such a neurological event. The article also reviewed various factors that could result in misdiagnosis or under-diagnosis. For example, the constellation of symptoms described could be overlooked in the face of more dramatic physical injury. Some patients may not become aware of, or admit to, the extent of their symptoms until they attempt to return to normal functioning (e.g., return to work).

Colorado Medical Society

Somewhat earlier, the Colorado Medical Society had been concerned about establishing guidelines for on-the-scene management of sports-related concussion.[12] This followed an alarming incident in which a 17-year-old, male, high school football player suffered catastrophic, diffuse brain swelling and death following two concussions without loss of consciousness occurring over a period of a week. This phenomenon is now referred to as the "second impact syndrome." The Colorado Medical Society Sports Concussion Guidelines included a system of grading the severity of concussion based on qualitative distinctions and symptom presentation. The grading system was necessary to determine specific guidelines regarding how to treat the athlete at the scene of the contest:

- Grade   I: Confusion without amnesia, no loss of consciousness.
- Grade II: Confusion with amnesia, no loss of consciousness.
- Grade III: Loss of consciousness.
- Prolonged unconsciousness, persistent mental status alterations, worsening post-concussion symptoms, or abnormalities on neurological examination require urgent neurosurgical consultation by transfer to a trauma center.

These guidelines advocated keeping the athlete out of the contest after a grade I concussion for at least 20 minutes while performing serial evaluations of neurological function. The player could then return to the game after 20 minutes if amnesia and other symptoms did not appear. However, the grade II concussion, in which amnesia does appear, would prevent the athlete's re-entry into the same event and require frequent examinations for signs of evolving intracranial abnormalities with return to practice only after a full week without symptoms.

A grade III concussion in which the athlete is rendered unconscious would require transportation from the field to the nearest hospital by ambulance with cervical spine immobilization if indicated. Neuroimaging of the brain would be recommended with unconsciousness or worsening post-concussion symptoms, focal neurological deficits, or persistent mental status alterations. With normal neurological findings, the athlete could be released and could return to practice only after two full weeks without symptoms.

American Academy of Neurology

Based on the Sports Concussion Guidelines published by the Colorado Medical Society, the Quality Standard Subcommittee of the American Academy of Neurology[13] produced a summary statement on the management of concussion in sports. In that summary statement, it was clearly asserted that concussion may or may not involve loss of consciousness and that confusion and amnesia were the hallmarks of concussion. They reviewed frequently observed features of concussion and also noted early (minutes and hours) and late (days to weeks) signs of concussion. The subcommittee also asserted that a grading scale would be useful in determining appropriate actions in response to concussive injury. Their "practice parameter" presented the following grading scale:

Grade I:

1. Transient confusion;
2. No loss of consciousness;
3. Concussion symptoms or mental status abnormalities on examination resolved in less than 15 minutes.

Grade II:

1. Transient confusion;
2. No loss of consciousness;
3. Concussion symptoms or mental status abnormalities on examination last more than 15 minutes.

Grade III:

1. Any loss of consciousness, either brief (seconds) or prolonged (minutes).

A list of recommendations for return to competition after concussion were listed as "practice options" depending on the grade (or severity) of the concussion. While the Colorado Medical Society Sports Concussion Guidelines developed its grading system on qualitative distinctions and symptom presentation (i.e., presence or absence of amnesia and/or loss of consciousness), the American Academy of Neurology system focused on a combination of qualitative and quantitative distinctions (i.e., the 15-minute cutoff) in determining severity of concussion. The issue of how to grade individuals whose symptoms last just under (or beyond) the time limit can become a problem in both determining the severity of concussion and in making appropriate decisions regarding follow-up evaluation and return to competition.

Diagnostic and Statistical Manual -- Fourth Edition

Psychiatry was the third discipline to attempt to diagnose and define PCS. Research criteria were published in the most recent edition of the American Psychiatric Association *Diagnostic and Statistical Manual—Fourth Edition (DSM-IV)*.[14] The *DSM-IV* research criteria for PCS requires the following:

> A history of head trauma that has caused significant cerebral concussion. LOC, PTA, or seizures are evidence of concussion.
>
> Evidence from neuropsychological testing or quantified cognitive assessment of impaired attention and memory.
>
> Three (or more) of the symptoms listed below should be present and persistent for at least three months:

1. Becoming fatigued easily.
2. Disordered sleep.
3. Headache.
4. Vertigo or dizziness.
5. Irritability or aggression on little or no provocation.
6. Anxiety, depression or affective lability.
7. Changes in personality (e.g., social or sexual inappropriateness).
8. Apathy or lack of spontaneity.

> Significant impairment of social or occupational functioning and significant decline from a previous level of functioning.
>
> Rule out: Dementia due to head trauma, Amnestic Disorder due to head trauma, Personality Change due to head trauma.

The Brain Injury Interdisciplinary Special Interest Group of the American Congress of Rehabilitation Medicine, however, published a number of concerns regarding the validity of the *DSM-IV* definition of post-concussional disorder.[15] For example, as has been previously noted in the original ACRM definition, as well as the Colorado Medical Society and American Academy of Neurology definitions, MTBI can certainly occur without loss of consciousness, PTA, or seizures. They also noted that cognitive symptoms may not be present and the patient may also have impairment of executive functions in addition to impaired attention and memory. They thought that only two symptoms should be required for diagnosis and that tinnitus and photophobia should be included in the symptom list. They felt the three-month criteria could prevent early intervention, and that the determination of "significant" impairment might be overly subjective. Finally, they asserted that there were also a number of additional psychiatric and physical disorders that would need to be ruled out.

Neuropsychological Definition

Dr. Ronald Ruff (a neuropsychologist) proposed another diagnostic system which involves discriminating between three types of MTBI, varying in symptom severity.[16] Dr. Ruff's diagnostic criteria attempt to bridge the gap between the ACRM definition (which specifies that a MTBI can result without loss of consciousness or PTA) and the more conservative *DSM-IV* criteria (which requires *either* PTA *or* loss of consciousness for inclusion) (Table 12-1).

Type I MTBI most closely resembles the ACRM definition. Type III MTBI follows most closely from the *DSM-IV* classification while Type II serves as a bridge between the two discrepant definitions.

The terms *concussion* and *MTBI* have been used interchangeably thus far. However, it is important to note that these are somewhat different concepts that carry with them different clinical implications. *Concussion* refers to a neurological event involving the impact of the head with an object or the rapid acceleration and deceleration of the head. *PCS* is the description of the signs and symptoms following a concussion. While concussion and PCS involve neurological substrates resulting in physical, cognitive, and behavioral abnormalities, there is no specific reference in these terms to brain injury. On the other hand *MTBI* refers specifically to a level of brain injury. While there is no doubt that brain injury is occurring in concussion, none-the-less the term MTBI implies permanency of damage, whereas concussion implies potentially reversible dysfunction. The ACRM suggests the term *post-concussion prodrome* for symptomatology under a three-month duration, and PCS for symptomatology beyond three months. The term MTBI is generally utilized when symptoms persist beyond an 18-month period, implying brain injury of a more permanent nature with symptoms less likely to resolve.

There are cases in which patients do not meet even the ACRM criteria for concussion based on the immediate effects of the accident on their behavior and cognition. However, these patients none-the-less present with a constellation of symptoms characteristic of PCS. In these cases, it is important not to automatically rule-out the possibility of concussion. Parker notes with regard to the definition of concussion, "although there is usually an alteration of consciousness, varying from a slight degree of disorientation to a relatively limited loss of consciousness, PCS is not contingent on actual alterations of consciousness"[2] He goes on to point out that, based on the forces involved, the pattern of trauma to the brain can vary and in some cases no alteration of consciousness occurs at the time of the accident. As will be noted later in this chapter, there are a variety of progressive, neuropathological processes that can ensue resulting in onset of symptoms within a period of 12 to 24 hours after the injury yet with no immediate onset of symptoms.

Table 12-1 Ruff MTBI Classification System

	Type I	Type II	Type III
LOC	Altered state or transient loss	Definite loss with time unknown or <5 min.	Loss 5–30 min.
PTA	1–60 sec.	60 sec–12 hr.	>12 hr.
Neurological Symptoms	One or more	One or more	One or more

Reprinted by permission from Ruff R.M. Discipline-specific approach versus individual care. In Varney NR, Roberts RJ (eds). *The Evaluation and Treatment of Mild Traumatic Brain Injury*, pp 99–113. Mahweh, NJ, Lawrence Erlbaum Assoc, 1999.

It is critical to note that the diagnosis of *MTBI* does not imply minimal consequences on the patient's functional ability. As noted previously by the National Institute of Health, traumatic brain injury, even when classified as mild, can result in a variety of significant impairments of cognitive, psychological, behavioral, social, and vocational functioning often resulting in catastrophic consequences in the patient's personal, social, and occupational life.[9] Parker notes, "The use of the diagnosis 'mild' brain injury is misleading insofar as it emphasizes lack of neuro and traumatic severity when indeed there may be a poor neurobehavioral outcome."[2]

BIOMECHANICS AND PATHOPHYSIOLOGY OF MTBI

Biomechanics of MTBI

In Parker's recent discussion of concussive brain trauma, he notes that brain injury results from a transfer of energy between an external mechanical event and soft tissue with limited elasticity.[2] When the capacity of the brain to move and be displaced internally is exceeded, temporary or permanent tissue damage occurs.

Parker summarizes the mechanical factors affecting the brain as follows:

1. the *magnitude* of the force applied
2. the *velocity* of the head relative to surrounding body and environmental structures
3. the *direction of force*
4. the *point of contact*
5. the *relative mobility* of the skull
6. the *angular and other directional components* of the velocity of the brain after trauma.

Lui notes that it is somewhat misleading to refer to "low-velocity impact" collisions as the implication is that low-velocity will result in minimal or minor injury.[4] Clearly, velocity is only one factor affecting potential injury. Another crucial determinant in the severity of the injury to a motor vehicle occupant is the degree and direction of force absorbed by the occupant. That is determined by the *relative change* in the velocity (acceleration/deceleration) of the occupant and the *interval* of the velocity change. The shorter the interval, the greater the force exerted on the occupant. Additionally, the *torque*, or tendency of the force to rotate the object is an additional important determinant in injury severity.

Liu[4] gives as an example a vehicle traveling 33 miles per hour and coming to a stop in one second. He considers the same vehicle going 3.3 miles per hour but abruptly stopping in 0.1 second. While the former example seems the more dramatic deceleration, in fact, the average acceleration and resultant force in both instances is identical.

In motor vehicle accidents, a poor understanding of biomechanics can result in misleading notions about the severity of an occupant injury, based on observing the body damage to the vehicle. While it is easy to conclude that there is a direct relationship between damage to the vehicle and injury to the occupant, this is not necessarily the case.

Dr. Nils Varney gives a cogent example of an armored car and a Mercedes Benz both hitting a wall at 35 miles per hour. The armored car suffers little body damage while the Mercedes crumples to the firewall.[17] While the Mercedes appears to be the more serious accident for the occupant, Varney points out that is likely that the occupant of the armored car is the more seriously injured party.

By analyzing the kinematics of the accident (that is, the study of the motion of the object), it becomes clear that the crumpling of the Mercedes dramatically increased the stopping distance of the vehicle and thereby extended the time interval of the deceleration. This, in turn, reduced the physical force operating on the occupant. Or, to put it another way, the force that was not absorbed by the armored car in the form of damage was transferred directly to that vehicle's occupant.

According to Liu, in motor vehicle accidents in which there is a hyperextension/hyperflexion or "whiplash" of the neck and head, the mechanism of brain injury is due to induced translational and rotational accelerations of the head.[4] Even in collisions apparently involving only linear forces (that is, a rear-end or head-on collision in which the occupant's body and head are facing forward) translational and angular rotational forces will be involved. This is because the head is attached to the neck and will rotate on the stalk of the neck with any induced motion.

In clinical case studies, clinical evidence of MTBI was documented in collisions in which acceleration forces were as low as 30g and forces as low as 20g were considered potentially unsafe.[5,18] In all examples, while there was definitive evidence of brain injury, there was no evidence of concomitant injury to the head. In the case of low speed collisions, the stopping distance becomes crucial in that, with very small stopping distances (or rapid acceleration in the case of rear-end impact), dangerous acceleration/deceleration can result even though the speed is low. The conclusion was that it appeared "highly unlikely" that individuals could withstand acceleration/deceleration forces beyond 34g without brain damage.

In many cases of whiplash secondary to motor vehicle collisions, the assumption is often made that only acceleration/deceleration forces were at play and that impact of the head did not occur. Many times patients will deny or simply not know whether an impact to the head occurred. However, in many accidents backward motion of the head results in an impact with the headrest. This will dramatically reduce the stopping distance of the head's backward motion. While reducing the hyperextension of the neck, this could increase the forces inside the cranium by reducing the time interval of the deceleration of the brain. It is, therefore, important to query the patient carefully regarding potential impact with the headrest.

Pathophysiology of MTBI

In discussing the pathophysiological mechanisms of brain injury, it is important to note that there are a number of injuries and mechanisms that more typically accompany moderate to severe brain injuries. Mechanisms such as intracerebral, acute subdural, extradural, and subarachnoid hematomas as well as cerebral edema and changes in blood volume and blood flow secondary to hemorrhage will not be discussed. The discussion will be limited, therefore, to those mechanisms underlying mild brain trauma.

Pathophysiological mechanisms of brain injury can be discussed in terms of both primary and secondary injury. Lezak notes that primary injury is the damage that occurs at the time of impact while secondary injury consists of the effects of the physiological processes set in motion by the primary injury.[19]

Primary injuries can further be differentiated into focal and diffuse lesions. A cursory analysis of the internal geography of the skull reveals bony ridges (sphenoid and temporal bones) as well as an irregular surface to the inferior frontal portion of the skull. The acceleration/deceleration forces described previously will result in the brain moving within the skull causing a compression of the frontotemporal areas against these irregular, bony surfaces resulting in focal areas of cerebral contusion. Frontotemporal regions of the brain will be more frequently contused than the occipitoparietal area because of this internal geography.[10] The contused area may occur at the coup and/or contre coup sites. The coup site is the area in which the head was struck. The contre coup site is the region of the brain exactly opposite the initial blow. In the latter case, a "rebound" effect occurs in which a compression wave causes the brain to be compressed against the opposite side of the skull. Coup/contre coup lesions usually result in specific behavioral changes that accompany closed head injuries.

Diffuse lesions in cases of MTBI usually occur as a result of the mechanism of diffuse axonal injury (DAI). The small stopping distances and rapid acceleration/deceleration intervals previously described result in a rapid rotational movement (or torque) of the brain inside the skull. Rapid acceleration/deceleration and rotational movement can result in damage at the level of the nerve cell. As the brain is composed of neuronal regions of different densities, layers of nerve cells in the brain will be propelled at different rates. Particularly at junctures between cortical and subcortical regions, axons may be "sheared." *Shear strain* is characterized by alterations in the shape of adjacent tissues due to alterations in the relative positions of these tissues caused by rotational movement. Shear strain can result in multiple microscopic lesions occurring simultaneously within the deep white matter of both cerebral hemispheres.[19] *Tensile strain* causes damage secondary to the elongation of neural tissues by the change in stretching force.

Axonal injury can also result from *cavitation* and *pressure waves*. Secondary to translational movement (when force is applied perpendicular to a mass with anterior-posterior movement) a compression wave is released causing compression of the frontal and temporal tips resulting in a contusion. In addition, a pressure gradient develops which can exceed the atmospheric pressure at one pole and drop the vapor pressure of the brain. Parker[2] notes that, "the liquid boils and changes rapidly to the gaseous state, causing instantaneous formation of gas bubbles with great violence, analogous to the sudden pressure changes in the center of an explosion."[2]

DAI frequently occurs in MTBI. It can occur without any direct impact to the head and requires only rapid acceleration/deceleration, such as in whiplash injuries secondary to the rapid hyperextension/hyperflexion of the neck. The secondary injuries occur as a result of physiological processes set into motion by the immediate effects of the primary injury on the brain. Brain swelling and associated dramatic increase in intracranial pressure can be a catastrophic outcome of MTBI as previously noted. Brain swelling is secondary, in part, to increased intravascular blood within the brain. The magnitude of brain swelling does not correlate with the severity of brain injury.[10] As noted earlier, catastrophic brain swelling can occur in association with consecutive concussions (second impact syndrome) involving no loss of consciousness.[12]

As noted in the National Institute of Health Consensus Statement, MTBI can result in damaging neurochemical changes to the basic molecules of metabolism, to mechanisms of the human cellular response to injury, and can increase the quantity of certain molecules that can be dangerous in excessive amounts.[9] These damaging changes in neurochemistry and metabolism have been referred to as a neurochemical "cascade."

Dixon, *et al.* describe many of these neurochemical "cascade" mechanisms in some detail.[20] Firstly, abnormal neurochemical agonist-receptor interactions related to excitotoxic processes can contribute to the pathophysiology associated with traumatic brain injury.[20] A massive release of neurotransmitters caused by a traumatically induced membrane depolarization can result in activation of muscarinic cholinergic and/or M-methyl-D-aspartate glutamate receptors. Increased levels of glutamate and aspartate appear to create irreversible damage to neurons and glia.[2] Secondly, soon after brain trauma, there is oxygen radical formation (i.e., high valence, unbound, and a highly reactive species of oxygen) which causes additional cellular injury. Thirdly, abnormalities in the axonal cytoskeleton such as blockages of axoplasmic transfer and accumulation of axonal materials can affect the ability of neurons to respond to and communicate with their environment. This could, in turn, have important functional consequences. After moderate traumatic brain injury, cytoskeletal damage was observed in the hippocampus in particular and this could be an important factor in the development of functional memory deficits.[20]

Mild to moderate traumatic brain injury can induce increases in acetylcholine and increased cholinergic activity can persist for some time following injury.[10] It is possible that excessive release of acetylcholine could result in excitotoxic disturbances to cholinergic neurons contributing to memory functions as cholinergic pathways in the brain play a crucial role in memory systems.[20] Increased activity of cholinergic neurons in the brainstem may be related to attentional deficits after concussion and chronic acetylcholine neurotransmission deficits may persist after traumatic brain injury. In terms of cognitive functioning, these alterations in neuro-networks and neurotransmitter systems (especially ones involving acetylcholine, dopamine, and serotonin) can dramatically affect both cognition and behavior.[10]

Dixon, *et al.* assert that, while mechanical forces are necessary to produce axonal injury, such injury may result in a "biochemical cascade of pathophysiological events initiated by the mechanical events rather than formed at the moment of injury."[20] Experimentally induced minor and moderate traumatic brain injury in cats resulted in focal, axonal damage in both the cerebral cortex and cerebellum. While there was no evidence of axonal tearing, reactive swellings or retraction balls could be seen within 12 to 24 hours of the traumatic event. It appeared that with mild to moderate injury, a focal compression or stretching of axons had occurred. Over time (one to three hours post-injury) this led to impairment of anterograde axoplasmic transport, local accumulation of organelles and axoplasm with the ultimate result of a focal swelling of the axons. By 12 to 24 hours post-injury, a swollen axoplasmic mass had formed and detached, constituting a classic retraction ball. Therefore, progressive post-traumatic change had been observed rather than an immediate tearing of the axon.[21]

Furthermore, once an axon is severed it can affect the undamaged neurons that make synaptic contact with it. Presynaptic terminals withdraw from the dendrites of the injured neuron and the cell body adjacent to the injured neuron undergoes retrograde transneuronal degeneration. In the postsynaptic neuron, similar anterograde transneuronal degeneration can occur. This is known as *diaschisis* or *long-distance neuronal impairment* and can contribute to the explanation of why a "minor" lesion may result in significant functional impairment.[2]

Axonal injury in human beings is therefore an "evolutionary process." These latter findings in particular confirm the importance of exercising caution in not immediately ruling-out PCS/MTBI in individuals who do not meet the diagnostic criteria (as has been previously defined) based on the immediate effects of the accident on the patient. There is a subset of patients who will begin to develop a constellation of concussive symptoms over time because of the secondary injury mechanisms described above.

PREDISPOSITION/VULNERABILITIES TO MTBI

Premorbid Neurological History

Individuals with premorbid conditions that affect the central nervous symptom are, for a variety of reasons, more vulnerable to the effects of a MTBI. The normal effects of aging result in more significant impact of any brain injury. Individuals over the age of 40 typically have poorer outcome than those who are younger.[22] Pre-existing conditions such as hypertension, diabetes, hyperlipidemia, and a significant history of alcohol abuse can leave an individual more susceptible to the effects of a concussion. Gualtieri suggests that a MTBI may affect such an individual to the degree that a severe brain injury would affect someone else.[23] The cognitive and neurobehavioral symptoms are more significant and persistent. Individuals with medical conditions such as epilepsy, multiple sclerosis, attention deficit disorder, and attention deficit hyperactivity disorder, as well as a variety of learning disabilities, mental retardation and cerebral palsy, are also more susceptible to the effects of PCS/MTBI. Elderly patients who are experiencing subclinical dementias may become clearly demented following a mild concussion.

It is now well established in the literature that brain injuries, even mild concussions, are cumulative. The history of a prior concussion, even if the individual is asymptomatic following that accident, predisposes him or her to having more significant deficits and a poorer outcome following a second neuro-trauma.[10] In clinical practice, this is often demonstrated by the following scenario: an individual has a history of a prior significant concussion. This person may have been symptomatic for a period of time but experienced a complete or near-complete recovery. He or she is then involved in a second, rather minor, motor vehicle accident, experiences minimal acceleration/deceleration forces to the head, and is now demonstrating rather significant symptoms of a full-blown PCS. This appears to occur because of the brain's reduced reserve capacity to initially manage and then recover from the second, albeit extremely mild, neuro-trauma.

Premorbid Psychological/Psychiatric History

Brain injuries in general and even MTBI's potentially compromise the course and treatment of a wide variety of psychological and psychiatric disorders. Gualtieri notes that there tends to be inverse relation to the severity of the psychiatric disorder, that is, mild anxiety disorders or mild chronic depressions can be more significantly exacerbated by a MTBI than a more major psychiatric disorder, such as schizophrenia or a bipolar disorder.[23] Ruff, *et al.* identified a variety of emotional risk factors associated with MTBI.[24] They reviewed four case studies of individuals that demonstrated pre-existing personality traits that compounded the symptom presentation associated with a MTBI. These included over-achievement, dependency, grandiosity, and borderline personality traits. The authors point out that MTBI can result in a significant breakdown in the individual's traditional psychological defense mechanisms and character style. The brain injury itself can result in compromised cognitive abilities that in turn compromises cognitive coping abilities such as intellectualization and compartmentalization. The injuries and resulting limitations can negatively affect self-confidence and self-esteem and this is particularly true if these were rather tenuous pre-accident.

If there is frontal involvement, which there often is in cases of MTBI, emotional regulation can be affected which results in lability or irritability. This, in turn, results in a sense of loss of control and the individual becoming more emotionally fragile. As a result, any premorbid personality traits or tendencies tend to be exacerbated and magnified. The authors further point out that this breakdown in psychological defense mechanisms can be further exacerbated by professionals, family members, and friends who question and/or dismiss the patient's symptoms. In the scenario presented above, the personality traits or characteristics that are relatively benign, functionally asymptomatic, or in some cases adaptive (e.g., over-achiever/workaholic) can become clearly maladaptive following a MTBI.

Genetic Predisposition

Recent research suggests that the genetic marker apolipoprotein E (Apo E) may provide information about an individual's vulnerability to traumatic brain injury. The Apo E genotype moderates the formation of beta-amyloid deposits that occur following DAI. Research suggests that individuals who are homozygous for the E-4 allele are found to experience more significant evidence of brain damage following traumatic brain injury.[7]

CO-MORBID FACTORS AFFECTING COGNITIVE FUNCTION FOLLOWING MTBI

An individual patient's cognitive status and neurobehavioral presentation can be compromised by factors apart from the organic sequelae of brain injury. These "co-morbid" factors can pre-exist the injury or, more frequently, are co-occurring conditions secondary to concomitant physical injury. Such factors can also be secondary to the distress of coping with physical impairments and social/occupational loss. The most frequently encountered co-morbid factors include severe psychological distress, pain, fatigue, medication effects, and level of motivation/effort.

Emotional Distress

Psychological distress in the form of either severe depression and/or anxiety can exacerbate cognitive dysfunction in general and neuropsychological test performance in particular. The *DSM-IV* clearly specifies that in major depressive episodes there can be reports of diminished ability to think, concentrate, and make decisions by either the patient or via the observations of the patient by others. Depression often co-occurs with MTBI and, when severe, is likely to reduce the patient's ability to process information efficiently and may also compromise both learning efficiency and attention/concentration. Depression can be reactive in nature and/or co-vary with the patient's pre-existing character structure or can occur as a result of the neurological injury.[10]

Depression and anxiety are obvious reactions to both cognitive and physical loss frequently accompanying MTBI. Kay, in his paper on minor head injury, discusses in some detail the devastating impact on the patient's sense of self, secondary to what appeared to be minor cognitive changes.[25] He notes that the individual's sense of emotional balance, sense of integrity, and personal "identity" can be critically disrupted following a MTBI. He notes that sense of self can be more devastated after mild, rather than more severe traumatic brain injury, because the deficits encountered after minor brain injury are unexpected and may not be apparent to anyone else. That is, without appearing or feeling any different, the individual is not able to perform with the same success. This can result in a loss of self-confidence and increasing self-doubt creating a significant degree of performance anxiety and depression.

Emotional stress and depression are more likely to develop when patients have passed through the early stages of recovery but do not experience the degree of recovery that they had hoped for. If disability persists and the prospect of return to a previous lifestyle becomes less likely, a more severe reaction can occur and the patient may become clinically depressed with associated feelings of hopelessness, helplessness, apathy, and a loss of will to continue with rehabilitation. Following repeated, unexpected failures, a sense of self-blame and guilt may result in further erosion of the individual's sense of self with resultant feelings of depression, grief and loss.[25] Individuals with a previous history of depression as part of their character will be more likely to enter this state and will need a higher degree of support.[26] Certainly, just because a patient has been diagnosed with a MTBI, does not mean that their level of reactive emotional distress will also be "mild" and this must be carefully evaluated.[27]

It is important to note that most PCS/MTBI patients do not present with an extreme level of emotional distress. For example, while it is clear that depressive symptoms are common following MTBI, major depressive episodes occur in only 20 to 30 percent of MTBI patients. For this subgroup of patients, depressive sequelae are likely to contribute to functional, cognitive and psychosocial disability.[28] In such individuals, formal neuropsychological assessment should be postponed. Early treatment intervention is critical and is likely to decrease the potential for chronic symptoms. It is important to treat depressive symptoms aggressively (with psychotropic medications, education, and psychotherapy) as they can mask the cognitive and behavioral sequelae associated with MTBI. Postponing treatment can create greater difficulties that will require more treatment and more cost in the future.[10]

The second, less obvious cause of depression in MTBI patients is the direct effect of neurological damage on the biochemical function of the central nervous system. In one study, CSF levels of serotonin (5-HT), Substance P (SP), and lipid peroxidation (LPx) products were measured in patients with traumatic brain injury and compared to controls. The levels of SP and 5-HT in patients with head trauma were lower than those found in controls.[10] Once again, early psychopharmacological intervention can be very helpful in minimizing depressive symptoms directly related to organic injury. Therefore, selective serotonergic re-uptake inhibitors (SSRIs), such as Prozac, Paxil, and Zoloft, are now commonly used as first-line antidepressant medications.[28] Celexa, the newest of the SSRI antidepressants, has also become popular with the neurologists and physiatrists with whom we work. Jay recommends a small dose of tricyclic antidepressant medication at night to help with sleep in addition to an SSRI in the morning in patients with traumatic brain injury.[10] For the minority of patients who experience extreme emotional distress, this needs to be treated and minimized before formal neuropsychological testing can be administered.

However, for the remainder of patients, who are not exhibiting severe depression or anxiety, their mild level of distress is not likely to either significantly compromise their cognitive function or their performance on neuropsychological testing when such testing is administered in an emotionally supportive and reassuring manner.[19] A study designed to evaluate the influence of depression upon neuropsychological test performance found that there were virtually no significant differences in neurocognitive test performance between three patient groups whose depression scale on the Minnesota Multiphasic Personality Inventory–Second Version (MMPI-2) had either remained stable, increased, or decreased. That is, the patients that became more depressed did not perform worse on cognitive testing.[29]

According to Reitan and Wolfson, "there appears to be strong evidence that emotional disorders do not directly result in poorer neuropsychological test performance." They assert that, "if neuropsychological tests are administered properly and cooperation and effort to perform well are elicited from the patient, the resultant test scores can be interpreted as indications of adequacy of brain function."[30]

Pain

Due to the fact that many patients who sustain a MTBI do so in conjunction with acceleration/deceleration forces affecting the head, neck and upper body, it is not surprising that a common co-morbid factor is pain. Pain is more likely to affect neuropsychological test performance and cognitive functioning as an internal distraction when it is acute and/or severe. Pain of this intensity primarily affects attention, concentration, information processing, and (to some degree) acquisition of new information. The effects of distractibility secondary to severe pain must be considered when interpreting neurocognitive deficits. Chronic pain is more likely to affect cognitive performance because of associated psychological distress. However, when psychological distress is managed, the impact of chronic pain on cognition appears to be minimal.[31]

A number of studies have suggested that pain is not likely to play a significant role in cognitive impairment or neuropsychological test performance if it is not acute or intense. For example, when a brief neuropsychological test battery was administered to 60 individuals with migraine headache, non-headache chronic pain, or MTBI, the frequency of impairment among the MTBI participants was significantly higher than normal. Furthermore, there was no significant difference between the performance of the headache and chronic pain patients and their performance was within normal limits. The results suggested that neither migraine headaches nor chronic nonmigraine pain is typically associated with meaningful cognitive impairment. Although some of the MTBI patients also reported pain symptoms, the cognitive limitations identified within the MTBI sample could not be attributed solely to this pain because the MTBI group performed more poorly than the two samples of pain patients. Even though a high percentage of the MTBI patients were involved in litigation, a comparable number of the chronic pain patients were seeking compensation as well.[32]

Another study reported that when MTBI patients were administered a cognitive battery and they were also asked to rate their headaches at the time of testing, no significant differences were found on any of the measures between subjects grouped by headache severity (none, mild, and severe).[33] Townsend and Mateer found no consistent relationship in a group of patients between level of reported pain secondary to degenerative joint disease and neuropsychological test results.[34]

Finally, a study of 409 patients objectively demonstrating good effort and divided into "no pain" and "high pain" groups revealed that, though the high-pain level group clearly had associated psychological distress, no measures of cognitive ability were affected. Similar negative results were reported for the same pain groups on several measures of verbal learning and memory. These results suggested that pain did not significantly impact measures of cognitive ability in a population of individuals objectively demonstrating good effort.[35]

Despite the above findings, it remains clear that severe levels of pain can potentially distract patients from the testing process, which in turn can negatively impact their performance. It is the responsibility of the neuropsychologist to assess a patient's pain level and ability to give reasonable effort to the testing before and during the evaluation process. Testing can often be divided into multiple sessions and frequent breaks can be given to accommodate the patient's pain. This in turn will maximize the chances for getting valid test scores.

Fatigue

An additional co-morbid factor that is commonly overlooked is patient fatigue. This is often secondary to sleep disturbance associated with pain or the brain injury itself. Organically based fatigue is also a common sequelae of MTBI. Clearly, a fatigued patient will perform sub-optimally in terms of daily cognitive tasks and neuropsychological test performance in particular. It is imperative that the physician intervenes early and aggressively in relation to problems with sleep disturbance. According to Wrightson and Gronwall, abnormal fatigue has a more direct effect on a patient's life than any other factor because it limits performance and increases the effect of other symptoms, creating a "downward spiral" of dysfunctioning.[26] Even when sleep has not been disturbed, patients may start the day with fairly good energy and suddenly find that they are struggling to keep going and also begin to struggle cognitively. Again, the neuropsychological testing can be divided into multiple sessions to accommodate a patient's fatigue. In most instances testing can be, and should be, discontinued and resumed at a later date should the patient's fatigue begin to impact test performance. In some instances, the neuropsychologist will want to postpone testing until the sleep and fatigue issues are addressed with medication and, in some instances, psychotherapy. As mentioned previously, the patient may be prescribed a tricyclic antidepressant medication in small dosages to address their sleep disorder or the patient may be administered Trazodone before bedtime because of its sedative side effects.[10] Trazodone also has the added benefit of potentiating the effect of an SSRI antidepressant if the patient is being treated for depression utilizing one of these medications. Ambien can also be a useful sleep aid for individuals who have sustained a MTBI.

Medication Effects

Kay notes that utilization of prescription medication may also interfere with cognitive performance.[31] He notes that the interpretation of the effects of medication on test performance can be rather complex. For example, many medications used at therapeutic levels, such as antidepressants and mood stabilizers, may actually serve to improve mental functioning yet these medications may also have side effects in some patients that could negatively affect their cognitive performance. Other medications (such as anxiolytics) are known to have negative effects on attention and memory yet the primary effects of anxiety reduction may relieve the more significant effects of severe anxiety on cognitive performance. In any case, Kay advises that the neuropsychologist be aware of which medications the patient is using and the potential impact on cognition. Furthermore, it is recommended that the impact of such medications on test performance be considered in the interpretation of the neuropsychological test results. If the patient is utilizing a medication that does sedate or otherwise negatively impacts cognition and it is a medication which is used on an as-needed basis, then the patient may be asked to avoid use of that medication just prior to and during the testing process.

Level of Effort

An individual's neurobehavioral presentation can, of course, be affected by sub-optimal motivation to perform well. The *DSM-IV* outlines a number of different psychiatric disorders whose sequelae involve a desire on the part of the patient to appear unhealthy and to perform sub-optimally.

Roughly, these disorders are divided into three categories. A subset of Somatoform Disorders (i.e., somatization disorder, undifferentiated somatoform disorder, and conversion disorder) have in common the unintentional production of medical complaints that either cannot be fully explained by a known general medical condition or are in excess of what would be expected from a known medical condition but in the absence of any external incentive. The Factitious Disorders have in common the intentional production of such complaints in the absence of external incentives. Usually the motivation for a factitious disorder is a desire to assume the sick role. Finally, there is the intentional production of false or grossly exaggerated physical or psychological symptoms motivated by clear external incentives, which is the essential feature of Malingering.

The specter of sub-optimal motivation and level of effort is particularly raised in medical-legal settings. However, the reality is that a small minority of patients complaining of post-concussive sequelae in medical legal settings are likely to be malingering. According to Jarvis and Barth, "it seems likely that relatively few of the people who claim deficits resulting from brain injuries are truly malingering, and most of them are probably so obvious that they are detected by attorneys who advise them to drop their claims."[36] Horn and Zaslar also assert that the incidence of gross malingering is probably quite low.[37]

Finally, Leininger and Kreutzer assert that there is no evidence to indicate that MTBI patients intentionally feign impairments or exaggerate difficulties on neuropsychological testing more than any other clinical population.[38] These authors suggest that the incidence of frank malingering in this diagnostic group is quite limited. While estimates of malingering on neuropsychological tests by individuals being evaluated for MTBI in the medical-legal context range anywhere from five to 50 percent, it is likely that these variations may be due to the setting in which the evaluation takes place (e.g., medical, medical-legal, forensic, Independent Medical Examination, rehabilitation), the nature of the referral sources, the procedures used to define or determine malingering, and the expectations and perspective of the examiner.[39]

As will be discussed later in this chapter, it is important for the examining neuropsychologist to rule-out sub-optimal motivation and level of effort as a potential confounding factor in the patient's neurocognitive presentation in general, and on neuropsychological test performance in particular. Because this issue is of such critical importance, it is recommended that the examining neuropsychologist employ a variety of modalities and methodologies to assess effort and motivation. It is recommended that a combination of behavioral observation methodologies as well as a variety of formal, objective measures of effort be employed to insure the veracity of the patient's clinical presentation and optimal test performance on formal neurocognitive testing.

In summary, neuropsychological testing is ultimately a measure of the patient's performance. A variety of factors have been described that have the potential of additionally compromising neurocognitive ability. It is important that such factors be accurately diagnosed and aggressively treated so that true cognitive problems can be identified and quantified. Formal neuropsychological testing can be postponed until these factors are eliminated or minimized. It is important to note that a substantial body of research appears to suggest that, when these factors are of limited intensity, an accurate diagnosis of neurocognitive sequelae can still be made. When these factors cannot be sufficiently minimized (as in the case of severe depression or high levels of pain), the neuropsychologist needs to adequately account for the potential effects of such co-morbid factors on the patient's neurocognitive test performance.

COMMON PCS/MTBI SYMPTOMS

The symptoms associated with PCS/MTBI are many and varied. It is helpful to conceptualize these symptoms as falling into four major categories:

- physical/somatic
- cognitive
- psychological/behavioral
- vision.

The argument has been made that the base rate for many PCS symptoms is quite high in the general population. The argument has also been made that many of these symptoms and problems can relate to other injuries or medical conditions. One way to help control for these variables is to specifically ask the patient to discuss symptoms that are new since the traumatic event or, if it is a problem that they have had previously (e.g., headaches), if there has been a notable exacerbation in either the frequency or intensity of that problem since the traumatic event. Should the clinician choose to use a symptom checklist, it should also be made clear to the patient that you are asking them to report new symptoms or significantly exacerbated symptoms since the traumatic event. The importance of structuring questions or questionnaires in this manner is reviewed in Ruff and Grant.[40] While there is no truly "classic" constellation of symptoms that identify a post-concussional disorder, there is now sufficient evidence supporting the idea that the symptoms often do have a predictable configuration.[41]

Physical

Patients who have sustained PCS/MTBI will frequently report a variety of physical symptoms and concerns. Headaches are a common post-concussive symptom and a comprehensive evaluation of the headache symptoms is clearly indicated. A thorough review of post-traumatic headaches is presented by Jay, Parker, as well as in Hines.[2,10,42] A variety of vestibular problems including dizziness, tinnitus, and balance problems are common in post-concussive patients. For a more thorough review of these symptoms, refer to Jacobson.[43] Motor coordination problems such as incoordination with the hands, dropping things more frequently, or disarticulation (such as stuttering or slurring) are common. Fatigue is by far one of the most common problems associated with PCS/MTBI. This is often described by the patient as both physical and cognitive fatigue. The patient will report that they become more tired more easily whether performing physical or cognitive activities. It is sometimes helpful to have the patient rate current stamina and endurance levels as compared to pre-injury levels. To some degree, the patient's fatigue may relate to sleep disturbance but in the absence of sleep problems it is common for individuals who have sustained MTBIs to report ongoing persistent problems with fatigue.

Additional physical problems that are often reported include alteration in sense of smell (increased or decreased) and alteration in sense of taste (again either increased or decreased). Post-concussive patients will often report odd or unusual tastes in their mouths. This often includes the taste of blood, metal or decayed food. These are classic symptoms of dysguesia. Phonophobia (noise sensitivity) is also an extremely common symptom. The patient will report being more sensitive to loud noises or noisy places. They will often describe becoming irritable or anxious in such situations. They will often report having difficulty filtering out background noise when in such a situation (the brain has difficulty habituating to the background noise and it continues to interfere with processing). Many patients will report persisting problems with nausea and/or vomiting. Intolerance to alcohol is also a common post-concussive symptom. Tactile functions such as the experience of tingling and weakness should be assessed. Blackout episodes or seizures are also fairly common.

Cognitive

It has widely been thought that PCS/MTBI would primarily result in rather isolated cognitive problems most notably in the areas of attention and concentration, short-term memory, and speed of processing. However, Barth, *et al.* and later Reitan and Wolfson have proposed that cognitive deficits following MTBI are much more widespread and diverse than previously thought.[44,45] As a result, when discussing cognitive problems with a patient, it is recommended that the questioning not be confined to the above areas. It is, however, well established that attention/concentration, short-term memory, and speed of cognitive processing are indeed common cognitive sequelae following MTBI. With regards to attention and concentration, gathering data related to the patient's ability to maintain mental focus (mind wandering or getting easily distracted), the patient's ability to maintain cognitive set, and also the ability to multitask (divide attention) is important. With regards to short-term memory, it is important to gather data about patients' ability to learn new information, as compared to prior to the accident. It is also critical to ask about their ability to retain that newly learned information over time. More frequently forgetting intentions, appointments, what is said to them, what they are doing if they are distracted, and repeating themselves are indicators of a short-term memory problem. If patients report having to rely more heavily on written notes, to-do lists, or organizational systems, this is a clear indication that they are indeed having difficulties with short-term memory in their day-to-day or work activities.

At times, individuals who have sustained a MTBI will report difficulty accessing remote information; however, in most instances they will report that cueing does help their memory. This suggests that they are having a problem with memory retrieval not that they have actually lost the memories. Slowed speed of cognitive processing is also common following MTBI. Patients will often report slowed speed of processing information as it is being presented. For example, if someone is talking too fast, they will have difficulty keeping up. In addition, they may also note that the slowed processing results in them taking longer to perform their day-to-day or work tasks.

A variety of language-based problems can also be seen following MTBI. These include difficulties with verbal fluency (word finding) and paraphasic errors in the individual's style of speech (i.e., saying the wrong word). Language and reading comprehension problems are also both quite common. Dysarthria and/or disruption of pragmatic language are less common but possible sequelae.

Executive dysfunction is common following MTBI.[46] Indeed, there are times when individuals who have sustained a MTBI will demonstrate deficits in executive functioning without significant impairment in other cognitive abilities. Executive function is defined as the neurocognitive operations that initiate and maintain purposeful, goal-directed behavior and enable adaptation to a range of environmental changes and demands as these unfold in time.[47] Obviously, this involves a wide variety of functions that become crucial when non-routine behavior or problem solving is involved. These functions are necessary when a situation requires flexibility, problem solving, planning and organization or shifting cognitive set. Some specific problems which patients report include difficulties with planning and organizing multi-step tasks, difficulties with problem solving and decision-making, problems initiating a task once it is planned, reduced motivation, making more frequent errors, and often not catching their own mistakes.

They often report difficulties staying on topic (tangentiality) or note that they are easily distracted by external stimuli. They may also demonstrate disinhibition in a variety of ways (e.g., saying or doing things that are inappropriate for various reasons that they would not have done or said prior to the injury). Family members often discuss this as a "change in personality." This type of disinhibition is often associated with orbitofrontal injury and is referred to in the literature as "frontal lobe syndrome."[2] In addition, the patient with executive dysfunction will also report disorganized or confused thinking. A wide variety of emotional and mood changes can occur associated with executive functioning.[28] It is important to note that even the most comprehensive neuropsychological testing will often miss significant executive dysfunction. Given the highly structured nature of the testing process, the fact that the patient is allowed to monotask and that there are no distractions or interruptions, the testing process simply does not "pull for" many of the executive functions. Data related to executive dysfunction is often best obtained from co-lateral data scores such as family members.

Psychological

Depression is common following MTBI. However, the nature, course and causes of the depression do not follow the typical patterns when compared to non-brain injured individuals. The depression may develop over time, especially if the individual experiences persisting deficits and resulting limitations. As a result, depression should be monitored throughout the course of the patient's treatment. Self-report symptoms that may relate to depression include feelings of sadness, crying more frequently or easily, active or passive suicidal ideation, reduced motivation, gastrointestinal disturbance, decreased libido, change in appetite (increased or decreased), anhedonia, and sleep disturbance. However, emotional lability (crying more frequently and easily) and sleep disturbance can exist as a part of the MTBI irrespective of depression. It is important to note that patients may experience some mild feelings of depression or sadness, which might best be described as dysthymia. As noted previously, depression that meets the *DSM-IV* Diagnostic Criteria for Major Depression occurs in only 20 to 30 percent of MTBI patients.[28]

McAllister and Flashman also note that mania can become a complication of MTBI as well.[28] Clinicians will often suspect a manic or hypomanic response based on reports of irritability/reduced frustration tolerance, affective or mood lability, increased psychomotor activity, disruption of sleep, disinhibited behavior, and poor judgment. Clearly, these are all problems that can relate directly to a MTBI and, if the symptoms are relatively constant, then these would best be diagnosed as a personality change secondary to traumatic brain injury. If the symptoms are episodic, then they may relate to a manic or hypomanic episode.

Because irritability and reduced frustration tolerance are such common sequelae of MTBI, some further elaboration is indicated. Patients will often describe being more "short-tempered or short-fused" since the injury. They will often note, "little things that never used to bother me before, now really get to me" or "I will go ballistic over nothing." In retrospect, patients will most often realize that they have over-reacted to the situation or stressor and then apologize to the family member, friend or co-worker. A general reduction in coping and stress management abilities is also commonly reported following MTBI.

Anxiety in a variety of forms is common following MTBI. The anxiety may relate to embarrassment associated with their cognitive deficits and resulting reduction in performance. When this occurs, generalized performance anxiety can develop. It is also important to note that substance abuse problems can develop following MTBI. If the individual had substance abuse problems prior to the injury, then these are often exacerbated by the injuries. However, even individuals who have never abused substances may begin over-using alcohol or drugs such as marijuana as a way of self-medicating their pain and/or depression.

When an individual is injured in an accident, the development of Post-Traumatic Stress Disorder (PTSD) or Specific Phobia will often occur. These are separate and distinct entities from the MTBI and warrant thorough evaluation and treatment. These will be discussed in a separate part of this chapter.

Vision

A wide variety of vision problems are common following traumatic brain injury, including MTBI. Politzer[48] notes that a large percentage of individuals who sustain traumatic brain injury will demonstrate deficits in binocular vision in the form of strabismus, phoria, ocular-motor dysfunction, and convergence, or accommodative abnormalities. In addition, they can also demonstrate visual problems suggestive of Post-Traumatic Vision Syndrome (PTVS) and/or Visual Midline Shift Syndrome (VMSS). Patients will often experience these problems functionally as double vision or blurred vision. They will often report visual scanning problems, such as losing their place when they read or missing things that they are looking for. They will often notice problems with depth perception (judging distance) and report events such as knocking objects over, missing them when they reach for them, or getting too close to stopped cars in front of them.

The ambient visual system can also be affected. The ambient visual system assists with spatial orientation and provides information required for balance, movement, posture, gait and coordination. Disruption of the ambient visual system will often result in patients reporting that they bump into things more frequently or tend to veer off center when walking or driving. They will report accommodative dysfunction by noting that their eyes are slow to focus when changing distance of gaze. When patients experience binocular vision dysfunction, they will often note that their eyes fatigue more easily when performing visually loaded tasks. Photophobia (light sensitivity) for bright sunlight and florescent lights is common. Patients will at times note the perception of movement in their peripheral vision when there is nothing there. This is a classic symptom of unilateral saccades (a unilateral eye-tracking motion). Another commonly reported visual problem is the perception of things moving that the patient knows are stationary. Decreased night vision is also commonly reported. Hemispatial inattentions are relatively common following MTBI and patients will often report missing things (e.g., bumping into things) predominantly on one side or the other. In more significant injuries, visual field or hemispatial field losses can occur.

Box 12-1 contains a PCS/MTBI symptom checklist. The reader is encouraged to copy and use this checklist in clinical practice.

Box 12-1 PCS/MTBI symptom checklist

Cognitive ("Thinking Skill") Problems
- Attention or concentration (mind wanders; easily distractible; cannot keep focus)
- Short-term memory loss, "forgetfulness", or trouble learning new things.
- Trouble remembering old things (remote memory)
- Finding the right word when talking
- Understanding what is said
- Understanding what is read
- Making decisions or solving problems
- Planning or organization
- Making more mistakes than usual
- Not catching mistakes
- Slower speed of thinking or takes longer to do tasks
- Transposing letters or numbers when writing
- Getting lost or disoriented (even in familiar places);
- Trouble alternating attention or "juggling" several things at once
- Disorganized or confused thinking

Physical Symptoms
- Dizziness
- Periods of "blacking out" or seizures
- Problems with coordination of hands, feet, or legs (drops things more; balance problems)
- Increased/decreased (circle one) sense of smell
- Increased/decreased (circle one) sense of taste
- Ringing in the ears
- Headaches
- Fatigue
- More sensitive to loud noises or noisy places
- Intolerance of alcohol
- Tingling or numbness (where?)
- Nausea/vomiting

Emotional Symptoms
- Feelings of sadness and depression
- Crying spells or weepiness
- Suicidal thoughts or intentions
- Decreased or increased emotion (circle one)

(continued)

Box 12-1 (Continued)

- Low motivation
- Decreased or increased sex drive (circle one)
- Decreased or increased appetite (circle one)
- Decreased interest in "fun" activities
- Difficulties with sleeping (getting to sleep or staying asleep)
- Irritability/easily frustrated
- Feelings of anxiety or fear
- Difficulties with relationships

Visual Problems

- Double vision
- Blurry vision
- Losing place when reads and/or misses things looking for
- Problems with depth perception (judging distance)
- Bumping into things more often
- Veering off center when walking or driving
- Eyes are slow to focus when changing distance of gaze
- More sensitive to bright light or florescent lights
- Eyes fatigue easily
- Perception of movement in peripheral vision when there is nothing there
- Perception of things moving that you know are stationary
- Decreased night vision

MEDICAL DIAGNOSTICS

Neuroimaging Techniques

Of the variety of neuroimaging techniques currently in use, one can broadly classify them into three general categories (purposes):

1. techniques designed to image gross structural changes in brain physiology such as computerized tomography (CT) and magnetic resonance imaging (MRI)
2. techniques designed to assess cerebral function rather than structure such as positron emission tomography (PET), single-photon emission computed tomography (SPECT), functional MRI (fMRI) scanning, and diffusion-weighted MR imaging
3. detecting chemical by-products of traumatic injury such as the magnetic response spectroscopy (MRS).

Neuroimaging techniques designed to image gross structural changes are generally found to be negative in patients with MTBI.[31] Typically, when patients are evaluated in the emergency room,

> ...CT scanning is the neuroimaging technique of choice because of its accuracy in detecting life-threatening, intracranial bleeding that necessitates rapid treatment. Although CT may detect intracranial bleeding, it does not seem to be sensitive to detecting smaller lesions lying adjacent to the skull or in other areas. On the other hand, MRI is more sensitive in detecting nonhemorrhagic

lesions, such as diffuse axonal injury (DAI), cortical contusions, and brainstem injury … unfortunately, CT, not MRI scans, is generally performed in emergency rooms during initial medical evaluation and treatment of MHIs.[1]

Hartlage notes that, while it may be more appealing to demonstrate x-ray, CT, or electroencephalography (EEG) evidence of brain abnormality, such procedures contribute very little to understanding an individual's functional status subsequent to MTBI.[49] He also notes that it is quite common for individuals who have sustained documented mild brain injury with well-documented residual sequelae, to show absolutely no evidence of abnormality on CT, x-ray, or standard EEG measures. Horn and Zasler also note that studies, such as CT scans of the brain and standard EEG, typically do not show abnormalities supportive of mild brain dysfunction and/or trauma.[37]

MRI, though clearly more sensitive than CT scanning, can nevertheless also fail to show significant structural abnormality in patients with MTBI. Bigler in a study comparing either CT or MRI scans obtained prior to a MTBI, to scans obtained during the chronic phase following MTBI (i.e., more than four months post-injury) demonstrated no quantitative changes.[50] In this clinical study, each patient served as their own control. No great structural atrophy or change in brain anatomy could be demonstrated as a consequence of MTBI in these subjects. As Bigler suggests, the relative insensitivity of CT and MRI scanning is predictable as MTBI typically does not result in gross structural changes in tissue. When gross structural changes are evident, the patient is more likely to suffer significantly greater gross mental status impairment. This will then lower the GCS score below 13, thus putting the patient in the range of moderate to severe brain injury. As has been discussed earlier, the locus of MTBI pathology is more typically at the microstructural and/or neurochemical level.

Neuroimaging techniques that assess cerebral function rather than gross structure are more likely to be sensitive to MTBI. PET scanning is the method of choice for measuring cerebral metabolism. In general, PET abnormalities more closely correspond to the site and extent of cerebral dysfunction noted on neurological and neuropsychological examinations. PET scanning has demonstrated that the frontal and temporal lobes are most vulnerable to traumatic brain injury in the face of negative CT or MRI scanning. PET scanning can image dysfunction of cerebral metabolism beyond visualized structural abnormalities.

For example, after an acceleration/deceleration motor vehicle accident accompanied by cervical and back pain, a child experienced neurobehavioral symptoms over the two years subsequent to the accident. After four years of ongoing symptoms, a more extensive work-up involving EEG and PET scanning was administered. The child had a negative standard EEG, but two positive ambulatory EEGs with epileptiform activity. The PET scan revealed marked hypometabolism (low metabolism of glucose) in both temporal lobes, which was consistent with neuropsychological test results that showed verbal and visual memory deficits in a child with high average intelligence.[10]

A study involving nine cases of individuals complaining of persistent neurocognitive deficits months or years post-accident was performed by Ruff, *et al.*[51] In each of these cases little or no evidence of brain damage could be demonstrated based on structural neuroimaging (CT and MRI), yet their neuropsychological examinations were positive. PET scanning of these patients documented neuropathology, particularly in the frontal and anteriotemporo-frontal regions. Additionally, there were no significant differences between the five cases with reported loss of consciousness versus the four cases without loss of consciousness. In this study, PET and neuropsychological test results provided converging evidence that MTBI (including those with no loss of consciousness) can lead to neuropathology in the absence of evidence from structural imaging. The other important aspect of this study is that, even though most individuals will recover from concussion in one to three months post-injury, there is a minority of patients who present six or even more months post-injury with persistent physical, mental, emotional, and psychosocial complaints. Further, this study noted that such patients can present with abnormalities in cerebral glucose metabolism suggesting ongoing central nervous system dysfunction in the face of negative CT and MRI scanning.

Mateer reports a retrospective study of 20 patients with MTBI (age 12 to 59 years at the time of the injury) designed to compare neuropsychological testing results, behavioral dysfunction, and PET neuroimaging.[39] The study was conducted one to five years post-injury. Results of PET scanning revealed abnormal local cerebral metabolic rates most prominent in the mid-temporal, anterior cingulate, precuneus, anterior temporal, right frontal, and corpus callosum brain regions. Abnormal local cerebral metabolic rates were significantly correlated with overall clinical complaints (most specifically attention and concentration) and were consistent with overall neuropsychological test results.

Examination of cerebral blood flow relative perfusion via SPECT scanning also appears quite promising. Studies with MTBI patients with SPECT scanning appears to be useful in demonstrating cerebral dysfunction in a morphologically normal brain and such dysfunction appears consistent with the clinical presentation of patients with chronic symptoms.

Jay reports a study involving 41 MTBI patients without loss of consciousness and with normal CT scans.[10] Twenty-eight of these patients had abnormal SPECT scans with focal areas of hypoprofusion. In 228 mild and moderate traumatically brain injured patients, abnormalities in SPECT scans were found in the basal ganglia and thalamus in 55.2 percent of those patients. Abnormalities were found in the frontal lobes in 23.8 percent, temporal lobes in 13 percent, parietal lobes in 3.7 percent, and insular and occipital lobes in 4.6 percent.

Mateer[39] report another study comparing SPECT, MRI, and CT scans in 43 adult patients with symptoms of persistent PCS. Fifty-three percent of these patients had abnormal SPECT scans and exhibited a total of 47 lesions while abnormal MRIs were present in only nine percent. CT scans were abnormal in only 4.6 percent of these patients. Authors of this study concluded that SPECT was more sensitive in detecting cerebral abnormalities in patients with persistent PCS symptoms than either CT or MRI.

Other techniques, such as perfusion MRI (pMRI) measuring blood volume, blood transit time, and blood flow, as well as functional MRI (fMRI), measuring changes in tissue perfusion based on changes in blood oxygenation, are also potentially useful techniques. For example, pMRI can demonstrate regions of acute ischemia before MRI lesions can be detected. Diffusion-weighted imaging (DWI) is sensitive to slow flow and thus to the random flow of hydrogen protons in water. DWI as well as pMRI may be useful during the acute and subacute phase of MTBI.

fMRI operates on the physiological property that when a brain region is working, it experiences a local increase in blood flow and blood oxygenation. Because oxygenated and deoxygenated blood have differing magnetic properties, the fMRI can detect changes in blood oxygenation.[52] fMRI may be more useful during the later chronic rehabilitation phase when medical and surgical conditions have stabilized.[1]

Other promising neuroimaging techniques beginning to be explored include:

- diffusion tensor imaging
- quantitative MR imaging morphology
- transcranial magnetic stimulation
- magnetoencephalography or magnetic source imaging.[52]

Diffusion Tensor Imaging is a recent extension of DWMR imaging. Because diffusion is hindered by the cell membranes in white matter, diffusion occurs mainly along the length of the axon. This technique can provide microstructural physiologic information on the integrity of white matter. Mapping white matter tracts should be possible with this technique.

Quantitative MR Imaging Morphology is a term for a large class of techniques used to measure the size of brain structures. The surface areas of a particular brain structure on a particular slice can be measured. Multiplying the area by slice thickness can derive volumes.

Transcranial Magnetic Stimulation (TMS) uses the principle of inductance to transmit electrical energy across the scalp using a wire coil and brief bursts of electricity through the coil. A magnetic field is produced orthogonal to the coil.

Magnetoencephalography (MEG) or Magnetic Source Imaging (MSI) measures electrical activity of the brain similar to electroencephalography. MEG, however, measures the magnetic field properties of the signal and magnetic signals suffer less attenuation than electrical signals when traversing the skull. MEG machines offer much better spatial resolution than EEG and better temporal resolution than any MRI technique.

Proton MR Spectroscopy (MRS) is a technique designed to detect neurochemical changes in the brain following a TBI. This technique has been available for some time but has recently become more accessible in clinical settings and more economical due to advances in computer software. Specifically, MR Spectroscopy measures alterations in myo-inositol, total creatinine, total choline, and, most importantly, N-acetylaspartate (NAA). NAA levels have been shown to fall rapidly and irreversibly with neuronal death and are, therefore, considered a marker of neuronal integrity.[53] Friedman and his colleagues cite numerous studies in which both NAA and creatinine levels have been shown to decrease in the frontal lobes of TBI patients who have poor outcomes, and decreased levels of NAA have been shown within the brainstem, subcortical white matter, and gray matter regions.

Sinson, *et al.* examined the NAA/creatinine ratio in the splenium of the corpus callosum of 30 TBI patients.[54] In the 10 patients with poorer outcome (as measured by the Glasgow Outcome Scale), the NAA/creatinine ratio was significantly lower than in the 20 patients with better outcomes. Friedman, *et al.*[53] found that reduced levels of white matter NAA and elevated levels of gray matter creatinine in TBI patients were associated with poorer composite neuropsychological performance as well as poorer performances on many individual neuropsychological tests.[54]

Electrophysiological Techniques

While some of the previously cited studies point to the relative lack of efficacy in standard EEG in detecting cerebral dysfunction in MTBI patients, quantitative digitalized electroencephalography (QEEG) appears more promising. QEEG assays neurophysiological deficits quantitatively. QEEG can be helpful in identifying mild injury to white matter that, if present, results in reducing the efficiency of communication between different parts of the cortex. Therefore, the quality of neurotransmission is diminished when axons are injured. QEEG measures the time delay between two regions of the cerebral cortex and the time needed to transmit information from one region to another. It is also able to assess the integrity of neuronal connections between the regions of the cortex. Information regarding differentiation of function can be evaluated by examining phase or the measure of lead or lag of shared rhythms between regions.[10]

One recent study examined the neuropsychological, physiological and behavioral functioning of 32 adult outpatients (aged 18 to 66 years) up to 65 months following a non-impact brain injury (i.e., whiplash). All subjects in the study were administered a flexible battery of cognitive tests. Although structural neuroimaging was not sensitive in detecting brain pathology, QEEG findings were abnormal in all the subjects evaluated. In particular, results demonstrated frontocentral slowing and increased spike wave activity. However, there was no correlation between the patients' cognitive and emotional-behavioral problems with the routine neurological examination, EEG, and structural neuroimaging (i.e., CT and MRI). The authors concluded that whiplash injury can produce wide-ranging circuitry dysfunction.[55]

With regard to evoked potentials, cortical auditory evoked responses (CAERs) may be better able to reflect the extent and degree of cerebral dysfunction than brainstem-evoked responses (BAERs), although evoked potentials in general are probably not sensitive enough to document physiological problems, even in patients with active symptoms. Jay reports two studies on evoked potentials in MTBI patients. In the first study, a group of 40 MTBI patients were evaluated with brainstem trigeminal and auditory-evoked potentials (BTEP and BAEP), as well as middle-latency auditory evoked potentials (MLAEP).[10] All three evoked responses showed markedly increased latencies at the initial evaluation indicative of disseminated axonal damage.

In the second study, 26 MTBI patients were evaluated via Brainstem Auditory Evoked Responses (BAERs), reaction time testing, and EEG.[10] Post-traumatic symptoms had persisted in half of the patients at six weeks and six months follow-up. There were decrements in BAER conduction time in half the group and the findings were felt to indicate three different patterns of recovery. Half the patients recovered within six weeks, a minority had persistent brainstem dysfunction over six months, and less than one-third of the patients showed symptom exacerbation with no evidence of brainstem dysfunction, possibly secondary to psychological and/or social factors.

Mental Status Methodologies

Mental status methodologies typically employed to assess brain injury both by paramedics at the scene and by physicians in the emergency room are generally inadequate in providing early diagnosis of PCS/MTBI. The typical methodologies employed involve informal assessment of orientation, brief formal assessment of gross mental status (e.g., mini-mental state exam [MMSE]), and evaluation of level of consciousness utilizing the GCS.

A review of the diagnostic guidelines for assessing PCS/MTBI, pathophysiology of MTBI, and neuroradiological research indicates that MTBI and associated brain dysfunction can occur without loss of consciousness or gross changes in mental status. Clearly, a measure designed to evaluate level of consciousness (e.g., GCS) is not going to be helpful in diagnosing brain injury in patients who have not lost consciousness. A study of 1,448 patients seen in the emergency room after MTBI revealed that limiting CT scans to patients with focal neurologic deficits with GCS scores less than 15 would have missed 56 positive scans and one patient who required emergent neurosurgical intervention.[56]

GCS findings can be misleading.[1] The total GCS score utilized as part of the clinical neurological examination in most emergency rooms masks important clinical details. Once again, it is not unusual to find individuals who have GCS scores of 13 to 15, less than 20 minutes loss of consciousness (or no loss of consciousness), less than 48 hours of hospitalization (or no physical complications) who show mild neuroimaging abnormality (e.g., skull fracture or small hematoma).[57] If the GCS is administered on the patient's admission into the emergency room and the score is 15, this does not exclude the possibility that the patient was non-responsive at the scene of the accident.[58] Therefore, GCS by itself does not capture the presence or absence of a MTBI and does not reflect the retroactive status of the patient at the scene. Rather, it describes the status at the time of administration.

A gross assessment of mental status, such as the MMSE, is going to be equally ineffective in detecting dysfunction in MTBI patients. Such patients may be grossly oriented to time, place, and person but they may, nevertheless, present with an alteration of consciousness (such as being dazed or confused). To determine whether these conditions are present, the evaluator would need to ask the appropriate questions, such as "do you feel you are thinking clearly?" or "are you feeling dazed or confused?" These specific questions are rarely asked either at the scene or in the emergency room.

The routine administration of the MMSE or the GCS will also not assess the presence of a PTA. To capture this, another instrument would need to be utilized such as the Galveston Orientation and Amnesia Test (GOAT). In addition to assessing orientation, the GOAT is able to estimate both loss of consciousness and PTA by asking the person to recall the last event prior to the accident that they can remember and the first event subsequent to the accident that they can remember. The determination of whether a patient is briefly unconscious, confused, or in a state of PTA immediately following the accident, is the key issue that needs to be addressed and evaluated. Ruff and Richardson primarily rely on the GOAT.[58] They typically proceed with the specific questions on the GOAT and then have patients review the accident in their own words, relaying all the information that they know about the accident.

NEUROPSYCHOLOGICAL ASSESSMENT

Referral Process

As a general rule of thumb, when a clinician has diagnosed a PCS/MTBI or strongly suspects that one exists, then it is best to refer for neuropsychological services sooner than later. While most neuropsychologists will not perform standardized testing until three to six months post-injury, there can be a number of services provided that will help the patient and family significantly. As will be noted later in the chapter, individual psychotherapy that focuses on education regarding the effects of PCS can help to reduce the patient's and family's overall distress related to the symptoms. Such treatment can validate that the symptoms do relate to a medical condition and that the injured family member is indeed not "going crazy." This type of validation can be extremely therapeutic. In addition, knowing that the potential for recovery is extremely high can also help to relieve the patient's and family's distress.

If the patient is continuing to try to work but is struggling vocationally, cognitive rehabilitation may be implemented. This treatment will help the patient develop strategies to compensate for residual cognitive problems at work and, in many instances, will help to maximize job performance and potential for keeping the job.

When referring to a neuropsychologist, the physician should include medical records regarding the patient and his or her impressions and initial recommendations. It is also helpful if the patient is prepared for referral to a neuropsychologist. Educating the patient as to why a physician is making the referral and what a neuropsychologist does can be quite helpful. We often receive referrals from physicians and, when asked if the patient knows why he or she has been referred, we often hear the response, "I don't know" or "I guess my doctor thinks I was going crazy."

Clinical Interview

Most neuropsychologists will begin the evaluation process with a clinical interview. One of the first steps in the interview process is obtaining a history of the accident. Typically, this portion of the interview will be structured around the events of the accident as well as the diagnostic criteria for PCS/MTBI, which have been previously discussed in this chapter. Establishing whether the patient experienced any loss of consciousness, alteration of consciousness or alteration of memories surrounding the events of the accident is important in helping to determine if the individual did indeed sustain a concussion. Often times, medical records are of no help regarding this issue and a neuropsychologist must rely on the patient's self-report. Ruff and Richardson note that use of the GOAT can be helpful in this regard.[58] The authors point out that it is rare that a qualified outside observer is present to document the presence of loss of consciousness and that, even if an observer is present, one often cannot observe altered consciousness such as a dazed, disoriented or confused status. In addition, with regards to the patient's memories before, during and after the accident, it is important to phrase your questions in a specific manner. Ruff and Richardson suggest that this set of questions be prefaced by stating the following:

> Since the accident, you have discussed various aspects with your lawyers, friends, families and various examiners and you may also have had the opportunity to review various records including police reports and other medical records. For the questions we are about to ask you, we would like you to rely on your independent recall without any reference to information that you have learned after the accident.[58]

In this way, the clinician is more likely to obtain accurate data about what the patient actually remembers versus what they have been told or "figured out." Specific questions related to memories leading up to, during and following the accident are a critical aspect of this portion of the interview. It is important to note that PTA is defined by the International Neuropsychology Society as "A period of anterograde amnesia in which new memories cannot be consistently made and recalled that follows recovery of consciousness in head injury or other neurological trauma."[59] Therefore, when establishing the period of PTA, it is important to try to identify when the patient's memories become *consistent* and ongoing, not just when they have their first memory post-accident.

When discussing the issue of altered consciousness with patients, be aware that they will often not use terms such as dazed, confused, or disoriented. They will often describe their state of altered consciousness as "everything was in slow motion;" "things seemed unreal;" "I was not thinking clearly;" "it was like I was there but I wasn't;" and so forth. Obviously, patients' perception of this sense of altered consciousness varies and it is important to get them to describe it in their own words and also attempt to identify how long the sense of altered consciousness persisted.

For a variety of reasons, it is important to attempt to establish a patient's baseline of functioning prior to the accident. Many neuropsychologists will attempt to obtain this type of information through use of an adult history questionnaire. Such questionnaires typically attempt to gather information about the person's educational, vocational, medical, psychological, and relationship histories prior to the accident. Because prior brain injuries and other neurological conditions present a significant risk factor for poor recovery following a concussion, this is important historical data to obtain. If patients have been involved in prior motor vehicle accidents, it is important to determine if the person meets the diagnostic criteria for a concussion related to that accident and if he or she experienced residual PCS following that accident. As has been noted previously, many concussions or MTBIs will often go undiagnosed and untreated and to the degree possible, it is important to retrospectively determine if the individual may have indeed experienced a prior concussion.

Another important aspect of the clinical interview relates to the patient's current PCS symptoms. Typically, neuropsychologists will not just rely on symptom checklists completed by the patient but will talk with the patient in some detail about each symptom, obtaining functional examples of how the problem manifests itself in day-to-day or work activities. As noted previously, many of the symptoms have a high base rate in the general population and/or these symptoms can relate to other conditions.

Therefore, it is important to ask questions related to symptoms in a very specific manner in order to control for the base rate phenomenon. The patient should be asked about new symptoms since the accident or, if certain symptoms were present pre-accident, whether those symptoms had been exacerbated either in terms of frequency or severity since the accident.

Clinical Psychological Screening

As part of a comprehensive neuropsychological test battery, most neuropsychologists will also attempt to assess the patient's emotional and psychological status. As part of the clinical interview, information will be gathered about the person's psychological and psychiatric history, if indeed such history exists. Attempts will be made to determine how the patient was functioning from an emotional and psychological perspective just prior to the accident as well as post-accident. Particular attention should be paid to feelings of depression, emotional lability, sleep disturbance, irritability/reduced frustration tolerance, sexual dysfunction, anxiety, and symptoms that may relate to PTSD or specific phobia related to the accident (to be discussed later in this section of the chapter).

In addition to the clinical interview, neuropsychologists will often also utilize more objective clinical measures of emotional and psychological status. These include measures such as in the MMPI-2, the Millon Clinical Multi-axial Inventory-3 (MCMI-3), the Beck Depression Inventory (BDI), the Beck Anxiety Inventory, or the Symptom Checklist-90 Revised (SCL90-R). Any objective test of personality or emotional status should be viewed as a self-report symptom checklist.[19] In these instruments, patients will describe their current symptoms and problems. On these tests the effects of actual impairment may be manifested through the patients' responses to items associated with cognitive or personality changes which relate directly to their injuries and resulting impairment.[19] As a result, caution must be utilized when interpreting the results of any such self-report questionnaire. It is important to be aware that these instruments were developed for use with clinical populations and, if the patient is responding affirmatively to a specific symptom, then it is assumed that that symptom relates to an emotional or psychological condition. However, following accidents that result in true physical and/or brain injury, the patient may respond affirmatively to certain symptoms because they relate to their injuries not because they are experiencing a psychological or psychiatric condition.

The MMPI-2 represents an excellent example of the above problem. The MMPI-2 contains 111 items that could relate directly to physical injuries or traumatic brain injuries. With regards to this issue, Lezak notes

> Since so many MMPI items describe symptoms common to a variety of neurological disorders, self-aware and honest patients with these symptoms may produce MMPI profiles that could be misinterpreted as evidence of psychiatric disturbance when they do not have a psychiatric or behavioral disorder.[19]

Lezak notes that the most commonly elevated MMPI scales for individuals who have sustained neurological injuries are Hs(1), D(2), Hy(3), Pt(7), and Sc(8).

For individuals who have sustained traumatic brain injury Pd(4) can also be elevated. The same problem exists with the MCMI-3. With regards to this issue, Neppe and Goodwin state:

> It should be pointed out that traditional interpretative approaches for the MMPI-2 and MCMI-3 are inadequate and often lead to erroneous conclusions when applied to the head trauma population. Too often, computerized printouts of MMPI-2 and MCMI-3 results are misused by clinicians unfamiliar with the dynamics of head trauma and those patients are assessed inaccurately. Interpretations of these psychological instruments should be made within the context of background information, details of the injury event, symptomatology, and co-lateral information.[60]

It has also been pointed out by McAllister and Flashman that there is significant overlap between the *DSM-IV* post-concussion disorder symptomatology and symptoms contained in the BDI.[28] Therefore, if a patient is responding to the BDI (or BDI-II) in an honest fashion, they may be acknowledging symptoms not necessarily because they are depressed, but because they have sustained a PCS/MTBI. Again, the clinician is admonished to perform an item-by-item analysis of the BDI as opposed to utilizing the total score without regard to the specific symptoms that the patient is acknowledging. The BDI-II contains items related to emotional lability, agitation, irritability, problems with decision-making, problems with concentration, fatigue, and disruption of sleep patterns which are all common symptoms associated with a PCS/MTBI. As a result, the BDI-II score could be significantly elevated not because of depression but because of post-concussive symptoms.

In summary, while more objective measures of emotional and psychological status are commonly used as part of comprehensive neuropsychological evaluations, the results from these instruments should be used with extreme caution. As a consumer of neuropsychological evaluations, it would be important to determine from the narrative report or from direct contact with the neuropsychologist if, indeed, these cautions and considerations were utilized when interpreting the results of such instruments.

Neuropsychological Testing

Cognitive Domains Assessed

As MTBI can result in either a focal or diffuse pattern of neurocognitive deficits, an objective assessment of neuropsychological functioning should be comprehensive. Consequently, all basic domains of neurocognitive functioning should be evaluated. Typically, these involve five general areas of function:

1. sensory-perceptual processes
2. motor functions
3. central processing functions
4. executive abilities
5. intellectual/academic abilities.

Neuropsychological testing assesses the integrity of the individual's sensory-perception in visual, auditory, and tactile modalities. In particular, gross sensory defects or more subtle signs of sensory inattention are critical in determining whether the patient's ability to accurately process information is going to be initially handicapped by sensory imperception or distortion.

Secondly, it is important to assess motor functioning, as impaired motor function will affect any cognitive or intellectual task requiring motor output. We recommend a thorough assessment of upper extremity motor strength, speed, and coordination. Additionally, it is important to assess the patient's ability to plan or program subtle sequences in motor movement, which is an important aspect of executive motor function. Deficits in areas of motor planning/programming are typically present in MTBI patients when the anterior portion of the cerebral cortex, and the premotor cortex, in particular, are affected. Ineffective motor planning will naturally affect the patient's upper extremity fine motor coordination and control.

Thirdly, a comprehensive evaluation of central processing functions is performed. At the simplest level, the patient's attention, concentration, and ability to register both auditory and visual information is assessed along with the speed with which that information can be processed. In addition, the patient's ability to efficiently learn new verbal/auditory and visual information is evaluated. The patient's ability to remember and recall newly learned information over varying time frames is also assessed. Incidental memory (or ability to remember new information without planning or forewarning) should be evaluated as well. Other cognitive abilities are also evaluated, such as the patient's basic receptive and expressive language functioning, as well as visual organization and constructional abilities.

It is also important to assess the patient's ability to perform a variety of executive skills that serve to coordinate and integrate the various individual cognitive abilities so that the patient may be able to perform tasks efficiently and accurately. These include:

- the ability to initiate and terminate activity
- planning, sequencing, and organizing
- the ability to generate words and ideas fluently
- the patient's ability to be flexible and adapt to changing situations
- the patient's ability to integrate information from various sources.

Related to executive function it is also important to assess the patient's higher-order reasoning abilities. This includes the patient's pragmatic judgment and abstract reasoning ability that allow the individual to make everyday decisions as well as see their decisions in the context of a larger perspective. In addition, the patient's ability to generate solutions to new or ambiguous problems is important to assess.

Finally, a thorough assessment of intellectual and academic skills is an important aspect of any comprehensive neuropsychological evaluation. This includes measures of the patient's verbal and nonverbal intellectual ability as well as specific academic skill levels in the areas of mathematical reasoning, spelling, and reading skill.

Levels of Data Analysis

Lezak notes that:

> one distinguishing characteristic of neuropsychological assessment is its emphasis on the identification and measurement of psychological deficits, for it is primarily in deficiencies and dysfunctional alterations of cognition, emotionality, and self-direction and management (i.e., executive functions) that brain damage is manifested behaviorally.[19]

There are four general ways in which deficits or impairments in cognitive functioning are identified in neuropsychological testing:

1. an assessment of the patient's level of performance
2. the pattern of performance
3. patterns of lateralization
4. pathognomonic signs of brain injury.

The patient's level of performance (e.g., whether the patient's performance in a particular cognitive domain or on a particular test is falling within or below expectation) is based on normative comparison standards. Just as normative comparison standards have been developed for various indices of physiological functioning (e.g., blood pressure, level of hemoglobin), a normative standard or norm for many cognitive functions and characteristics have also been developed. For many cognitive functions, variables such as age, gender, and education can significantly affect test performance; such variables are, therefore, often taken into account in developing such normative data. An individual's test performance in any of these cognitive domains is then compared with what is expected on the basis of how neurologically normal individuals who are matched along these variables typically perform. Therefore, a pattern of performances that fall significantly below the level expected, given that person's demographic characteristics, can suggest impaired ability in those areas of functioning. However, a description of that individual's functioning in terms of normative comparison standards will shed little light on the extent or pattern of the patient's impairments unless there is some assessment of the patient's probable premorbid functioning.

There are a variety of methods that help to establish the patient's premorbid ability. Certainly, obtaining information about the patient's pre-injury developmental, educational, and occupational functioning can provide some important clues. Unfortunately, it is rarely the case that objective data documenting the patient's premorbid cognitive functioning is available. When this material is unavailable or inadequate, one can utilize the Best Performance method in which the patient's highest score or set of scores on the test battery, serves as the best estimate of premorbid cognitive ability.

The Best Performance method rests on several assumptions.[19] First, there is one performance level that best represents each person's cognitive abilities and skills generally. Second, marked discrepancies between the levels at which a person performs different cognitive functions or skills probably gives evidence of disease, developmental anomalies, cultural deprivation, emotional disturbance, or some other condition that has interfered with the full expression of that person's cognitive potential. And third, for cognitively impaired persons, the least depressed abilities are the best remaining behavioral representations of the original cognitive potential.

The Best Performance method can be critical in evaluating the presence of neurobehavioral impairment in an individual when used in concert with the level of performance analysis. For example, a patient may score in the average or low average range on a variety of learning and memory tests but also generate IQ scores that are in the very superior range. This statistically significant discrepancy could suggest that an average performance is actually deficient in an exceptionally bright person.

In addition to level of performance, the pattern of impaired performances in an individual is important in determining the presence or absence of a cognitive deficit and the nature of the deficit. For example, as stated earlier, because of the internal architecture of the skull and the biomechanics of MTBI, it is more typical that the inferior frontotemporal aspects of the cerebral cortex suffer the greatest degree of impairment. As a result, we would expect neurobehavioral functions associated with those areas of the cortex to be impaired more frequently in the neuropsychological test protocols of MTBI patients. A pattern of impaired scores affecting frontal lobe functions, such as attention and concentration, speed of information processing, and executive skills as well as functions associated with the medial temporal lobes, particularly learning and memory ability, are more typically affected in MTBI patients.

Then, patterns of lateralized dysfunction are evaluated. Lateralization, demonstrating significantly different sensory and motor functioning on the two sides of the body, as well as significantly different performances in cognitive skills typically associated with the left (as opposed to the right) hemisphere of the cerebral cortex, support inferences with regard to lateralized brain dysfunction.

Finally, the presence of pathognomonic signs, particularly on tests of sensory-perception, motor, and language functioning, also assist a neuropsychologist in making inferences with regard to presence, localization, and lateralization of brain dysfunction following MTBI. The interpretation of neuropsychological test data involves simultaneous analysis of data at each of these levels and a diagnosis of MTBI is made based on this multi-level analysis.

Fixed vs. Flexible Batteries

There are four general approaches to neuropsychological assessment:

1. standard or fixed batteries
2. flexible batteries
3. the "process" approach
4. micro-computer-based neuropsychological batteries.

The two most widely used standard/fixed batteries are the Halstead-Reitan Battery (HRB) and the Luria-Nebraska Neuropsychological Battery (LNNB). The HRB is the most widely used standardized battery. The tasks were originally developed by Dr. Ward Halstead and were later modified and standardized by his graduate student, Dr. Ralph Reitan.[61] As it exists today, the HRB consists of five tests producing seven scores.

Several supplemental tests and one of the Wechsler Intelligence scales, as well as academic testing, are also commonly used in conjunction with the HRB. The LNNB is based on methods developed by the Russian psychologist, Dr. Alexander Luria. These items were first introduced by Christenson in 1975 and further developed by Golden, *et al.* in 1980.[62,63] The LNNB produces 11 scales entitled, "motor, rhythm, tactile, visual, receptive language, expressive language, writing, reading, arithmetic, memory, and intelligence."

When utilizing a flexible battery approach, the neuropsychologist will choose existing standardized neuropsychological tests that have proved to be valid and reliable in the diagnosis of brain function. The neuropsychologist will typically choose tests that have been found to be sensitive to cognitive abilities most affected by MTBI. This type of battery can range from an extremely comprehensive assessment of brain function to more minimal screening-type batteries. Obviously, screening batteries are less sensitive and accurate than comprehensive testing.

In our view, for MTBI patients, it would be most appropriate to perform a standard battery such as the HRB and then supplement that testing with additional standardized tests to evaluate more fully frontal lobe function (which includes many of the executive skills), memory function, visual-perceptual abilities, and information-processing abilities commonly affected by MTBI. The obvious disadvantage to such a battery is the length of time involved to administer the tests, which will typically range from six to eight hours. However, in our clinical experience, this is by far the most desirable approach to evaluating an individual who has suffered a MTBI. It is the most comprehensive, sensitive, and accurate method of neuropsychological assessment. Such an approach provides a high degree of validity and standardized normative data are available. Many of the tests are normed demographically for age, gender and education.[64,65] In addition, the wealth of data obtained is extremely helpful in developing a cognitive rehabilitation program for the patient and in making vocational and other treatment recommendations.

The "process approach" to neuropsychological assessment places greater emphasis on the patient's approach to the neuropsychological tasks than on standardized, quantitative performance. This approach incorporates both standardized neuropsychological tests as well as tests developed by the clinician during the process of the evaluation to evaluate specific problem areas qualitatively. While this type of approach does utilize some standardized testing, it also includes substantial subjective interpretation of performance by the examiner. In addition, the content of the testing is often based on the patient's self-report of deficits. Unfortunately, there are often times when the MTBI patient has impaired self-monitoring and may have reduced self-awareness and, therefore, lacks sufficient insight into his or her deficits. Overall, the process approach has multiple disadvantages and should be avoided in the assessment of patients with MTBI.

Several computerized cognitive test batteries are also available. While the automated batteries have several advantages, such as ease of transport, standardized administration, consistency of administration, and cost efficiency related to administering, scoring and analyzing the test data, they also present several disadvantages. They often lack clinical norms, do not thoroughly assess all areas of cognitive functioning, can encourage inappropriate interpretation, important behavioral and observational data are missed, and a subset of the population remains computer phobic.[66]

READING AND UNDERSTANDING NEUROPSYCHOLOGICAL EVALUATION REPORTS

As treating clinical neuropsychologists, the authors will often receive questions from our referral sources related to our test results, conclusions and recommendations. Several of these questions come up on a regular basis and we would like to discuss those here in the hope that it will give the reader a more in-depth understanding of the data contained in a typical neuropsychological report.

The most widely used fixed neuropsychological test battery in the United States is the Expanded Halstead-Reitan Neuropsychological Test Battery (HRB). This battery produces three index scores, which are derived from individual scores in the test battery. The Halstead Impairment Index (HII) is generated from seven of the scores. The average impairment rating (AIR) is generated from 12 of the scores and the general neuropsychological deficit scale (GNDS) is generated from 42 of the scores. In cases of MTBI, it is not uncommon that all of these index scores are within normal limits yet the neuropsychologist will conclude that the individual is demonstrating specific cognitive deficits consistent with a MTBI.

It is important to be aware that these index scores were never designed to be sensitive to the more subtle or localized cognitive effects of MTBI. They were designed to be sensitive to an acute brain injury, a widespread injury to the brain, or a rapidly progressive neurological condition. Mateer[39] states, "recognize that few of the major neuropsychological tests and none of the major test batteries was designed specifically to identify the cognitive and adaptive problems experienced by individuals with MTBI." Ruff and Richardson state:

> an impairment index in essence assumes that the sum total of deficits across the test battery is sensitive for capturing brain damage. If the battery is designed to capture the degree of diffuse damage, this assumption may have validity. However, no index has been designed for the specific deficits caused by MTBI.[58]

They go on to note:

> It is the cluster of deficits that is essential; a cumulative approach is not wrong but far less powerful. Thus, a pattern analysis across a test profile that emphasizes the evaluation of attention, memory, learning, and executive functions appears to us as equally or more sensitive since these are the cognitive domains that are particularly affected after MTBI.[58]

It is important to be aware that none of the index scores includes scores from tests designed to assess short-term memory, speed of information processing, and many of the tests sensitive to executive dysfunction.[39] Clearly, these are cognitive abilities frequently affected by MTBI and this explains why the index scores can be within normal limits yet the patient demonstrates specific deficits, inconsistencies or relative weaknesses suggestive of a MTBI. In summary, our referral sources (and at times IME evaluators) will recognize that the index scores are within normal limits and conclude that there is no significant cognitive impairment. Clearly, in many of the cases this would be an inaccurate conclusion.

Most comprehensive neuropsychological evaluations incorporate an IQ measure. The most frequently used tests are the Wechsler Adult Intelligence Scale-Revised (WAIS-R) and the Wechsler Adult Intelligence Scale-III (WAIS-III). Based on the results, often times neuropsychologists will note that it appears that the overall IQ scores have been reduced from their pre-injury level. At times, referral sources will question this conclusion as there is a common myth that traumatic brain injuries will not affect IQ scores. This certainly begs the question, "how could a mild TBI negatively impact IQ?" Lezak[19] notes that virtually all 11 subtests of the WAIS-R can be negatively affected by brain injury based on the nature, extent and localization of the brain injury.

Raskin, *et al.* analyzed the results of neuropsychological testing conducted on a group of 148 individuals who met the ACRM diagnostic criteria for MTBI.[67] They note that there was no correlation between the duration of loss of consciousness and any neuropsychological or emotional variable. Impairment was defined as performance greater than one standard deviation below the age-adjusted normative mean for the test. It is important to note that some percentage of the group scored in the impaired range on each of the 11 WAIS-R subtests. The percentages were as follows:

- Information – 16 percent
- Digit Span – 12 percent
- Vocabulary – 12 percent
- Comprehension – 10 percent
- Similarities – 10 percent
- Arithmetic – 7 percent
- Picture Completion – 7 percent
- Digit Symbol – 7 percent
- Picture Arrangement – 6 percent
- Object Assembly – 6 percent
- Block Design – 2 percent.

These findings would suggest that performance on virtually any of the 11 subtests of the WAIS-R can be negatively impacted by MTBI.

Parker and Rosenblum utilized a sample of 33 individuals who had sustained MTBIs due to whiplash incurred in motor vehicle accidents.[68] On the average, the individuals were evaluated at 20 months post-injury and all were administered the WAIS-R. Pre-injury estimated IQs were obtained through tables based on the standardization population for the WAIS-R. On the average, the group demonstrated a loss of full scale IQ of 14.2 points; verbal IQ loss was 6 points on the average; and performance IQ loss was 15.6 points on the average. It is important to note that 14 points represents almost a full standard deviation decrease in full scale IQ. The study supports previous studies that have clearly identified that Performance IQ is more significantly affected by brain injury than is Verbal IQ.

Often in the course of a neuropsychological evaluation report, reference will be made to the *pattern* of symptoms suggested by the testing. We often receive questions related to what is meant by a common symptom pattern. For patients who have sustained a MTBI, there are two such patterns.[69] When diffuse injury is the primary mechanism of injury involved, then the patient will typically demonstrate deficits in overall slowed speed of processing, decreased capacity for processing information, an overall decreased efficiency in productivity, problems with execution in tasks, and difficulty integrating mental processes.

The authors go on to note that a second common symptom pattern in MTBI is one of focal injuries. This occurs when the soft brain tissue is abrased by bony ridges that protrude from the base of the skill primarily in the frontal and temporal regions. These individuals will demonstrate a rather classic frontotemporal pattern of deficits on neuropsychological testing. Deficits will often be noted in the areas of planning, organizing, attention, concentration, problem solving and decision-making, and verbal and visual short-term memory. The authors go on to note that focal injuries can co-exist with diffuse injuries causing a wide array of possible deficits on neuropsychological testing.

As has been noted throughout this chapter, MTBI will often result in more subtle cognitive dysfunction, which for a variety of reasons may not be clearly detectable on standardized neuropsychological testing. In the course of our reports, we will often utilize the term "relative weakness" and our referral sources often ask about the use of this term. This concept is nicely summarized by Ruff and Richardson.[58] They state:

> none-the-less, group means cannot be the sole basis for determining neuropsychological deficits for individual patients. For example, it is conceivable that, if someone had been functioning above the 90th percentile and after MTBI this declines to the 50th percentile, the test results would still fall in the average range (i.e., 50th percentile). Thus, for each individual a reduction is always relative and an "average" result does not necessarily prove that a specific patient has not experienced a decline.[58]

Therefore, particularly in cases of MTBI, the method of data analysis known as the Best Performance method is often utilized. This method was reviewed previously in this chapter and involves comparing specific test scores to other test scores within the test battery; especially those that are expected to correlate highly. In addition, the neuropsychologist will evaluate behavioral observations of the patient during testing as well as historical data, such as educational and work history, to establish an expected baseline of cognitive functioning.

Lezak[19] notes that, given reasonably normal development of physical and cognitive abilities, there is one performance level that best represents each person's cognitive abilities and skills generally. She goes on to note that for individuals who have sustained cognitive injury, the least depressed abilities in the neuropsychological testing are the best remaining indicators of original cognitive potential. When there is significant discrepancy between a test score and expected baseline levels, then for that individual that score may indicate a deficit. A functional example would be, if Verbal IQ was tested at the 90th percentile and verbal learning and retention were tested at the 40th percentile, this would represent a relative decline of verbal learning and retention abilities as these scores would be expected to correlate fairly highly when the tests are administered to a non-brain injured individual. It is also important to note that, based on the areas of relative weakness; the individual may experience a significant functional or vocational impairment. For example, an engineer whose visual constructional and visual analytic abilities were in the superior range prior to an injury may now score in the low average range on tests of these abilities. While statistically the scores are within normal limits, this individual would not be able to continue to function at a competitive level as a professional engineer.

It is also important for the consumer of a neuropsychological evaluation to understand that the testing is performed in a highly artificial environment. In order to maintain the standardization of test administration, the tests must be administered in a quiet room with no distractions or interruptions. Many of the tests are power tests and are, therefore, untimed. In addition, at no time are patients expected to multitask. They are able to maintain their focus on one task at a time, work to completion, and then they move on to the next. Ruff and Richardson note that:

> given that tests must be standardized, the examiner provides very clear-cut instructions minimizing distractions by testing in a quiet room. Patients may perform fairly well, for example on attention tests, in such an artificial testing environment. However, in everyday life, the patient may be working in an office cubicle with lots of distracting noises occurring all day and the demands on attention in such an environment may be substantially different. Thus, test scores do not always translate perfectly to the difficulties experienced in everyday life.[58]

This issue is discussed in some detail by Sbordone and Guilmette.[70] They conclude their discussion by stating:

> more importantly, the patient's quantitative test performance under such conditions may significantly underestimate the patient's cognitive and behavioral impairments and result in inaccurate predictions about the patient's ability to return to work or school, live independently, or function effectively within the community.[70]

This underscores the importance of attending to scores within the neuropsychological test battery that, while not frankly impaired, may represent a relative decline for that individual. It also underscores the importance of attending to the self-report of the patient and family regarding ongoing functional deficits and limitations that are observed in more "real-life" circumstances.

Feedback Session

As a standard part of most clinical neuropsychological evaluations, patients and, if they desire, their families will receive feedback regarding their test results. Most patients typically find the feedback session to be extremely beneficial as in most cases it will confirm the presence of the cognitive problems that they have experienced. In addition, it gives the neuropsychologist an opportunity to review their areas of cognitive strength. The feedback session is often used by the neuropsychologist as the first opportunity to begin to educate the individual and family about the effects of PCS/MTBI so that they can better understand and not overreact to the problems. If the individual is early post-injury, it also gives the neuropsychologist an opportunity to reinforce the fact that substantial recovery is expected. This is also the time that the neuropsychologist will present the treatment plan and enlist the patient's and family's involvement in recommended treatment. The authors commonly receive feedback from their patients and families that the feedback session is something of a "double-edged sword." While it is somewhat distressing to learn that they have sustained a PCS/MTBI, they are relieved to know that there is an explanation for the symptoms that they are experiencing and that there is something that can be done to assist them in their recovery.

TREATMENT/REHABILITATION

Multidisciplinary Approach to Treatment

The typical MTBI patient is most likely going to suffer from a diverse set of functional deficits and early intervention is critical. As the National Institute of Health Consensus Statement reported, the consequences of traumatic brain injury often influence human functions along a continuum.[9] These range from altered physiological functions to neurological and psychological impairments, to medical problems and disabilities that affect not only the individual with traumatic brain injury but the patient's family, friends, community and society in general. As a result, treatment of the MTBI patient will, by necessity, be a multidisciplinary endeavor.

The direct physical concomitants of the injury will often require chiropractic, physical, massage and/or occupational therapies in addition to the physiatrist. Visual problems associated with deficits in either central visual processing or oculomotor dysfunction will require neuro-ophthalmological or neuro-optometric treatment. Frequently occurring disturbances of the inner ear subsequent to the physical trauma may result in vestibular dysfunction, dysequilibrium and hearing problems such as phonophobia and these will require otological evaluation. Emotional sequelae usually require psychotherapeutic and/or psychiatric intervention. If the patient ultimately faces vocational jeopardy or dislocation, vocational rehabilitative services will be necessary. Of course, neuropsychological evaluation and cognitive rehabilitation will also be required to address the individual's cognitive dysfunction.

Psychotherapy

The personal suffering secondary to physical and cognitive impairment almost necessarily requires psychotherapeutic intervention. Prigatano defines psychotherapy as:

> . . . teaching patients to learn to behave in their own best self-interest, not selfish interests, by slowly helping patients to observe aspects about their behavior that they may not fully recognize and by providing patients with practical guidelines and suggestions for how to cope with specific problems. The goal is to see the big picture of the patient's life before they can deal with the specific effects of the brain injury. Psychotherapy is about achieving a greater understanding of one's self and one's behavior in order to be better able to make choices that do not complicate the patient's adjustment to life. It offers the patient an opportunity to avoid pain and suffering by making appropriate choices.[71]

Individual Psychotherapy

Individual psychotherapy for MTBI patients includes educating them about the injury itself and its emotional sequelae, as well as assisting them in coming to terms with their losses. Emotional sequelae, which are typical of physical injury in general and brain injury in particular, include depression, questions of identity in the face of lost abilities, compromise of coping mechanisms, generalized and performance anxiety, irritability/ anger/emotional lability, and specific phobia/PTSD symptoms. Patients' emotional recovery varies over time and can be divided into three stages.

Stage 1 typically occurs from the point of injury through the first year afterward. Patients experience a great deal of confusion about what has happened to them. Not only are they unsure of their own abilities and injuries, they frequently have difficulty understanding and processing the explanations given them by their health care providers. They are certain, though, that they are not the same and it is at this point that we often hear them ask, "am I going crazy?" It is also not unusual for patients to present with flat affect and such slowness of information processing at this stage that they appear to be in a "brain fog" that will eventually lift. In this stage, the patient begins the grieving process that continues on various levels throughout the rehabilitation process and beyond. The losses or potential losses facing them include:

- cognitive abilities
- emotional control
- identity and self-esteem
- job or change in occupation status
- roles in the home
- relationships, social status and intimacy
- autonomy and control over their own time
- financial losses
- future plans.

A common theme we hear is, "I miss the person I used to be. I wish I had my old life back." Patients take stock of all they have lost, which often compounds the depression, anxiety, and irritability they experience. Treatment in Stage 1 consists of educating patients about MTBI and the recovery process, and providing a supportive environment where their feelings of loss, depression, and fear can be examined, processed, and normalized.

Stage 2 of individual psychotherapy generally occurs in the 12 to 18 months post-injury. In this phase, patients work to cope with their losses and compensate for them. Coping mechanisms they utilized prior to the injury are often compromised, so they now have to work to establish new ones and learn to live more effectively given their limitations. This is where the true work of rehabilitation occurs. The psychotherapist assists patients in establishing new and realistic expectations of themselves in their various roles and helps them learn to focus on the positive traits and abilities they still have. Fatigue and the brain injury itself make it difficult to cope with the inevitable frustrations of the rehabilitation process, and patients are often impulsive, distractible and irritable. Teaching anger management techniques, better environmental management, and cognitive-behavioral skills assists patients to manage these emotions and to gain perspective.[72] Anxiety and depression may persist in this stage, particularly if patients experience ongoing financial pressures due to job loss or change, and if physical, cognitive, and/or emotional or psychosocial or sexual difficulties persist. Patients may begin to question their prognosis and wonder, "will I ever get better, back to normal?" It should be noted that feelings of victimization, loss of control, and anxiety can be compounded by the litigation process if patients are so involved, and must be treated with proper medication management and teaching relaxation/stress management and assertiveness skills.

In *Stage 3*, typically 18 to 24 months post-injury, MTBI patients usually reach maximum medical improvement from a neuropsychological standpoint. Psychotherapy then assists patients to deal with the finality of losses, review the gains that have been made, and plan for a different future perhaps than the one envisioned pre-injury. Grief issues are re-examined and put into perspective as patients come to make essential sense of what has happened to them. They continue to adjust to the changes in their lives and to adapt to live more effectively. As patients review the rehabilitation and healing process, a stronger sense of self (albeit changed) emerges and there is often the desire to give back to the brain injury community and to help others recently injured.

Specific Phobias and PTSD are also issues that are addressed in individual psychotherapy. They are most commonly seen in Stage 1, but may persist into Stage 3 and beyond if left untreated. According to one report, PTSD is seen in up to one-third of all accident victims.[73] As defined in the *DSM-IV*, the patient exposed to a traumatic event can re-experience that event in one (or more) of the following ways:

1. recurrent or intrusive distressing recollections of the event
2. recurrent distressing dreams of the event
3. acting or feeling as if the traumatic event were recurring
4. intense psychological distress at exposure to internal or external cues that symbolize or resemble an aspect of the traumatic event
5. physiological reactivity at exposure to internal or external cues that symbolize or resemble an aspect of the traumatic event.

Additionally, the patient exhibits persistent avoidance of stimuli associated with the trauma as indicated by three (or more) of the following:

1. efforts to avoid thoughts, feelings or conversations associated with the trauma
2. efforts to avoid activities, places or people that arouse recollections of the trauma
3. inability to recall an important aspect of the trauma
4. markedly diminished interest or participation in significant activities
5. feeling of detachment or estrangement from others
6. restrictive range of affect
7. sense of a foreshortened future.

Finally, the patient may exhibit persistent symptoms of increased arousal (not present before the trauma) as indicated by two (or more) of the following:

1. difficulty falling or staying asleep
2. irritability or outbursts of anger
3. difficulty concentrating
4. hypervigilance
5. hyperstartle responses.

Where a patient may not present with a full-blown PTSD syndrome, they may present with symptoms of a phobic reaction specific to the circumstances under which the accident occurred. In this case, exposure to the phobic stimulus or situation produces an immediate anxiety response. *DSM-IV* refers to this as a *Specific Phobia*. This can take the form of a situationally-bound or situationally-predisposed panic attack. The individual usually recognizes that the fear is excessive or unreasonable, and the situation is either avoided or else is endured with intense anxiety or distress. The avoidance, anxious anticipation, and the fear of the situation significantly interfere with the person's normal routine, occupational or academic functioning, social activities or relationships, or there is marked distress about having the phobia.

While a number of psychotherapeutic interventions have been utilized in treating Specific Phobias and PTSD, one of the most effective treatment modalities has been Eye Movement Desensitization and Reprocessing (EMDR), a technique developed by Dr. Francine Shapiro.[74] The technique involves the desensitizing effect of repeated eye movements (i.e., visually scanning across mid-line) on memories and thoughts regarding the traumatic event. The rapid, repeated eye movement accelerates the individual's ability to re-process and re-integrate information regarding the event without the emotional trauma attached. EMDR rapidly changes the impact of these memories and thoughts, which in turn, alters the symptom presentation. Research related to a single event trauma (such as a motor vehicle accident), as well as our clinical experience, suggests the complete or near complete resolution of the trauma is frequently achieved in relatively few sessions, usually four to six. For patients with PTVS problems, alternating tactile, and/ or auditory stimulation are as effective as the visual scanning-stimuli. It is our experience that patients' other therapies are more effective when PTSD and Specific Phobia are resolved, preferably in Stage 1 treatment.

Conjoint/Family Therapy

For most MTBI patients, the combination of physical and cognitive deficits result in a deterioration of social relationships and a disruption of family dynamics in particular. Disruption in familiar patterns of interaction in the marital and family system often requires psychotherapeutic intervention involving spouses and family members. Research has indicated that the prevalence of depression and anxiety in family members, especially spouses, of individuals with brain dysfunction is higher than 40 percent.[75]

Family intervention should involve the education of family members as to the typical cognitive, emotional, and behavioral sequelae of MTBI, the causes of these symptoms and ways of managing them. Intervention should also create opportunities for family members to convey their own feelings of loss, anger, fear, and frustration in response to the patient's illness. Pragmatic attempts to reorganize the family roles and responsibilities should be addressed so that the family system can compensate for what the patient is no longer able to do, or do well. Finally, bolstering communication skills between the patient and family members (and among family members) is also critical if the family is to adjust adequately.

Supportive Group Psychotherapy

It can also be quite helpful for the MTBI patient to participate in a supportive group environment with other similarly injured patients. Supportive group settings can counter the inevitable sense of isolation that these patients often experience. Supportive group environments also promote the practice of effective coping styles, identify common sources of frustration and create a supportive community on which the patient can rely.

Cognitive Rehabilitation

Early cognitive rehabilitation intervention is essential to the effective treatment of the MTBI patient. Cognitive rehabilitation typically involves a two-pronged approach. First, an effort is made to introduce compensatory strategies into an individual's daily life designed to maximize functioning. It is particularly critical to introduce compensatory strategies as early as possible post-injury. This is particularly indicated if the individual is struggling at work or at school and is facing loss of a job or a significant drop in grades. The first goal of the cognitive rehabilitation process is to stabilize and maintain patients' functioning in the environment where they were prior to the accident. A variety of intrinsic and external cueing strategies as well as organizational strategies can be introduced to attempt to replace cognitive functions that were automatically available prior to the accident.

The second goal of cognitive rehabilitation is to attempt to restore or remediate cognitive functions compromised by the injury. These techniques may involve exercises and skill building training sessions that have no pragmatic relationship with the patient's everyday life but serve to remediate cognitive domains compromised by the brain injury. Sohlberg and Mateer[76] developed a procedure known as Attention Process Training (APT) to help remediate problems with information processing. For remediation of memory functions, Sohlberg and Mateer suggested a three-part approach involving attention process training, prospective memory training, and the use of external compensatory devices simultaneously. Raskin[46] discusses a variety of techniques designed to remediate higher-order cognitive functions including executive skills. Such techniques involve direct retraining of executive systems and metacognitive training approaches.

Vocational Rehabilitation

While the initial goal of cognitive rehabilitation, particularly the introduction of compensatory strategies, is to maintain or prevent deterioration of occupational functioning, and to avoid job loss, often this is not possible. Despite efforts at compensation, the patient may simply be unable to maintain adequate job performance. This can occur because the patient's productivity or accuracy has been compromised, or the patient is no longer able to maintain adequate social relationships at work, or is not able to work the required number of hours because of fatigue.

This is not surprising as most vocational environments commonly place demands on endurance, sustained attention, the ability to deal with distractions, memory, and organizational skills. Weaknesses in these areas, of course, are familiar features of PCS/ MTBI. The combination of disruptions in these cognitive domains coupled with mental and physical fatigue, and perhaps persistent pain and other physical limitations severely diminish the patient's ability to cope effectively in the workplace.[77]

It is important that the physician assess the patient's vocational status in the initial stage of treatment, particularly if the patient is continuing on the job. This is especially critical as cognitive disturbances are more likely to be noticed in the work environment where the patient is presented with specific cognitive demands. The following questions might be helpful for the physician in the assessment of the patient's vocational status:

- "Are you making more mistakes at work?"
- "Are you making unusual mistakes that you wouldn't have made before the accident?"
- "How are you getting along with your co-workers?"
- "What is your productivity like at work?"
- "What feedback have you been getting from your supervisor?"

When the patient has been out of work and the physician is evaluating their readiness to return to work, the following factors should be considered:

- chronic fatigue due to general deconditioning and effortful cognitive processing
- chronic pain
- impaired balance and coordination
- visual difficulties.[77]

Additionally, it is important for the physician to consider ongoing cognitive deficits, interpersonal and psychosocial problems, and the patient's emotional coping abilities. All of these factors are likely to combine and interact with each other and compromise a successful return to work. In many cases, patients will be unable to return to work at their former occupations because of the combination of any or all of the above factors. In that case, a vocational rehabilitation evaluation and a process of vocational retraining and alternative vocational placement may be necessary.

The vocational assessment process involves formal testing designed to assess vocational strengths and limitations, as well as occupational interests and needs. Thorough educational and work histories are also obtained. When the prior job is no longer viable, job development and placement should emphasize the identification of alternatives for future employment. Transferable skills are assessed and training is initiated to assist the individual in learning to develop new skills. The feasibility of vocational alternatives is assessed with treatment providers providing significant input regarding vocational restrictions/limitations. If the patient is to return to a previous job site either in the same job or at a lower skill level, interfacing with the employer, supervisor, and co-workers can facilitate appropriate job re-entry so that individuals in the workplace can develop appropriate expectations for the returning employee.[77]

VESTIBULAR EVALUATION AND TREATMENT

Jacobson notes that, because the auditory and vestibular systems contain delicate structures, it is not uncommon for pathophysiological changes to occur from the same forces that resulted in the PCS/MTBI.[43] It is, therefore, common for individuals presenting with PCS/MTBI to have associated problems with the vestibular system. Common symptoms include tinnitus, ear fullness and pressure, hearing loss, and dysfunction of the vestibular system causing vertigo and dysequilibrium. Referral to an otolaryngologist for evaluation and treatment of these disorders is often necessary.

Frequently, MTBI patients will also complain of phonophobia (also known as "acustophobia") and difficulty filtering out background noise. It is quite common in concussive patients for the auditory gating mechanism of the central nervous system to be disrupted. This system is designed to naturally filter-out extraneous noise from the patient's awareness. As a result, patients often complain not only of sensitivity to noise, but of feeling overwhelmed by the volume and quantity of auditory stimuli. We have found it very helpful to refer such patients for noise attenuation earplugs. These earplugs are specifically designed to filter-out background noise allowing the patient to hear proximal auditory stimuli. The patients can utilize the earplugs as needed to compensate for deficits in auditory gating. They can also utilize the earplugs to manage their exposure to auditory stimuli in environments in which there is a high degree of ambient noise in order to gradually retrain the brain to filter-out extraneous auditory stimuli. The ER 15/25 earplugs, also known as "musician's" earplugs, are one option.

PSYCHIATRIC INTERVENTION

As has been previously noted in this chapter, emotional disturbance and mood destabilization are central and frequent features of PCS/MTBI. For moderate to severe levels of depression and/or irritability, the use of selective serotonergic reuptake inhibitors (SSRIs) are often helpful in reducing levels of depression and effectively controlling irritability in many of these patients. Psychiatric consultation may also be helpful when problems of impulse control and aggressive behavior become particular areas of concern. The use of mood stabilizers may be indicated in these cases.

Additionally, the psychiatrist can be particularly helpful in those cases where hypo-arousal significantly limits functional ability. The administration of Ritalin, for example, can be helpful in such individuals. Wrightson and Gronwall recommend initial dosage mid-morning with a second dosage in the afternoon.[26] Many patients find the medication worthwhile and report a significant increase in the number of productive hours they have for work or academic activities. Provigil is another psychostimulant medication which has been helpful in improving wakefulness, attention and concentration.

VISUAL DEFICITS AND REHABILITATION FOLLOWING MTBI

Politzer notes that vision is our dominant sense and it has been estimated that 80 to 85 percent of our perception, learning, and cognitive activities are, to some degree, mediated through vision.[48] Padula, *et al.* state, "The majority of individuals that recover from a traumatic brain injury will have binocular function difficulties in the form of strabismus, phoria, ocular dysfunction, convergence, and accommodative abnormalities."[78] Padula further notes that this abrupt change in ocular-motor function can result in significant problems with double vision.[79] He states, "This condition of diplopia can severely affect recovery from depth judgment, object localization, ability to match visual information with kinesthetic, proprioceptive, and vestibular experience, thereby affecting balance, coordination, and movements."[79] There are two integrated visual systems.[48] One is the ambient process that appears to occur at the mid-brain where vision is matched with kinesthetic, tactile, proprioceptive, and vestibular processes. The other is focal, which relates to the ability to localize on a specific visual detail. VMSS results from dysfunction of the ambient visual process.[79] Padula states, "It is caused by distortions of the spatial system causing the individual to misperceive his or her position in the spatial environment. There results a shift in the concept of perceived visual midline so that it does not correspond with the actual physical, neuro-motor midline."[79] Padula, *et al.* describe a simple test that can be performed without specialized equipment to screen for a possible visual midline shift.[80] Politzer goes on to note that PTVS has also been associated with traumatic brain injury and:

> is a constellation of signs and symptoms felt to represent another dysfunction between the ambient and the focal processes and PTVS patients tend to be overwhelmed by details and movement around them. It is as though their peripheral (ambient) visual system has become hypervigilant rather than operating on a more subconscious or automatic level. Peripheral visual stimulation becomes disorienting as attention is continually drawn to any motion or stimulus.[48]

PTVS and VMSS can both result from whiplash injury. Padula states:

> Given a neurological event such as a traumatic brain injury (this includes a mild whiplash), multiple sclerosis, cerebral-vascular accident, etc., the ambient visual process can lose its ability to match information with other components of the sensory-motor feedback loop. Even a whiplash as mentioned can cause significant dysfunction at the level of the mid-brain. Thomas has calculated that at the level of the foramen magnum as much as 14,000 pounds of internal force is exerted on the spinal cord with a minimal 10 mile per hour rear-end collision.[80]

Politzer reviews a variety of other vision problems that can be associated with PCS/ MTBI including deficits in binocular vision.[48] He states, "binocular vision refers to using both eyes together. It comprises convergence and divergence. Convergence is the ability of the eyes to work together tracking an object as it approaches the individual and divergence is the ability to track an object as it moves away."[48] The types of visual problems discussed above can result in a wide variety of self-reported vision problems by the patient who has sustained a PCS/MTBI. For the patient reporting these types of vision problems, referral for evaluation and treatment is indicated and can potentially be extremely beneficial. Various treatment modalities include vision therapy, use of corrective lenses, prisms and yoked prisms.[48]

It is our clinical experience that significant gains are frequently observed when these vision problems are properly diagnosed and treated. This is also true for the physiatry colleagues that we work with on a regular basis. In a recent report, one of our local physiatrists wrote about a patient who had the potential for excellent recovery but was not making recovery:

> I think the answer to the question is a problem with visual orientation. On testing, he has an obvious midline shift that is perpetuating these myofascial problems due to his abnormal visual orientation. This is fortunately a correctable situation. I believe that, once it is corrected, the therapies that have improved the situation in the past but not been maintained will hopefully be maintained and he can get beyond this ongoing problem. It is awful to think that this relatively young man will have to deal with chronic myofascial symptoms indefinitely and I do not think he does. With appropriate treatment

through visual rehabilitation/prism lenses, I believe there will be considerable improvement in his situation. The situation with his vision is directly related to the automobile trauma. It is commonly seen. It is also commonly missed. It is not unusual for a patient to be undiagnosed even for years after an accident since the patients are able to compensate to a certain degree and usually have fairly subtle specific visual complaints.

PHYSIATRIST'S ROLE IN MTBI REHABILITATION

The role of physical medicine is, of course, critical to the rehabilitation process. In many cases, as the medical director of the treatment team, the physiatrist will serve as the "glue" holding the team together as a cohesive entity rather than a disparate group of independently operating professionals.

In this regard, because the treatment of these patients is multidisciplinary, the physiatrist should be aware of the potential of iatrogenically induced stress simply due to the number and volume of treatments in which patients may be engaged. Patients often feel as if their lives are dominated by their treatment schedule and this can serve to further undermine their quality of life. Patients may feel as if they are unduly "intruded upon" by their treaters. Because patients may not volunteer this information, the physiatrist should inquire. While aggressive, multidisciplinary treatment is ideal in more quickly ameliorating the problems faced by patients, it may be necessary for patients to prioritize treatments and postpone some treatments. The physiatrist can play a major role in helping patients prioritize their many therapies/appointments. It is critical that the physiatrist insure good communication among the treatment providers. It is also important to refer to providers who have demonstrated timely and efficient communication patterns as part of their practice.

As noted earlier, pain is going to be a central component in the clinical picture for most patients. Physical pain can be an ongoing, central, co-morbid factor in compromising the patient's cognitive status and overall functional capacity. It will be a key factor in determining whether the patient will be formally evaluated neurocognitively. Therefore, the physiatrist's role in treating the causes of the patient's physical discomforts, as well as providing relief from that discomfort, is essential. The physiatrist should keep in mind the potential usefulness of ancillary treatments such as relaxation training, biofeedback therapy, and psychotherapy directed at pain management, in improving patients' capacity for coping with their discomfort.

Secondary to physical discomfort and emotional distress, or as a direct result of the PCS/MTBI, patients will often present with significant sleep disturbance. Fatigue, as stated earlier, frequently represents as a troublesome co-morbid issue. It is the physiatrist who will have the central role in treating fatigue and sleep disturbance. From our perspective, it is critical to evaluate sleep patterns early on in treatment and to aggressively treat sleep disorder with MTBI patients. The physiatrist may want to proceed in a four-tier process beginning with herbal/homeopathic remedies such as Kava Kava, Valerian Root, or Melatonin. If these are not found to be effective, the physiatrist can then proceed to prescription medications such as: (1) tricyclic antidepressants; (2) a serotonergic medication with pronounced sedative side effects such as Trazodone; and (3) Ambien until the patient demonstrates a consistently adequate sleep pattern.

Finally, as noted earlier, the physiatrist will be central in determining when (and if) the patient should return to work. If return to work is to be considered, it is important to consider not only the patient's physical capacity, but also to consider fatigue, cognitive status, balance and coordination, emotional/psychological status, and visual functioning in making the determination. In many cases, we advise a graduated return to work based on a careful assessment of these factors to maximize the probability of a successful transition back into the workplace.

CASE STUDY

Referral Information

Mr JD was a 54-year-old, right-handed, white male with 13 years of formal education. His physiatrist referred him for neuropsychological evaluation three months following a motor vehicle accident. He was the passenger in the front seat of a small sedan. He was wearing a seatbelt and shoulder harness. The driver of the vehicle was attempting to pull onto the highway from a parking lot and there was a truck approaching in the right-hand lane. The truck began a right-hand turn into the parking lot and the driver of the vehicle proceeded across the highway. There was a small sedan traveling on the left side of the truck and the truck blocked the view of that vehicle. As Mr JD's vehicle pulled into the roadway, they were hit broadside on the driver's side front quarter panel. It was estimated that the other vehicle was traveling at approximately 40 to 50 miles per hour. They were hit with enough force to cause their vehicle to rotate one-and-a-half times. Therefore, there were significant rotational forces involved in this accident. Mr JD did experience a whiplash injury but did not sustain a blow to the head in the course of the accident. He did not lose consciousness but he did experience altered consciousness in the form of being dazed and confused post-accident. He made the observation, "I was about to pass out and felt very woozy." He also noted, "I kept fading out." The altered consciousness persisted until the time of the arrival of the ambulance.

The accident occurred at approximately 9 am. Mr JD had just dropped his car off at the garage but has no memory for getting up and getting ready that morning and had no memory for driving his vehicle to the garage. He also has no memory for driving from the garage to the point of the accident. This would suggest some retrograde amnesia. He does have a memory for the sound of the impact, rotation of the vehicle and seeing the hood crumple towards him. There is then a brief gap in his memory and his memories for the rest of the day are quite vague and incomplete. He made the observation that his memories for the rest of the day were "all a blur." He experienced some nausea and dizziness post-accident.

Mr JD continued to experience a variety of physical, visual, cognitive, and emotional coping problems consistent with a closed head injury resulting in a PCS at 3 months post-accident. By the time of referral, he had already received treatment for his physical injuries by the referring physiatrist, an internal medicine physician, and a chiropractor. He had also been receiving individual psychotherapy from a licensed clinical psychologist familiar with trauma and closed head injury and he was utilizing Celexa as an antidepressant and Ambien as a sleep aid at the time of referral. Both medications were working well.

It is important to note that, once the insurance company received the initial screening report recommending neuropsychological testing, they immediately scheduled Mr JD for an independent medical evaluation (IME) with both a physiatrist and a neuropsychologist. This action on the part of the insurance company was neither surprising nor unusual and neuropsychological testing was placed on hold pending the results of those IMEs. What was pleasantly surprising and quite unusual was that both independent medical evaluators agreed totally and completely with the treating providers: The IME physiatrist diagnosed a PCS resulting in cognitive deficits. The IME neuropsychologist diagnosed a MTBI and both independent evaluators agreed that neuropsychological testing was indicated. They both agreed that a period of cognitive rehabilitation was also indicated, medically necessary, and accident related. Mr JD's clinical psychologist had diagnosed PTSD related to the accident. Both independent evaluators also agreed with this diagnosis and agreed that the individual psychotherapy that he was receiving was also indicated, medically necessary, and accident related. Therefore, in this case study, there was no argument that Mr JD had, indeed, sustained a closed head injury in the accident resulting in a PCS and was also experiencing PTSD for driving related to the accident.

Background Information

Mr JD was a high school graduate and he was an above average student. He attended community college and was within 6 semester hours of completing an Associate's of Arts (AA) degree. Because he had not completed this degree, for the purposes of neuropsychological testing, he was given credit for 13 years of formal education. He did not have a history of any learning disabilities, involvement with special education or ever having been held back a grade.

Work History

After graduation from high school, he worked in a factory for two years. He then served in the United States Navy for four years as a machinist mate and his rank at discharge was E5. He then worked for seven years in retail sales as a salesman and department manager followed by eight years as a jeweler. For the 12 years prior to the accident, he worked as an independent insurance broker.

Medical History

Mr JD did not have a history of alcohol abuse or dependence. His medical history was essentially unremarkable as was his neuropsychological and neurological history. He had never had any prior concussions or head injuries, periods of unconsciousness for any reason, epilepsy, toxic exposure, or neurological illnesses. Mr JD's prior psychological history is notable for a brief period of individual psychotherapy for approximately five months, a year before the accident. Issues that he addressed in therapy included his home life as a child, diet, and weight loss. He found the treatment to be quite helpful. It was evident that he was not experiencing any diagnosable psychological or psychiatric conditions at the time of the motor vehicle accident.

At the time of the accident, his business was doing extremely well and his client base was growing on a steady basis. His marriage and family relationships were stable, positive and happy.

Self-reported Symptomatology

Mr JD reported some ongoing intermittent pain in his neck, right shoulder, and back. He also was experiencing two headaches per week. He noted that at worst the pain was at a moderate level and usually less. He was noting some ongoing balance problems associated with dizziness. He reported ongoing problems with phonophobia. When in a noisy or loud environment, this caused him to feel irritable and anxious. In addition, he had difficulty filtering out background noise. He was also noting significant ongoing problems with fatigue. He found that he was becoming more tired more easily, whether performing physical or cognitive activities.

He was experiencing a wide variety of vision problems. He was noting ongoing blurred vision and he felt that his distance acuity was worse than prior to the accident. He was noting difficulties with visual scanning such as losing his place when he read and missing things that he was looking for. He was aware that his eyes were slow to focus, suggesting problems with accommodation. He was noting ongoing photophobia for both sunlight and florescent lights. His eyes fatigued easily when reading or doing computer work. At times, he would note the perception of movement in his peripheral vision when there was nothing there. As noted in the body of the chapter, this is a classic symptom of unilateral saccades (a unilateral eye-tracking motion).

From an emotional and psychological standpoint, he was acknowledging some intermittent mild feelings of depression. He had also noted problems with emotional lability. Following the accident, he tended to cry more frequently and easily. He also experienced significant sleep disturbance post-accident. He had difficulties getting to sleep and staying asleep and the sleep disturbance was unrelated to his physical pain. As noted above, he had been prescribed Celexa for his depression and Ambien as a sleep aid. He was experiencing ongoing problems with nausea post-accident and had lost approximately 20 pounds. He was experiencing difficulties with irritability and decreased frustration tolerance. He was finding that he became easily upset and angry over small things that would not have bothered him previously. He reported occasional verbal outbursts but realized that he was overreacting to situations after the fact.

From a cognitive standpoint, Mr JD was experiencing ongoing problems with attention and concentration. He was finding that his mind wandered more easily and that he was easily distracted. He also reported events that likely related to cognitive set loss (loss of mental focus mid-task or mid-conversation). He was also experiencing problems with multitasking. He was having difficulty alternating his attention between several tasks and could no longer attend to several things simultaneously. He felt that his most significant cognitive problem was short-term memory loss. He would often forget his intentions, appointments, what was said to him, what he read, and what he had done or said. He was finding that cueing typically did not help his memory, suggesting that there was a problem with memory consolidation. He was using written notes, organizational systems, and a variety of compensations for the memory deficit. He was also reporting difficulties with verbal fluency and reading comprehension. He felt his speed of information processing was much slower than prior to the accident. He reported that problem solving and decision-making were more difficult. He was also noting problems with planning, organizing, and logical sequencing of multi-step tasks. When writing, he was tending to transpose letters.

Based on the initial screening/interview, it was evident that Mr JD did meet the diagnostic criteria for a PCS/MTBI established by the American Congress of Rehabilitation Medicine.[11] He also met the diagnostic criteria for a grade II concussion established by the American Academy of Neurology (Table 12-2).[13]

Interpretation of Test Results

Because of the IMEs required by the insurance company, neuropsychological testing had to be postponed for Mr JD. It was ultimately conducted at seven months post-accident. As discussed in the body of the report, it is common for individuals who have sustained a MTBI to perform within normal limits on the index scores. In this case, Mr JD's HII and AIR were both well within normal limits. However, his GNDS, the index, which takes into account the greatest number, and widest variety of tests, suggested a mild level of generalized cerebral dysfunction. Mr JD also demonstrated specific neuropsychological deficits, inconsistencies, or relative weaknesses suggestive of residual and more localized cerebral dysfunction, most notably in the frontal, bilateral temporal, and right parietal regions of the brain.

An analysis of his WAIS-R scores suggested a significant variability among the 11 subtests. His scale score range was nine and Lezak considers scale score variability of five or greater to be non-random and indicative of organicity.[19] His percentile range was 10th percentile to 93rd percentile. This represents a 2.8 standard deviation variability, which is highly significant.

As noted in the body of the chapter, executive dysfunction is common following MTBI. Research suggests that this most likely relates to frontal lobe involvement. Mr JD demonstrated significant executive dysfunction as evidenced by his inconsistent sustained attention and concentration abilities, which ranged from the 28th to the 99th percentile. His speed of auditory information processing was far below expectation, ranging from the 25th to the 34th percentiles. These scores represent an excellent example of a relative cognitive weakness. While statistically these scores are considered to be "within normal limits," when compared to his other above average test scores, as well as his academic and work histories, these scores are below expectation for Mr JD. In addition, he did report slowed speed of cognitive processing in his day-to-day and work activities.

His ability to generate solutions to new and ambiguous problems, as measured by the Category Test, was in the borderline range at the 21st percentile. Planning, organizing, and logical sequencing abilities, as measured by the Picture Arrangement subtest of the WAIS-R, was in the borderline range at the 28th percentile. Figural fluency, as measured by the Ruff Figural Fluency Test (unique designs score) was in the borderline range at the 16th

Table 12-2 Test results

INDEX SCORES – Age 54   Education = 13 years   Dominant   hand = right

Index	Raw	T	Percentile	Level
Halstead Impairment Index (HII)	0.3	56	73rd	Above Average (Heaton)
Average Impairment Rating (AIR)	1.0	53	72nd	High Average (Heaton)
General Neuropsychological Deficit Scale (GNDS)	30		6th	Mild Impairment

INTELLIGENCE

Wechsler Adult Intelligence Scale – Revised

	IQ Score	WAIS-R		Heaton	
		Percentile	Range	Percentile	Range
FSIQ	110	75th	High Average	50th	Average
VSIQ	115	84th	High Average	66th	High Average
PSIQ	102	55th	Average	28th	Borderline

WAIS-R Subtests

	SS	Age	Heaton			SS	Age	Heaton	
			Per-centile	Level				Per-centile	Level
INFO	11	12	38th	Average	PC	8	10	25th	Borderline
DIGIT	10	10	38th	Average	PA	8	10	28th	Borderline
VOCAB	15	15	93rd	Above average	BD	12	13	76th	Above average
ARITH	11	12	42nd	Average	OA	6	8	10th	Mild
COM	11	11	46th	Average	DS	10	12	69th	Above average
SIM	14	15	90th	Above average	(DS memory 9/9; WNL)				

Percentile Range = 10th to 93rd (2.8 standard deviation variability)

SS Range = 9 (3.0 standard deviation variability.)

ACADEMIC

Peabody Individual Achievement Test (PIAT)

	Raw	Grade Equivalent	Std %	Heaton Percentile	Level
Math (PIAT-R)	95	12.9+	77th		
Reading recognition	81	12.9+	87th	98th+	Above average
Reading comprehension	75	12.8+	77th	46th	Average
Spelling	80	12.9+	93rd	86th	Above average

(*continued*)

Table 12-2 continued

HALSTEAD REITAN TESTS

	Raw Score		T	Heaton		RNG Level
				Percentile	Level	
Category test	Errors: 71		42	21st	Borderline	2
TPT Dom	Time 10.0 min.	Blocks: 6	35	7th	Mild	3
TPT Ndom	Time 6.3 min.	Blocks: 10	46	34th	Low average	3
TPT both	Time 5.0 min.	Blocks: 10	43	25th	Borderline	3
TPT total	Time 21.3	Blocks: 26	39	13th	Mild	3
TPT memory	Correct: 7		45	31st	Low average	1
TPT location	Correct: 5		56	73rd	Above average	1
Rhythm	Errors: 0		78	98th+	Above average	0
Speech	Errors: 7		44	28th	Borderline	1
Tapping Dom	58.4		64	92nd	Above average	1
Tapping NDom	47.5		52	58th	Average	1
Trails A	56 sec.	Errors: 0	34	5th	Mild/moderate	3
Trails B	73 sec.	Errors: 0	52	58th	Average	1
Pegs D	66 sec.	Drops: 0	58	79th	Above average	0
Pegs ND	82 sec.	Drops: 2	44	28th	Borderline	1

SPEECH AND LANGUAGE

Reltan-Indiana Aphasia Screening:	Raw	T	Percentile	Heaton Level
	4	50	50th	Above average
	(NOTE: Dyscalculia was evident on this aphasia screening test.)			

Boston Aphasia Screening Test:	Raw	T	Percentile	Heaton Level
Complex Sentences	10/12 Easy 8/8 Hard 8/8	35	7th	Mild

Thurstone Verbal Fluency:			T	Percentile	Heaton Level
Part A: 48	Part B: 18	Total: 66	65	93rd	Above average

Ruff Figural Fluency Test	Raw	Percentile	Level
Error Ratio	.1689	20th	Borderline
Unique Designs	71	16th	Borderline
Perseverative Errors	10	54th	Average
Strategy Based Designs	7		
Total Strategies	2		

(continued)

Table 12-2 continued
VISUAL PERCEPTUAL

	Raw	T	Percentile	Level
Spatial Relations	2	58	79th	Above average
Rey-Osterreith Copy	29		<1st	Impaired
Hooper Visual Organization Test	21.5		19th	Borderline
Key Copy (RKSPE)				Impaired

SENSORY/PERCEPTUAL
Reitan/Klove Sensory Perceptual Examination

	Right	Left		Right	Left
FA	0	0	Tactile suppressions	0	0
FNW	0	0	Auditory suppressions	0	2
FORM	0	0	Visual suppressions	0	0

	Raw	T	Percentile	Level
TFR-R	6.6	66	95th	Above average
TFR-L	6.1	66	95th	Above average

	Raw	T	Percentile	Heaton Level
SP-R	0	68	96th	Above average
SP-L	3	43	25th	Borderline
Total	3	51	54th	Average

Digit Vigilance Test

	T	Percentile	Heaton Level
Time: 344 sec.	57	76th	Above average
Errors: 65	16	<1st	Severe

Line Bisection Test

# Significant to right:	0
# Significant to left:	2
(Significant = 1.0 cm or greater off center)	

(*continued*)

Table 12-2 continued

MOTOR

Behavioral Dyscontrol Scale

	Motor Psv.	Disinhibition	R/L Confusion	Echopraxic	Sequencing	Learning
Errors	0	1	0	0	0	0
Score:	19	Range: Within normal limits				

Dynamometer

	Raw	T	Percentile	Heaton Level
Dominant:	40 kg	43	25th	Borderline
Nondominant	45 kg	50	50th	Average

MEMORY

Test:	1	2	3	4	5	DR	%Loss	T	%ile	Heaton Level
Story Memory	8	11	15.5			8	48.4	21	<1st	Moderate/severe
Figure Memory	14	20				8	60	27	1st	Moderate
Story Learning				5.17				34	5th	Mild/moderate
Figure Learning				10				48	42nd	Average

Buschke Verbal Selective Reminding Test: (Larabee norms)

	Raw	Percentile	Level
Long Term Recall	91	10%	Mild
Long Term Storage	95	7%	Mild
Cumulative LTR	81	18%	Borderline
$\frac{1}{2}$ Hour Delayed Recall	10	28%	Borderline
Cued Recall = 11	MC recall =12	Intrusive errors = 1	

Rey-Osterreith Complex Figure (Meyers & Meyers norms):

	Raw	Percentile	Level
Copy	29	<1%	Severe
Immediate Recall	18	31%	Low average
$\frac{1}{2}$ Hour Delayed Recall	13	4%	Mild/moderate
Percent Loss		27.8%	Mild

(continued)

Table 12-2 continued

OTHER
PASAT (Levin Version)

	Raw	Percentile	Level
Trial 1	41	28th	Borderline
Trial 2	35	34th	Low average
Trial 3	27	25th	Borderline
Trial 4	22	28th	Borderline

STROOP

	Raw	Percentile	Level
Interference	−1	46th	Average

Wisconsin Card Sorting Test

	Raw	T	Percentile	Heaton Level
PSV Responses	17	50	50th	Average
Categories 6/6	Lost Sets 0			

SYMPTOM VALIDITY TESTS
Tombaugh Test of Memory Malingering (TOMM)

Raw	Level
50/50	Non-significant

Hiscock Type Digit Recognition Test

Raw	Level
36/36	Non-significant

Rey II 15-Item Memory Malingering Test

Raw	Level
12/15	Non-significant

percentile. His copy of a complex figure was poorly planned and organized suggesting a clear frontal quality to the construction.

Left temporal lobe dysfunction was suggested by language comprehension being mildly impaired at the 7th percentile. His ability to learn large amounts of new meaningful verbal information presented in paragraph form (Story Memory Test) was mildly to moderately impaired at the 5th percentile. Retention of this type of information following a four-hour delay period was severely impaired at 1st percentile. Mr JD lost 48.4 percent of the information that he had previously learned. Learning of new rote verbal information, as measured by the Buschke Verbal Selective Reminding Test (long-term storage score) was mildly impaired at the 7th percentile. Retention of newly learned rote verbal information following a 30-minute delay period was in the border-line range at the 28th percentile.

Right temporal lobe dysfunction was suggested by a mild impairment of his ability to retain visual information following a 30-minute delay period. On the Rey-Osterreith Complex Figure Test, he lost 27.8 percent of the information that he had previously learned. Retention of newly learned visual information following a four-hour delay period (Figure Memory Test) was moderately to severely impaired at the 1st percentile. Mr JD lost 60 percent of the information that he had previously learned over the four-hour delay period.

Right parietal lobe dysfunction was suggested by visual analysis, synthesis and organization without a visual model present (Object Assembly subtest of the WAIS-R) being mildly impaired at the 10th percentile. Complex visual organization, as measured by the Hooper Visual Organization Test, was in the borderline range at the 19th percentile. His copy of a key figure suggested a borderline to mild constructional dyspraxia. Copy of the Rey-Osterreith figure suggested a mild constructional dyspraxia.

Additional neuropsychological deficits of note included psychomotor problem solving in the right hand being mildly impaired at the 7th percentile. This would suggest some left parietal involvement. Dyscalculia was noted on an aphasia-screening test. Attention to salient visual detail, as measured by the Picture Completion subtest of the WAIS-R, was in the borderline range at the 25th percentile. Visual scanning accuracy was severely impaired at 1st percentile. On the Digit Vigilance Test, his visual scanning speed was in the above average range. This test was re-administered a second time and Mr JD was asked to slow his rate of scanning and focus on accuracy. While his scanning speed score dropped to the low average range, his visual scanning accuracy remain mildly impaired at the 10th percentile. A mild right hemispatial inattention was evident on the Line Bisection Test. He demonstrated an inferior (downward) midline shift on the Padula Visual Midline Screening Test.[82]

MMPI-2 and BDI-II Interpretation

Mr JD was administered the MMPI-2 as well as the BDI-II at the time of neuropsychological testing. His BDI-II score was 21, which is considered to be in the moderate range. However, his score was notably elevated as a result of his responding affirmatively to a variety of symptoms that more likely relate to his MTBI. These include ongoing problems with fatigue, concentration, irritability, sleep disturbance, problems with decision-making, agitation, and emotional lability. When this factor was taken into account, Mr JD's corrected BDI-II score was nine, which is non-significant or suggestive of only minimal feelings of depression. This is consistent with his self-report of minimal, if any, feelings of depression at the time of testing.

Mr JD's MMPI-2 profile was as follows:

- Scale 1 (Hs) = 77
- Scale 7 (Pt) = 74
- Scale 3 (Hy) = 71
- Scale 2 (D) = 70
- Scale 8 (Sc) = 67.

With the MMPI-2, any T-score greater than 65 is considered to be clinically significant. As noted previously in the chapter, there is a large body of research that clearly indicates that individuals who have sustained some type of neurological injury such as a traumatic brain injury will often demonstrate elevations on Scales 1, 2, 3, 7 and 8. This is true even for cases of MTBI.[81] As noted previously in the report, following a neurological injury, many of the physical, visual, cognitive and emotional coping problems that the individual experiences will load heavily on these five clinical scales. Therefore, the MMPI-2 profile must be interpreted cautiously, taking this factor into account.

Mr JD's elevation on Scale 2 (the Depression Scale) could be interpreted as representing some minimal feelings of depression. However, further analysis of the MMPI-2 reveals that his Depression Content Scale was not elevated. On the five Harris-Lingoes Subscales only two were elevated: the subjective depression subscale and the mental dullness subscale. Clearly, the mental dullness subscale was elevated as a result of his cognitive dysfunction associated with the MTBI. A critical item analysis reveals that indeed he is acknowledging some subjective feelings of sadness, "most of the time, I feel blue (true)"; "I am happy most of the time (false)"; and "I very seldom have spells of the blues (false)." However, there are no other indications of significant depression. Therefore, the MMPI-2 is best interpreted as representing some minimal feelings of depression and would best be described as feelings of sadness.

His elevation on Scale 7 could suggest some mild feelings of anxiety. Neither of his PTSD scales was significantly elevated. His Anxiety Content Scale was not significantly elevated. A critical item analysis reveals that Scale 7 was most likely elevated as a result of his responding affirmatively to problems associated with sleep disturbance and restlessness, decreased ability to work, and some gastrointestinal distress (which appears to relate directly to the head injury). He did respond affirmatively to feeling "high strung" and feeling a higher level of "tension." Therefore, his elevation on Scale 7 would suggest at most some minimal feelings of heightened stress and tension.

His elevations on Scales 1 and 3 suggest that he was acknowledging a variety of ongoing physical problems and concerns. A critical item analysis reveals that he is acknowledging ongoing problems with concerns associated with his health, tingling and numbness, neck pain, faint spells, dizziness, blank spells, fatigue, and sleep disturbance. Each of these clearly relate to his physical and traumatic brain injuries.

Further critical item analysis reveals that he is acknowledging ongoing cognitive problems, including generalized mental confusion as well as specific problems with attention and concentration and short-term memory. Further, he is acknowledging problems with emotional lability, irritability, and reduced frustration tolerance. Overall, Mr JD's MMPI-2 profile was totally consistent with his physical and traumatic brain injuries.

Summary and Recommendations

The neuropsychological deficits, inconsistencies, and relative weaknesses noted on testing were felt to be totally consistent with a closed head injury resulting in a PCS sustained in the motor vehicle accident. Mr JD was evaluated at seven months post-injury. Some additional cognitive recovery was anticipated and a neuropsychological re-evaluation was recommended at 18 months post-injury as a way to monitor his progress.

By the time of testing, he had reported good resolution of the blurred vision, double vision, visual scanning problems, and photophobia. He was still reporting ongoing problems with accommodation and eye fatigue. The testing revealed a significant visual scanning deficit, a mild right hemispatial inattention, and an inferior (downward) visual midline shift. As a result, referral was made to a neuro-optometrist for further evaluation and treatment.

It was recommended that Mr JD continue his individual psychotherapy focusing on the treatment of his depression and PTSD symptoms, as per his psychologist's recommendations. At the time of the original screening evaluation, it had been recommended that Mr JD obtain a pair of noise attenuation earplugs. He had seen an audiologist and had obtained the ER 15/25 earplugs (aka Musician's Earplugs). He noted that they had been working extremely well as a way to compensate for his phonophobia.

Mr JD had been referred for cognitive rehabilitation following the screening interview. He had received cognitive rehabilitation with a neuropsychologist. He found that treatment to be extremely helpful. A large focus of the treatment had been on helping him develop strategies to compensate for his residual cognitive deficits in his day-to-day and work activities.

Mr JD had been working as an independent insurance broker at the time of the accident. He reported that he had an excellent administrative assistant and that she had assumed the bulk of the responsibility for monitoring and servicing active clients. Mr JD noted that on several occasions post-accident he had attempted to return to insurance sales (i.e., generating new business) and each time he had encountered significant problems from a cognitive standpoint. He reported that he would often forget to take necessary materials to meetings and would often forget to follow up with client's requests and questions. He had made numerous significant errors, which he would not have made prior to the accident (e.g., leaving a client's children off a health policy). He was experiencing extreme difficulties with multitasking and he noted that, when several things were going on in the environment at the same time, he was unable to focus, which in turn led to significant errors. He was also noting ongoing problems with irritability and decreased frustration tolerance on the job. He found that he had little patience for clients with whom he was working and actually "snapped" at people on several occasions. He noted that this was quite unlike him, as prior to the accident, he was extremely patient with his clients. Other significant errors included giving wrong quotes to clients and writing up policies with wrong numbers (e.g., benefit limits and so forth).

Therefore, at the time of testing, it was evident that Mr JD was unable to work in his job as an independent insurance broker generating new business. It was felt that, should he continue to try to do so, he may significantly jeopardize his reputation in the community. The recommendation was made that he continue his medical leave of absence and that his cognitive rehabilitation continue to focus on strategies that he could use to compensate for his residual deficits in his work activities. Given the significance of some of his cognitive deficits at seven months post-injury, it was felt that his ability to return to work as an independent insurance broker remained guarded.

CONCLUSIONS

The primary aim of this chapter was to focus on the relationship between whiplash injury and PCS/MTBI. Clearly, concussion concomitant with whiplash can and does occur frequently. We established that concussions can occur in low velocity motor vehicle accidents and reviewed the biomechanical factors important in evaluating the nature of such accidents. We stressed the importance of early diagnosis and intervention in these cases to avoid a "negative spiral" wherein physical, cognitive, psychological, social, and economic forces combine to exacerbate the patient's condition. In summary, the following issues should be emphasized.

1. MTBI is often misdiagnosed or undiagnosed. It can often present without loss of consciousness or disorientation and commonly utilized radiological techniques (CT and MRI) and neurological evaluation tools (GCS and gross mental status exam) are inadequate in evaluating these more subtle signs and symptoms.
2. PCS/MTBI can occur under conditions of rapid acceleration/deceleration without impact to the head.
3. The pathophysiology of MTBI is at the microstructural level and results in changes in cerebral function without evidence of gross structural damage.
4. A variety of pre-existing factors can increase an individual's vulnerability to the effects of MTBI.
5. A variety of co-morbid factors can serve to compromise the patient's cognitive function and clinical presentation. Efforts need to be made to carefully elucidate these factors, and then eliminate, minimize or account for such factors when evaluating the patient's clinical presentation.
6. PCS encompasses a wide range of symptoms including physical, cognitive, psychological, and visual sequelae. Regarding the cognitive symptoms Kassels *et al.* conducted a meta-analysis of 22 neuropsychological studies on whiplash patients. They concluded that, "These results indicate that the subjective complaints about cognitive deterioration, as reported by many whiplash patients, can be consistently and objectively demonstrated with the help of standardized neuropsychological tests."[82]
7. Early referral to neuropsychology is essential in providing timely evaluation. In addition, this referral will often serve as the precursor for beginning both psychotherapy and cognitive rehabilitation.
8. The neuropsychological assessment process should comprehensively evaluate the complete array of cognitive domains. Neuropsychological assessment should be

performed in a step-wise process involving initial interviewing and screening and, if necessary, proceeding to formal testing. Such assessment should include a careful, multi-modal evaluation of motivation and level of effort. It should be performed under the supervision of a neuropsychologist who can demonstrate specialized training and experience in neuropsychology.

9. The treatment team is, by necessity, multidisciplinary. It will involve a physiatrist as team leader, but will also involve disciplines such as psychotherapy, cognitive therapy, neuro-ophthalmology or neuro-optometry, neuro-otology, vocational rehabilitation, and psychiatry if needed.

SUGGESTED READING

Professionals

1. Varney NR, Roberts RJ (eds). *The Evaluation and Treatment of Mild Traumatic Brain Injury*, Mahwah, NJ, Lawrence Erlbaum Assoc, 1999.
2. Jay GW (ed). *Minor Traumatic Brain Injury Handbook: Diagnosis and Treatment*. New York, CRC Press, 2000.
3. Parker RS. *Concussive Brain Trauma: Neurobehavioral Impairment and Maladaption*. New York, CRC Press, 2001.
4. Wrightson P, Gronwall D. *Mild Head Injury: a Guide to Management*. New York, Oxford University Press, 1999.
5. Raskin SA, Mateer CA. *Neuropsychological Management of Mild Traumatic Brain Injury*. New York, Oxford University Press, 2000.

Patients

1. Denton GL. *Brainlash: Maximize Your Recovery from Mild Brain Injury*. Niwot, CO, Attention Span Books, 1996.
2. Stoler DR, Hill BA. *Coping with Mild Traumatic Brain Injury: A Guide to Living with the Problems Associated with Brain Trauma*. New York, Avery Publishing Group, 1998.
3. Osborn CL. *Over My Head: a Doctor's Account of Head Injury from the Inside Looking Out*. Denver, CO, The Peripatetic Publisher, 1998.

REFERENCES

1. Uzzell BP. Mild head injury: much ado about something. In Varney NR, Roberts RJ (eds). *The Evaluation and Treatment of Mild Traumatic Brain Injury*, pp 1–13. Mahwah, NJ, Lawrence Erlbaum Assoc, 1999.
2. Parker RS. *Concussive Brain Trauma: Neurobehavioral Impairment and Maladaption*, p 25. Boca Raton, CRC Press, 2001.
3. Gennarelli TA, Segawa H, Wald U, *et al.* Physiological response to angular acceleration of the head. In Grossman RG, Gildenberg PL (eds). *Head Injury. Basic and Clinical Aspects*, pp 129–140. New York, Raven Press, 1982.

4. Liu YK. Biomechanics of 'low-velocity impact' head injury. In Varney NR, Roberts RJ (eds). *The Evaluation and Treatment of Mild Traumatic Brain Injury*, pp 49–62. Mahwah, NJ, Lawrence Erlbaum Assoc, 1999.

5. Varney NR, Varney RN. Brain injury without head injury: some physics of automobile collisions with particular reference to brain injuries occurring without physical trauma. *Appl Neuropsychol* 1995; 2: 47.

6. Ommaya AK, Faas F, Yarnell P. Whiplash injury and brain damage. *JAMA* 1968, 204(4)z: 285.

7. Malec JF. Mild traumatic brain injury: scope of the problem. In Varney NR, Roberts RJ (eds). *The Evaluation and Treatment of Mild Traumatic Brain Injury*, pp 15–37. Mahwah, NJ, Lawrence Erlbaum Assoc, 1999.

8. Bazarian JJ, Wong T, Harris M, *et al*. Epidemiology and predictors of post-concussive syndrome after minor head injury in an emergency population. *Brain Inj* 1999; 13(3): 173.

9. *NIH Consensus Development Panel on Rehabilitation of Persons With Traumatic Brain Injury.* Rehabilitation of persons with traumatic brain injury. *JAMA* Sep 8 1999; 282(10): 974.

10. Jay GW. *Minor Traumatic Brain Injury Handbook: Diagnosis and Treatment.* Boca Raton, CRC Press, 2000.

11. American Congress of Rehabilitation Medicine. Definition of mild traumatic brain injury. *J Head Trauma Rehabil* 1993. 8(3): 86–87.

12. Kelly JP, Nichols JS, Filley CM, *et al*. Concussion in sports: guidelines for the prevention of catastrophic outcome. *JAMA* 1991; 266(20): 2867.

13. Quality Standards Subcommittee—American Academy of Neurology. Practice parameter: the management of concussion in sports (summary statement). *Neurology* 1997; 48: 581.

14. *American Psychiatric Association Diagnostic and Statistical Manual*—Fourth Edition (DSM-IV). Washington, DC, American Psychiatric Assoc, 1994.

15. Malec JF. DSM-IV postconcussional disorder: recommendations. *J Neuropsychiatry Clin Neurosci* 1996; 8(1): 113.

16. Ruff RM. Discipline-specific approach versus individual care. In Varney NR, Roberts RJ (eds). *The Evaluation and Treatment of Mild Traumatic Brain Injury*, pp 99–113. Mahwah, NJ, Lawrence Erlbaum Assoc, 1999.

17. Varney NR. *Mild traumatic brain injury: separating facts versus interpretation.* Orlando, 20th Annual National Academy of Neuropsychology Meeting, Nov 2000.

18. Varney RN, Roberts RJ. Forces and accelerations in car accidents and resultant brain injuries. In Varney NR, Roberts RJ (eds). *The Evaluation and Treatment of Mild Traumatic Brain Injury*, pp 39–47. Mahwah, NJ, Lawrence Erlbaum Assoc, 1999.

19. Lezak MD. *Neuropsychological Assessment*, 3rd ed. New York, Oxford University Press, 1995.

20. Dixon CE, Taft WC, Hayes RL. Mechanisms of mild traumatic brain injury. *J Head Trauma Rehabil* 1993, 8(3): 1.

21. Povlishock JT, Coburn TH. Morpho-pathological changes associated with mild head injury. In Levin HS, Eisenberg HM, Benton AL (eds). *Mild Head Injury*, pp 37–53. New York, Oxford University Press, 1989.

22. Vollmer DG, Torner JC, Jane JA, *et al*. Age and outcome following traumatic coma: why do older patients fare worse? *J Neurosurg Report Traumatic Coma Data Bank* 1991; 75. 37–49.

23. Gualtieri CT. The pharmacologic treatment of mild brain injury. In Varney NR, Roberts RJ (eds). *The Evaluation and Treatment of Mild Traumatic Brain Injury*, pp 411–419. Mahwah, NJ, Lawrence Erlbaum Assoc, 1999.

24. Ruff RM, Camenzuli L, Mueller J. Miserable minority: emotional risk factors that influence the outcome of a mild traumatic brain injury. *Brain Inj* 1996; 10(8): 551.

25. Kay T. *Minor head injury: an introduction for professionals.* Washington, DC, National Head Injury Foundation, 1986; CEM 86–039. 2.

26. Wrightson P, Gronwall D. *Mild Head Injury—a Guide to Management,* New York, Oxford University Press, 1999.

27. Hartlage LC, Wilson DD, Roth JS. *Relationship between neuropsychological impairment severity and specific emotional sequelae.* San Antonio, TX, National Academy of Neuropsychology Meeting, Nov 1999.

28. McAllister TW, Flashman LA. Mild brain injury and mood disorders: casual connections, assessment, and treatment. In Varney NR, Roberts RJ (eds). *The Evaluation and Treatment of Mild Traumatic Brain Injury*, pp 347–373. Mahwah, NJ, Lawrence Erlbaum Assoc, 1999.

29. Cancelliere A, Livshits R. *Evidence that depression does not influence neuropsychological test performance.* San Antonio, TX, National Academy of Neuropsychology Meeting, Nov 1999.

30. Reitan RM, Wolfson DW. Emotional disturbances and their interaction with neuropsychological deficits. *Rev Neuropsychol* 1997; 7(1): 3.

31. Kay T. Interpreting apparent neuropsychological deficits. what is really wrong? In Sweet JJ (ed). *Forensic Neuropsychology Fundamentals and Practice*, pp 145–183. Lisse, The Netherlands, Swets and Zeitlinger, 1999.

32. Bell BD, Primeau M, Sweet JJ, *et al.* Neuropsychological functioning in migraine headache, non-headache chronic pain, and mild traumatic brain injury patients. *Arch Clin Neuropsychol*, 1999, 14(4): 389.

33. Tsushima WT, Newbill W. Effects of headaches during neuropsychological testing of mild head injury patients. *Headache* 1996; 36(10): 613–615.

34. Townsend L, Mateer CA. The effects of pain intensity on tasks of attention and memory. *Can J Psychol* 1997; 28(2a): 127.

35. Allen LM, Green P, Eimer BN. *The effect of pain on neurocognitive measures in patients demonstrating good effort, part two: data on measures of psychopathology and commonly used neuropsychological tests.* San Antonio, TX, National Academy of Neuropsychology Meeting, 1999.

36. Jarvis PE, Barth JT. *The Halstead Reitan neuropsychological battery. a guide to interpretation and clinical application*, p 305. Charlottesville, VA, University of Virginia Psychological Assessment Resources, 1994.

37. Horn LJ, Zaslar ND. *Medical Rehabilitation of Traumatic Brain Injury*, pp 134, 161. Philadelphia, Hanley & Belfus, 1996.

38. Leininger BE, Kreutzer JS. Neuropsychological outcome of adults with mild traumatic brain injury: implications for clinical practice and research. *Physical Medicine and Rehabilitation. State Art Rev* 1992; 6(1): 169.

39. Mateer CA. Assessment issues. In Raskin SA, Mateer CA (eds). *Neuropsychological Management of Mild Traumatic Brain Injury*, pp 39–69. New York, Oxford University Press, 2000.

40. Ruff RM, Grant I. Postconcussional disorder. background to DSM-IV and future considerations. In Varney NR, Roberts RJ (eds). *The Evaluation and Treatment of Mild Traumatic Brain Injury*, pp 315–325. Mahwah, NJ, Lawrence Erlbaum Assoc, 1999.

41. Brown SJ, Fann JR, Grant I. Postconcussional disorder: time to acknowledge a common source of neurobehavioral morbidity. *J Neuropsychiatry Clin Neurosci* 1994; 6(1): 15.

42. Hines ME. Posttraumatic headaches. In Varney NR, Roberts RJ (eds). *The Evaluation and Treatment of Mild Traumatic Brain Injury*, pp 375–410. Mahwah, NJ, Lawrence Erlbaum Assoc, 1999.

43. Jacobson EJ. Auditory/vestibular symptoms, evaluation and medico-legal considerations. In Jay GW. *Minor Traumatic Brain Injury. Diagnosis and Treatment*, pp 283–310. Boca Raton, CRC Press, 2000.

44. Barth JT, Macciocchi SN, Giordani B, *et al.* Neuropsychological sequelae of minor head injury. *Neurosurgery* 1983; 13(5): 529.

45. Reitan RM, Wolfson D. *The Halstead-Reitan Neuropsychological Test Battery: Theory and Clinical Interpretation*, 2nd ed. Tucson, Neuropsychology Press, 1993.

46. Raskin SA. Executive functions. In Raskin SA, Mateer CA. *Neuropsychological Management of Mild Traumatic Brain Injury*, pp 113–133. New York, Oxford University Press, 2000.

47. Hart T, Schwartz MF, Mayer N. Executive function: some current theories and their applications. In Varney NR, Roberts RJ (eds). *The Evaluation and Treatment of Mild Traumatic Brain Injury*, pp 133–148. Mahwah, NJ, Lawrence Erlbaum Assoc, 1999.

48. Politzer T. Vision function, examination and rehabilitation in patients suffering from traumatic brain injury. In Jay GW. *Minor Traumatic Brain Injury. Diagnosis and Treatment*, 311–328. Boca Raton, CRC Press, 2000.

49. Hartlage LC. Forensic aspects of mild brain injury. *Appl Neuropsychol* 1997; 4(1): 69.

50. Bigler ED. Neuroimaging in mild TBI. In Varney NR, Roberts RJ (eds). *The Evaluation and Treatment of Mild Traumatic Brain Injury*, pp 63–80. Mahwah, NJ, Lawrence Erlbaum Assoc, 1999.

51. Ruff RM, Crouch JA, Tröster AI, *et al*. Selected cases of poor outcome following a minor brain trauma: comparing neuropsychological and positron emission tomography assessment. *Brain Inj* 1994; 8(4): 297.

52. Prigatano GP, Johnson SC. *Neuroimaging studies and recovery of function after brain injury. implications for neuropsychological rehabilitation*. Orlando, 20th Annual National Academy of Neuropsychology Meeting, Nov 2000.

53. Friedman SD, Brooks WM, Jung RE, *et al*. Proton MR spectroscopic findings correspond to neuropsychological function in traumatic brain injury. *Am J Neuroradiol* 1998; 19: 1879.

54. Sinson G, Bagley LJ, Cecil KM, *et al*. Magnetization transfer imaging and proton MR spectroscopy in the evaluation of axonal injury: correlation with clinical outcome after traumatic brain injury. *Am J Neuroradiol* 2001; 22: 143.

55. Henry GK, Gross HS, Herndon CA, *et al*. Non-impact brain injury. neuropsychological and behavioral correlates with consideration of physiological findings. *Appl Neuropsychol* 2000; 7(2): 65.

56. Borczuk P. Predictors of intracranial injury in patients with mild head trauma. *Ann Emerg Med*, 1995; 25: 731.

57. Barth JT, Varney RN, Ruchinskas RA, *et al*. Mild head injury: the new frontier in sports medicine. In Varney NR, Roberts RJ (eds). *The Evaluation and Treatment of Mild Traumatic Brain Injury*, pp 81–98. Mahwah, NJ, Lawrence Erlbaum Assoc, 1999.

58. Ruff RM, Richardson AM. Mild traumatic brain injury. In Sweet JJ (ed). *Forensic Neuropsychology. Fundamentals and Practice*, pp 315–338. Lisse, The Netherlands, Swets and Zeitlinger, 1999.

59. Loring DW (ed). *International Neuropsychological Society Dictionary of Neuropsychology*. New York, Oxford University Press, 1999.

60. Neppe VM, Goodwin GT. Neuropsychiatric evaluation of the closed head injury of transient type (CHIT). In Varney NR, Roberts RJ (eds). *The Evaluation and Treatment of Mild Traumatic Brain Injury*, pp 149–208. Mahwah, NJ, Lawrence Erlbaum Assoc, 1999.

61. Reitan RM, Wolfson D. *The Halstead-Reitan Neuropsychological Test Battery. Theory and Clinical Interpretation*. Tucson, Neuropsychology Press, 1985.

62. Christensen A. *Luria's Neuropsychological Investigation*. New York, Spectrum, 1975.

63. Golden CJ, Hammeke TA, Purisch AD. *The Luria-Nebraska Neuropsychological Battery Manuals*. Los Angeles, Western Psychological Press, 1980.

64. Heaton RK, Grant I, Mathews CG. *Comprehensive Norms for an Expanded Halstead-Reitan Battery*. Odessa, FL, Psychological Assessment Resources, 1991.

65. Heaton RK. *Comprehensive Norms for an Expanded Halstead-Reitan Battery. a Supplement for the Wechsler Adult Intelligence Scale-Revised*. Odessa, FL, Psychological Assessment Resources, 1992.

66. Hartman DE. *Neuropsychological Toxicology. Identification and Assessment of Human Neuro-toxic Syndromes*, 2nd ed. New York, Plenum Press, 1995.

67. Raskin SA, Mateer CA, Tweeten R. Neuropsychological evaluation of mild traumatic brain injury. *Clin Neuropsychol* 1998; 12: 21.

68. Parker RS, Rosenblum A. IQ loss and emotional dysfunctions after mild head injury incurred in a motor vehicle accident. *J Clin Psychol* 1996; 52(1): 32.

69. Lee KE, Cox RH. Neuropsychology for the non-neuropsychologist: special guidance for working with persons with mild TBI (MTBI). In Jay GW. *Minor Traumatic Brain Injury. Diagnosis and Treatment,* pp 265–282. Boca Raton, CRC Press, 2000.

70. Sbordone RJ, Guilmette TJ. Echological validity: prediction of everyday and vocational functioning from neuropsychological test data. In Sweet JJ (ed). *Forensic Neuropsychology. Fundamentals and Practice,* pp 227–254. Lisse, The Netherlands, Swets and Zeitlinger Publishers, 1999.

71. Prigatano GP. *Principles of Neuropsychological Rehabilitation.* New York, Oxford University Press, 1999.

72. Hovland D, Mateer CA. Irritability and anger. In Raskin SA, Mateer CA (eds). *Neuropsychological Management of Mild Traumatic Brain Injury,* pp 187–201. New York, Oxford University Press, Publishers, 2000.

73. Teasell RW, McCain GA. Clinical spectrum and management of whiplash injuries. In Tollison CD, Satterthwaite JR (eds). *Painful Cervical Trauma. Diagnosis and Rehabilitative Treatment of Neuromusculoskeletal Injuries,* pp 292–318. Philadelphia, Williams & Wilkins, 1992.

74. Shapiro F. *Eye Movement Desensitization and Reprocessing: Basic Principles, Protocols and Procedures.* New York, Guilford Press, 1995.

75. Raskin SA, Stein PN. Depression. In Raskin SA, Mateer CA (eds). *Neuropsychological Management of Mild Traumatic Brain Injury,* pp 157–170. New York, Oxford University Press, 2000.

76. Sohlberg MM, Mateer CA. Effectiveness of an attention training program. *J Clin Exp Neuropsychol* 1987; 9(2): 117–130.

77. Hurt GD. Vocational rehabilitation. In Raskin SA, Mateer CA (eds). *Neuropsychological Management of Mild Traumatic Brain Injury,* pp 215–230. New York, Oxford University Press, 2000.

78. Padula WV, Shapiro JB, Jasin P. Head injury causing post-trauma vision syndrome. *N Eng J Optom* Dec 1988; 12: 16.

79. Padula WV. Neuro-optometric rehabilitation for persons with a TBI or CVA. *J Optom Vision Dev* 1992; 23(4): 5.

80. Padula WV, Argyris S. Traumatic vision syndrome and visual midline shift syndrome. *Neurorehabil* 1996; 6: 165.

81. Cripe LI. Use of the MMPI with mild closed head Injury. In Varney NR, Roberts RJ (eds). *The Evaluation and Treatment of Mild Traumatic Brain Injury,* pp 291–314. Mahwah, NJ, Lawrence Erlbaum Assoc, 1999.

82. Kessells RP, Aleman A, Verhagen WI, *et al.* Cognitive functioning after whiplash injury. a meta-analysis. *J Int Neuropsychol Soc* 2000; 6(3): 271–278.

13

Opioid Analgesia

Jack L Rook

A subset of chronic pain patients might benefit physically, functionally, and emotionally from the use of opioid analgesic maintenance therapy for management of chronic unrelenting pain. In the past, the use of opioids for CNMP was a controversial issue. For every physician who believed that narcotic analgesics were indicated for patients with chronic pain, objective pathologic processes, and failure of conservative and sometimes even surgical interventions, there were numerous opponents (medical and lay people, government agencies) who believed that such management was detrimental to the patient and to society. These beliefs developed for a number of reasons: the topic of pain management was poorly addressed in most medical schools and knowledge of opioid pharmacology was lacking in the medical community. As a result, opioids with a half-life of only 2 to 3 hours were given on an every 4- to 6-hour schedule, leaving patients to endure several hours of uncontrolled pain. Attempts by patients to increase dosage or frequency in such situations was perceived as abuse or drug-seeking behavior, when in effect it represented the patient's response to waning levels of medication and breakthrough pain.

Under-treatment of pain was the rule until the past few years. Indeed, many physicians went to great lengths to avoid the use of opioids. Multiple pharmacologic combinations with poorly tolerated medications, costly pain clinics, multiple surgical procedures, spinal-cord stimulator implantation, and neuroablative procedures (e.g., rhizotomy, sympathectomy, neurectomy) were formerly considered preferred treatments as opposed to around-the-clock opioid analgesic maintenance therapy.[1]

Reservations regarding the use of opioids often focus on the risk of opioid toxicity, although typically the development of addiction is overestimated. Knowledge of salient terminology (e.g., *addiction, tolerance, dependence, pseudoaddiction*) is generally deficient throughout the medical community and society. However, for physicians, it is the perceived risk of sanctions by governmental and medical agencies that has the greatest effect on prescribing practices.[2] Although no statutory limitations apply to the treatment of pain with opioid drugs,[3] many physicians perceive an unacceptable degree of risk in prescribing these drugs for patients with CNMP. Perceived sanctions might include investigation by the US Drug Enforcement Agency, a state medical board, or local peer review committees. Also, concern arises over liability if the patient does become iatrogenically addicted. Such perceived risks have a powerful conscious or subconscious effect on the prescribing habits of virtually all physicians. Physicians choosing to undertake prescription of opioid maintenance therapy for CNMP should follow a series of strict prescribing guidelines. Over the past few years, it has become the "standard of care" to provide patients with optimal pain management measures—including the appropriate use of opioid analgesics.[4,5]

FUNCTION OF OPIOIDS IN RELIEVING PAIN

Stimulation-Produced Analgesia

The concept that there was an independent and specific CNS network that modified pain sensation was first suggested by the observation that electrical stimulation of the midbrain in rats selectively suppressed responses to painful stimuli.[6,7] This phenomenon—stimulation-produced analgesia—was reproduced in humans when neurosurgeons placed electrodes in homologous sites and demonstrated how electrical stimulation produced a striking reduction of severe pain.[8–10] The periaqueductal gray area (PAG) and the rostroventral medulla (RVM) are regions in which electrical stimulation is highly effective in producing analgesia.[11–14] Both PAG and RVM are believed to be part of a descending pain modulatory network.

Opiates produce analgesia by a direct action on the CNS. In animal studies, microinjection of small amounts of narcotics into the brain stem can produce potent analgesia.[15,16] Similarly, application of opioids to the outer layers of the spinal cord has an additive analgesic effect.[17] Opiate-sensitive systems at both spinal cord and brain stem levels clearly seem to contribute to the narcotic analgesic effect.[18] Opiate analgesics such as morphine are believed to relieve pain by activating this descending pain modulatory network.

Opiate Receptors

The analgesia produced by opiate drugs depends on their ability to bind with opiate receptors on neuronal cell membranes. The opioid receptor function is described in terms of a *lock-and-key phenomenon*. Opiates bind to their receptors with varying affinity; the stronger the attachment, the greater the analgesic potency of the drug. For example, codeine (a mild narcotic), binds weakly to opioid receptors, whereas morphine, a drug with greater analgesic potency, has greater affinity for the same receptor.[19–22]

Dense concentrations of opiate-binding sites have been localized to the amygdala, hypothalamus, midbrain (PAG), medulla (RVM, nucleus raphe magnus), and spinal cord dorsal horn.[18–21] All of these regions are felt to be part of the descending pain-modulatory network. However, opioids produce a variety of *other* biological actions, aside from analgesia, including respiratory depression, pupillary constriction, decreased body temperature, and decreased gastrointestinal tract motility and constipation. These effects result from the presence of opiate receptors in tissues not involved in analgesia (e.g., medullary respiratory center, hypothalamus, intestines).[18] Four specific classes of opioid receptors have been identified: mu (μ), kappa (κ), delta (δ), and sigma (σ). The μ receptor seems to play a critical role in analgesia.

TERMINOLOGY

For the clinician who manages chronic pain patients with opioid analgesics, the terms *addiction, tolerance, dependence*, and *pseudoaddiction* must be understood. Addiction, a psychosocial phenomenon, differs from tolerance and physical dependence, which are due to pharmacological and biological properties of opioid analgesics. A patient can be tolerant or dependent on an opioid without being addicted to it. In general, the term addiction is used carelessly in clinical practice. Many physicians have an overwhelming fear of turning their patients into narcotics addicts. This fear, in conjunction with the fear of potential legal ramifications should addiction ensue, often leads to gross undertreatment of chronic pain. Although addiction is a potentially serious complication of opioid therapy, recent surveys suggest that in patients without a prior history of substance abuse, there is only a small risk of abuse behaviors following the short- or long-term administration of opioids.

Addiction

Addiction or *psychological dependence*, has been defined as a behavioral pattern of drug use characterized by overwhelming or compulsive use of a drug, the securing of its supply, and the high tendency to relapse after withdrawal.[23] More recently, the American Medical Association Task Force described addiction as a chronic disorder characterized by "the compulsive use of a substance resulting in physical, psychological, or social harm to the user and continued use despite that harm."[24] Loss of personal control over drug use distinguishes the addict from the patient who is merely physically dependent. Portenoy provides a definition of addiction relevant to the pain patient to whom opioid drugs are administered:[2]

> Addiction in the chronic pain patient can be defined as a psychologic and behavioral syndrome characterized by: (a) an intense desire for the drug and overwhelming concern about its continued availability (psychologic dependence); (b) evidence of compulsive drug use (unsanctioned dose escalation, continued dosing despite significant side effects, use of drug to treat symptoms not targeted by the therapy, or unapproved use during periods of no symptoms); and/or (c) evidence of one or more of a group of associated behaviors, including manipulation of the treating physician or medical system for the purposes of obtaining additional drugs (altering prescriptions, for example), acquisition of drugs from other medical sources or from a non-medical source, drug hoarding or sales, or unapproved use of other drugs, particularly alcohol or other sedatives/hypnotics during opioid therapy.

Pseudoaddiction

Addiction needs to be differentiated from the term *pseudoaddiction*, which refers to an iatrogenic syndrome characterized by abnormal behaviors that develop as a consequence of inadequate pain management. The natural history of pseudoaddiction includes progression through three characteristic phases including inadequate prescription of analgesics to manage the patient's pain, escalation of analgesic demands by the patient associated with behavioral changes to convince others of the pain's severity, and a crisis of mistrust between the patient and the health care team. The behavioral changes seen in pseudoaddiction can be alleviated through appropriate and timely analgesic administration to control the patient's level of pain.[25]

Addiction and pseudoaddiction are behavioral phenomena. The terms tolerance and dependence are biological sequelae resulting from the pharmacologic properties of opioids.

Tolerance

Tolerance can be defined as the need for higher doses of an opioid over time to maintain the same analgesic effect.[26] Tolerance to various opioid effects develops at different rates. Fatigue, nausea, and subtle cognitive dysfunction typically subside after the first two to three weeks of opioid therapy. Constipation may resolve over time, but it usually continues to be an ongoing problem, necessitating dietary changes or medical treatment. Tolerance to analgesia, the critical issue for therapy, is usually a slow process in CNMP patients with stable disease pathology. The literature suggests that patients with CNMP can usually be maintained on relatively stable doses of opioids for prolonged periods.

Dependence

Lastly, physical *dependence* is a pharmacologic property of the opioids characterized by the occurrence of an abstinence syndrome (withdrawal syndrome) after abrupt discontinuation of the drug or administration of an antagonist.[24,26–28] This term does not imply the aberrant psychological state or behaviors of the addicted or drug-abusing patient. Likewise, the term addiction should *not* be applied to patients who demonstrate only the potential for withdrawal.[2,29]

INDICATIONS FOR OPIOID ANALGESIC MAINTENANCE THERAPY

It is not uncommon for a physician to be presented with a patient whose quality of life, emotional status, and functional abilities have significantly deteriorated as a result of chronic pain. Often, unemployment, deconditioning, insomnia, frequent doctor or emergency-room visits, extensive diagnostic workup, and failed surgical procedures are other associated problems when a physician takes on a new chronic pain patient.

It is impossible to characterize those CNMP patients for whom opioid therapy is either particularly suited or contraindicated.[30] However, certain generalizations can be made. For example, chronic opioid treatment should be considered if it can improve the patient's quality of life, decrease overall health care costs, help patients to avoid potentially dangerous surgical procedures to alleviate pain, and if side effects from the opioids can be minimized.

After taking a comprehensive history, the physician might consider opioid therapy if it appears that:

- the patient has an appropriate diagnosis to justify the use of chronic opioids
- reasonable conservative measures have already failed to alleviate the pain
- functional abilities, quality of life (including quality of sleep), and level of depression can be improved
- use of the medical system (visits to emergency rooms, hospitalizations for pain management, additional or repeated medical testing) can be reduced, thereby decreasing health care costs.

Generally, researchers agree that chronic opioid therapy would not be justifiable if it further impaired function.[2] Ideally, function should improve with effective analgesia. However, if cognitive impairment, excessive sedation, and mood disturbances interfere with activity, the opioid should be switched, the dosage lowered, and occasionally, opioid therapy should be discontinued altogether.

Prior history of addiction to or abuse of prescription drugs (e.g., narcotics, benzodiazepines), alcohol, or street drugs should be viewed as a relatively strong contraindication for the use of prescribed opioids for CNMP.[2,31] If opioids are prescribed, informed consent, regular follow-up, close scrutiny of medication usage, and a contract stating that the drug will be discontinued at the first sign of abuse behavior, are often effective in keeping such patients from abusing the prescribed opioid.

The rapid development of tolerance with progressively escalating doses may make the use of opioids impractical. In general, the CNMP patient with unchanging pathology should remain comfortable for prolonged periods on relatively stable doses of opioids.[2] Rapid development of tolerance may be an early signal of psychological dependence.

PHARMACOLOGIC PROPERTIES OF OPIOIDS

The pharmacologic effects of opioids are based on their ability to bind to stereospecific opioid receptors; the greater the binding ability (affinity), the more potent the analgesic qualities of the drug. Three major categories of opioid receptors have been described, designated μ, κ, and δ. The putative effects mediated by these three main classes of receptors were delineated by Martin in 1976 (Table 13-1).[32]

The μ and κ receptors are concerned with analgesia. Mu receptors exert their effects principally at a supraspinal level. Agonist action at μ receptors results in both the analgesia and euphoria commonly associated with opioids. Other consequences of μ receptor activity include respiratory depression, meiosis, and reduced GI motility.[33]

Kappa receptors exert their analgesic effect at the spinal cord level. The outer layers of dorsal horn gray matter have dense concentrations of κ receptors, although κ receptors are found within the brain. Stimulation of kappa receptors causes less intense meiosis and respiratory depression than μ stimulation. Instead of euphoria, κ agonists produce dysphoria and sedation.[33] Because of these properties, κ agonists are felt to have lower potential for abuse than opioids with strong μ affinity.

Table 13-1 Three major categories of opioid receptors have been designated mu, kappa, and delta

Mu (μ)	kappa (κ)	delta (δ)
Miosis	Miosis	—
Supraspinal analgesia	Spinal analgesia	—
Euphoria	Sedation	Dysphoria
—	—	Hallucinations
—	—	Delusions
Respiratory depression	Respiratory depression	Respiratory stimulation
Physical dependence	—	Vasomotor stimulation

Reprinted by permission from Rook JL: Opioid analgesia. In Cassvan A, Weiss LD, Weiss JM, Rook JL, Mullens SU (eds). *Cumulative Trauma Disorders*, p186, Table 12-3. Boston, Butterworth-Heinemann, 1997.

Opioids affect the CNS (analgesia, sedation, euphoria, decreased hypothalamic hormone secretion, pupillary changes, depression of respiratory drive, suppression of cough, and effects on the nausea and vomiting centers in the brainstem), cardiovascular system, and GI tract.[20,34,35] The relief of pain is felt to occur by activation of the opioid-mediated descending pain inhibitory pathways. At the spinal cord level, opioids inhibit transmission of substance P from the primary nociceptors. There is also direct inhibition of second order pain transmission cells.[18,36–40]

Effects on the Hypothalamus

Morphine acts in the hypothalamus to inhibit the release of gonadotropin-releasing hormone (GnRH) and corticotropin-releasing factor (CRF), thus decreasing circulating concentrations of luteinizing hormone (LH), follicle stimulating hormone (FSH), and ACTH. As a result of decreased pituitary trophic hormones, plasma testosterone and cortisol concentrations will decline. In females, the menstrual cycle may be disrupted. However, with chronic administration, tolerance to the effect of opioids on the hypothalamic-releasing factors develops, resulting in normalization of menstrual cycles in woman, and circulating testosterone in men.[41,42]

Pupils

Morphine and most μ and κ opioid agonists cause pupillary constriction (meiosis) by an excitatory action on the nucleus of the oculomotor nerve. A pathognomic sign of opioid toxicity or overdosage is pinpoint pupils.[43]

Respiration

Morphine-like opioids depress respiration by a direct inhibitory effect on brainstem respiratory centers. The primary mechanism involves a reduction in the responsiveness of brainstem respiratory centers to carbon dioxide, and a depression of pontine and medullary centers involved in regulating respiratory rhythmicity. Therapeutic doses of opioids depress all phases of respiratory activity (rate, minute volume, and tidal exchange) and may also produce irregular breathing. In man, death from opioid poisoning is nearly always due to respiratory arrest.[20]

Cough

Morphine and related opioids also depress the cough reflex. This occurs, at least in part, by a direct effect on a cough center in the medulla.[43]

Nauseant and Emetic Effects

Nausea and vomiting produced by morphine and other μ agonist opioids are unpleasant but common side effects that result from the drugs' direct stimulation of the emesis center in the medulla. Certain individuals never vomit after morphine, whereas others do so each time the drug is administered. The nausea and vomiting is worse if the patient is ambulatory, suggesting a vestibular component.[43] In addition to the central actions, opioids decrease gastric motility, leading to abdominal bloating, discomfort, and increased risk of vomiting.

Cardiovascular System

Therapeutic doses of morphine-like opioids produce peripheral, arteriolar and venous dilatation. Peripheral edema, orthostatic hypotension and/or fainting may occur in some patients.[44]

Gastrointestinal Tract

In the stomach, relatively low doses of morphine decrease gastric motility, thereby prolonging gastric emptying time. Progressive gastric distension can further aggravate the centrally-induced nausea, and can increase the likelihood of esophageal reflux. Prolonged gastric emptying may retard absorption of orally administered medications.[44]

In the small intestine, morphine diminishes biliary, pancreatic, and intestinal secretions and delays digestion of food. The viscosity of bowel contents increases as water is more completely absorbed and intestinal secretions are decreased. This contributes to the problem of constipation.[45,46]

In the large intestine, four processes contribute to opioid-induced constipation.

1. Propulsive peristaltic waves are diminished or abolished in the colon.
2. The resulting delay in passage of feces causes considerable desiccation which further retards its advance through the colon.
3. Anal sphincter tone is greatly augmented.
4. The reflex anal sphincter relaxation response to rectal distension is reduced.[43,47]

ROUTES OF ADMINISTRATION

Opioids can be administered through a variety of routes including oral, rectal, intramuscular, intravenous, sublingual, subcutaneous, transdermal, via nasal inhalation, epidural, and intrathecal. Each patient's analgesic requirements may be different due to varying pathology, their individual perception of pain, how rapidly tolerance develops, and how efficiently the medication is metabolized. To properly prescribe opioids, physicians need to have a good working knowledge of the various preparations available, the medication's strength, duration of action, common side effects, typical dosages, mode of metabolism, and cost.

MORPHINE

Morphine remains the standard against which other opioid analgesics are measured. Morphine is a purified alkaloid obtained from opium. Many semisynthetic derivatives are made by relatively simple modifications of the morphine molecule.[43] Morphine is available for oral, rectal, intramuscular, intravenous, sublingual, epidural, and intrathecal administration.

With most opioids, including morphine, the effect of a given dose is less after oral than parenteral administration, due to variable but significant first pass metabolism in the liver. For example, it requires 60 mg of oral morphine to get similar blood levels as 10 mg of an intramuscular or subcutaneous dose. After oral or parenteral administration of morphine, its duration of analgesic action lasts somewhere in the range of 4 to 6 hours. The drug's half-life is 2 hours, and depending on the situation, its analgesic potency may be insufficient to control pain after only 2 or 3 hours. Therefore, patients treated with oral or parenteral morphine may require regular and frequent doses to maintain adequate analgesia.[44]

Morphine is available as a slow release oral preparation. Sustained-release morphine sulfate (SRMS) is available in 15, 30, 60, 100, and 200 mg tablets. Duration of action is in the range of 8 to 12 hours, so b.i.d. to t.i.d. dosing is possible. A dosage of 60 mg of SRMS b.i.d. would be the equivalent of taking 20 mg of oral morphine every 4 hours (6 doses per day). Certainly, b.i.d. dosing would be much more convenient.

Some key features of morphine sulfate, its sustained-release derivative, and other opioid preparations can be found in Table 13-2. Each drug has different features with respect to analgesic potency, duration of action, routes of administration, metabolism, combinations with nonopioid analgesics, receptors stimulated, side effects and toxicities. The opioids in Table 13-2 are categorized as having mild, intermediate, or strong analgesic potency.

SIDE EFFECTS

The physiological effects of opioids are described in Box 13-1. Important side effects, which may interfere with opioid treatment of chronic nonmalignant pain, include

Table 13-2 Common opioid analgesics

Generic Name	Trade names	Routes of administration	Half-life	Duration of action	Receptors stimulated	Metabolism	Advantages	Disadvantages
A. Mild Opioids:								
1. Propoxyphene hydrochloride (HCl): Propoxyphene napsylate	Darvon (propoxyphene HCl), Darvon Compound-65 (propoxyphene HCl, aspirin, caffeine), Darvon-N (propoxyphene napsylate 100 mg), Darvocet-N (propoxyphene napsylate (50 mg, 100 mg), acetaminophen 650 mg)	p.o.	6–12 hours	4–6 hours	Primarily μ	Liver and kidney		
2. Codeine	Tylenol 2 (15 mg codeine phosphate, 300 mg acetaminophen), Tylenol #3 (30 mg codeine phosphate, 300 mg acetaminophen), Tylenol #4 (60 mg codeine phosphate, 300 mg acetaminophen)	p.o., IM	4–6 hours	2–4 hours	Primarily μ	Liver and kidney	a. High oral to parenteral potency (in terms of total analgesia, codeine is about 60% as potent when given orally as when it is injected intramuscularly).	a. Short duration of action necessitates frequent dosing.

(continued)

Table 13-2 continued

Generic Name	Trade names	Routes of administration	Half-life	Duration of action	Receptors stimulated	Metabolism	Advantages	Disadvantages
							b. The abuse liability of codeine is lower than that of morphine. c. Suppresses cough (with dosages as low as 10–20 mg)	b. Dosage is limited by its combination with Tylenol. Maximum dosage should be about 12 per day because of the Tylenol
3. Pentazocine HCl	Talwin (pentazocine lactate), Talwin Compound (pentazocine HCl, aspirin 325 mg), Talwin NX (pentazocine hydrochloride and naloxone hydrochloride), Talacen (pentazocine HCl, acetaminophen 650 mg)	IM, subcutaneous, p.o.	4–7 hours	4–5 hours	Liver and kidney	Receptors stimulated: Pentazocine is a strong κ agonist and a weak antagonist or partial agonist of μ receptors	a. Because of the μ antagonist or partial agonist effects, there is less abuse potential. b. The action at κ receptors produces an analgesic effect. c. The addition of naloxone (opioid receptor antagonist) in Talwin NX dissuades against parenteral abuse of the drug	a. In higher dosages, pentazocine increases heart rate and blood pressure. It is therefore contraindicated in patients with coronary artery disease and hypertension. b. Pentazocine is irritating to subcutaneous and muscle tissues. c. Repeated injections over long periods of time will result in fibrosis and possible contractures

| 4. Hydrocodone bitartrate | Anexsia 5/500 (hydrocodone 5 mg, acetaminophen 500 mg), Anexsia 7.5/650 (hydrocodone 7.5 mg, acetaminophen 650 mg), Lorcet 10/650 (hydrocodone 10 mg, acetaminophen 650 mg), Lortab 2.5, 5 or 7.5/500 (hydrocodone 2.5, 5 or 7.5 mg and acetaminophen 500 mg), Vicodin (hydrocodone 5 mg, acetaminophen 500 mg), Vicodin ES (hydrocodone 7.5 mg, acetaminophen 750 mg), Vicodin HP (hydrocodone 10 mg, acetaminophen 660 mg) Norco (hydrocodone 10 mg, acetaminephen 325 mg) | p.o.; 5–10 mg (1–2 tablets) | 4–5 hours | 4 hours | Liver and kidney | Primarily μ | a. Antitussive qualities | a. Dosage limited by presence of Tylenol. b. Short duration of action |

(continued)

Table 13-2 continued

Generic Name	Trade names	Routes of administration	Half-life	Duration of action	Receptors stimulated	Metabolism	Advantages	Disadvantages
B. Intermediate Opioids: 1. Oxycodone HCl	Percodan (oxycodone 5 mg, aspirin 325 mg), Percocet (oxycodone 5 mg, Tylenol 325 mg), Tylox (oxycodone 5 mg, Tylenol 500 mg)	p.o.; 5–10 mg		4–5 hours	Liver and kidney	Primarily μ	a. Now available without acetaminophen in immediate release and sustained release preparations. The sustained release derivative, Oxycontin, is available in 10, 20, 40, 80, and 160 mg doses with b.i.d. or t.i.d. dosing for convenience. Without Tylenol, there is no ceiling dosage	a. With above preparations, the dosage is limited by Tylenol or aspirin (i.e. maximum of 8–12 tablets per day)
C. Strong Opioids: 1. Morphine sulfate	MS Contin, Oramorph SR, Roxanol, MSIR		6–8 hours for SRMS; 2–3 hours for MSIR		Opioid receptors stimulated: $\mu++$, $\kappa+$, $\delta+$	Morphine is metabolized in the liver and excreted in the kidneys. Small amounts of morphine will persist in the feces and urine for several days after the last dose	Sustained analgesia with less frequent dosing (SRMS)	Side effects (nausea, vomiting, and constipation), and cost (SRMS)

Drug	Trade/generic	Route			Metabolism	Receptor	Advantages	Disadvantages
2. Methadone HCl	Dolophine, methadone	IM, p.o.	15–40 hours	4–24 hours.	Biotransformation in the liver. Metabolites are excreted through the kidney and bile	μ+++, κ+	a. Inexpensive. b. Long duration of action. c. Often well tolerated with good analgesia and few side effects. d. Efficacy by the oral route. e. Because of its long duration of action, it is useful in treatment of addiction and detoxification.	a. Needs to be titrated slowly until optimal dosage is reached. Because of its long half-life, repeated doses may build up with increased sedation and confusion after a few days. b. In the United States, special controls on methadone have been enacted in an effort to prevent its unregulated large-scale use in the treatment of opioid addiction. c. Patients and physicians frequently do not want to use methadone because of its connotations with the addict population, despite its analgesic potency.

(continued)

Table 13-2 continued

Generic Name	Trade names	Routes of administration	Half-life	Duration of action	Receptors stimulated	Metabolism	Advantages	Disadvantages
3. Hydromorphone HCl	Dilaudid.	p.o. (2 and 4 mg tabs), rectal (3 mg), IM, subcutaneous.	2–3 hours	4–6 hours.	Liver and kidney.	Primarily μ.	a. Good, short-term analgesia.	a. Short duration of action. b. From personal experience, more subject to abuse.
4. Meperidine HCl	Demerol, Mepergan (meperidine 50 mg/Phenergan 25 mg).	IM, IV, subcutaneous, p.o.	3–4 hours	4–6 hours.	Liver and kidney.	Primarily μ.		a. Poor oral absorption (the oral to parenteral potency ratio is lower that than of codeine). b. Short duration of action. c. Large doses repeated at short intervals can produce tremors, muscle twitches, dilated pupils, hyperactive reflexes, and convulsions. These excitatory symptoms are due to the accumulation of normeperidine, a breakdown product of Demerol which has a half-life of 15–20 hours and is a CNS *excitant*.

		Duration	Metabolism	Receptor	Comments
					d. Since normeperidine is eliminated by both kidney and liver, decreased renal or hepatic function increases the likelihood of such toxicity.
5. Levorphanol tartrate	Levo-Dromoran. IM, IV, subcutaneous, p.o. (2 mg tabs)	6–8 hours	Liver and kidney	Primarily μ	a. Repeated administration at short intervals, may lead to accumulation of drug in plasma a. Clinical reports suggest that it produces less nausea and vomiting than morphine in sensitive patients. b. Long duration of action
6. Fentanyl	Sublimaze, Duragesic transdermal system	IM, IV, epidural, intrathecal, transdermal (Duragesic patches —25, 50, 75 and 100 μg/hr)	Duragesic patches last 72 hours. IM, IV or epidural/intrathecal administration only lasts 1–2 hours.	Liver and kidney	μ+++, κ+, δ+

a. Steady serum levels for prolonged periods with each patch.
b. Fentanyl is a selective μ agonist and is estimated to be 80 times as potent as morphine as an analgesic.
c. Its lipophilic qualities make it useful for transdermal application, and, when used with epidural or intrathecal routes, it does not migrate as far in the CSF as morphine, and provides potent analgesia for shorter periods

a. Cost of the transdermal patches.
b. Not available in oral form.[43,50,53]

Reprinted by permission from Rook JL. Opioid analgesia. In Cassvan A, Weiss LD, Weiss JM, Rook JL, Mullens SU (eds): *Cumulative Trauma Disorders*, pp 190, Table 12-4. Boston, Butterworth-Heinemann, 1997.

Box 13-1 The physiological effects of opioids.

CNS effects:
- analgesia
- sedation
- euphoria, tranquility, alterations of mood
- dysphoria (with κ stimulation)
- subtle cognitive impairment
- decreased hypothalamic hormone secretion
- pupillary changes (meiosis)
- depressed respiratory drive
- cough suppression
- stimulation of medullary emesis center

Cardiovascular System:
- peripheral arteriolar and venous dilatation

GI Tract:
- prolonged gastric emptying
- decreased biliary, pancreatic, and intestinal secretions
- constipation

Reprinted by permission from Rook JL. Opioid analgesia. In Cassvan A, Weiss LD, Weiss JM, Rook JL, Mullens SU (eds). *Cumulative Trauma Disorders*, p 196, Table 12-5. Boston, Butterworth-Heinemann, 1997.

respiratory depression, nausea, vomiting, constipation, sedation, and subtle cognitive impairment.

Almost all opioids produce adverse reactions, but those that do occur are generally manageable and nonhazardous.[30] Dangerous reactions such as respiratory depression occur rarely, if at all, in the literature on opioids and CNMP. The pain itself seems to have a stimulating effect on medullary centers for respiration. Nevertheless, this potential complication needs to be kept in mind, particularly with patients who have respiratory compromise (COPD, asthma, pneumonia, congestive heart failure, pneumonectomy patients). In such cases, opioids should be titrated slowly, with serial checking of arterial blood gases or pulse oxymetry. Sleep studies might be helpful in looking for the development of abnormal respiratory patterns, sleep apnea, and decreased oxygen saturation during sleep.

A combination of other adverse reactions such as fatigue, nausea, vomiting, and dizziness may also occur in the initial phase of opioid therapy. However, these effects often subside during the course of therapy.[30] In the case of persistent nausea, one of the following suggestions might prove helpful:

- waiting a few weeks after initiation of treatment to see if tolerance develops to this side effect
- switching to a different opioid which may be better tolerated
- trying the medication either with food or on an empty stomach. Opioids produce gastroparesis and the progressive buildup of food contents in the stomach may worsen nausea

- the regular use of low-dose metoclopramide (Reglan) may help promote gastric emptying if gastroparesis is contributing to the problem
- H_2 blockers and/or a proton pump inhibitor may prove helpful
- administering the opioid in combination with Phenergan or Vistaril will decrease nausea and these medications have the added effect of potentiating opioid analgesics.

Prevention of constipation is obligatory for patients managed on chronic opioids. This is one common side effect to which patients usually do not become tolerant.[30] Treatment measures would include adding fiber to the diet, stool softeners, and laxatives.

There is great concern that opioids might produce changes in cognition that might hamper rehabilitation and cause a deterioration of functional status. However, there seems to be a rather rapid development of tolerance to the subtle cognitive impairment produced by opioid drugs. This has been demonstrated in a study of cancer patients and clinical experience in the management of these patients suggests that chronic opioid administration is usually compatible with normal cognitive and psychologic functioning. None-the-less, it is true that occasional patients report persistent mental clouding sufficient to impair function.[2,48]

GUIDELINES FOR OPIOID MAINTENANCE THERAPY FOR NONMALIGNANT PAIN

The physician needs to have documentation of the patient's diagnoses. In addition, there should be mention of how the pain has affected the patient's quality of life, ability to function, sleep, and ability to engage in vocational or avocational pursuits. There needs to be documentation that all reasonable conservative measures have been tried and failed (physical therapy, TENS, psychological counseling, biofeedback, neurological blocks, epidural steroids, non-opioid analgesics, etc.).

Two important concepts that govern the use of opioids in the CNMP patient include: (1) By-the-ladder; (2) By-the-clock; approach to administration. The "by-the-ladder" approach to medication management of cancer and non-cancer pain has been outlined by the World Health Organization.[49] It states that there should be a step-wise approach to treatment of chronic pain, and that one of the steps might include the use of opioids (Figure 13-1).

The use of regularly scheduled doses (by-the-clock) should be applied in virtually all chronic opioid therapy. Most of the orally administered opioids have short half-lives and short durations of action. In many patients, use of these opioids provides only 2 to 3 hours of effective analgesia. Therefore, an every 4- to 6-hour dose regimen will result in one to several hours of breakthrough pain. A 4-time-per-day, "as required" opioid administration schedule with weak opioids, may produce a pseudoaddiction, in which recurrent pain produces drug seeking. The discontinuous use of analgesics results in dysphoria, increased pain, and craving for pain relief. This phenomenon is prevented by administration of the opioid on a regular basis at a dose that provides for pain prophylaxis and the prevention of breakthrough pain. The long-acting opioid derivatives

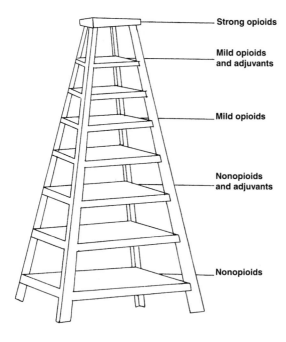

Strong opioids

Mild opioids
and adjuvants

Mild opioids

Nonopioids
and adjuvants

Nonopioids

Figure 13-1 The analgesic ladder. Reprinted by permission from Rook JL. Opioid analgesia. In Cassvan A, Weiss LD, Weiss JM, Rook JL, Mullens SU (eds). *Cumulative Trauma Disorders*, p 196, fig 12-3. Boston, Butterworth-Heinemann, 1997.

are particularly helpful in this regard. Longer acting opioids (SRMS, levorphanol, oxycontin, fentanyl patches, methadone) can be given less frequently. This results in better and more accurate compliance by the patient, fewer number of pills required per month, steady analgesia, and less chance of breakthrough pain.

A psychological screen is recommended prior to initiation of opioid treatment. Thorough evaluation of family history, social history, previous psychiatric history, and previous history of substance abuse (tobacco, alcohol, caffeine, illegal drugs), will enable the psychologist or psychiatrist to place the patient in a "potential risk for addiction" category of low, moderate, or high. Patients in the moderate to high-risk categories may still be candidates for chronic opioid therapy. However, they need to be watched closely for abuse behaviors and rapid development of tolerance.

In addition, the presence and severity of depression is readily identified in these psychological intake reports. Appropriate counseling and medications for patients identified as having major depression is critical so as to avoid an individual's use of opioids to "help forget about their worries," a situation that can lead to higher opioid dosages than actually called for by the individual's analgesic requirements. It is recommended that patients sign a consent form or contract upon initiation of chronic opioid therapy for nonmalignant pain (Figure 13-2).

Each patient with CNMP will have their own analgesic requirements, rates of drug absorption and metabolism, allergies, side effects, and previous histories of opioid use. Therefore, analgesic requirements will vary from case to case, even if similar diagnoses are involved. If a patient is to be changed from short-acting opioids to one of the longer acting preparations, equi-analgesic dose charts should be used (Table 13-3).[50,51]

Consent for Chronic Opioid Analgesic Maintenance Therapy

I, _____, consent to the use of chronic opioid/narcotic analgesic medications for the management of my chronic pain syndrome.

- I understand that a small percentage of patients on such therapy can develop psychological dependence to the opioids.
- I understand the following definitions:
  Addiction or psychological dependence refers to a set of aberrant behaviors marked by drug craving, efforts to secure its supply, interference with physical health or psychosocial function, and recidivism after detoxification.
  Tolerance refers to a decrease in the effect of a given narcotic over time.
  Dependence refers to the appearance of a withdrawal syndrome on abrupt cessation of the narcotic drug.
- I understand that the use of alcohol is not recommended while I am on chronic therapy.
- For female patients of childbearing age: I understand that a newborn will be physically dependent on opioids if these medications are taken chronically during the pregnancy.
- I agree to the medications as prescribed.
- I agree to receive my narcotic medications from only Dr. _____

_____
Date

_____
Patient (signature)

_____
Physician (signature)

Figure 13-2 Consent form for chronic opioid maintenance analgesic therapy. Reprinted by permission from Rook JL. Opioid analgesia. In Cassvan A, Weiss LD, Weiss JM, Rook JL, Mullens SU (eds). *Cumulative Trauma Disorders*, p 197, fig 12-4. Boston, Butterworth-Heinemann, 1997.

When starting treatment with opioid naive patients, low doses of weak preparations given around the clock should be used initially. There should be upwards titration until the patient experiences analgesic relief or unacceptable side effects. Frequent followup to evaluate the titration process is necessary in the early stages.

The physician needs to gauge side effects versus the beneficial analgesic qualities of the particular opioid. If the patient's functional level decreases, switch to a different drug, and if necessary discontinue opioid treatment completely and seek out other alternatives for pain management.

Watch closely for the appearance of abuse behaviors:

- frequent loss or theft of medications
- the patient's purse or luggage was stolen with the medications inside
- medications left out-of-town when returning from a trip
- calling in for medications early on a frequent basis
- rapid escalation of dose due to claims of tolerance, especially after a steady state dosage had provided sufficient analgesia for a prolonged period of time.

Table 13-3 Equianalgesic dose chart for oral (a) and transdermal (b) opioids. In (a), daily opioid dosage will be approximated to 15 mg, 30 mg and 60 mg of sustained release morphine sulfate (SRMS). In (b) oral morphine dose will be approximated to the Duragesic (fentanyl) transdermal system.

Medication	(a) Converting to SRMS 15 mg b.i.d.	Converting to SRMS 30 mg b.i.d.	Converting to SRMS 60 mg b.i.d
Tylenol #4 (codeine 60 mg)	6/day	12/day	*
Oxycodone 5 mg	6/day	12/day	*
Oral morphine	—	10 mg p.o. q.4h.	20 mg p.o. q.4h.
Hydromorphone	1 mg p.o. q.4h.	3 mg p.o. q.4h.	8 mg p.o. q.6h.
Methadone	10 mg p.o. b.i.d.	10 mg p.o. q.6h.	20 mg p.o. q.6h.
Meperidine	50 mg p.o. q.3h.	100 mg p.o. q.3h.	200 mg p.o. q.3h.
Levorphanol	—	2 mg p.o. q.6h. 4 mg p.o. q.6h.	

(b) Oral Morphine (mg/day)	Duragesic Dosage (mcg/hr)
45–134	25
135–224	50
225–314	75
315–404	100

*Cannot go above 12/day due to acetaminophen toxicity.
Reprinted by permission from Rook JL. Opioid analgesia. In Cassvan A, Weiss LD, Weiss JM, Rook JL, Mullens SU (eds). *Cumulative Trauma Disorders*, p 198, tables 12-6 & 12-7. Boston: Butterworth-Heinemann, 1997.

Such behaviors may also be indicative of iatrogenic pseudoaddiction, and each case needs to be evaluated carefully before punitive measures (cessation of opioids, discharge from care) are taken.

Refer patients for detoxification if addiction develops. Adjuvant medications will often potentiate the effects of opioid drugs. Catapres (clonidine) potentiates opioids, has its own analgesic qualities, and through central mechanisms it decreases sympathetic outflow, thereby minimizing withdrawal symptomatology as the opioid wears off or during detoxification. Tricyclic antidepressants, caffeine, and antihistamines may also potentiate the effects of opioids.

The prescribing physician should have thorough knowledge of the patient's overall medical condition. Opioids may be contraindicated, or lower doses required in patients with severe medical conditions, chronic renal failure or end stage renal disease, liver disease, or the elderly. Always consider cost of the medication.

Once the patient has been titrated to a steady state dosage, monthly followup to evaluate degree of analgesia, side effects, and functional status is recommended. Selected patients who have shown particular stability with their dosage for prolonged periods, can be seen at less frequent intervals. If any concerns arise about a particular patient and their use of opioids, get a second medical opinion, ideally from another physician with experience in the management of chronic pain.[2,31]

Recommended Prescribing Practices

Adherence to state and federal regulations goes a long way in protecting your medical practice from becoming a source of drug diversion and prescription drug abuse. You can also protect your practice by safeguarding blank prescription pads, prescribing controlled substances judiciously, and being on the lookout for patient scams. Forgery is a major source of drug diversion. Prescriptions are forged on prescription blanks stolen from physicians' offices, hospitals, and clinics. Whole pads or single sheets may be stolen. Forgers also alter legitimate prescriptions by changing the refill instructions or quantity to be dispensed, or by erasing the name of the drug prescribed and replacing it with a controlled substance. Specific suggestions for preventing diversion and abuse of *controlled substances* include the following.

- Do not leave prescription pads in unattended examination rooms, office areas, or anywhere they can easily be picked up.
- Stock only a minimum number of pads. When not in use, store surplus stock in a secure drawer or cabinet where they cannot be easily stolen.
- Report any prescription pad theft to the local police, the local pharmacy network, and state board of pharmacy.
- Write complete prescriptions with signature and appropriate date. Include the full name of the patient, and your name, address, and phone number.
- Do not pre-print your DEA registration number on your personalized blanks. Have a line present on the blank onto which your DEA number can be written as needed.
- Indicate the number of units and strengths to be dispensed by writing the number, and then spelling out the number of units, e.g. "10 (ten)."
- Indicate the number of refills for the prescription. If the acceptable number is zero, write "0" in the appropriate blank.
- Never sign prescription blanks in advance.
- Do not write for more than one controlled substance on a single blank; pharmacists must file prescriptions separately for scheduled drugs.
- Patiently, personally, and promptly respond to all calls from pharmacists who verify prescriptions for controlled substances. A corresponding responsibility rests with the pharmacist who dispenses the prescription order.
- Physicians may not order prescriptions to dispense narcotic drugs for detoxification or maintenance treatment of a person who is dependent on narcotic drugs unless separately registered with DEA, FDA, and state department of health as a narcotic treatment program.
- Prescribing, distributing, or giving schedule II controlled substances to a family member or to oneself except on an emergency basis should be avoided.
- There are prescription pads available that when photocopied bring out the word "Void." This will protect against photocopy forgery.

Clues for screening drug abusers.

Current behavior:
- must be seen right away; very agitated; "Found you in the phone book"
- makes a late afternoon (often Friday) appointment
- calls or comes in after regular hours
- must have a specific narcotic drug or other controlled substance right away
- gives evasive or vague answers to questions regarding medical history
- reluctant or unwilling to provide reference information
- traveling through town, visiting friends or relatives/not a permanent resident
- does not give a primary or referring physician
- states that specific non-narcotic analgesics do not work or that they are allergic to them
- lost or stolen prescription needs replacing.

Medical history:
- may admit to excessive use of coffee, cigarettes, alcohol, or other prescription drugs
- history of frequent trauma, burns, or breaks
- general debilitation.

Social history:
- repeated automobile accidents and/or drunk driving arrests
- difficulty with employment
- child abuse or severe family problems.

Psychological history:
- mood disturbances
- suicidal thoughts
- lack of impulse control
- thought disorders.

Physical examination:
- overt debilitation not related to medical problem
- physical findings out of proportion to patient's complaints
- unsteady gait
- slurred speech
- inappropriate pupil dilatation or constriction
- unexplained sweating or chills
- inappropriate lapses in conversation
- cutaneous signs of drug abuse (skin tracks and related scars on the neck, axilla, forearm, wrist, hand, foot, and ankle). Such marks usually are multiple, hyperpigmented and linear. New lesions may be inflamed
- "pop" scars from subcutaneous injections; abscesses, infections or ulcerations (this may be infective or chemical reactions to injections).[52,53]

REFERENCES

1. *Use of opioids in chronic noncancer pain-a multidisciplinary continuing education program.* Perdue Pharmaceuticals L.P., Norwalk, CT 06850-3590.

2. Portenoy RK. Chronic opioid therapy in non-malignant pain. *J Pain Symptom Manage* 1990;5.S: 46.

3. Haislip GR. Impact of drug abuse on legitimate drug use. In CS Hill, WS Fields (eds). *Advances in Pain Research and Therapy*, vol 11, p 205. Drug Treatment of Cancer Pain in a Drug-Oriented Society. New York, Raven, 1989.

4. Marcus DA. Treatment of not malignant chronic pain. *Amer Fam Physician*, 2000 61(5)1331, 1345. 25A.

5. Starr C. Opioid analgesia. an essential tool in chronic pain. *Patient Care*, 1998; 32(12): 47.

6. Fields HL, Basbaum AI. Brain stem control of spinal pain transmission neurons. *Ann Rev Physiol* 1978; 40: 217.

7. Mayer DJ, Price DD. Central nervous system mechanisms of analgesia. *Pain* 1976; 2: 379.

8. Richardson DE, Akil H. Pain reduction by electrical brain stimulation in man. *J Neurosurg* 1977; 47: 178.

9. Baskin DS, Mehler WR, Hosobuchi Y, *et al.* Autopsy analysis of the safety, efficacy, and cartography of electrical stimulation of the central gray in humans. *Brain Res* 1986; 371: 231.

10. Hosobuchi Y, Adams JE, Linchitz R. Pain relief by electrical stimulation of the central gray matter in humans and its reversal by naloxone. *Science* 1977; 197: 183.

11. Zorman G, Hentall ID, Adams JE, *et al.* Naloxone-reversible analgesia produced by microstimulation in the rat medulla. *Brain Res* 1981; 219: 137.

12. Abols JA, Basbaum AI. Afferent connections of the rostral medulla of the cat: a neural substrate for midbrain medullary interactions in the modulation of pain. *J Comp Neurol* 1981; 201: 285.

13. Beitz AJ. The organization of afferent projections to the midbrain periaqueductal gray of the rat. *Neuroscience* 1982; 7: 133.

14. Mantyh PW. The ascending input to the midbrain periaqueductal gray of the primate. *J Comp Neurol* 1982; 211: 50.

15. Leavens ME, Hill CS Jr, Cech DA, *et al.* Intrathecal and intraventricular morphine for pain in cancer patients: initial study. *J Neurosurg* 1982; 56: 241.

16. Nurchi G. Use of intraventricular and intrathecal morphine in intractable pain associated with cancer. *Neurosurgery* 1984; 15: 801.

17. Yeung JC, Rudy TA. Multiplicative interaction between narcotic agonists expressed at spinal and supraspinal sites of antinociceptive action as revealed by concurrent intrathecal and intracerebro-ventricular injections of morphine. *J Pharmacol Exp Ther* 1980; 215: 633.

18. Fields HL. Central nervous system mechanisms for control of pain transmission. In Fields HL (ed). *Pain*, p 99. New York, McGraw-Hill, 1987.

19. Chang K-J. Opioid receptors: multiplicity and sequelae of ligand-receptor interactions. In Conn RA (ed). *The Receptors*, vol 1, p 1. Orlando, Academic, 1984.

20. Martin WR. Pharmacology of opioids. *Pharmacol Rev* 1984; 35: 283.

21. Snyder SH, Matthysse S (eds). Opiate receptor mechanisms. *Neurosci Res Program Bull* 1975; 13: 1.

22. Kosterlitz HW. Opiate actions in guinea pig ileum and mouse vas deferens. *Neurosci Res Program Bull* 1975; 13: 68.

23. Jaffe JH. Drug addiction and drug abuse. In Gilman AG, Goodman LS, Rall TW, *et al.* (eds). *The Pharmacological Basis of Therapeutics*, 7th ed, p 532. New York, Macmillan, 1985.

24. Rinaldi RC, Steindler EM, Wilford BB, *et al.* Clarification and standardization of substance abuse terminology. *JAMA* 1988; 259: 555.

25. Weissman DE, Haddox JD. Opioid pseudoaddiction—an iatrogenic syndrome. *Pain* 1989; 36: 363.

26. Dole VP. Narcotic addiction, physical dependence, and relapse. *N Engl J Med* 1972; 286: 988.

27. Martin WR, Jasinski DR. Physiological parameters of morphine dependence in man—tolerance, early abstinence, protracted abstinence. *J Psychol Res* 1969; 7: 9.
28. Bruera E, Macmillan K, Hanson JA, *et al.* The cognitive effects of the administration of narcotic analgesics in patients with cancer pain. *Pain* 1989; 39: 13.
29. Virik K, Glare P. Pain management in palliative care—morphine and the new opioids in 2000. *Aust Fam Physician* 2000; 29(12): 1167.
30. Zenz M, Strumpf M, Tryba M. Long-term oral opioid therapy in patients with chronic non-malignant pain. *J Pain Symptom Manage* 1992; 7: 69.
31. College of Physicians and Surgeons of British Columbia. *Guidelines for management of chronic non-malignant pain.* Vancouver, BC. College of Physicians and Surgeons of British Columbia, 1993.
32. Martin WR, Eades CG, Thompson JA, *et al.* The effects of morphine and nalorphine-like drugs in nondependent and morphine-dependent chronic spinal dog. *J Pharmacol Exp Ther* 1976; 197: 517.
33. Pfeiffer A, Brantl V, Herz A, *et al.* Psychotomimesis mediated by opiate receptors. *Science* 1986; 233: 774.
34. Martin WR, Sloan JW. Neuropharmacology and neuro-chemistry of subjective effects, analgesia, tolerance, and dependence produced by narcotic analgesics. In Martin WR (ed). *Handbook of Experimental Pharmacology, vol 45. Drug Addiction I. Morphine, Sedative/Hypnotic and Alcohol Dependence*, p 43. Berlin, Springer-Verlag, 1977.
35. Duggan AW, North RA. Electrophysiology of opioids. *Pharmacol Rev* 1983; 35: 219.
36. Glazer EJ, Basbaum AI. Axons which take up (3H) serotonin are presynaptic to enkephalin immunoreactive neurons in cat dorsal horn. *Brain Res* 1984; 298: 389.
37. Ruda MA. Opiates and pain pathways. Demonstration of enkephalin synapses on dorsal horn projection neurons. *Science* 1982; 215: 1523.
38. Fields HL, Emson PC, Leigh BK, *et al.* Multiple opiate receptor sites on primary afferent fibers. Nature 1980; 284: 351.
39. Hiller JM, Simon EJ, Crain SM, *et al.* Opiate receptors in culture of fetal mouse dorsal root ganglia (DRG) and spinal cord. Predominance in DRG neurites. *Brain Res* 1978; 145: 396.
40. Mudge AW, Leeman SE, Fischbach GD. Enkephalin inhibits release of substance P from sensory neurons in culture and decreases action potential duration. *Proc Natl Acad Sci USA* 1979; 76: 526.
41. Howlett TA, Rees LH. Endogenous opioid peptides and hypothalamo-pituitary function. *Annu Rev Physiol* 1986; 48: 527.
42. Grossman A. Opioids and stress in man. *J Endocrinol* 1988; 119: 377.
43. Jaffe JH, Martin WR. Opioid Analgesics and antagonists. In Gilman AG, Goodman LS (eds). *The Pharmacological Basis of Therapeutics*, p 485. New York, McGraw-Hill, 1990.
44. Goldstein A. Opioid peptides: function and significance. In Collier HOJ, Hughes J, Rance MJ, *et al.* (eds). *Opioids. past, present and future*, p 27. London, Taylor & Frances, 1984.
45. Duthie DJR, Nimmo WS. Adverse effects of opioid analgesic drugs. *Br J Anaesth* 1987; 59: 61.
46. Dooley CP, Saad C, Valenzuela JE. Studies of the role of opioids in control of human pancreatic secretion. *Dig Dis Sci* 1988; 33: 598.
47. Manara L, Bianchetti A. The central and peripheral influences of opioids on gastrointestinal propulsion. *Ann Rev Pharmacol Toxicol* 1985; 25: 249.
48. Bruera E, Macmillan K, Hanson JA, *et al.* The cognitive effects of the administration of narcotic analgesics in patients with cancer pain. *Pain* 1989; 39: 13.
49. World Health Organization. *Cancer pain relief.* Geneva, World Health Organization, 1986.
50. *Physician's Desk Reference*, 48th ed. Montvale, NJ, Medical Economics, 1994.
51. *Dosing Conversion Reference.* East Norwalk, CT, The Perdue Frederick Co, 1991.
52. *Colorado Guidelines of Professional Practice for Controlled Substances—Physicians.* Denver, Colorado Department of Health, 1993.
53. Roth SH, Fleischmann RM, Burch FX, *et al.* Around-the-clock, controlled-release oxycodone therapy for osteoarthritis-related pain. placebo-controlled trial and long-term evaluation. *Arch Intern Med* 27, 2000, 160(6): 853.

14

Spinal Cord Stimulation

Jack L Rook

In 1967, Dr. Norman Shealy published an article describing a new technique for the management of chronic intractable pain.[1] The process used radio frequency-induced electrical stimulation of the spinal cord via electrodes implanted over the dorsal columns. This original technique was termed *dorsal column stimulation.* Over time, the term *spinal cord stimulation* (SCS) came to be used to describe this technique. The original surgical procedure was cumbersome, involving subarachnoid implantation of a monopolar electrode via laminectomy.[2]

Since that time, the field of SCS has grown immensely with major advances in various areas. Electrodes previously placed intrathecally are now placed in the epidural space, resulting in fewer complications. The open technique (i.e., surgically implanted electrodes via laminotomy) for electrode implantation has been replaced by a percutaneous technique done under fluoroscopic guidance. Electrodes have evolved from monopolar to multipolar to dual multipolar leads. Multipolar electrodes cover larger areas of the spinal cord for stimulation purposes. Advances in computer technology, miniaturization of circuitry and hardware, and improvements in the biochemistry of hardware have led to more reliable and more comfortable equipment. Careful screening procedures now used result in better outcome data.[3]

PATIENT SELECTION CRITERIA

SCS may prove helpful in treating a variety of painful conditions. However, it is important to adhere to a number of general patient selection criteria.

Characteristics of the Patient

As SCS is a costly procedure, patients must be selected carefully. If rigid criteria for selection are followed, 60 to 80 percent efficacy can be expected with spinal neuro-augmentation.[4–11] For SCS to be considered, documentation should state that all reasonable conservative pain management techniques for the patient have failed. Also, the typical prospective patient would express a desire to avoid extensive surgical procedures. Most protocols for SCS require patients to detoxify from opioid analgesics prior to consideration for the procedure. At the very least, successful stimulation in patients on opioids should lead to gradual tapering of the analgesic. SCS could be considered as an alternative to neuro-ablative procedures and extensive surgeries.

Psychopathologic elements contributing to or causing the pain must be determined through careful screening that includes a thorough psychological evaluation and appropriate testing (e.g., the Minnesota Multiphasic Personality Inventory, Wahler Symptom Inventory, Zung Scale, Beck Depression Index, Behavioral Analysis of Pain, McGill Pain Questionnaire). Patients with a somatoform pain disorder should not be considered for the SCS procedure. Depression, common in chronic pain, may actually lessen with successful SCS. Underlying psychopathologic components must be treated before any consideration of spinal neuro-augmentation.

The pain should not be complicated by nor contribute to any secondary gain, either emotional or financial. For some patients involved in litigation, magnified pain behaviors may be present, driven consciously or subconsciously in an effort to effect final settlement. Ideally, complicated legal issues and litigation should be resolved before implantation. Obviously, this contingency is not always possible. Patients with drug-seeking behavior or substance abuse should be excluded from consideration until detoxification and sobriety are well established.

Last, patients must have realistic expectations regarding results from the SCS procedure. They must understand that SCS may reduce but not necessarily eliminate the pain, that SCS is not a cure for the underlying problem, that permanent implantation will be considered only if trial stimulation provides *significant* pain relief, and that careful and regular follow-up will be necessary for a postoperative period.[3,12,13]

Characteristics of the Pain

The more localized the pain in the extremity, the better the response will be; a unilateral painful extremity will respond better to stimulation than both extremities. Bilateral extremity pain will respond to stimulation, but the electrode must be located in the midline. Trunk pain is not treated well by SCS. The more diffuse the pain problem, the less successful the procedure will be. Stimulation trials still may be indicated even if patients do not fulfill these criteria.[3,5–7,12–29] The literature supports the use of SCS in the management of peripheral causalgia and reflex sympathetic dystrophy syndrome (RSDS).[30–35]

Over the years, hundreds of articles about SCS have been published. More recent literature consistently reports a decrease in subjective pain intensity in the majority of patients undergoing the procedure, a decrease in their oral narcotic requirements, and an increase in their functional and working capacity. Also commonly accepted is that SCS has become an easily implemented, low-morbidity technique for treatment of properly selected intractable chronic nonmalignant pain (CNMP) patients. In benign chronic pain problems, stimulation is superior to many other methods, especially destructive surgery. It is expected that applications for SCS will continue to expand with improvements in technology and with more widespread understanding and acceptance of the methods involved.[4–11]

TECHNIQUE

Trial Stimulation

Trial stimulation is necessary to:

- determine whether the patient will respond to spinal cord stimulation
- help the patient to decide whether to proceed with the implantation procedure
- avoid the needless, high cost of direct implantation of a permanent system if the quality of analgesia is insufficient or poor
- help the surgeon to determine the optimum site for electrode positioning and optimal SCS programmable unit parameters before undertaking a permanent procedure.

Major components necessary for trial stimulation include the electrode lead (monopolar or multipolar), an extension wire, and a power source. Multipolar leads provide more precise stimulation. Permanent leads also can be used (although at greater cost) if the anticipation is that the patient ultimately will undergo a permanent placement procedure.

The patient undergoes a trial stimulation procedure as an outpatient. An intravenous line is started, and the patient is given pretrial antibiotic coverage and is placed in the prone position. Some sedation may be used, but the patient must remain lucid and able to answer questions about the location of the paresthesias created by stimulation.

After iodophor solution preparation, the patient receives a local anesthetic-field block at the site of epidural needle insertion. At the appropriate inter-space, a large (15- to 16-gauge) needle is inserted into the epidural space. Needle and subsequent electrode position are visualized fluoroscopically. The test lead is placed through the needle and is advanced into the epidural space. Patience is required for proper positioning of the electrode, as the electrically induced paresthesias need to cover the painful dermatomes. For bilateral stimulation, the lead electrodes should be as close as possible to the midline (i.e., lying adjacent to the dorsal median sulcus). For unilateral stimulation, the electrode can be placed near the dorsolateral sulcus (Figure 14-1).

Pain relief is not absolutely necessary at this point. If it does occur, outcome will most likely be excellent. If it does not occur, analgesia may be achieved on an outpatient basis once optimal radio frequency-stimulation parameters are found. When appropriate paresthesias are created, the epidural needle is removed with special care so as not to dislodge the lead electrode. The electrode position is verified again with the fluoroscope. A suture fixes the lead to the skin.

After the procedure, the patient may be sent home with a temporary unit attached to the lead electrode. The lead can remain in place for 7–10 days, during which the patient will experience the electrically induced paresthesias and gauge the pain relief. Stimulator parameters may need adjustment on a daily basis. After the 10-day trial, the patient should be able to determine whether to proceed with permanent implantation. If permanent implantation is chosen, the test lead is removed, and the permanent implantation process proceeds. If permanent leads were used for the trial, they are left in place, and the implantation process is completed.[3,12,36–40]

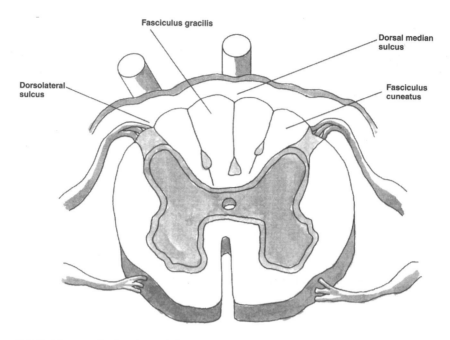

Figure 14-1 Electrode lead position. For unilateral stimulation, the electrode can be placed near the dorsolateral sulcus. For bilateral stimulation, single-lead electrodes should be as close as possible to the midline, or dual electrodes can be placed in the more lateral positions. Reprinted by permission from Rook JL. Spinal cord stimulation. In Cassvan A, Weiss LD, Weiss JM, Rook JL, Mullens SU (eds): *Cumulative Trauma Disorders*, p 214, fig 14-1. Boston, Butterworth-Heinemann, 1997.

Permanent Implantation

Permanent implantation is performed in the operating room with strict sterile technique and antibiotic coverage. Once again, the patient will require conscious sedation. As noted earlier, the temporary lead from trial stimulation is removed; however, if a permanent lead was used initially, it is left in place, and the procedure is completed. If a new permanent lead is required, it is inserted with the previously outlined technique, with fluoroscopic guidance and the patient's interpretation of the electrically induced paresthesias. Once optimal lead positioning is found, the permanent lead is anchored by suture to the supraspinous ligament.

Then the patient goes under general anesthesia following which he/she is placed in the lateral decubitus position for implantation of the spinal cord stimulator pulse generator (SCSPG) (Figure 14-2). Possible locations for the SCSPG include the anterolateral chest for leads placed in the cervical or upper thoracic area and the abdomen or buttocks for lower-extremity stimulation leads. A large subcutaneous pocket is created for insertion of the SCSPG.

Next, a subcutaneous tunnel is created to run from the pocket to the midline back incision. An extension wire placed in the tunnel connects the lead wire to the SCSPG unit.

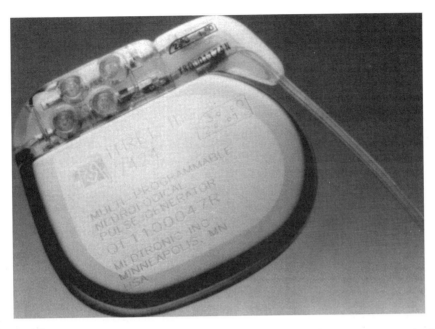

Figure 14-2 The spinal cord stimulator pulse generator. The Medtronic ITREL II pulse generator delivers electrical impulses via an insulated lead electrode. (Courtesy of Medtronic, Inc., Minneapolis, MN.) Reprinted by permission from Rook JL. Spinal cord stimulation. In Cassvan A, Weiss LD, Weiss JM, Rook JL, Mullens SU (eds): *Cumulative Trauma Disorders*, p 215, fig 14-2. Boston, Butterworth-Heinemann, 1997.

The patient is awakened. The system is activated and tested for integrity. If stimulation is satisfactory, the wounds are irrigated, closed, and dressed, and the patient is transferred to the recovery room.[3,12,41]

Postimplantation Care

The SCSPG has a number of programmable parameters, and optimal settings vary from patient to patient. Such settings must be determined for each patient, through trial and error, after implantation. Some patients need very little stimulation for pain relief; others require continuous stimulation with high-voltage requirements.

The programmable parameters include pulse amplitude, or intensity of the stimulus (0–10.5 V); pulse frequency (2–130 Hz); pulse width (60–450 microseconds); and stimulation cycles (on: 0.1–64.0 seconds; off: 0.4 seconds–17 minutes). SCS units (both internally and externally controlled systems) are available. Stimulation parameters for the ITREL system are set by the clinician via a desktop programming console and a hand-held programmer (Figures 14-3 and 14-4). With external systems, an implanted receiver receives signals from a belt-mounted transmitter.

During the early postoperative period, physician guidance is necessary for parameter adjustment of both internal and external systems. However, with external systems, the

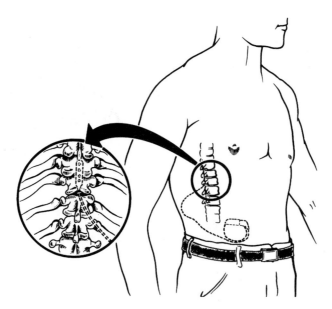

Figure 14-3 The Medtronic ITREL implantable spinal cord stimulation system has a completely internalized pulse generator and one quadripolar lead. (Courtesy of Medtronic, Inc., Minneapolis, MN.) Reprinted by permission from Rook JL. Spinal cord stimulation. In Cassvan A, Weiss LD, Weiss JM, Rook JL, Mullens SU (eds): *Cumulative Trauma Disorders*, p 216, fig 14-3. Boston, Butterworth-Heinemann, 1997.

goal is for patients to become independent in turning the unit off and on, and in changing parameters (amplitude, frequency, and pulse width) by using the portable external programmer. During the postoperative period, attempts are made to find the lowest possible parameter settings that simultaneously provide pain relief and preserve battery life. Patients are encouraged to turn off or turn down the parameters of the SCSPG when pain is well controlled.

Patients should be checked regularly until wounds are well healed and sutures are removed. They are given a number of responsibilities.[3,42]

- Avoidance of stooping, bending, twisting, and lifting for the first six to eight weeks after surgery to maintain proper electrode position during the period it is most prone to dislodge.
- Avoidance of chiropractic treatment for six to eight weeks and sparing, cautious treatments after that time.
- Avoidance of wetting the transmitter (assuming use of an external transmitter device), which is not waterproof.
- Avoidance of magnetic resonance imaging scans.
- Gradual return to daily activities (traveling, sex, and vocational and avocational pursuits) as tolerated and based on the improved quality of analgesia.

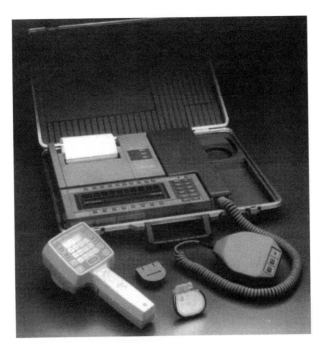

Figure 14-4 Stimulation parameters for the ITREL system are set by the clinician using a desk-top programming console and a hand-held programmer (bottom left). The desktop programming console (top) also programs the pulse generator and provides printouts of information from it. (Courtesy of Medtronic, Inc., Minneapolis, MN.) Reprinted by permission from Rook JL. Spinal cord stimulation. In Cassvan A, Weiss LD, Weiss JM, Rook JL, Mullens SU (eds): *Cumulative Trauma Disorders*, p 216, fig 14-4. Boston, Butterworth-Heinemann, 1997.

GOALS OF TREATMENT

Researchers generally agree that, when applied to appropriate patients by trained practitioners, realistic goals of treatment include 60 to 70 percent efficacy, 50 to 75 percent pain relief when efficacious, reduction in narcotic-analgesic intake, improvement in activity levels and quality of life, and elimination of need for further surgery.[4–11,13]

COMPLICATIONS

Problems and complications associated with SCS implantation include failure, infection, lead migration, electrode damage, and battery failure. Even selecting patients through a careful screening process does not guarantee the efficacy of SCS. According to the literature, failure rates of 20 to 40 percent can be expected.[4–11]

Infection, the most serious complication, occurs in 1.5 to 10 percent of cases.[43] It can involve the epidural space or the SCSPG pockets. Epidural infection, characterized by increasing blood pressure, fever, chills, and leukocytosis mandates aggressive treatment that includes electrode removal, appropriate cultures, and intravenous antibiotics. If infection is untreated, sepsis, spinal cord injury, meningitis, and even death can result. If infection is treated appropriately, long-term morbidity is rare, and the electrode or SCSPG can be replaced at a later time.

Lead migration is common, especially in active individuals. Lead migration will require opening of the back wound for repositioning of the lead. Battery failure is inevitable over time. Continuous high-voltage stimulation will cause a more rapid drain on the lithium cell, whereas patients who turn the unit off when resting, use the lowest possible parameters (without sacrificing pain relief), and use intermittent (cycling mode) stimulation will slow battery depletion. Battery replacement requires a minor surgical procedure.

Lead fractures, although uncommon, may occur if electrodes are mishandled or traumatized during implantation. A more common occurrence is disruption of the insulating sheath around the leads with abnormal stimulatory patterns or complete cessation of stimulation. Such problems necessitate lead removal and reimplantation.[3]

CONCLUSION

For some patients with chronic nonmalignant pain, spinal cord stimulation could represent a particularly attractive alternative to treatment options that often include living with the pain, ongoing sympathetic blockade, neuro-ablative/neurolytic procedures, long-term opioid intake, or further surgical attempts at correcting underlying pathologic conditions.

For the procedure to be successful, patients must be selected carefully, depression must be treated optimally, and opioids must be tapered as much as possible. Centralized disease with diffuse body pain will not respond as well as will localized pain confined to a single extremity. Success of SCS depends also on the patient not having serious psychopathologic characteristics identified on psychological screening procedures.

For appropriate patients, SCS is a nondestructive, reversible, low-morbidity procedure. Patients can be screened for response prior to implantation of a permanent system.

REFERENCES

1. Shealy CN, Mortimer JT, Reswick J. Electrical inhibition of pain by stimulation of the dorsal column: preliminary clinical reports. *Anesth Analg* 1967; 46: 489.
2. Shealy CN, Mortimer JT, Hagfors NR. Dorsal column electroanalgesia. *J Neurosurg* 1970; 32: 560.
3. Robb LG, Spector G, Robb M. Spinal cord stimulation neuroaugmentation of the dorsal columns for pain relief. In Weiner RS (ed). *Innovations in Pain Management—A Practical Guide for Clinicians*, p 33. Orlando, FL, Deutsch Press, 1993.
4. North RB, Ewend MG, Lawton MT, *et al.* Spinal cord stimulation for chronic, intractable pain. superiority of "multichannel" devices. *Pain* 1991; 44: 119.
5. Meglio M, Cioni B, Rossi GF. Spinal cord stimulation in management of chronic pain. a nine-year experience. *J Neurosurg* 1989; 70: 519.

6. Racz GB, McCarron RF, Talboys P. Percutaneous dorsal column stimulator for chronic pain control. *Spine* 1989; 14: 1.

7. Spiegelmann R, Friedman WA. Spinal cord stimulation. a contemporary series. *Neurosurgery* 1991; 28: 65.

8. North RB, Ewend MG, Lawton MT, *et al.* Failed back surgery syndrome: 5-year follow-up after spinal cord stimulator implantation. *Neurosurgery* 1991; 28: 692.

9. DeLaPorte C, Siegfried J. Lumbosacral spinal fibrosis (spinal arachnoiditis). *Spine* 1983; 8: 593.

10. Kumar K, Wyant GM, Ekong CE. Epidural spinal cord stimulation for relief of chronic pain. *Pain Clin* 1986; 1(2): 91.

11. Ray CD. Implantation of spinal cord stimulators for relief of chronic and severe pain. In Cauthen JC (ed). *Lumbar Spine Surgery. Indications, Techniques, Failures, and Alternatives*, 2nd ed, p 350. Baltimore, Williams & Wilkins, 1988.

12. North RB, Kidd DH, Zahurak M, *et al.* Spinal cord stimulation for chronic, intractable pain: experience over two decades. *Neurosurgery* 1993; 32: 384.

13. Medtronic, Inc. *Spinal cord stimulation—background and efficacy.* Minneapolis. Medtronic, Inc., 1991.

14. Kumar K, Nath R, Wyant GM. Treatment of chronic pain by epidural spinal cord stimulation: a 10-year experience. *J Neurosurg* 1991; 75: 402.

15. Law JD. Targeting a spinal stimulator to treat the "failed back surgery syndrome." *Appl Neurophysiol* 1987; 50: 437.

16. Meilman PW, Leibrock LG, Leong FTL. Outcome of implanted spinal cord stimulation in the treatment of chronic pain: arachnoiditis versus single nerve root injury and mononeuropathy. *Clin J Pain* 1989; 5: 189.

17. Ray CD, Burton CV, Lifson A. Neurostimulation as used in a large clinical practice. *Appl Neurophysiol* 1982; 45: 160.

18. Sweet W, Wepsic J. Stimulation of the posterior columns of the spinal cord for pain control. *Clin Neurosurg* 1974; 21: 278.

19. Burton C. Dorsal column stimulation: optimization of application. *Surg Neurol* 1975; 4: 171.

20. Clark K. Electrical stimulation of the nervous system for control of pain. University of Texas Southwestern Medical School experience. *Surg Neurol* 1975; 4: 164.

21. de Vera JA, Rodriguez JL, Dominguez M, *et al.* Spinal cord stimulation for chronic pain mainly in PVD, vasospastic disorders of the upper limbs and failed back surgery. *Pain* 1990; Suppl 5: 81.

22. Erickson DL, Long DM. Ten-year follow-up of dorsal column stimulation. In Bonica JJ (ed). *Advances in Pain Research and Therapy*, vol 5, p 583. New York, Raven, 1983.

23. Hoppenstein RL. Electrical stimulation of the ventral and dorsal columns of the spinal cord for relief of chronic intractable pain. *Surg Neurol* 1975; 4: 187.

24. Long DM, Erickson DE. Stimulation of the posterior columns of the spinal cord for relief of intractable pain. *Surg Neurol* 1975; 4: 134.

25. Long DM, Erickson D, Campbell J, *et al.* Electrical stimulation of the spinal cord and peripheral nerves for pain control. *Appl Neurophysiol* 1981; 44: 207.

26. Nielson KD, Adams JE, Hosobuchi Y. Experience with dorsal column stimulation for relief of chronic intractable pain. *Surg Neurol* 1975; 4: 148.

27. Young RF, Shende M. Dorsal column stimulation for relief of chronic intractable pain. *Surg Forum* 1976; 27: 474.

28. Brandwin MA, Kewman DG. MMPI indicators of treatment response to spinal epidural stimulation in patients with chronic pain and patients with movement disorders. *Psychol Rep* 1982; 51: 1059.

29. Daniel M, Long C, Hutcherson M, *et al.* Psychological factors and outcome of electrode implantation for chronic pain. *Neurosurgery* 1985; 17: 773.

30. Hassenbusch SJ, Stanton-Hicks M, Walsh J, *et al. Effects of chronic peripheral nerve stimulation in stage iii reflex sympathetic dystrophy (RSD).* Cleveland, Cleveland Clinic Foundation, 1992.

31. Racz GB, Lewis R, Heavner JE, *et al.* Peripheral nerve stimulator implant for the treatment of causalgia. In Stanton-Hicks M (ed). *Pain and the Sympathetic Nervous System.* Norwell, MA. Kluwer Academic, 1990.
32. Schwartzman RJ. New treatments for reflex sympathetic dystrophy. *N Eng J Med* 2000; 343(9): 654.
33. Claeys LGY. Correspondence: reflex sympathetic dystrophy. *N Eng J Med* 2000; 343(24): 1811.
34. Kemler MA, Barendse GAM, Van Kleef M, *et al.* Spinal cord stimulation in patient with chronic reflex sympathetic dystrophy. *N Eng J Med* 2000; 343(9): 618.
35. Kemler MA, Barendse GAM, Van Kleef M, *et al.* Pain relief in complex regional pain syndrome due to spinal cord stimulation does not depend upon vasodilation. *Anesthesiologist* 2000; 92:1653.
36. Erickson DL. Percutaneous trial of stimulation for patient selection for implantable stimulating devices. *J Neurosurg* 1975; 43: 440.
37. Hoppenstein R. Percutaneous implantation of chronic spinal cord electrodes for control of intractable pain: preliminary report. *Surg Neurol* 1975; 4: 195.
38. Hosobuchi Y, Adams JE, Weinstein PR. Preliminary percutaneous dorsal column stimulation prior to permanent implantation. *J Neurosurg* 1972; 37: 242.
39. North RB, Fischell TA, Long DM. Chronic stimulation via percutaneously inserted epidural electrodes. *Neurosurgery* 1977; 1: 215.
40. Zumpano BJ, Saunders RL. Percutaneous epidural dorsal column stimulation. *J Neurosurg* 1978; 46: 459.
41. North RB. Spinal cord stimulation for intractable pain: indications and technique. In Long DM (ed). *Current Therapy in Neurological Surgery,* vol 2, p 297. Toronto, Decker, 1988.
42. Medtronic, Inc. *Understanding your X-TREL spinal cord stimulation system.* Minneapolis, Medtronic, 1991.
43. Law JD. *The failed back syndrome treated by percutaneous spinal stimulation.* Presented at the American Association of Neurosurgeons Annual Meeting, 1986, San Diego, CA.

15

Intrathecal Opioid Pump Implantation

Jack L Rook

Since the discovery of opioid receptors in the outer layers of the spinal cord, the intrathecal space has become a popular route for application of exogenous opioid drugs. This technique may provide potent analgesia to the suffering patient, usually with few systemic side effects. Some patients with chronic nonmalignant pain may be appropriate candidates for placement of an intraspinal opioid pump. Potential candidates should have tried all reasonable forms of treatment, both conservative and invasive, and found them ineffective. Trials with adequate doses of oral opioids should be attempted before opioid pump implantation. However, some patients are unable to achieve adequate analgesia via the oral route, or side effects from the opioids (nausea, vomiting, sedation, confusion, and other forms of cognitive impairment) make oral administration impractical. Such patients may benefit from placement of an opioid pump. Use of the spinal route can be justified only if it results in pain relief greater than that achieved from conventional routes associated with less troublesome or fewer unwanted effects.

In the superficial dorsal horn, μ and κ receptors predominate. For an opioid to be effective in producing analgesia when applied to the spinal cord, it must bind with μ and κ receptors. Opiates with both μ and κ agonist activity currently used for intrathecal application include morphine, methadone, hydromorphone, and fentanyl. Each drug varies with respect to analgesic potency and distance traveled within the cerebrospinal fluid (CSF) before exerting its effect.

Hydrophilic opioids such as morphine tend to remain in the CSF for prolonged periods, migrate cephalad and caudally in the subarachnoid space, and result in a less intense quality of analgesia, a longer duration of action, and a larger analgesic area (encompassing more spinal segments) than that of the more lipophilic agents. A potential major problem in intrathecal administration of a hydrophilic opioid is cephalad migration of the drug into the brain, producing depression of respiratory centers in the medulla. If this effect occurs, respiratory depression may be quite delayed, perhaps occurring 8 to 12 hours after intrathecal morphine bolus injection (owing to the drug's slow transit within the CSF). Careful monitoring of vital signs during early trials with intrathecal opioids is important.[1–5]

The more lipophilic an opioid is, the more rapidly it will leach out of the water phase of the CSF and enter the spinal cord. Thus, the highly fat-soluble opioid fentanyl tends to have a rapid onset of action, and if it is not carried very far from the site of injection, the

Table 15-1 Varying qualities of hydrophilic versus lipophilic intrathecal opioids

Quality of Drug	Morphine	Fentanyl
Intensity of effect	−	+
Number of spinal segments	+	−
Chance for respiratory depression	+	−
Fat solubility	−	+
Duration of action	+	−

− = lesser; + = greater.

Reprinted by permission from Rook JL. Intrathecal opioid pump implantation. In Cassvan A, Weiss LD, Weiss JM, Rook JL, Mullens SU (eds). *Cumulative Trauma Disorders*, p 204, Table 13-2. Boston, Butterworth-Heinemann, 1997.

subsequent analgesic effect will tend to be more intense and limited to relatively few spinal segments (Table 15-1).[1]

Intrathecal opioids distribute between epidural and intrathecal CSF, epidural fat, epidural blood vessels, and the spinal cord (Figure 15-1). Opioids distribute between the CSF and spinal cord according to their lipid solubility. Poorly lipid-soluble agents spread rostrally, possibly reaching intracranial structures.[1]

TECHNIQUE OF OPIOID PUMP IMPLANTATION

The first step in considering implantation of an opioid pump is to identify a potential candidate for the device. Generally, patients with chronic nonmalignant pain should have failed all reasonable approaches to pain management, including optimal doses of oral opioids, before implantation of an infusion pump. Once an appropriate candidate has been identified, a trial of intrathecal opioids can commence. Patients with a favorable analgesic response may wish to proceed with infusion pump placement.

The next step is to provide the patient with appropriate education about the surgical procedure, potential beneficial effects, side effects and complications, and the need for regular follow-up. Postoperatively, follow-up is quite frequent, as the opioid must be titrated to an optimal dosage. Once a steady state has been reached, monthly follow-up to monitor analgesic efficacy and to refill the infusion pump reservoir is necessary.

At this point, the infusion pump and catheter can be implanted. The opioid can be delivered by either continuous-infusion (Infusaid, Shiley-Infusaid Inc., Norwood, MA) or programmable (SynchroMed Infusion Pump, Medtronic, Inc., Minneapolis, MN) devices. Each system consists of several parts surgically implanted into the patient's body: an infusion pump, catheter, and filling port.

The infusion pump is a round, metal disc approximately 1 in. thick and 3 in. in diameter and weighing approximately 6 oz (Figure 15-2). It stores and releases prescribed amounts of medication. A computer-like external programmer can be used by physician or nurse to readjust the prescription flow rate (Figure 15-3). In the center of the pump is a raised portion that helps the treating physician to find the filling port. A self-sealing rubber

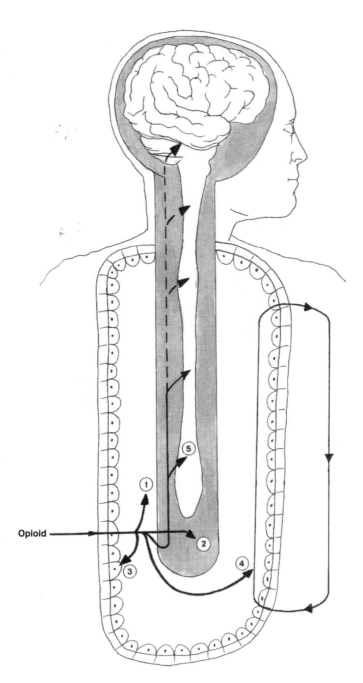

Figure 15-1 Pharmacokinetics of the epidural space. Epidural opioids distribute among epidural (1) and intrathecal (2) cerebrospinal fluid, epidural fat (3), epidural blood vessels (4), and the spinal cord (5). (Adapted from Wall PD, Melzack R. *Textbook of pain*, 2nd ed, p 745. New York, Churchill Livingstone, 1989) Reprinted by permission from Rook JL. Intrathecal opioid pump implantation. In Cassvan A, Weiss LD, Weiss JM, Rook JL, Mullens SU (eds). *Cumulative Trauma Disorders*, p 206, fig 13-2. Boston, Butterworth-Heinemann, 1997.

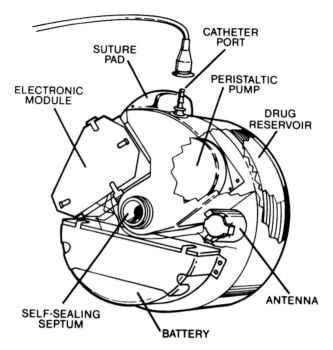

CATHETER PORT
SUTURE PAD
PERISTALTIC PUMP
ELECTRONIC MODULE
DRUG RESERVOIR
SELF-SEALING SEPTUM
ANTENNA
BATTERY

Figure 15-2 The Medtronic SynchroMed Infusion Pump. (Courtesy of Medtronic, Inc., Minneapolis, MN.) Reprinted by permission from Rook JL. Intrathecal opioid pump implantation. In Cassvan A, Weiss LD, Weiss JM, Rook JL, Mullens SU (eds). *Cumulative Trauma Disorders*, p 207, fig 13-3. Boston, Butterworth-Heinemann, 1997.

septum is located in the middle of this filling port. At appropriate intervals, the physician inserts a needle through the septum to refill the pump. Last, a catheter leading from the infusion pump delivers medication to the intrathecal space.

The infusion pump is designed to deliver a controlled amount of medication to the intrathecal space. The opioid binds to μ and κ receptors in the spinal cord dorsal horn, exerting an analgesic effect. The device is implanted surgically, usually by a neurosurgeon. Initially, the surgeon makes a subcutaneous pocket to receive the reservoir portion of the pump and then creates a tunnel leading from the pump to the spinal canal. A catheter inserted through the tunnel connects the pump with the intrathecal space. Once the catheter and pump are in place, the wounds are closed (Figure 15-4).

The patient needs regular physician follow-up indefinitely. Initially, flow-rate titration follow-up is frequent. After that, return visits may vary from weekly to monthly for refill of the pump reservoir. The patient is instructed to:

- comply with all physician follow-up appointments
- watch for any swelling, redness, or pain near the incision (which may indicate the presence of infection and would necessitate prompt treatment with antibiotics, drainage, or even pump removal)

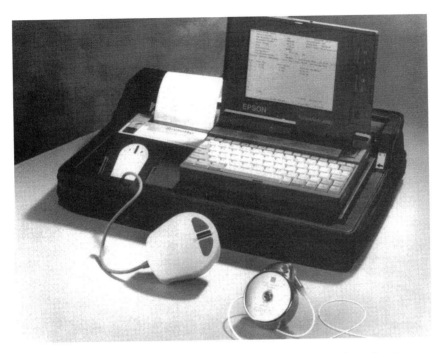

Figure 15-3 The SynchroMed infusion system from Medtronic, Inc., was the world's first commercially available implantable, programmable system. It consists of an implantable drug pump and a desktop programmer. Once implanted, the pump is programmed externally via radio signals to dispense the intrathecal opioid. (Courtesy of Medtronic, Inc., Minneapolis, MN.) Reprinted by permission from Rook JL. Intrathecal opioid pump implantation. In Cassvan A, Weiss LD, Weiss JM, Rook JL, Mullens SU (eds). *Cumulative Trauma Disorders*, p 208, fig 13-4. Boston, Butterworth-Heinemann, 1997.

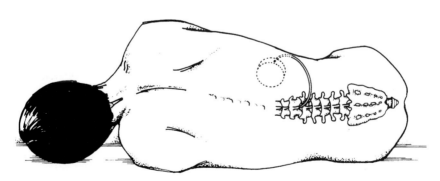

Figure 15-4 The surgically implanted morphine infusion pump. (Courtesy of Medtronic, Inc., Minneapolis, MN.) Reprinted by permission from Rook JL. Intrathecal opioid pump implantation. In Cassvan A, Weiss LD, Weiss JM, Rook JL, Mullens SU (eds). *Cumulative Trauma Disorders*, p 208, fig 13-5. Boston, Butterworth-Heinemann, 1997.

- avoid activities that afford a chance of a blow to the pump
- watch for any unusual reactions to or side effects of the infused medication
- notify the physician in advance of prolonged vacations so that refills can be arranged
- ensure that family members are aware of the device so that they can provide assistance in an emergency.[6–10]

SIDE EFFECTS AND COMPLICATIONS OF OPIOID PUMP IMPLANTATION

As with any surgical therapy, opioid pump implantation entails a slight risk of infection. If infection does occur, immediate and aggressive treatment is indicated (antibiotics, incision and drainage, and possibly removal of the unit). If treatment is not optimal, infection can spread along the catheter to the intrathecal space, possibly resulting in meningitis. Once the incision has healed, the pump and injection site require no special care, and the chances for infection are minimal, especially if proper sterile technique is used during the periodic refill injections.

Problems can occur with the unit itself (Box 15-1). The catheter could become plugged or kinked, may leak, or may dislodge. Such problems require surgical correction. The battery powering the pump will deplete every few (three to seven) years. As with any complicated device, a component may fail, necessitating pump replacement.[7]

Respiratory depression is the most feared side effect of pump implantation. If delayed respiratory depression does occur, it can be treated promptly with the opioid antagonist naloxone.[1,2–5,11] A potentially serious complication is the development of scar tissue at the catheter tip which could cause spinal cord injury with paraparesis or paraplegia.[12,13]

Box 15-1 Side effects and complications of opioid pump implantation

Complication of surgery:
- infection

Problems with the pump:
- kinked catheter
- rundown battery
- device component failure
- scar tissue formation at catheter tip

Reactions to medication:
- respiratory depression
- urinary retention
- pleuritis
- nausea or vomiting
- development of tolerance

Reprinted by permission from Rook JL. Intrathecal opioid pump implantation. In Cassvan A, Weiss LD, Weiss JM, Rook JL, Mullens SU (eds). *Cumulative Trauma Disorders*, p 209, table 13-3. Boston, Butterworth-Heinemann, 1997.

Other potential problems with intrathecal opioids include urinary retention, pruritus, nausea and vomiting, and the development of tolerance.[8,14] Tolerance to analgesia varies from case to case. If it occurs, pump flow rate can be titrated appropriately. However, if tolerance develops too rapidly, requiring pump refills more than once weekly, other forms of pain control may have to be considered.[1,6,15–17]

REFERENCES

1. Bromage PR. Epidural anesthetics and narcotics. In Wall PD, Malzack R (eds). *Textbook of Pain*, p 744. London, Churchill Livingstone, 1989.
2. Bromage PR. The price of interspinal narcotic analgesia: basic constraints [editorial]. *Anesth Analg* 1981; 60: 461.
3. Camporesi EM, Nielsen CH, Bromage PR, *et al*. Ventilatory CO_2 sensitivity following intravenous and epidural morphine in volunteers. *Anesth Analg* 1983; 62: 633.
4. Yaksh TL. Spinal opiate analgesia: characteristics and principles of action. *Pain* 1981; 11: 293.
5. Doblar DD, Muldoon SM, Albrecht PH, *et al*. Epidural morphine following epidural local anesthesia. effect on ventilatory and airway occlusion pressure responses to CO_2. *Anesthesiology* 1981; 66: 423.
6. Penn RD, Price JA. Chronic intrathecal morphine for intractable pain. *J Neurosurg* 1987; 67: 182.
7. Medtronic, Inc. *Ease of pain, ease of mind. The synchromed infusion system—patient information*. Minneapolis, Medtronic, Inc, April 1990.
8. Auld AW, Maki-Jokela A, Murdoch DM. Intraspinal narcotic analgesia in the treatment of chronic pain. *Spine* 1985; 10: 777.
9. Coombs DW, Saunders RL, Gaylor MS. Continuous epidural analgesia via implanted morphine reservoir. *Lancet* 1981; 2: 425.
10. Coombs DW, Saunders RL, Gaylor M, *et al*. Epidural narcotic infusion reservoir: implantation technique and efficiency. *Anesthesiology* 1982; 56: 469.
11. Glynn CJ, Mather LE, Cousins MJ, *et al*. Spinal narcotics and respiratory depression. *Lancet* 1979; 2: 365.
12. Aldrete JA, Vascello LA, Ghaly R, Tomlin D. Paraplegia in a patient with an intrathecal catheter and a spinal cord stimulator. *Anesthesiology* 1994; 81(6): 1542.
13. Cabbell KL, Taren JA, Sagher O. Spinal cord compression by catheter granulomas in high-dose intrathecal morphine therapy. Case report. *Neurosurgery* 1998; 42(5): 1176.
14. Kirkpatrick AF, Herndon MP. Intrathecal morphine in chronic pain management. *Anesthesiology*. 2000; 93(6): 1553.
15. Woods WA, Cohen SC. High-dose epidural morphine in a terminally ill patient. *Anesthesiology* 1982; 56: 311.
16. Greenberg HS, Taren J, Ensminger WD, *et al*. Benefit from and tolerance to continuous intrathecal infusion of morphine for intractable cancer pain. *J Neurosurg* 1982; 57: 360.
17. Coombs DW, Saunders RL, Lachance D, *et al*. Intrathecal morphine tolerance: use of intrathecal clonidine, DADLE, and intraventricular morphine. *Anesthesiology* 1985; 62: 358.

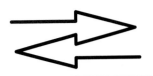

Subject Index

Abbreviations: MTBI: mild traumatic brain injury; PCS: post-concussive syndrome; RSDS: reflex sympathetic dystrophy syndrome; WDRN: wide dynamic-range neurons. All entries refer to low speed, rear end collisions unless otherwise stated.

A

A-alpha mechanoreceptor sensory fibers, 53, 253
  down-regulation of pain, RSDS
      pathophysiology, 280
Abdomen
  CT scans, 76–77
  MRI scans, 79
Abduction external rotation (AER) position, 140, 141, 255
Abductor pollicis brevis muscle, 256
Abductor pollicis longus tendon, 91
  inflammation *See* DeQuervain's tenosynovitis
Acceleration (acceleration force), 10
  definition, 6
  errors, impact on kinetic energy, 7
  force relationship/equation, 10
  impact speed relationship, 15
  low, brain injury evidence, 306
  rotational, effect on vestibular mechanism, 70
  translational and rotational in whiplash, 306
Acceleration/deceleration forces, 298, 306
  diffuse axonal injury (DAI), 307
  frontotemporal brain injury, 307
  PET scans after, 322
Accelerometer, 17
Accident reports, 6
Accidents *See* Motor vehicle accidents
Accommodative dysfunction, 319
Acetabulum, 171
Acetaminophen (Tylenol), 242
N-Acetylaspartate (NAA), 324
N-Acetylaspartate (NAA)/creatinine ratio, 324–325
Acetylcholine, increase, in MTBI, 308
Achilles bursa, pain due to, 47
Achilles bursitis/tendonitis, 160–161

Achilles tendon, 156
  injuries, 47, 160
  tear/rupture, 160
Acromioclavicular fibers, tears, 116
Acromioclavicular joint strain, 116–117
Acromion
  anatomy, 111
  bursitis, 47
Action potentials, nerve, 81
Activities of daily living, G-forces and, 13–14, 17
Acupuncture
  chronic cervical radiculopathy, 147
  RSDS treatment, 288
Acustophobia (phonophobia), 317, 345, 350, 359
Adapin *See* Doxepin (Adapin, Sinequan)
Addiction, drug *See* Drug addiction
A-delta fibers (thin myelinated), 52–53, 253
  ascending pain pathway to nucleus caudalis, 218
  mechanical nociceptors, 52–53
  mechanothermal nociceptors, 53
  reflex sympathetic dystrophy syndrome, 277, 278
  termination in dorsal horn, 54, 55
Adhesive capsulitis *See* Shoulder, frozen (adhesive capsulitis)
Adjuvants, pain management, 242–243
Adrenal insufficiency, tests, 74
Adrenergic receptors/blockers
  alpha *See* Alpha-adrenergic antagonists; Alpha-receptors
  beta *See* Beta blockers; Beta-receptors
Adson's maneuver, 118, 140
Afferent fibers, 53
Aids, walking *See* Walking aids
Alcohol, intolerance, 317

Allodynia, 51, 154, 255
  definition, 271
  pathophysiology, 277
  in reflex sympathetic dystrophy syndrome, 271
Alpha-adrenergic antagonists, 276
  common drugs, 283
  reflex sympathetic dystrophy syndrome, 281
  urinary incontinence, 180–181
Alpha-receptors, 276
  stimulation, 276–277
Ambien, 347, 349
Ambulation *See* Gait
Amerge (naratriptan hydrochloride), migraine
    (vascular headache), 223
American Academy of Neurology, 302
American Congress of Rehabilitation Medicine,
    300–301, 303, 304
American Medical Association, 235
Amitriptyline (Elavil), 239
  migraine (vascular headache)
    prophylaxis, 228
    treatment, 222
  neurogenic pain management, 246
Amnesia *See also* Memory
  post-traumatic *See* Post-traumatic amnesia (PTA)
  retrograde, MTBI, 348
  sports-related concussion grading, 301
Analgesic ladder, 242, 383, 384
  opioids, 383–384
Analgesics
  chronic pain management, 242
    opioids *See* Opioid analgesia
  combination, migraine (vascular headache),
    223, 225
  depression management in chronic pain, 238
  migraine (vascular headache), 223, 225
  oral, 242
  RSDS treatment, 289
"Anal wink" reflex test, 184–185
Anatomical "snuffbox," 92, 94, 98
Anesthetic/steroid injection *See also* Steroid
    injections
  acromioclavicular joint strain, 116
  subacromial, 112
Anger management, 340
Angiograms, thoracic outlet syndrome, 141
Animal studies, 18
  acceleration/deceleration force effects, 298–299
  neurochemical cascade in brain injury, 308
  pain pathways, 218
Ankle brace, 160

Ankle joint, 155–161
  anatomy, 155–156
    ligaments, 155, 157
    nerves, 155–156
    tendons, 156
  chronic pain, 159
  eversion injuries, 158
  injuries, 157–161
    bone avulsion, 157
    fractures, 157
    ligament tears, 157, 158
    RSDS after, 269
    sprains, 157–158
    tarsal tunnel syndrome *See* Tarsal tunnel
      syndrome
  injury mechanisms, 156–157
  inversion stress and inversion strain, 157–158
  osteoarthritis, 159–160
  range of motion, 49
  tenderness, 160
Ankylosing spondylitis, diagnostic tests, 73
Annulus fibrosus, 193
  collagen fibers, 193, 195, 198
    bulging, 206
    excessive motion and tears, 198
  disc bulging effect, 206, 209
  flexibility, 193, 198
  lamellae, 193, 195
  tears, 26, 193, 209
    in hyperextension injuries, 42
Antecubital fossa, 99, 104
Anterior cruciate ligament, 161, 163, 166
  testing, 166, 168
Anterior draw sign, 166, 168
Anterior horn cells, activation in RSDS, 279
Anterior longitudinal ligament, 196
  injuries, 46
  lumbar spine, 182
  pain sensitivity, 203
  tears in hyperextension injuries, 41–42
Anterior scalene muscle, tenderness, 140
Anterior tarsal tunnel syndrome, 258
Anterolisthesis, 210
Anticonvulsants
  migraine headache prophylaxis, 227, 228
  neurogenic pain management, 245–246, 262
  RSDS treatment, 289
  side effects, 245
Antidepressants
  in depression, 237, 238
  headache prophylaxis, 227

Antidepressants (*Continued*)
  SSRIs *See* Selective serotonin reuptake inhibitors (SSRIs)
  tricyclic *See* Tricyclic antidepressants
Antidromic conduction (nerve), 123
Antiemetics, migraine (vascular headache) treatment, 223, 226
Antihistamines, chronic pain management, 243
Antihypertensive agents, 244
Anti-inflammatory agents
  ankle osteoarthritis, 160
  cervical radiculopathy, 146
  chronic pain management, 242
  "dashboard knee," 165
  epicondylitis, 103
  hand or wrist ligament tears, 98
  hand or wrist tendonitis, 93
  interdigital neuroma, 153
  nonsteroidal *See* Nonsteroidal anti-inflammatory drugs (NSAIDs)
  plantar fasciitis, 153
  side effects, 242
Antinuclear antibody (ANA), 73
Anxiety
  after MTBI, 311, 319, 340
    effect on cognitive function, 311
  chronic pain perception, 238
Anxiolytics, effect on cognitive testing, 314
Apley's compression (grinding) test, 169, 170
Apolipoprotein E (Apo E) genotype, 310
Aponeurosis *See* Plantar fascia
"Apprehension sign," 114, 115
Arcade of Frohse, 137
  transection, 139
Arm, abduction, rotator cuff muscles role, 107
Armored car, 306
Arthritis
  degenerative *See* Osteoarthritis
  rheumatoid, diagnostic tests, 73
Arthrography
  hand and wrist ligament tears, 97
  rotator cuff tear, 117
  rotator cuff tendonitis, 113
Arthroscopic surgery
  "dashboard knee," 165
  meniscal tears, 170
Arthroscopy, subacromial, 112
Aseptic necrosis, hip joint, 50, 174–175
Aspartate, in brain injury, 308

Aspiration
  bursitis, 103–104
  ganglion, 95–96
Aspirin, 242
Assistive devices, walking *See* Walking aids
Atlas, 142, 199
Atrophy, reflex sympathetic dystrophy syndrome, 272
Attentional deficits, 308, 317, 350
Attention Process Training (APT), 343
Auditory information processing, assessment, 351
Autonomic fibers, median nerve, 129
Autonomic system *See also* Sympathetic nervous system
  imbalance, reflex sympathetic dystrophy syndrome, 272, 276
Axillary nerve, 120
Axis, 142, 199, 200
  dens, fractures, 75
Axons
  diffuse injury, 307, 336–337
  injury, as "evolutionary process," 309
  shear strain and injuries, 307
  tearing, 308
    transneuronal degeneration, 309

B

Baclofen, 243
  RSDS treatment, 289
Bactrien test, 129
Balance, 68–71
  development, 68, 70
  problems after MTBI, 350
  vestibular and neck proprioceptive systems, 70–71
Barium enema, 77
Beck Anxiety Inventory, 329
Beck Depression Inventory (BDI), 329
  case study interpretation, 357–358
  overlap with symptoms of PCS, 330
Behavioral deficits, underestimation by neuropsychological tests, 335, 337, 338
Behavioral features, reflex sympathetic dystrophy syndrome, 272
Behavioral therapy, tension-type headache, 216
Benzodiazepines, in sleep disturbance, 239
Best Performance method, 332–333, 337
Beta blockers
  acute RSDS treatment, 281
  common drugs, 283
  contraindications, 228

Beta blockers *(Continued)*
  migraine headache prophylaxis,
      227, 228
  side effects, 228
Beta-receptors, 276
Bias, 2
  evaluation of causation and, 4
Biceps brachii, anatomy, 108
Biceps reflex, diminished in C5 radiculopathy,
    146
Biceps tendon
  acute inflammation, 111, 113–114
  anatomy, 105, 108
  injuries, 47, 50
  long head, 105
Bicipital groove, 105
Bicipital tendonitis, 111, 113–114
Bier block
  diagnostic, 275–276
  RSDS treatment, 282–283
  technique, 283
Biofeedback
  migraine (vascular headache), 229
  pelvic floor muscles, 180
  RSDS treatment, 289
  tension-type headache, 216
Biomechanics, 1–38
  causation and *See* Causation
  concepts, 5–8
  definition, 1
  factors increasing injury potential, 27–28, 29
  during gait, 64
  G-forces *See* G-force (gravity)
  injury potential evaluation *See* Injury potential
      evaluation
  mild traumatic brain injury (MTBI),
      305–306
  physicians' understanding, 6
  risk factors for injury and, 29–30
  spinal injury, 198–199
  terminology, 1–2
  testing methods, 17–18
    problems, 18
Biomechanics experts, 1
  goals, 21
Biomechanics field, origin, 1
Blackouts, 317
Bladder
  dysfunction, 182, 184, 186, 208
    treatment, 189
  nerve supply, 186, 187

Blood flow
  cerebral, evaluation after MTBI, 323
  changes, reflex sympathetic dystrophy, 260–261,
      270
  hand, carpal tunnel syndrome, 129
  thoracic outlet syndrome, 141
Blood tests, 73–74
  reflex sympathetic dystrophy syndrome, 275
Blood vessels, vascular headache
    pathophysiology, 221
Bone
  avulsion, ankle, 157
  demineralization, 80
  fractures *See* Fractures
  pain, 42, 48
  sesamoid, 161
Bone scanning, 80
  ankle osteoarthritis, 160
  neurogenic pain in foot, 155
  occult fractures, 80, 98
    foot, 154
  reflex sympathetic dystrophy syndrome, 275
  sacroiliac joint dysfunction, 178
  triple-phase, 80, 275
    angiogram and blood pool phases, 275
Bone spurs (osteophytes), 75
  acromion, 111, 113
  after disc degeneration, 207
  ankle osteoarthritis, 160
  lumbar radiculopathy, 186
  vertebral, 204
Boston Aphasia Screening Test, 353
Botulinum toxin (Botox), thoracic outlet
    syndrome, 141–142
Bowel dysfunction, 182, 184, 186, 208
Brachial plexopathy *See* Thoracic outlet syndrome
Brachial plexus, 253
  anatomy, 120, 139–140, 202, 269
  entrapment, 121–122, 139–142, 258 *See also*
      Thoracic outlet syndrome
  evaluation, 123
  irritation, 45, 50, 51, 118
    hypersensitivity of distal peripheral nerves,
        258
Brachioradialis reflex, diminished in C5
    radiculopathy, 146
Bracing before accident *See* Lower extremity
    bracing; Upper extremity bracing
Brain injury
  cumulative effects, 301, 308, 309
  frontotemporal region, 307

Brain injury (Continued)
  low impact forces causing, 297–299
  mild See Mild traumatic brain injury (MTBI)
Brainstem, projections to spinal cord, 56
Brainstem-evoked responses (BAERs), 325
Brain swelling, 307–308
Bretylium, 283
Bruxism, 43
Bulbocavernous ("anal wink") reflex test, 184–185
Bumpers (car)
  goals of manufacturers, 11–12
  not protective for occupants, 12
  standards (2.5 and 5.0 mile/hour), 11, 12
Bumpers (vehicle), design, 8, 11, 28
Bupropion hydrochloride (Wellbutrin), 248
  contraindications, 248
Bursa
  Achilles, 47
  ankle, 156
  calcaneal, 156
  hip, 171
  knee, 168
  olecranon, 99
  pes anserine, 168
  retrocalcaneal, 156
  subacromial See Subacromial bursa
Bursectomy, 173
Bursitis
  Achilles, 160–161
  acromion, 47
  aspiration, 103–104
  elbow, 103–104
  knee, 47, 168–169
  olecranon, 103–104
  pain, 47
  subacromial See Subacromial bursitis
  trochanteric, 173
Buschke Verbal Selective Reminding Test, 355, 357

C
Cadaver studies, 18
  load values after collisions, 15
  stress–strain curve studies, 18–19
  whiplash injury mechanism, 20
Cafergot, migraine (vascular headache), 223
Caffeine
  chronic pain management, 243
  content of specific foods, 224
  daily intake, 223
  excessive intake, 223
  mechanism of action, 243

Caffeine (Continued)
  migraine (vascular headache), 223
  withdrawal headaches due to, 223
Calcaneal bursa, 156
Calcification See also Bone spurs
  after disc degeneration, 207
Calcitonin gene-related polypeptide (CGRP)
  release
    inhibition, 223
    by serotonin, 220
  vascular headache, 218
Calcium channel blockers See also Verapamil
  migraine (vascular headache)
    prophylaxis, 227, 228
    treatment, 222
  RSDS treatment, 281
Capsaicin cream
  neurogenic pain management, 262
  RSDS treatment, 289
Capsule See Facet capsule; Joint capsule
Carbamazepine (Tegretol)
  migraine headache prophylaxis, 228
  neurogenic pain management, 245, 262
Carbon dioxide, accumulation in muscle, 45
Cardiovascular system, opioids side effects,
    373, 382
Carotid sheath, 284, 286
Carpal bones, 89
Carpal tunnel, 90, 121
  anatomy, 90–91, 126
Carpal tunnel syndrome, 121, 125–131, 258
  complications, 130–131
  diagnostic tests, 129
  electrodiagnostic testing, 86, 129
  neurogenic pain, 51, 130–131
  physical examination, 127, 255
  post-traumatic, 92, 93, 126
  symptoms, 126–127
  treatment, 129–130
    steroid injection, 263
    surgery, 130
Cartilage degeneration, 49
Case closure, chronic pain clinic work, 240–241
Casting
  ankle fractures, 157
  hand and wrist ligament tears, 98
Catecholamine receptors, 276
Cauda equina, 182, 200
Causalgia, 267, 392 See also Reflex sympathetic
    dystrophy syndrome (RSDS)
"Causalgic personality," 272

Causation, 3–5
  definition, 3
  disputed, 4
  evaluation, 3
    steps, 3–4
Cause and effect relationship, 3–4
Cavitation, axonal injury, 307
Celecoxib (Celebrex), 242
Celexa (citalopram hydrobromide), 247, 348
Central nervous system (CNS), 51, 200, 253
  opioid side effects, 382
Cerebral blood flow, evaluation after
    MTBI, 323
Cerebral contusions, acceleration/deceleration
    forces causing, 299
Cerebral hypometabolism, 322
Cerebrospinal fluid (CSF), opioid distribution,
    401–402, 403
Cervical discs, 142
  comparison with lumbar, 194–195, 197
  herniation, 208
    prevention, 142
Cervical epidural steroid injections, cervical
    radiculopathy, 146–147
Cervical facet joints See Facet joints
Cervical immobilization, cervical radiculopathy, 146
Cervical muscles, chronic contraction, 216
  tension-type headaches, 215
Cervical myofascial pain syndrome, 217
Cervical nerve roots, 120, 142–143, 253
  C1 and C2, 200
  C5, 256
  C8, 201
  clinical workup to exclude lesions, 145
  dermatomes and myotomes, 143
  impingement See also Cervical radiculopathy
    investigations, 145
  muscles innervated, 143, 144
  pain, 52
Cervical radiculopathy, 52, 142–147, 259
  acute, 146–147
  C5, 145–146
  C6, 145, 146
  C7, 145, 146
  C8, 146
  chronic, 147
  electrodiagnostic testing, 145
  MRI and CT imaging, 145
  radiography, 145
  specific syndromes, 145–146
  treatment, 146–147

Cervical spinal cord, protective structures,
    199–200
Cervical spine
  absence of motion after injury, healing
    reduction, 30
  anatomy, 142–145, 191, 199–200
  compression during rear end collisions,
    21–22
    tolerance reduction, 21
  gait relationship, 65–66
  hyperextension injury, muscle tears, 41–42
  loading, injury potential, 21–22
  lower, hyperextension, 21, 22
  lumbar spine comparison, 194–195, 197
    similarities, 65
  malalignment, thoracic outlet syndrome due to,
    140
  minor injuries definition, 23
  motion during whiplash, 21, 22
  radiography, 75
  range of movement, 191, 199
    planes of motion, 142, 191
  restricted motion, proprioceptive
    dysfunction, 70
  rotation with extension, injury, 26, 27–28
  seven-segment model, 64
  sigmoid (S-shaped) curve See Sigmoid
    (S-shaped) curve
  upper, hypoflexion, 21, 22
  venous system, water hammer effect, 25
Cervical vertebrae, anatomy, 142, 191
Cervical vertigo, 45
Cervicogenic head pain, C2 ganglion
    decompression, 26
C-fibers (unmyelinated), 52–53, 253
  ascending pain pathway to nucleus
    caudalis, 218
  nociceptors, 53
  reflex sympathetic dystrophy syndrome,
    277, 278
  termination in dorsal horn, 54, 55
Chemical sympathectomy, 287–288
Chiropractic treatment, lumbar radiculopathy,
    189
Cholinergic activity, increased in MTBI, 308
Chondromalacia, 49, 50
Chondromalacia patella See "Dashboard knee"
Chronic injury, prediction from initial
    symptoms, 28
Chronic nonmalignant pain (CNMP) See Chronic
    pain/chronic pain syndromes

Chronic pain/chronic pain syndromes, 23, 39–40, 43, 233–251 *See also specific pain syndromes*
  bilateral, spinal cord stimulation, 392
  delayed recovery, 235–236
  depression with *See* Depression
  development, 59
  disability due to, 234–235
    management, 235
  factors contributing to, 31–32
  financial/employment costs, 40, 234
  MTBI comorbidity, 312–313 *See also* Mild traumatic brain injury (MTBI)
  muscular/ligamentous injuries, 40–41, 235
  myofascial pain syndrome *See* Myofascial pain syndrome
  nervous system involvement, 41
  perception, anxiety/depression effect, 238
  pharmacological management, 242–248
    adjuvant drugs, 242–243
    in neurogenic pain *See* Neurogenic pain
    opioids *See* Opioid analgesia
  reduced pain tolerance, 40
  scenarios for, 40–41
  sleep disturbance *See* Sleep disturbance
  symptoms, 55, 233–234
  treatment
    mandates, 234
    spinal cord stimulation *See* Spinal cord stimulation (SCS)
  under-treatment, 367
  wide dynamic-range neuron (WDRN), 55
Chronic pain clinic, 239–241
  indications for, 241
  program and treatment provided, 241
Chronic regional pain syndrome *See* Reflex sympathetic dystrophy syndrome (RSDS)
Citalopram hydrobromide (Celexa), 247, 348
Claudication, neurogenic, 208
Clinical interview, neuropsychological *See* Neuropsychological assessment
Clinical psychological screening, 329–330
Clonazepam (Klonopin)
  neurogenic pain management, 245–246
  for sleep disturbance, 238, 239
Clonidine
  neurogenic pain, 244, 262
  transdermal patch, 244
Coccyx, 175
  anatomy, 191
Codeine, 375–376

Cognitive abilities *See also* Cognitive function
  assessment, 331
  not included in some neuropsychological tests, 335
  underestimated by neuropsychological tests, 335, 337, 338
Cognitive deficits
  assessment, 330–331
  case study, 298
  mild traumatic brain injury causing, 337
    DSM-IV definition of MTBI, 303
  pain effect on, 312–313
  PCS/MTBI symptoms, 317–318
Cognitive function
  central processing, assessment, 331
  factors affecting after MTBI *See under* Mild traumatic brain injury (MTBI)
  opioid-induced changes, 383
Cognitive processing speed, reduced, 317, 351
Cognitive rehabilitation, after MTBI, 343
  case study, 349, 359
Cognitive testing, 86, 331
Cognitive therapy, tension-type headache, 216
Cold packs, RSDS treatment and, 288
Cold-water stress test, 80–81, 274
Collagen, in annulus *See* Annulus fibrosus
Collagen, type III, 24
Color (of extremity)
  changes in RSDS, 272
  sympathetic nervous system abnormality, 255, 272
Colorado Medical Society, 301–302
Common peroneal nerve, entrapment, 258
Compazine (prochlorperazine), migraine (vascular headache), 223
Complex regional pain syndrome (CPRS)
  type I *See* Reflex sympathetic dystrophy syndrome (RSDS)
  type II, 267
Compound motor action potential (CMAP), 81, 82, 124
  cubital tunnel syndrome, 136
  nerve conduction velocity calculation, 125
  radial tunnel syndrome, 138
  thoracic outlet syndrome, 141
Computerized motion capture and analysis (CMCA), 64
Computerized tomography (CT, CAT scan), 75–77
  advantages/disadvantages, 76
  cervical radiculopathy, 145
  contrast, 76

Computerized tomography (CT, CAT scan)
   (Continued)
   CT numbers, 76
   films after motor vehicle accidents, 76–77
   lumbar radiculopathy, 186
   mild traumatic brain injury, 321–322
   principle, 75–76
   procedure, 76
   sacroiliac joint dysfunction, 178
Concentration deficits, 317, 350
Concussion See also Post-concussive
   syndrome (PCS)
   definition, 304
   grading, 301
   sports-related, 301–302, 302
   susceptibility to effects, 309
Confusion, after MTBI, 340, 348
Consciousness See also Concussion
   altered, in neuropsychological interview, 328
   level, evaluation, 326
   loss, neuropsychological interview, 327–328
Constipation, opioid-induced, 370, 373
   prevention, 383
Contrast baths, RSDS treatment and, 288
Conus medullaris, 200
Coping mechanisms, for losses after MTBI, 340
Coracoacromial ligament, 105, 107
Coracohumeral ligament, 105
Cortical auditory evoked responses
   (CAERs), 325
Corticosteroids See also Steroid(s)
   benefits in water hammer mechanism of
      injury, 25
   RSDS treatment, 289
Cortisol, assays, 74
Cortisol stimulation test, 74
Costochondral joints, thoracic, injuries, 50
Costs
   chronic pain, 40, 234
   depression, 236
   employment See Employment costs
   motor vehicle accidents, 4
   rear end collisions, 4
   RSDS treatment, 289–290
Cough reflex, depression by opioids, 373
Counseling
   chronic pain clinic, 240, 241
   in depression, 237
Coup/contre coup lesions, 307
"Coupled motion" concept, 65–66
Cranial fractures, 42, 48

Crash tests
   cadavers, 18
   human volunteers, 18
   hybrid dummy, 17
Crashworthiness of vehicles, 1, 6
   effect on injury potential, 28
Cruciate ligaments, 161, 163, 166
   testing, 166, 168
Crumple zones (of cars), 11
   comparison with armored car, 306
Cubital tunnel syndrome, 121, 135–137, 258
   clinical features, 135–136
   diagnostic workup, 136
   injuries causing, 135
   physical examination, 136
Cueing, 317, 350
   strategies, cognitive rehabilitation after
      MTBI, 343
Cyclobenzaprine (Flexeril)
   fibromyalgia syndrome, 243
   in sleep disturbances, 239

D

"Dashboard knee," 41, 50, 161, 164–166
   reflex sympathetic dystrophy syndrome after,
      269
Daubert rule (702-Daubert rule), 3
Deceleration force See also Acceleration/
   deceleration forces
   injury potential determination, 9
Deceleration time, 306
Deep heating See Ultrasound
Deep peroneal nerve, 149
Deformation
   definition, 6
   load, 7 See also Stress–strain curve
   loading causing, 19
   plastic, definition, 8
Delta fibers See A-delta fibers (thin myelinated)
Delta-t ($\triangle t$), 6
   time increase and injury potential less, 9, 10–11
      increase by collision damage, 13
Delta-v ($\triangle v$), 6, 10
   accident severity indication, 10
   calculation and factors included, 10–11
Deltoid ligament (medial collateral ligament),
   155
   injuries, 158
Deltoid muscle, 107, 110
   shoulder stability, 111
Depakote See Valproate (Depakote)

Depression, 237–238 *See also* Antidepressants
  chronic pain clinic, 240, 241
  chronic pain syndrome, 233, 246
  effect on cognitive function after MTBI, 311
  management, 237, 238, 246–248
  MTBI and, 311, 312, 318, 340
    case study, 357–358
    causes, 312
  opioid analgesia and, 384
  pathophysiology, 237–238
  screening, 236
  symptoms, after MTBI, 311, 318
  treatment in RSDS, 289
Depth perception, visual, 319
DeQuervain's tenosynovitis, 47, 94–95
  treatment, 95
Dermatomes, 256
  cervical nerve roots, 143
  lumbosacral nerve roots, 182, 185
Descending pain modulatory pathways *See* Pain
  pathways, descending modulatory
Desensitization techniques
  neurogenic pain, 261–262
  repeated eye movement and, 342
Desipramine (Norpramin), 239
  migraine headache prophylaxis, 228
Desyrel *See* Trazodone (Desyrel)
Detoxification
  after overmedication, 240
  opioids, 386
    before spinal cord stimulation, 391–392
Diagnosis, as first step in causality determination,
  3, 4
*Diagnostic and Statistical Manual - Fourth
  Edition (DSM-IV)*, 303, 304, 318
Diagnostic workup, 73–87 *See also individual
  imaging methods*
  blood tests, 73–74
  cognitive/psychological testing, 86
  computerized tomography, 75–77
  electrodiagnostic testing, 81–86 *See also*
    Electrodiagnostic testing
  to exclude cervical nerve root lesion, 145
  MRI scanning, 77–79
  radiography (x-rays), 74–75
  radionuclide imaging, 79–80
  thermography, 80–81
Diaschisis, 309
Diethylenetriamine pentaacetic acid (DTPA),
  technetium-99m, 79
Diffuse axonal injury (DAI), 307, 336–337

Diffuse head pain syndrome, 24
Diffuse myofascial pain syndrome, 22
Diffusion tensor imaging, 324
Diffusion-weighted imaging (DWI), mild traumatic
  brain injury, 323
Digital nerves, 90
Digit Vigilance Test, 354, 357
Dihydroergotamine (D.H.E. 45), migraine
  (vascular headache), 222, 223
Dihydroergotamine mesylate (Migranol), migraine
  (vascular headache), 223
Dilantin *See* Phenytoin (Dilantin)
Dimercaptosuccinic acid (DMSA), technetium
  99M, 79
Diplopia (double vision), 319, 345
Disability
  chronic pain causing *See* Chronic pain/chronic
    pain syndromes
  as societal problem, 236
Disc(s) *See* Intervertebral disc (IVD)
Discectomy
  cervical radiculopathy, 147
  lumbar radiculopathy, 189
Discogenic pain, 26–27
Disinhibition, 318
Displacement, definition, 6
Dizziness, 316
  paracervical muscle spasm causing, 45
Doctor/patient relationship, 235
Doppler ultrasound, thoracic outlet syndrome, 141
Dorsal column stimulation *See* Spinal cord
  stimulation (SCS)
Dorsal horn, 54, 202, 253
  ascending pain pathway, 54, 253
  descending modulatory pain system, 254
  medullary (nucleus caudalis), 218
  nociceptive neuron inhibition, 56, 58
Dorsalis pedis artery, 150
Dorsal root ganglion, 26–27
  C2, 26
  decompression, 26
  sensitivity to mechanical/chemical changes, 26
Dorsal roots, hematoma, 25–26
Dorsal ulnar cutaneous nerve, 89, 90
Dorsolateral funiculus (DLF), 56
"Double crush syndrome," 258
"Double hump" (Bactrien) sign, 129
Doxepin (Adapin, Sinequan), 239
  migraine headache prophylaxis, 228
Drag factor *(F)*, 12, 27
"Drop arm test," 117

Drug addiction
definition, 369
history, opioid analgesia and, 371
opioids, 371
detoxification, 386
screening, features, 388
Drugs *See also individual drugs/drug groups*
caffeine content, 224
effect on cognitive testing, 314
modification, chronic pain clinic, 240
withdrawal
caffeine, headaches due to, 223
clonidine minimization of effects, 244
Dynorphin peptides, 59
Dysarthria, 317
Dyscalculia, 357
Dysgeusia, 316–317

E

Ear, inner, 70
Earplugs, 345, 359
Edema
brawny, 271
reflex sympathetic dystrophy syndrome, 271
Education
family, after MTBI, 342
patients *See* Patient education
Efferent fibers, 53
Elasticity, definition, 7
Elavil *See* Amitriptyline (Elavil)
Elbow joint/region, 99–105
anatomy, 99–100
ligaments, 99
nerves and muscles, 100
injuries causing RSDS, 269
injury mechanisms, 100–105
epicondylitis, 102–103
forearm myofascial pain, 100–102
fractures, 104
ligament strains, 104–105
nerve entrapment, 104
olecranon bursitis, 103–104
nerve conduction block at, 127
range of motion, 49, 99
Elbow pain, 47, 100–105
chronic, after fractures, 104
neurogenic, 105
Electrodiagnostic testing, 81–86 *See also*
Electromyogram (EMG); Nerve conduction
velocity (NCV)
advantages, 83–84

Electrodiagnostic testing *(Continued)*
carpal tunnel syndrome, 129
cervical radiculopathy, 145
cubital tunnel syndrome, 136
disadvantage, 84
Guyon's canal syndrome, 134
neurogenic pain in foot, 155
pronator syndrome, 133
radial tunnel syndrome, 138
reflex sympathetic dystrophy syndrome, 275
superficial radial nerve entrapment, 137
tarsal tunnel syndrome, 158
thoracic outlet syndrome, 141
upper extremity, 145
Electroencephalography (EEG), in MTBI, 322
Electromyogram (EMG), 81, 122
cervical radiculopathy, 145
cubital tunnel syndrome, 136
Guyon's canal syndrome, 134
indications, 122
lumbar radiculopathy, 186
neurogenic pain, 260
procedure, 83, 122
pronator syndrome, 133
tarsal tunnel syndrome, 158
time frame (optimal) in nerve entrapments,
122
Electrophysiological testing, mild traumatic brain
injury, 325
Emotional changes, after MTBI, 318–319,
320–321
Emotional disorders, neuropsychological testing
and, 312
Emotional response
to MTBI, 310, 311, 339
recovery, 339–341
to pain, 254
Employment *See also entries beginning
vocational*
demands from/of (after MTBI), 343
rehabilitation after MTBI and, 343–344
return to work, after MTBI, 344, 348
Employment costs
chronic pain/chronic pain syndromes, 40, 234
mental illness and depression, 236
musculoskeletal disorders, 235
Endorphins, 59, 254
Energy
absorbing structures in vehicles, 13
of collision, conservation, 10
conservation, 10, 30

Energy *(Continued)*
  conserving system, shoulder-pelvis counter-
    rotation, 65
  definition, 6
  expenditure in gait, 66–67
  kinetic *See* Kinetic energy
  photon, 76
  potential, conversion from/to kinetic
    energy, 65
  transfer mechanisms in rear end collisions, 8
Engineering, concepts, 6–8
Engineers, physicians vs, 6, 31, 32
Enkephalins, 59
Epicondylitis, 102–103
  definition, 102
  lateral, 101, 102–103, 138
  long-term complications, 103
  medial, 102–103
Epidural infection, spinal cord stimulation
  complication, 397–398
Epidural space, opioid pharmacokinetics,
  401–402, 403
Equal and opposite law, 13
Ergot, migraine (vascular headache), 222
Ergotamine derivatives, migraine (vascular
  headache), 223, 226
Ernest Johnson Fourth Finger Test, 129
Erythrocyte sedimentation rate (ESR), 73–74
Erythromelalgia, 267 *See also* Reflex sympathetic
  dystrophy syndrome (RSDS)
Evoked potentials, assessment, 325
Executive function
  assessment, 331
  deficits, after MTBI, 303, 318, 351
  definition, 318
Exercise(s)
  home program, lumbar radiculopathy, 189
  Kegel, 180
  RSDS treatment and, 288
  stretching *See* Stretching exercises
Expert witnesses, vii
Extension-flexion injuries, 6
Extensor hallucis longus, innervation, 182
Extensor indicis proprius muscle, 138
Extensor muscles, wrist, 100
Extensor pollicis brevis tendon, 91
  inflammation *See* DeQuervain's
    tenosynovitis
Extensor tendons, hand and wrist, 91
Eye Movement Desensitization and Reprocessing
  (EMDR), 342

F

FABER test, 178, 213
Facet arthropathy, 207, 208, 209
Facet capsule, 198
  compression resistance, 22
  ligament injuries, 46
  pain sensitivity, 22, 30
Facet joints, 196, 198
  cervical, 142, 198, 199
    lower, pinching, 23
    lower vs upper, 21, 22
  in disc degeneration, 207
  gliding, 21
  hyperextension injuries, 204
  injuries, 50, 199
  lumbar spine, 182, 198
  pain sensitivity, 21, 30
  separation by joint space, 206
Facial muscles, pain, 217
Factitious Disorders, 315
Family discord
  chronic pain syndrome, 233
  MTBI predisposition and, 310
Family therapy, MTBI treatment, 342
Fat, body, MRI or CT scans, 76, 77
Fatigue
  diagnostic tests, 74
  MTBI comorbidity, 313–314, 316,
    340, 347
Femoral condyles, 161, 162
Femoral nerve, 182, 253
Femur, 161, 171
Fentanyl, 381, 401–402
Fetus, radiation hazard, 75
Fibrillation potential, 83, 85–86
Fibromyalgia syndrome, 41, 43
  "tender points," 43
  treatment, 243
Fibula, 155
Fight-or-flight response, 276
Fingers
  anatomy, 89
  locking in flexed position, 96, 97
  "pencil-pointing," 271
  pinching with thumb, weakness, 134, 136
  trigger, 96–97
Finite element modeling method, 17
Finkelstein's test, 94
Flexeril *See* Cyclobenzaprine (Flexeril)
Flexor muscles, wrist, 100

Flexor retinaculum
  carpal tunnel, 92
  tarsal tunnel, 158
Flexor tendons
  in carpal tunnel, 126
  hand and wrist, 91
    trigger finger, 96
Fluoxetine hydrochloride (Prozac), 247
Foot, 149–155
  anatomy, 149–150
    arteries, 150
    bones/joints, 149, 150
    nerves, 149, 151
  chronic pain
    interdigital nerve damage, 152
    plantar fasciitis, 153
  drop, 182
  injury mechanisms, 150–151
  pain, tarsal tunnel syndrome, 158
  pathological conditions after accidents, 151–155
    fractures, 154
    interdigital neuroma, 151–153
    neurogenic pain, 154–155
    plantar fasciitis, 153
    reflex sympathetic dystrophy, 154–155
Foramina *See* Neural foramen
Force(s) *See also* G-force (gravity)
  acceleration *See* Acceleration (acceleration
    force)
  calculation, 15
  definition, 7
  direction and degree, MTBI biomechanics, 305
  equation, 10
  evaluation by direction (of source), 5
  multi-vector planes in rear end collisions, 16, 17
  Newton's third law of motion, 13
  rules of comparison, violation, 14, 16
Forearm
  anatomy, 100
  discomfort, 102
  muscles, 100–101
    spasm and epicondylitis due to, 102
  myofascial pain, 100–102
    treatment and complications, 102
  myofascial spasm, pronator syndrome, 132
Forgery, prescriptions, 387
Forward motion, perceived by occupant, 5
Forward torso bending, 68, 69
Fractures
  ankle joint, 157
  bone pain, 42, 48

Fractures *(Continued)*
  complications, 98, 104
    shoulder, 116
  compression *See* Vertebral compression fractures
  cranial, 42, 48
  dens of axis, 75
  elbow, 104
  foot, 154
  hand or wrist, 98
  hip joint, 174
  humeral head, 115–116
  humerus, 139
  internal fixation
    humeral head, 116
    vertebral, 204
  knee, 171
  lower extremity, 42
  occult (hairline)
    foot, 154
    radionuclide imaging, 80, 98, 154
  open and closed types, 104
  pars interarticularis *See* Spondylolysis
  radiography, 75
  RSDS after, 269
  shoulder, 115–116
  spinal, 48
  sternal, 42
  treatment, 104
    hand/wrist, 98
    immobilization, 98
  upper extremity, 48
Froment's sign, 134, 136
Frontal lobe syndrome, 318
Frontotemporal lesions, features/assessment, 333
Frontotemporal pattern of deficits, 337
Frontotemporal regions, injury, 307
Frozen shoulder *See* Shoulder, frozen (adhesive
  capsulitis)
Frustration tolerance, reduced after MTBI, 319, 359
Fry rules (701-Fry rule), 3
Functional capacity assessment (FCA), 241
Functional capacity evaluation (FCE), 241
Functional limitations, chronic pain syndrome, 233
Functional MRI (fMRI), mild traumatic brain injury,
  323, 324
F values (drag factor), 12, 27
F-waves, 125
  definition, 124
  median, prolongation, 133
  ulnar, prolongation, 136, 141
  upper extremity, 123

G

Gabapentin (Neurontin), 228–229
  migraine headache prophylaxis, 228
  neurogenic pain management, 262
Gadolinium DPTA, 78
Gaenslen's test, 178, 213
Gait
  alterations
    interdigital neuroma, 153
    knee bursitis/tendonitis, 169
    knee ligament injuries, 167
  balance and, 68–71 See also Balance
  compensatory (after injury), pelvic injuries, 176
  forward torso bending (forward carriage), 68, 69
  functional asymmetry, 67–68
    patterns, 68
  head rotations during, 71
  head tilt and lower extremity muscle activity, 70
  kinetic chain and, 64–65
  lateral torso bending (lateral carriage), 68
  limb lift phase, 67
  lower extremity weight and lifting load during, 67, 68
  phases, 66–67
  repetition and symmetry, 66–68
  shoulder-pelvis counter-rotation, 65, 66
  spine relationship, 65–66
  steps per minute, 67
  steps (cycles) per walking hour, 67
  trunk position and neck reflexes, 70
  vestibular and neck proprioceptive systems, 70–71
Gait analysis, 63–72
  video See Video gait analysis
"Gait control hypothesis," pain, 262
Galveston Orientation and Amnesia Test (GOAT), 326, 327
Gamma camera, 79
Gamma radiation, 79
Ganglion (fluid collection), 95–96
  aspiration, 95–96
  complications, 96
Ganglion, sympathetic, 283–284, 285
Ganglion blocks, 283
  sympathetic, 283–287
Gastric motility, opioid-induced decrease, 373
Gastrointestinal tract, opioids side effects, 373, 382
Gaze stability, during ambulation, 71
General Neuropsychological Deficit Scale (GNDS), 335, 351

G-force (gravity), 6–7, 13–17
  Allen's theories, 13–14
    arguments against/problems, 14, 16–17
  calculation, 13–17
    activities of daily living and, 13–14, 16
  crush distance relationship, 11
  reasons for inappropriateness to rear end collisions, 13–14, 16–17
  single plane, problem, 17
  tolerance, human factors affecting, 15
Glasgow Coma Scale (GCS), 299, 326
Glenohumeral joint, 105, 107
  capsule, 105, 107
Glenohumeral ligaments, 105, 107
Glenoid fossa, 105, 106
Glenoid labrum, 105
Glial injury, 308
Glutamate, in brain injury, 308
Gluteal pain, 179
Gluteus maximus, 176
Gluteus medius, 171, 175
Gravity See G-force (gravity)
Greater occipital nerves, 24, 26, 44, 52, 143
  irritation, headache, 44
Grieving process, for losses after MTBI, 340, 341
Group psychotherapy, MTBI treatment, 342–343
Guanethidine, 283
Guyon's canal, 90, 121
  anatomy, 91, 133
Guyon's canal syndrome, 133–134, 258
  diagnosis and treatment, 134

H

Halstead Impairment Index (HII), 335
Halstead-Reitan Battery (HRB), 333–334, 335, 353
Hamstring muscle, tight, 186
Hamstring tendons
  injuries, 47
  pain, 184
Hand and wrist, 89–99 See also Fingers; Wrist
  anatomy, 89–92
    bones, 89, 90
    joints, 89
    ligaments, 89
    nerves, 89–90
    tendons, 91, 92
  blood flow, carpal tunnel syndrome, 129
  injuries due to motor vehicle accidents, 93–99
    fractures, 98
    ganglion, 95–96
    ligament tears, 89, 97–98

Hand and wrist *(Continued)*
  injuries due to motor vehicle
      accidents *(Continued)*
    RSDS, 99
    strained ligaments, 97
    tendonitis, 93–94
    trigger finger, 96–97
  injury mechanisms, 92–93
  muscles, 100
  sensory abnormality, carpal tunnel syndrome, 128
  sensory testing, carpal tunnel syndrome, 127–128
  weakness
    carpal tunnel syndrome, 127
    pronator syndrome, 132
Head
  acceleration, neck circumference effect,
      15–16, 27
  acceleration G force variability, 15
  angular stabilization
    inertial guidance, 71
    visual and vestibular reference, 70–71
  CT scans, 76
  impact with headrest, 306 *See also* Headrest
  inertia, lag time for movement, 7, 9
  injury, pain, 41 *See also* Headache
  MRI scans, 78
  position at impact, injury potential, 27
  posterior tilt, lower extremity muscle activity, 70
  rotations
    decreased in normal subjects, 71
    during locomotion, 71
    whiplash, 306
Headache, 43–44, 215–231, 259
  causes, 215
  effect on neuropsychological testing, 313
  mixed, 44
  MTBI comorbidity, 313
  occipital nerve irritation, 44, 52, 143,
      215–216, 259
  pathophysiology, 43–44, 52
  post-concussive symptom, 316
  secondary to temporomandibular joint
      dysfunction, 44, 216–218
  tension-type, 215–216
  vascular (migraine) *See* Migraine (vascular
      headache)
  withdrawal, after high caffeine intakes, 223
Headrest
  impact and effect on deceleration time, 306
  injury potential affected by, 28, 30
Heel spurs, 153

Hemarthrosis, knee, 171
Hematoma, dorsal roots, 25–26
Hemispatial inattention, 320
Herbal remedies, sleep disturbance in MTBI, 347
Hip abductor muscles, 176
Hip extensors, 176
Hip flexors, 171, 176
Hip joint/region, 171–175
  abduction, 171, 176
  anatomy, 171, 172
    muscles, 175
  arthroplasty, 175
  chronic pain, 174, 175
  degenerative arthritis, 174
  injuries, 50
    mechanisms, 172–173
  pain, 175
    in sacroiliac joint dysfunction, 178
  pathological conditions after accidents, 50,
      173–175
    aseptic necrosis, 50, 174–175
    fractures, 174
    hip strain, 173–174
    myofascial pain, 175
    trochanteric bursitis, 173
  range of motion, 49
  stretching exercises, 174
Hippocampus damage, 308
Histamine, 53
HLA B27 antigen, 73
Home exercise program, lumbar
    radiculopathy, 189
Homeopathy, sleep disturbance in MTBI, 347
Hooper Visual Organization Test, 354, 357
Hormones, opioids effect on, 372
Horner's syndrome, 284
Hot packs, RSDS treatment and, 288
Human tolerance to injury *See* Tolerance to injury
Humeral groove, 139
Humeral head, fracture, 115–116
Humerus, fractures, radial nerve
    entrapment with, 139
Hybrid dummy crash tests, 17
Hydrocodone bitartrate, 377
Hydrogen nuclei, MRI, 77
Hydromorphone hydrochloride, 380, 401
5-hydroxytryptamine (5-HT) *See* Serotonin
Hyperabduction test
  abduction external rotation (AER) position, 140,
      141, 255
  positive (shoulder), 118

Hyperextension
    facet joints injuries, 50
    hyperflexion–hyperextension injury, 21, 22, 41
    spine, 199, 203–204
    wrist *See* Wrist, hyperextension
Hyperflexion, spine, 198–199, 203, 209
    facet joint injuries, 50
Hyperflexion–hyperextension injury (whiplash),
        21, 22, 41 *See also* Whiplash
Hypersensitivity, to pain, 43
Hypnosis, RSDS treatment, 289
Hypnotics
    in chronic pain, 239
    depression management, 238
    for sleep disturbance, 238, 239
Hypoarousal, after MTBI, 345
Hypometabolism, cerebral, 322
Hypothalamus, opioids effect on, 372
Hypothenar muscle, atrophy, 133
Hypothyroidism, tests, 74
Hypoxia, muscle, 45

I

Ice applications
    hand or wrist tendonitis, 93–94
    migraine headache treatment, 229
Iliac bones, 175
Iliopsoas muscle, 175, 176
Imipramine (Tofranil), 239
Immobilization
    fracture treatment, 98
    shoulder capsule strain, 114
Impairment rating, 240, 241
Impulse, definition, 7
Independent medical evaluation (IME), case study
        of MTBI, 349
Inderal (propanolol), migraine (vascular
        headache), 222
Inertia, 7
    lag time for head/neck, 7, 9
    Newton's first law of motion, 9
Infection
    intrathecal opioid pump implantation
        complication, 406
    spinal cord stimulation complication, 397–398
Inflammation, pain management, 242
Information processing, slowed, after MTBI,
        340, 351
Infrared imaging technique, 80–81
Infraspinatus muscle, 110
Infusaid pump, 402

Injury evaluation, 2
Injury exposure, definition as first step in causality
        determination, 3
Injury mechanisms, 21–23, 30–31
    elbow *See* Elbow joint/region
    foot, 150–151
    hand and wrist, 92–93
    knee, 161–164
    myofascial/myoneuronal entrapments,
        24–25
    neurovascular entrapments, 25
    pelvis, 176
    rectus capitis posterior minor muscle, 24
    shoulder, 111
    S-shaped curve of cervical spine, 21–23
    water hammer theory of neuromas, 25–26
Injury potential
    cervical spine loading, 21–22
    despite vehicle damage absence, 10, 12
    determination from deceleration force, 9
    factors increasing, 27–28, 29
    headrest affecting, 28, 30
    neck rotation, 26, 27–28
    not determined from vehicle damage, 29
    preparedness effect, 17, 28
    primary direction of force effect, 28
    reduced by accident time increase, 9,
        10–11
Injury potential evaluation, 17–20, 29
    stress–strain curve, 18–20
    tissue damage, 17
Injury predictive factors, 16
Injury rates
    motor vehicle accidents, 4, 5
    rear end collisions, 4, 5
Insurance companies/agents, vii *See also*
        Reconstructionist (of accidents)
    case study of MTBI and, 349
Intellectual/academic abilities, assessment, 331
Interdigital nerve
    anatomy, 149, 151–152
    entrapment, 52
    foot, 52, 149
    injuries, 151–153
Interdigital neuroma, 151–153, 259
Internal focus of control, 235
International Neuropsychology Society, 328
Interneurons, anterior horn cell activation, 279
Interosseii, atrophy, 133
Interspinous ligaments, 182, 196, 203
    tears, 209

Intervertebral disc (IVD)
    anatomy, 193–195, 196 *See also* Annulus
        fibrosus; Nucleus pulposus
    bulging, 198, 207, 208, 209
    cervical *See* Cervical discs
    degeneration, 205–208
        appearance, 207
        consequences, 206–207
    function as shock-absorber, 193, 206
    herniation, 195, 208–209, 259
    lumbar *See* Lumbar discs
    lumbar vs cervical, 194–195, 197
    normal appearance, 207
    as source of spinal pain, 26
Intrathecal opioid pump implantation, 289,
    401–407
    cephalad migration of opioid, 401, 406
    indications, 401, 402
    infusion pumps, 402, 404, 405
        continuous-infusion, 402
        programmable, 402, 404, 405
    morphine vs fentanyl, 401, 402
    side effects and complications, 406–407
    technique, 402–406
        flow-rate titration follow-up,
            404, 406
        implantation position, 405
Involuntary activities, 200
Iodine contrast
    for CT, 76
    hypersensitivity, 76
Iontophoresis, epicondylitis, 103
IQ measurement, 336, 352
Irritability, after MTBI, 319, 359

J

Jaw, malalignment, 217
Jerk, 7
Joint *See also individual joints*
    "ball and socket," 171
    definition/anatomy, 48
    degrees of motion, 49
    as focus of pain, 49
    injuries of specific joints, 49–50
    pain, 48–50
        causes, 49
    sutures, 48
    synarthrodial, 48, 196
    synovial (diarthrodial), 48, 198
Joint capsule, 48
    sacroiliac joint, 175

Joint Commission for the Accreditation of Hospital
    Organizations (JCAHO), 234
Jolt, 7

K

Kegel exercises, 180
Kinematic models, 64–65
Kinetic chain, 64–65
    compensatory postures/movements, 68, 69
    position during ambulation, 68, 69
Kinetic energy, 6, 7, 27
    concepts relating to, 14
    conversion to/from potential energy, 65
    definition, 7
    increased for occupants by vehicle deformation
        failure, 15, 29, 30, 31
    vehicle size effect, 27
Klonopin *See* Clonazepam (Klonopin)
Klove Sensory Perceptual Evaluation, 354
Knee
    anatomy, 161, 162 *See also* Patella; *specific
        ligaments*
        bursas, 168
        ligaments, 161, 163, 166
        menisci, 161, 164
    bracing, 167, 170
    "dashboard" *See* "Dashboard knee"
    effusion, 164, 166
    giving way, 166
    hemarthrosis, 171
    injury mechanisms, 50, 161–164
        direct impact injuries, 164
    instability, 166, 167
    pain, "dashboard knee," 164
    pathological conditions after accidents, 50,
        164–171
        bursitis/tendonitis, 47, 168–169
        chondromalacia patella *See* "Dashboard
            knee"
        fractures involving, 171
        ligament strain/sprains, 166–167
        torn meniscus, 169–170
    popping, 166, 169
    range of motion, 49
    valgus/varus stress testing, 166, 167

L

Lactic acid, 45
Language, testing, 353
Language-based problems, 317–318
Large intestine, opioids side effects, 370, 373, 383

Lateral antebrachial cutaneous nerve, 100, 104, 120
Lateral collateral ligament
    ankle, 155
    knee, 161, 163, 166
        tears/strains, 166–167
        testing, 166, 167
Lateral epicondylitis, 101, 102–103, 138
Lateralization, dysfunction patterns, 333
Lateral plantar nerve, 149
Lateral recess stenosis, 207, 208
Lateral retinacular ligament, 161
Lateral torso bending, 68
Latissimus dorsi, 110
Law of conservation of momentum/energy, 10
Leg length discrepancy, 175
Lesser occipital nerves, 44, 52, 143
Level of effort, 314–315
Levorphanol tartrate, 381
Libido, decreased, chronic pain syndrome, 233
Lidocaine, 245
    oral agents, 245, 262
Ligament(s), 40, 48
    anatomy, 46
    ankle, 155, 157
    elbow, 99
    hand and wrist, 89
    knee, 161, 163, 166
    lumbar spine, 182
    shoulder, 105, 107
    spinal, 195–196, 198
Ligament injuries
    ankle, 157–158
    pain, 46–47
    strains
        ankle, 157
        definition, 157
        elbow, 104–105
        hand and wrist, 97
        hip, 173–174
    tears, 40–41, 46
        ankle, 157, 158
        anterior longitudinal ligament, 41–42
        complications, 98
        hand and wrist, 89, 97–98
        interspinous ligaments, 209
        lunotriquetal ligament, 97
        medial collateral ligament (knee), 166–167
        scapholunate ligament, 97
Ligamentum flavum, 182, 196, 202
Ligamentum lacinatum, 156

Limping, chronic
    aseptic necrosis of hip, 175
    "dashboard knee," 166
    hip strains, 174
    interdigital neuroma, 153
    plantar fasciitis, 153
    sacroiliac joint dysfunction, 179
Line Bisection Test, 354, 357
Lipid peroxidation, depression in MTBI due to changes, 312
Litigation aspects
    after MTBI, 340
    spinal cord stimulation and, 392
Livingston's vicious cycle, 279
Load
    definition, 7
    simulated collisions, cadaver studies, 15
Load deformation
    curve See Stress–strain curve
    definition, 7
Lock-and-key phenomenon, opiate receptors, 368
Longus coli, 25
Lordosis-kyphosis-lordosis curve, 66
Low back pain, 65
    facet arthropathy pain, 208
    structures involved, 203
Low back strains, 179
Lower extremity See also specific anatomical regions
    fractures, 42
    injuries causing RSDS, 269
    innervation, 256
    joint injuries, 50
    ligament injuries, 46
    muscle activity linked to posterior head tilt, 70
    muscles, nerve root innervation, 182, 184
    nerve entrapments, 51–52, 86, 258
    neurological examination, 184–185
    pain, 149–190
        causes, 42
    tendon injuries, 47
    weakness, 209
    weight and lifting load during ambulation, 67, 68
Lower extremity bracing (in accidents), 41
    Achilles bursa trauma, 47
    ankle injuries, 156
    foot injuries, 150–151
    fractures and bone pain, 42, 48
    hip injuries, 172
    knee injuries, 164

Lower extremity bracing
 (in accidents) *(Continued)*
 ligament injuries, 46
 pelvic injuries, 176
Low impact, rear end collisions, vii
Lumbar discs, 182
 comparison with cervical, 194–195, 197
 herniation, 208
Lumbar epidural steroid injections, 188
Lumbar laminectomy, 189
Lumbar nerve roots *See also* Lumbosacral
 nerve roots
 L4, nerve block, 261
 L4/L5 impingement, 182
 L5, 201–202
 pain, 52
Lumbar plexus, 183, 253
Lumbar radiculopathy, 52, 181–189, 259 *See also*
 Lumbosacral radiculopathy
 clinical features, 182, 184
 diagnostic workup, 186
 treatment, 188–189
Lumbar spinal nerve, 182
Lumbar spine
 anatomy, 181–182, 191
 cervical spine comparison, 194–195,
 197
 similarities, 65
 "functional unit" (three-joint complex),
 182
 instability, assessment (x-ray), 75
 ligaments, 182
 movement, 182
 pathology, 65
 radiography, 75
 range of movement, 191
 stability, 182
Lumbar traction, 188
Lumbar vertebrae, 181, 191
 anatomy, 206
Lumbosacral angle, 210
Lumbosacral nerve roots, 181, 182, 253 *See also*
 Lumbar nerve roots
 muscles innervated, 182, 184
 nerve blocks and, 188
Lumbosacral plexus, 183, 202
Lumbosacral radiculopathy, 86, 185–186 *See also*
 Lumbar radiculopathy
 bladder dysfunction, 186
 treatment, 188–189
Lunotriquetal ligament, tears, 97

Luria-Nebraska Neuropsychological Battery
 (LNNB), 333–334
Luschka, joints, 142
Luschka, recurrent nerve, 202

M

Magnetic resonance imaging (MRI), 77–79
 advantages, 77–78
 carpal tunnel syndrome, 129
 cervical radiculopathy, 145
 disadvantages, 78
 films after motor vehicle accidents, 78–79
 functional (fMRI), in MTBI, 323, 324
 lumbar radiculopathy, 186, 188
 mild traumatic brain injury, 322
 MR silent tissues, 77
 perfusion (pMRI), in MTBI, 323
 principle, 77
 procedure and preparation for, 78
 rotator cuff tear, 117
 safety issues, 78
Magnetic source imaging (MSI), 324
Magnetoencephalography (MEG), 324
Malingering, 315
 incidence, 315
Mania, after MTBI, 318–319
Manipulation under anesthesia, shoulder,
 119
Mass
 force relationship, 10, 27
 vehicles, 27
Massage therapy, vertebral body fractures, 204
Masseter muscle, 217
 chronic contraction, 217–218
 paracervical myofascial pain referred to,
 46, 217
Maxalt (rizatriptan benzoate), migraine (vascular
 headache), 223
Maximum medical improvement, 240
McMurray test, 169, 170
Medial collateral ligament
 ankle *See* Deltoid ligament
 knee, 161, 163, 166
 tears/strains, 166–167
 testing, 166, 167
Medial plantar nerve, 149
Medial retinacular ligament, 161
Median nerve, 89, 90
 anatomy, 89, 90, 121, 125–126
 course and branches, 90, 121, 131
 autonomic fibers, 129

Median nerve *(Continued)*
  conduction velocity assessment
    motor, 124
    sensory, 123
  at elbow, 100
  entrapment, 51, 121, 257–258
    at carpal tunnel *See* Carpal tunnel syndrome
    in proximal forearm *See* Pronator syndrome
    sites, 121, 132
  functions, 126
  irritation, forearm myofascial pain, 101
  lesions, 256
  mixed motor/sensory nerve, 89, 126, 129, 131
  origin from C4-T1 nerve roots, 126
  segmental stimulation technique, 129, 130, 131
  sensory latency, 129
Medical probability, of causation of injury, 3, 4
Medication *See* Drugs
Medico-legal aspects *See also* Litigation aspects
  case closure, chronic pain clinic work, 240–241
  causation evaluation, 3, 4
  sub-optimal motivation aspect, 315
Medtronic ITREL II pulse generator, 395, 396, 397
Medtronic SynchroMed Infusion Pump, 402, 404, 405
Medulla, descending modulatory pain system, 254
Memory *See also* Amnesia
  assessment, 355
  remediation, rehabilitation after MTBI, 343
  short-term, defects, 317, 350
Menisci, knee, 161, 164
  tears, 169–170
Mental capability, borderline, chronic pain clinic and, 241
Mental illness, costs, 236
Mental state assessment, mild traumatic brain injury, 326
Meperidine hydrochloride, 380–381
Meprobamate, 243
Metacarpal bones, 89
Metaxalone (Skelaxin), 243
Methadone hydrochloride, 379, 401
Methocarbamol (Robaxin), 243
Metoclopramide (Reglan)
  migraine (vascular headache), 223
  opioid-induced nausea, 383
Mexiletine (Mexitil)
  neurogenic pain management, 245, 262
  side effects, 245
Midbrain, stimulation, stimulation-produced analgesia due to, 56

Middle-latency auditory evoked potentials (MLAEP), 325
Migraine (vascular headache), 44, 218–222, 259
  causes, 218
  drug treatment, 222–229
    injectable and inhalable, 226
    mechanism of action, 222
    preventive, 223, 227–229
    symptomatic, 222–223, 225–227
  foods to avoid, 229
  frequency/course, 222
  nonpharmacologic treatment, 229
  pathophysiology, 218–222
  pre-existing history, 215
Migrating pain syndrome, 234
Mild traumatic brain injury (MTBI), 297–365 *See also* Post-concussive syndrome (PCS)
  acceleration/deceleration forces causing, 298, 306
  biomechanics, 305–306
  case study, 348–360
    history and background, 349–350
    interpretation of test results, 351, 357
    MMPI-2 and BDI-II interpretation, 357–358
    recommendations, 359–360
    referral information, 348–349
    symptoms, 350, 351, 356, 358
    test results, 352–356
  co-morbid factors affecting cognitive function, 310–315
    drugs affecting, 314
    emotional distress, 311–312
    fatigue, 313–314, 316, 340, 347, 350
    pain, 312–313, 347, 350
    sleep disturbances, 313–314, 316, 347, 350
    sub-optimal motivation (level of effort), 314–315
  cumulative effects of brain injury, 301, 308, 309
  definitions, 300–305
    American Academy of Neurology, 302
    American Congress of Rehabilitation Medicine, 300–301, 303, 304
    Colorado Medical Society, 301–302
    DSM-IV, 303
    neuropsychological, 303–304
    Ruff classification system, 304
  diagnosis, 321–326
    comparison of techniques, 322, 323
    electrophysiological, 325
    insensitivity of CT and MRI, 322

Mild traumatic brain injury (MTBI) *(Continued)*
  diagnosis *(Continued)*
    mental state methodologies, 326
    neuroimaging, 321–325
  effect on IQ scores, 336
  evidence, 298
  importance of asking questions, 299–300,
    316, 326
  importance of early diagnosis/treatment, 300
    cognitive rehabilitation, 342, 343
  incidence, 299
  losses resulting from, 340
  low impact, rear end collisions causing, 297–299
  neuropsychological assessment, 327–335 *See
    also* Neuropsychological assessment
  pathophysiology, 306–309
    axonal injury and transneuronal
      degeneration, 309
    diffuse axonal injuries, 307
    focal vs diffuse injuries, 307
    neurochemical cascade, 308
    primary injuries, 307
    secondary injuries, 307–308
  predisposition/vulnerability, 309–310
    genetic, 310
    premorbid neurological history, 309
    premorbid psychiatric history, 310
  significant cognitive impairment due to, 305
  symptoms, 316–321
    case study, 350, 351, 356, 358
    checklist, 320–321
    cognitive, 317–318, 320
    confusion after, 340, 348
    patterns (diffuse/focal), 336–337
    physical, 316–317, 320
    psychological, 318–319, 320–321
    vision, 319–320, 321, 345–347, 350
  treatment/rehabilitation, 339–348
    cognitive rehabilitation, 343
    iatrogenically-induced stress due to, 347
    multidisciplinary approach, 339
    physiatrist's role, 347–348
    psychiatric, 345
    psychotherapy *See* Psychotherapy
    vestibular evaluation/treatment, 344–345
    visual rehabilitation, 345–347
    vocational rehabilitation, 343–344
  underdiagnosis and misdiagnosis, 299–300,
    328
Millon Clinical Multi-axial Inventory-3 (MCMI-3),
  329, 330

Mimocausalgia *See* Reflex sympathetic dystrophy
  syndrome (RSDS)
Mini-mental state exam (MMSE), 326
Minnesota Multiphasic Personality Inventory–
  Second Version (MMPI-2), 312,
  329, 330
  case study interpretation, 357–358
Mirtazapine (Remeron), 248
  depression management, 248
MMPI-2 *See* Minnesota Multiphasic Personality
  Inventory–Second Version (MMPI-2)
Models, 14-segment, 64, 65
Momentum
  definition, 7–8
  equation, 10–12
  law of conservation, 10
Monoamine oxidase inhibitors (MAO), 246
Mood changes, after MTBI, 318
Morphine, 374 *See also* Opioid analgesia
  administration routes, 374
  intrathecal, 401
  mechanism of action, 368
  metabolism and half-life, 374
Morphine sulfate, 374, 378
  sustained-release (SRMS), 374, 378
Morton's neuroma, 52
Motor coordination problems, 316
Motor functioning, assessment, 330, 331, 355
Motor nerves, testing, 255–256
  lower extremity, 184
  upper extremity, 143
Motor planning, ineffective, 331
Motor vehicle accidents
  categorization by PDOF, 5
  costs, 4
  frontal, inertia and Newton's first law, 9
  pain types due to, 41–44
  preparation effect on injury potential, 17, 28
  primary direction of force (PDOF), 4, 5
  severity
    indication by $\triangle v$, 10
    reduction by use of G-force
      (inappropriately), 14
  side impact, torquing injuries, 42
  as uncontrolled events, daily living activities
    not comparison, 16
Movement, increased, pain down-regulation,
  262, 280
Movement receptor activation, neurogenic pain
  management, 262
MTBI *See* Mild traumatic brain injury (MTBI)

Multidisciplinary team
  chronic pain clinic, 239–240
  MTBI treatment/rehabilitation, 339, 347
Muscle(s)
  anatomy, 44
  atrophy, prevention, 262
  blood supply impairment, 45
  contraction, 44, 45
    motor nerve conduction velocity, 81, 82, 83
    myofascial pain syndrome, 236
    repetitive during ambulation, 68
  elbow, 100
  forearm, 100–101, 102
  hand and wrist, 100
  hip joint, 175
  pelvic floor, 180
  pelvis, 176, 179
  shoulder joint, 110
  spasm See Muscle spasm
  spine, 203
  strains, pain, 44
  tears
    chronic pain, 40
    strains causing, pain, 44
  toxic metabolite accumulation, 45
Muscle relaxants
  chronic pain management, 243
  drugs included, 244
  mechanism of action, 243
Muscle spasm, 45
  cycle, RSDS, 279
  epicondylitis, 102
  in fibromyalgia syndrome, 43
  forearm, 101
  headache due to, 43, 44
  muscle shortening, 45
  in myofascial pain syndrome, 42
  pain mechanism, 45
  paracervical, 45
  paracervical suboccipital muscles, 43–44
  as protective reflex, 45
  reactive, spinal, 209
  rotator cuff tendonitis complication, 113
  shoulder region, 50, 119
  spinal, 203
  tension-type headaches, 215
  treatment, 243
  trochanteric bursitis, 173
Musculocutaneous nerve, 120
Mutations, 75
Myelin, 253

Myelinated fibers
  large See A-alpha mechanoreceptor sensory
    fibers
  thin See A-delta fibers (thin myelinated)
Myelogram
  cervical radiculopathy, 145
  lumbar disc herniation, 209
  lumbar radiculopathy, 186
Myofascial pain
  hip, 175
  migration, 236
Myofascial pain syndrome, 42, 45–46
  cervical, 217
  chronic pain, 236–237
  clinical features, 236
  paracervical, 45, 46
  pelvis, 179–180
  shoulder, 118
  suboccipital region, 46
  treatment, 237
  "trigger points," 42, 236
Myogenic thoracic outlet syndrome See Thoracic
    outlet syndrome, myogenic
Myotomes, 182
  cervical nerve roots, 143
  lumbosacral nerve roots, 182

N

NAA/creatinine ratio, 324–325
Nail changes, thoracic outlet syndrome, 141
Naloxone, 406
Naratriptan hydrochloride (Amerge), migraine
    (vascular headache), 223
National Institute of Health Consensus Statement,
    308
Nausea/vomiting, 317
  drug treatment, 223, 226
  opioids causing, 373, 382–383
Neck
  circumference
    effect on head acceleration, 15–16, 27
    as risk factor for injury potential, 27
  inertia, lag time for movement, 7, 9
  injuries, cervical myofascial trigger points, 43
  pain
    after whiplash, 23
    mechanical, 65
    in women vs men, 16–17
  proprioception, 70
    disruption in whiplash, 70
  rotation, injury potential, 26, 27–28

Neck muscles
    functions, 70
    injury causing headaches, 43–44
    tears in hyperextension injuries, 41–42
Neck reflexes, trunk position association, 70
Nefazodone hydrochloride (Serzone), 247
Neospinothalamic tract (NSTT), 55–56, 57, 253, 279
    localization of pain impulses, 254
Nerve(s)
    elbow, 100
    entrapment *See* Peripheral nerve entrapment
    foot, 149, 151
    hand and wrist, 89–90
    peripheral *See* Peripheral nerve(s)
    regeneration, 51
    transection/damage, 51
Nerve blocks
    interdigital neuroma, 152
    lumbar radiculopathy, 188
    neurogenic pain
        assessment, 261
        in foot, 155
        management, 263–264
Nerve conduction velocity (NCV)
    antidromic conduction, 123
    distal latencies, 122
    lumbar radiculopathy, 186
    nerve damage effect, 260
    orthodromic, 123, 222
    upper extremity, 145
        vs lower extremity, 122, 260
Nerve conduction velocity (NCV), assessment, 81
    carpal tunnel syndrome, 129
    motor, 81, 82, 83, 124
        calculation, 125, 126
    neurogenic pain, 260
    principle, 122
    procedure, 122–123
    sensory, 81, 84, 85, 124–125
        calculation, 125
    upper extremity, 122–125
    at wrist, carpal tunnel syndrome, 129, 130, 131
Nerve roots *See* Spinal nerve roots
Neural foramen, 142, 182, 202
    cervical, 142
    lumbar, 182
    narrowing due to disc degeneration, 207
    stenosis, 207, 258–259
Neuralgia, occipital, 44, 52
Neurapraxia, 125, 127, 133, 136

Neurectomy, 153, 263
Neuritis, interdigital, 52
Neuroablative procedures, 263
Neurochemical cascade, brain injury, 308
Neurocognitive functioning, areas and testing, 330–331
Neurogenic claudication, 208
Neurogenic pain, 51–52, 253–265
    from carpal tunnel syndrome, 130–131
    elbow, 105
    foot injuries, 154–155
    medication, 244–246, 262
        anticonvulsants, 245–246, 262
        clonidine, 244, 262
        mexiletine, 245, 262
        tricyclic antidepressants, 246, 262
    pathophysiology, 253–254
    physical examination, 255–257
    symptoms and signs, 51, 154, 254–255
    tarsal tunnel syndrome, 159
    treatment, 261–264
        foot pain, 155
        interdigital neuroma, 153
        lumbar radiculopathy, 189
        physical/occupational therapy, 261–262
        tarsal tunnel syndrome, 159
        TENS and stimulation devices, 262–263
    upper extremity nerve entrapments, 130–131, 257–259
    workup, 259–261
Neurogenic problems, in motor vehicle accidents, 257–259
    entrapments *See* Peripheral nerve entrapment
    headache *See* Headache
    nerve root irritation, 258–259
    neuroma *See* Neuroma
    radiculopathy *See* Cervical radiculopathy; Lumbar radiculopathy
Neuroimaging
    categories of techniques, 321
    mild traumatic brain injury, 321–325
    new techniques, 324–325
Neurological examination
    lower extremity, 184–185
    upper extremity, 143–145
Neurolysis, 153, 263
Neuroma, 51, 259
    interdigital, 151–153, 259
    Morton's, 52
    water hammer theory, 25–26
Neuronal impairment, long-distance, 309

Neurontin (gabapentin), 228–229
Neuropsychological assessment, 86, 297–365
  case study, 351–360
    result interpretation, 351, 357
  clinical interview, 327–329
    baseline functioning, 328
    history of accident, 327
    preface to questions, 328
  clinical psychological screening, 329–330
    cautions on use/interpretation, 329, 330
  drugs affecting, 314
  headache effect, 313
  MTBI, 327–335
    PET scanning comparison, 323
  pain effect on, 312–313
  postponing, reasons, 315
  reading and interpretation of reports,
      335–338
    case study, 351, 357
    feedback session, 338
    "relative weakness" meaning, 337
  referral process, 327
  ruling out sub-optimal motivation, 315
  testing See Neuropsychological tests/testing
  underestimation of cognitive deficits, 335, 337,
      338
Neuropsychological tests/testing, in MTBI,
    330–334
  choice of tests/batteries, 334
  cognitive domains assessed, 330–331
  computerized batteries, 334
  emotional disorders effect, 312
  fixed batteries, 333–334, 335
    disadvantages, 334, 335
  fixed vs flexible batteries, 333–334
    process approach, 334
  index score sensitivity, 335
  levels of data analysis, 332–333
  pattern of symptoms revealed, 336–337
  standardization of environment for, 338
  ways for identification of deficits,
      332–333
    level of performance, 332–333
    pathognomonic signs, 333
    patterns of lateralized dysfunction, 333
    patterns of performance, 333
Neurotin, neurogenic pain management, 245
Neurotransmitters See also specific
    neurotransmitters
  release, brain injury, 308
Neurovascular entrapments, 25

Newton's laws of motion, 9–17
  first law, 9
  second law, 10–13
  third law, 13
Night vision, decreased, 320
Nociception, spinal, 203
Nociceptive fibers, 52–53 See also A-delta fibers
    (thin myelinated); C-fibers (unmyelinated)
Nociceptive impulses, 253–254
  ascending pathways, 52–54, 218 See also Pain
      pathways
  decreased by TENS, 262
  to nucleus caudalis, 218, 219
  reduced by increased proprioceptive input,
      262, 280
  RSDS pathophysiology, 277, 278
  supraspinal, 218–219, 220
Nociceptors
  primary, 52, 53
  spinal, 202, 203
  stimuli depolarizing, 53
  substances released from, 53
  transduction, 53
Nociceptor-specific pain transmission cell
    (NSPTC), 54, 55
  in nucleus caudalis, 218
  in RSDS, 277, 278
Nocturnal paresthesia, 51, 84
  carpal tunnel syndrome, 127
  elbow pain, 105
  thoracic outlet syndrome, 140
Noise
  background, difficulties after MTBI, 317, 345
  sensitivity (phonophobia), 317, 345, 350, 359
Noise attenuation earplugs, 345, 359
Nonsteroidal anti-inflammatory drugs (NSAIDs),
    242
  myofascial pain syndrome, 237
  RSDS treatment, 289
Noradrenergic pain modulatory pathway, 56, 58
Norepinephrine
  antidepressant mechanism of action, 246, 247
  depression pathophysiology, 238
  dorsal horn neuron inhibition, 56, 58
  release, endorphin action, 254
  sympathetically maintained pain (SMP),
      280–281
  vasoconstriction due to, 276, 281
Norpramin See Desipramine (Norpramin)
Nortriptyline (Pamelor), 239
  migraine headache prophylaxis, 228

Nuclear imaging *See* Radionuclide (nuclear) imaging
Nuclear magnetic resonance (NMR), 77
Nucleus caudalis, 218
    nociceptive impulses to, 218, 219
    second-order pain transmission cells, 218, 219
Nucleus pulposus, 193, 196
    insensitivity to pain, 202
    lumbar region, 195
    protrusion, 198
Numbness, lumbar radiculopathy, 182

O

Obturator nerve, 182
Occipital-atlas articulation, 199
Occipital nerves, 44, 52
    greater *See* Greater occipital nerves
    irritation, 259
        headache, 143, 215–216
        nociceptive pathway, 218
    lesser, 44, 52, 143
Occipital neuralgia, 44, 52, 215–216, 259
Occupants, of vehicle
    acceleration response variation, 15, 16
        validity/reliability reduction, 16
    biovariability, 20, 29
    perceived forward motion, 5
Occupational therapy
    carpal tunnel syndrome, 130
    cubital tunnel syndrome, 136
    elbow, ligament strains, 105
    epicondylitis, 103
    forearm myofascial pain, 102
    hand or wrist fractures, 98
    hand or wrist tendonitis, 93
    myofascial pain syndrome, 237
    rotator cuff tear, 117
    shoulder capsule strain, 114
    superficial radial nerve entrapment, 137
Olecranon, 99
Olecranon bursa, 99
Olecranon bursitis, 103–104
Opiate receptors, 368–369
    classes, 368–369
    delta (δ), 369, 371, 372
    distribution, 58, 368, 371, 401, 404
    kappa (κ), 369, 371, 372, 401, 404
    lock-and-key phenomenon, 368
    mu (μ), 369, 371, 372, 401, 404

Opioid(s)
    abstinence (withdrawal) syndrome, 370
    actions (non-analgesic), 368
    activation of descending pain modulatory system, 56, 58–59, 368, 372
    addiction (psychological dependence), 369
        detoxification, 386
    CNS systems sensitive to, 368
    dependence, 370
    detoxification, 386
        before spinal cord stimulation, 391–392
    distribution in CSF, 401, 402, 403
    half-life, 367, 374
    hydrophilic, 401, 402
    intermediate, 378
    lipophilic, 401–402
    long-acting, 384
    mechanism of action, 368–369
    mild, 375–377, 385
    pharmacokinetics, epidural, 401–402, 403
    pharmacological properties, 371–373
    pseudoaddiction, 369–370, 383
        iatrogenic, 386
    stimulation-produced analgesia, 368
    strong, 378–381 *See also* Morphine
    tolerance, 370
        intrathecal administration, 407
        rapid development, 371, 383
    toxicity, 367
Opioid analgesia, 367–390 *See also* Morphine
    abuse behaviors, 385
        screening and features, 388
    abuse prevention, 387–388
    administration routes, 374
    "as required," 383
    by-the-clock, 383–384
    by-the-ladder, 383, 384
    consent before, 384, 385
    contraindications, 386
    discontinuous use, adverse effects, 383
    equi-analgesic dose charts, 384, 386
    follow up, 386–387
    guidelines, 383–388
    indications, 370–371
    individual requirements, 384
    intrathecal *See* Intrathecal opioid pump implantation
    migraine (vascular headache), 223, 225–226
    oral, before intrathecal, 401
    oral and transdermal doses, 384, 386

Opioid analgesia *(Continued)*
  parenteral, migraine (vascular headache), 223
  perceived risks, 367–368
  prescribing recommendations, 387–388
  pump implantation *See* Intrathecal opioid pump implantation
  reservations over use, 367, 371
  RSDS treatment, 289
  screening prior to initiation, 384
  side effects, 374, 382–383
    dangerous reactions, 382
    monitoring, 385
    nausea/vomiting, 373
  terminology and definitions, 369–370
Opioid peptides, endogenous, 56, 58–59
Orthodromic conduction (nerve), 123, 222
Orthotics
  Achilles bursitis/tendonitis, 160
  interdigital neuroma, 153
  plantar fasciitis, 153
Osteoarthritis (degenerative arthritis), 75
  ankle joint, 159–160
  hip, 174
Osteophytes *See* Bone spurs
Osteoporosis, in RSDS, 270, 272, 274
  bone scans, 275
Otoliths, 70
Overmedication, chronic pain, 240
Oxycodone hydrochloride, 378
Oxygen radicals, formation in brain injury, 308

P
Padula Visual Midline Screening Test, 357
Pain, 39–61
  acute, 39
  acute traumatic, 40
  back *See* Low back pain
  bone, 42, 48
  breakthrough, inadequate opioids, 367, 383–384
  chronic *See* Chronic pain/chronic pain syndromes
  chronicity, factors contributing, 31–32
  definition, 39
  diffuse, 52, 59
  distribution, 30
  down-regulation by A-alpha proprioceptive fibers, 280 *See also* Pain pathways, descending modulatory
  drug management *See* Analgesics
  emotional response, 254

Pain *(Continued)*
  forearm myofascial, 100–102
  "gait control hypothesis," 262
  hypersensitivity, 43
  joint *See* Joint, pain
  lancinating (electrical shooting)
    C5 radiculopathy, 145–146
    from carpal tunnel syndrome, 131
    lumbar radiculopathy, 182
    neurogenic pain, 255
    radial nerve entrapment, 139
  localization, neospinothalamic tract role, 254
  localized immediately after accident, 59
  lower extremity *See* Lower extremity, pain
  management skills, 240
  mapping, 23
  migrating syndrome, 234
  modulation, pathways, 56
  MTBI comorbidity, 312–313, 347
    case study, 350
  neurogenic *See* Neurogenic pain
  neuropsychological effects, 312–313
  pathophysiology *See* Pain pathways
  psychological influences, 39
  receptors, spinal, 202, 203
  referral patterns, 23
    "trigger points" in myofascial pain syndrome, 42, 236
  soft tissue, 44–47
    bursitis, 47
    ligament injuries, 46–47
    muscle spasms *See* Muscle spasm
    myofascial pain *See* Myofascial pain syndrome
    strains, 44
    tendon injuries, 47
  subjective nature, 39
  types caused by motor vehicle accidents, 41–44, 44–52
  upper extremity *See* Upper extremity, pain
  as "warning signal" of potential injury, 39
  "wind up" of pathways, 41, 43
  worsening/migrating, 52
"Pain cocktail," 240
Pain fibers, 52 *See also* A-delta fibers (thin myelinated); C-fibers (unmyelinated)
Pain pathways, 52–59
  ascending, 52–54, 218, 219, 221, 253
    activation and RSDS pathophysiology, 277–279
  within brain, 55–56, 219, 254

Pain pathways *(Continued)*
  descending modulatory, 56, 58, 254
    opiate activation, 56, 58–59, 368, 372
  inhibition of first/second order cells, 254
  localization, neospinothalamic tract role, 254
  to nucleus caudalis, 218, 219
  second-order pain transmission cells, 54, 55, 59, 218, 253
    inhibition by opioids, 372
  third-order pain transmission cells, 55–56
Pain sensitive structures, 21, 30
  in low speed collisions, 22
  spine, 202–203, 209
Pain syndromes, 26–27 *See also individual pain syndromes*
Paleospinothalamic tract (PSTT), 55, 57, 59, 253, 279
  emotional response to pain, 254, 279
Panic attacks, after MTBI, 342
Paracervical suboccipital muscles, spasm, 43–44, 45
Paraphasic errors, 317
Parasympathetic system, energy conservation, 276
Paresthesia, nocturnal *See* Nocturnal paresthesia
Parietal lobe dysfunction, tests, 357
Paroxetine hydrochloride (Paxil), depression management, 247
Pars interarticularis, 193
  fracture *See* Spondylolysis
Passenger, injuries
  elbow, 100
  foot, 151
  wrist and hand, 93
Patella, 161, 162
  injuries, 50
Patella grind test, 164, 165
Patella ligament, 161
Patella tendon, 168
  inflammation, 168–169
Patella tracking brace, 165
Patient education
  disability management in chronic pain, 235
  effects of post-concussive syndrome, 327
  individual psychotherapy in MTBI, 339
  intrathecal opioid pump implantation, 402
Patients
  doctor/patient relationship, 235
  external focus of control, 235
  internal focus of control, 235
  perception as victims, 234
  rights to appropriate medical care, vii, 2

Patrick test, 174, 178, 213
Paxil (paroxetine hydrochloride), depression management, 247
Peabody Individual Achievement Test (PIAT), 352
Pectoralis major muscle, 110
Pectoralis minor muscle, 25, 110
Pectoral muscles, 110
Pedicles, vertebral, 193
Pelvic diaphragm, 181
Pelvic floor muscles, 180, 181
  strengthening exercise, 180
Pelvic floor strain, 180–181
Pelvic plexus, 182, 183
Pelvic splanchnic nerve (PSN), 187
Pelvic stabilization program, 214
Pelvis, 175–181
  anatomy, 175–176, 176
    muscles, 176, 179
  chronic pain, 178
  CT scans, 76
  injury mechanism, 176
  MRI scans, 79
  pathological conditions after injury, 176–181
    myofascial pain syndrome, 179–180
    pelvic floor strain, 180–181
    sacroiliac joint dysfunction, 177–179
Pentazocine hydrochloride, 376
Performance, level, assessment, 332–333
Performance, patterns, 333
Perfusion MRI (pMRI), in MTBI, 323
Peri-aqueductal gray matter (PAG), 56, 59, 368
Peripheral myofascial entrapment, 24
Peripheral nerve(s), 253
  anatomy, 53, 253
    upper extremity, 90, 120–122
  hypersensitivity in brachial plexus irritation, 258
  injuries
    causing RSDS, 269
    clinical presentation, 84
    electrodiagnostic testing, 84, 86
  large vs small fibers, damage, 255
  regeneration, 51
  transection/damage, 51
Peripheral nerve entrapment, 51
  clinical features, 122
  electrodiagnostic testing, 84, 86, 122–125 *See also* Electromyogram (EMG); Nerve conduction velocity (NCV)
  lower extremity, 51–52, 258
  steroid injection, 263
  treatment, anticonvulsants, 245–246

Peripheral nerve entrapment (Continued)
    upper extremity, 51, 119–147, 257–258 See also
        Median nerve; Ulnar nerve entrapment
    forearm/elbow, 102, 104
    sites, 121
Peripheral nervous system, 51
Peroneal nerves, 149
    entrapment, 51–52, 258
Personality diathesis, reflex sympathetic dystrophy
    syndrome, 272
Personality traits, effect on MTBI, 310
Pes anserine bursa, 168
Phalanges
    foot, 149
    hand, 89
Phalen's maneuver, 127, 128
    carpal tunnel syndrome, 127, 255
Phenergan See Promethazine (Phenergan)
Phentolamine test, reflex sympathetic dystrophy
    syndrome, 275, 276
Phenytoin (Dilantin)
    migraine headache prophylaxis, 228
    neurogenic pain management, 245
Phobias, 319, 341
    after MTBI, 342
Phonophobia, 317, 345, 350, 359
Photon energy, 76
Photophobia, 303, 319–320
Phrenic nerve, 143
Physiatrists, role in MTBI rehabilitation, 347–348
Physicians
    accident reports for, 6
    doctor/patient relationship, 235
    engineers vs, 6, 31, 32
    evaluation of causation, 3
    information requirement for reports
        vehicle speed estimation, 10
        vehicle type/mass, 10
    record-keeping for evaluation of causation, 4
    responsibilities, 6
        cautions on use of G-forces, 14, 15
    understanding of biomechanics/engineering, 6
Physiologic diathesis, reflex sympathetic
    dystrophy syndrome, 272
Picture Arrangement subtest, of WAIS-R, 351
Pins and needles (tingling), 51, 84
Piriformis muscle, 176, 177, 179, 211
    chronic spasm, 179
    tight, 177–178, 179
Piriformis-stretching program, 179
Piriformis syndrome, 52, 179

Plantar fascia, 150, 152, 153
    inflammation, 153
Plantar fasciitis, 153
Plantar nerves, 149
Plastic deformation, definition, 8
Pons (dorsal lateral pons), descending modulatory
    pain system, 254
Positron-emission tomography (PET) scanning, in
    MTBI, 322
    comparison of tests, 323
Post-concussion prodrome, 304
Post-concussive syndrome (PCS), 297 See also Mild
    traumatic brain injury (MTBI)
    definition, 304
    DSM-IV definition, 303
    importance of asking questions on, 299–300,
        316, 326
    incidence, 299
    overlap with symptoms in Becks Depression
        Inventory, 330
    residual, from prior accidents, 328
    symptoms, 316–321
Posterior cruciate ligament, 161, 163, 166
    testing, 166, 168
Posterior draw sign, 166, 168
Posterior interosseous nerve, 120, 137
    injuries, 138
    tenderness, 138
Posterior longitudinal ligament, 194–195, 196
    cervical region, 142
    injuries, 46
    lumbar spine, 182, 196, 208
    pain sensitivity, 203
    tapering in lumber region, 196, 208
Posterior tibial artery, 150
Post-traumatic amnesia (PTA), 301, 326
    definition, 328
    period, importance of establishing, 328
Post-Traumatic Stress Disorder (PTSD), 319
    after MTBI, 319, 341–342
    avoidance of stimuli and symptoms, 341
    case study interpretation, 358
    definition (DSM-IV), 341
Post-Traumatic Vision Syndrome (PTVS),
    319, 346
Posture
    erect, balance See Balance
    stability, role of vision after whiplash, 71
    upside-down standing, vision role, 70–71
Potential energy, conversion from/to kinetic
    energy, 65

Prescribing, opioids, 387–388
  abuse prevention, 387–388
Prescription forgery, 387
Pressure wave, axonal injury, 307
Primary direction of force (PDOF)
  collision categorization, 5
  effect on injury potential, 28
  motor vehicle accident types, 4, 5
Problem solving, 318
  deficit after MTBI, 357
Prochlorperazine (Compazine), migraine (vascular headache), 223
Promethazine (Phenergan)
  migraine (vascular headache), 223
  opioid-induced nausea, 383
Pronator muscle, innervation, 145
Pronator syndrome, 51, 121, 131–133, 258
  clinical features and examination, 132–133
  complications, 133
  electrodiagnostic testing, 133
  injuries associated, 132
  neurogenic pain, 51, 258
  treatment, 133
Pronator teres muscle, 131
Propanolol (Inderal), migraine (vascular headache), 222
Propoxyphene hydrochloride, 375
Propoxyphene napsylate, 375
Prostaglandins, 53
Proton MR spectroscopy (MRS), 324
Protriptyline, migraine headache prophylaxis, 228
Prozac (fluoxetine hydrochloride), 247
Psychiatric disorders
  effect on MTBI, 310
  sub-optimal motivation due to, 314–315
Psychiatric management, after MTBI, 345
Psychological aspects
  chronic pain development, 32
  reflex sympathetic dystrophy syndrome, 272
Psychological screening, clinical, 329–330
  cautions on use/interpretation, 329, 330
Psychological testing See Neuropsychological assessment
Psychosocial issues, delayed recovery, 236
Psychotherapy
  definition, 339
  mild traumatic brain injury, 339–343
    case study, 359
    conjoint/family therapy, 342
    individual, 327, 339–342, 348

Psychotherapy (Continued)
  mild traumatic brain injury (Continued)
    stages in individual therapy, 340–341
    supportive group, 342–343
  RSDS treatment, 288–289
Pterygoid muscle, 217
  paracervical myofascial pain referred to, 46
  trigger points, 217
Pubic symphysis, 175
Pulses, foot, 150
Pupils, opioids effect on, 372

Q
Quadriceps muscle, 163
  innervation, 182
Quadriceps tendon, 163
  injuries, 47
Quality of life, loss, chronic pain syndrome, 234
Quantitative digitalized electroencephalography (QEEG), 325
Quantitative MR imaging morphology, 324
Quebec whiplash study, 25, 28
Questionnaires, self-report, 329

R
Radial groove, 120
Radial nerve
  branches, 137
  course, 120, 137
  at elbow, 100
  entrapment, 51, 258 See also Radial tunnel syndrome
    at elbow, 104
    at humeral groove, 139
    sites, 121
  lesions, 256
  origin, 137
Radial pulse, obliteration, 140, 141
Radial tunnel, 137
  anatomy, 100
Radial tunnel syndrome, 51, 137–139, 258
  clinical history, 138
  electrodiagnostic testing, 138
  treatment and complications, 138–139
Radiation, hazards, 75
Radiculitis, 208
Radiculopathy, 208, 259
  cervical See Cervical radiculopathy
  definition, 208
  development, after compression fracture, 205
  herniated discs and, 208–209

Radiculopathy *(Continued)*
    lumbar *See* Lumbar radiculopathy
    lumbosacral *See* Lumbosacral radiculopathy
    symptoms, 209
    treatment, anticonvulsants, 245
Radiography, 74–75
    advantages, 74
    cervical radiculopathy, 145
    "dashboard knee," 165
    disadvantages, 74–75
    films required after motor vehicle accidents, 75
    lumbar radiculopathy, 186
    open mouth view, 75
    principle, 74
    reflex sympathetic dystrophy syndrome, 274
    stress x-rays
        acromioclavicular joint strain, 116
        hand and wrist ligament tears, 97
    views required, 75
Radionuclide (nuclear) imaging, 79–80
    advantages/disadvantage, 79
    contraindications, 79
    procedure, 79–80
    triple-phase bone scanning *See* Bone
        scanning
Radionuclides, 79
Radiopharmaceuticals, 79
Rear end collisions, costs, 4
Reasoning abilities, assessment, 331
Reconstructionist (of accidents), 3
    disputes over tolerance and vehicle damage,
        10, 13
    G-force estimation with low impact speeds, 15
    occupant unreliability, perceived forward
        motion, 5
    stress–strain curve information not used, 20
    time increase and acceleration decrease,
        10–11
    time increase and injury potential reduced, 9,
        10–11
    use of G-force inappropriately, 14
Reconstruction of accidents
    errors, 30
    invalidity of retrospective prediction, 31
    variability problem, 2
Recovery, delayed, 235–236
Rectus capitis posterior minor muscle, 24
Recurrent nerve of Luschka, 202
Referral, to neuropsychologist, 327
Reflex algodystrophy *See* Reflex sympathetic
    dystrophy syndrome

Reflex sympathetic dystrophy syndrome (RSDS),
    51, 267–296
diagnosis, 273–276
    radiography, 274
    radionuclide scanning (bone scans), 80, 275
    thermography, 80–81, 274
emotional reactions, 279
epidemiologic features, 268–270
foot injuries, 154–155
hand and wrist injuries, 99
injuries precipitating, 268–269
investigations, 261
pathophysiology, 267, 269
    causes, 269, 270
    features, 276–280
    WDRN involvement, 279
pathophysiology theories, 277–280
    A-alpha proprioceptive pain modulation, 280
    anterior horn cell activation, 279
    ascending pain pathway activation, 277–279
    nociceptive afferent system activation, 277,
        278
    sympathetic efferent system injury, 277, 278
physiologic and personality diathesis, 272
prevalence, 272
psychological/behavioral features, 272
stages, 270–271
    acute, 270
    atrophic, 271
    dystrophic, 270
    pathophysiologic hypothesis, 277
    treatment for specific stages, 281
sympathetic nervous system hyperactivity, 255,
    270
symptoms/signs, 154–155, 255, 271–272
    pain, 271, 279
    summary, 273
terminology and alternative names, 267–268
treatment, 281–290 *See also* Stellate ganglion
    block
    Bier blocks, 282–283
    costs, 289–290
    miscellaneous treatment modalities,
        288–289
    physical therapy, 288
    spinal cord stimulation, 392
    summary, 282
    sympathectomy, 287–288
    sympathetic ganglion blocks, 283–284, 285
    sympatholytic medications, 281–282
vasomotor abnormalities, 260–261, 270

Reflex testing, 255–256
    lower extremity, 184–185
    upper extremity, 144
Reglan *See* Metoclopramide (Reglan)
Reitan-Indiana Aphasia Screening, 353
Relaxation training, RSDS treatment, 289
Reliability, definition, 2
Remeron *See* Mirtazapine (Remeron)
Remote information, difficulties in accessing,
    317
Reserpine, 283
Respiratory depression
    intrathecal opioid pump implantation
        complication, 406
    opioid-induced, 372–373, 382, 401
Respiratory system, opioids effect on, 372–373
Restlessness, nocturnal, 238
Restrictions (patient), determination, 240, 241
Retrocalcaneal bursa, 156
Retrolisthesis, 210
Rey-Osterreith Complex Figure Test, 355, 357
Rheumatoid arthritis, diagnostic tests, 73
Rheumatoid factor, 73
Rhizotomies, 263
Rib, first
    in entrapment syndromes, 25
    resection, reflex sympathetic dystrophy
        syndrome after, 269
Ritalin, after MTBI, 345
Rizatriptan benzoate (Maxalt), migraine (vascular
    headache), 223
Road surface drag factor *(F)*, 12, 27
Robaxin (methocarbamol), 243
Roentgenography *See* Radiography
Rofecoxib (Vioxx), 242
Rostroventral medulla (RVM), 56, 368
Rotation
    head *See* Head, rotations
    neck/cervical spine, injury potential, 26,
        27–28
    torquing injuries in collisions, 42
Rotational forces, 306
    spinal injury, 198
Rotator cuff, musculotendinous junction (critical
    zone), 117
Rotator cuff muscles, 107, 109, 110
    abduction of arm function, 107
    injuries, 107
Rotator cuff tears, 117–118
    complications, 118
    persistent pain, 117

Rotator cuff tendon, 107
    anatomy, 107, 109
    injuries, 47
Rotator cuff tendonitis, 47, 113
    treatment and complications, 113
Ruff Figural Fluency Test, 351, 353
Rules 701 and 702, 3

S

Saccades, unilateral, 320, 350
Sacral nerve root, lesions, 184–185
Sacroiliac joint, 175, 176, 177
    anatomy, 211
    functions, 211
    injuries, 50
    ligament injuries, 46
    pain, 177
    strains, 177
    subluxation, 211
Sacroiliac joint dysfunction, 177–179, 211,
    213–214
    complications, 179
    physical examination, 177–178, 213
    symptoms, 211, 213
    treatment, 178–179, 213–214
Sacroiliac joint elastic belt, 214
Sacrum, 175
    anatomy, 191
Scalene anesthetic block, 141
Scalene muscle, 25
    spasm, thoracic outlet syndrome due to, 140
    tears in hyperextension injuries, 41–42
    in whiplash injury, 45
Scalenus anticus syndrome, 140
    physical examination, 140–141
Scaphoid fractures, 98
Scapholunate ligament, tears, 97
Scapula, 105
Scapulohumeral movement, 110, 111
Scapulothoracic movement, 110, 111
Scar tissue, 24
    chronic pain, 40
    healed muscle tears, 44
    ligament tears, 46
    muscle spasm, 45
    nerve root irritation, 209
    neuroma, 259
Sciatic nerve, 177, 182, 211
    entrapment, 52
Sciatic pain, 184
Scintillations, gamma radiation, 79

Seat belt loading, injuries, 20
"Second impact syndrome," 301, 308
Sedatives, for sleep disturbance, 238, 239
Seizures, bupropion hydrochloride (Wellbutrin)
        causing, 248
Selective serotonin reuptake inhibitors (SSRIs),
        238, 246–247
    after MTBI, 312, 345
    chronic pain syndrome and depression, 246–247
    in depression after MTBI, 312
    headache prophylaxis, 227
    metabolism and dosages, 247
    side effects, 247
Self, sense of, after MTBI, 311, 341
Semicircular canals, 70
Semispinalis muscle, 24
Sensitivity, definition, 1
Sensory nerve action potential (SNAP), 81, 85, 124
    cubital tunnel syndrome, 136
    radial tunnel syndrome, 138
    thoracic outlet syndrome, 141
Sensory nerves, 202
Sensory perception processes, assessment, 330,
        331, 354
Sensory receptors, 53
Sensory testing, 255–256
    lower extremity, 184
    upper extremity, 144, 256
Serological tests, 73–74
Serotonergic pain modulatory pathway, 56, 58
Serotonergic system, ascending, vascular
        headaches, 218, 221
Serotonin
    antidepressant mechanism of action, 246, 247
    binding to 5-HT receptors, 220
        release of other neurotransmitters, 220–221
    depression in MTBI due to changes, 312
    depression pathophysiology, 238
    dorsal horn neuron inhibition, 56, 58
    release
        endorphin action, 254
        inhibitors/prevention, 222
        vascular headache, 220
Serotonin receptors
    5-HT$_1$, agonists, 223
    5-HT$_{1D}$, inhibition of neurotransmitter release,
        220
    antagonists, 222
    classes, 220
Sertraline hydrochloride (Zoloft), 246–247
Serzone (nefazodone hydrochloride), 247

Sesamoid bone, 161
"Shaken baby syndrome," 298
Shear, definition, 8
Shear strain, axonal injury, 307
Shoulder, 105–119
    anatomy, 105–111 See also Rotator cuff muscles
        ligaments, 105, 107
        muscles, 110
        tendons, 105, 107, 108, 109
    flexion, abduction external rotation (AER)
        position and, 141
    fractures, 115–116
    frozen (adhesive capsulitis), 112, 113,
        118–119
        after inadequate treatment of shoulder strain,
        114
        thoracic outlet syndrome complication, 142
    immobilization, acromioclavicular joint strain,
        116
    impact injuries, 111
    impingement, 49–50, 111
    injuries, 49–50, 50, 112–119
    injury mechanisms, 111
    ligaments, 105, 107
        injuries, 46–47
    manipulation under anesthesia, 119
    MRI scans, 79
    muscle injuries, 118
    muscle spasm, 50
    pathological conditions after accidents, 112–119
        See also Shoulder pain
        acromioclavicular joint strain, 116–117
        bicipital tendonitis, 113–114
        bursitis, 112
        capsule strain, 114–115
        capsule tear, 115
        fractures, 115–116
        myofascial pain syndrome, 118
        rotator cuff tendonitis, 113
    "popping" in, 115
    positive impingement sign, 112, 114
    range of motion, 49, 105, 110
        limitations/loss, 118–119
        scapulohumeral movement, 110, 111
    stability, 107, 110, 111
    subluxation, 115
        repeated, 115
    tendinitis, 47
    trigger points, 118
Shoulder-hand syndrome, 268 See also Reflex
        sympathetic dystrophy syndrome (RSDS)

Shoulder harness
  acromioclavicular joint strain due to, 116
  shoulder capsule strain, 114
  shoulder injuries due to, 111
Shoulder pain *See also individual shoulder injuries/conditions*
  bicipital tendonitis, 113–114
  frozen shoulder, 119
  subacromial bursitis, 112
  tendon injuries, 47
  thoracic outlet syndrome, 140
  at tip
    acromioclavicular joint strain, 116
    rotator cuff tear, 117
    rotator cuff tendonitis, 113
Shoulder-pelvis counter-rotation, 65, 66
Shoulder region, muscle spasm, 50
Sick role, 315
Sigmoid (S-shaped) curve, cervical spine, 9, 21, 22, 23, 30
  compression/loading affecting, 21, 22
Sinequan *See* Doxepin (Adapin, Sinequan)
Single photon emission computed tomography (SPECT), 79, 323
Skelaxin (metaxalone), 243
Skid marks, 13
Skill building, training, after MTBI, 343
Skills, transferable, assessment, 344
Skin, changes in RSDS, 272
Skull fractures, 42, 48
Sleep disturbance
  chronic pain, 43, 233, 238–239, 254
    restlessness, 238
    tricyclic antidepressants, 238–239
  fatigue after MTBI, 313–314, 316, 347
    case study, 350
    management, 347, 348–349
Sling
  acromioclavicular joint strain, 116–117
  shoulder capsule strain, 114
Small intestine, opioids side effects, 373
Smell, sense, alterations, 316
Socialization, chronic pain clinic, 240
Soma, abuse, 243
Somatoform Disorders, 314–315
Somatosensory cortex, 56, 57, 254, 279
Somatosensory evoked potentials (SSEPs)
  lumbar radiculopathy, 186
  neurogenic pain, 260
Spasticity, baclofen treatment, 243
Specificity, definition, 1

SPECT imaging, 79, 323
"Speed from distance and drag," 12
Speed of vehicle *See* Vehicle speed
Spinal canal, stenosis, 207, 208
Spinal cord, 200–203
  anterolateral quadrant, 54, 55
  block, 284
  brain stem projections, 56
  compression, 208
  gray matter, laminae, 54
  injury, vertebral compression fractures, 48
  termination at T12, 182, 200
Spinal cord stimulation (SCS), 391–400
  complications, 397–398
  electrode placement, 391, 393, 394
  goals, 397
  infections after, 397–398
  lead fractures, 398
  lead migration, 398
    prevention advice, 396
  neurogenic pain management, 262–263
  patient responsibilities after, 396
  patient selection criteria, 391–392
    pain characteristics, 392
    patient characteristics, 391–392
  permanent, indications, 391–392, 393
  realistic expectations of, 392
  RSDS treatment, 289
  technique, 393–396
    open technique, 391, 394
    permanent implantation, 394–395
    postimplantation care, 395–396
    trial stimulation, 393
Spinal cord stimulator pulse generator (SCSPG), 394–395
"Spinal engine," 66
Spinal facet joints *See* Facet joints
Spinal ganglion, bruising injury, 25
Spinal injection studies, 23
Spinal ligaments, 195–196, 198
Spinal nerve, 182, 193
  bruising, 25
Spinal nerve roots, 200–202
  cervical *See* Cervical nerve roots
  entrapment, 258–259
  injury in disc degeneration, 207, 259
  irritation, 258–259
  lumbar *See* Lumbar nerve roots
  lumbosacral *See* Lumbosacral nerve roots
  naming, 200–201
  sheaths (dura), 203

Spinal pain, 191–214
  causes, 204–214
    intervertebral disc degeneration,
      205–208
    sites, 203–204
    soft tissue and bony, 209–210
    structures sensitive to, 202–203
    types, in disc degeneration, 207–208
    vertebral body fracture causing, 204–205
Spinal stenosis, 207, 208
Spine
  anatomy, 191–198 *See also* Cervical spine;
    Lumbar spine
  compression during rear end collisions,
    21–22
  CT scans, 76
  excessive flexion, 50, 198–199, 203, 209
  flexibility, 198
  fractures, 48
  "functional unit" (three-joint complex), 182, 193,
    196
  fusion, 189
  hyperextension, 199, 203–204
  injury biomechanics, 198–199
  instability, 208
  ligament injuries, 46
  lordotic curvature, 191, 192
  mechanics, 65–66
  MRI scans, 78
  muscles, 203
  pain sensitive structures, 202–203, 209
  range of movement, 191
  segment models, 64–65
  segments, 191
    "coupled motion" concept, 65–66
Spinothalamic tracts, 54, 55, 253, 277, 279
Spinous processes, 193
  fractures, 48
Splints
  carpal tunnel syndrome, 130
  cockup (wrist), 102
  hand or wrist ligament, 97, 98
  hand or wrist tendonitis, 93
  wrist, 102
Spondylolisthesis, 210, 212
  grading, 210, 212
  at L5-S1, 210, 213
Spondylolysis, 75, 193, 210, 211, 212
Spondylosis, 210
Sports-related concussion, 301–302, 302
Sport utility vehicles (SUV), 10

Sprains
  ankle joint, 157–158
  knee, 166–167
Spurling maneuver, 144–145, 256
Standardization/standardized approach, 1–2, 2
Steering wheel, gripping, injuries due to, 50
  wrist and hand injuries, 92
    ligament strains, 97
Stellate ganglion, 284
  anatomy, 284, 286
Stellate ganglion block, 284–287
  complications, 284
  diagnostic, 275–276
  principle, 284
  protocol, 286–287
Sternal fractures, 42
Sternocleidomastoid (SCM) muscle, 24–25
  tears in hyperextension injuries, 41–42
  tenderness, 25
  in whiplash injury, 45
Steroid(s) *See also* Corticosteroids
  hand or wrist tendonitis, 93
  migraine (vascular headache) treatment, 223,
    226
  oral, lumbar radiculopathy, 188
Steroid blocks, proximal, 263–264
Steroid injections *See also* Anesthetic/steroid
    injection
  Achilles bursitis/tendonitis, 160–161
  ankle osteoarthritis, 160
  carpal tunnel syndrome, 130, 263
  cervical epidural, cervical radiculopathy,
    146–147
  cubital tunnel syndrome, 136
  elbow ligament strains, 105
  frozen shoulder, 119
  hand or wrist ligament strains, 97
  hip strains, 174
  interdigital neuroma, 153
  knee bursitis/tendonitis, 169
  lumbar epidural, 188
  lumbar radiculopathy, 189
  peripheral nerve entrapment, 263
  rotator cuff tendonitis, 113
  sacroiliac joint dysfunction, 178
  shoulder capsule strain, 114–115
Stiffness properties, 20
Stimulation-produced analgesia, 56
  opioids, 368
Straight leg raising test, 184, 185–186,
    256–257

Strain
definition, 8
shear, of axons, 307
tensile, 307
Strains (ligament) *See* Ligament injuries, strains
Stress, definition, 8
Stress loading, RSDS treatment and, 288
Stress management
migraine (vascular headache), 229
reduced after MTBI, 319
RSDS treatment, 289
tension-type headache, 216
Stress–strain curve, 8, 18–20
elastic area, 8, 19
failure rates of different structures, 20
information derived from, 20
plastic area, 8, 19
yield point, 19
Stress testing, reflex sympathetic dystrophy, 80–81, 261, 274
Stretching exercises
epicondylitis, 103
hip, 174
Subacromial bursa, 107
compression, 49–50
Subacromial bursitis, 47, 112
treatment and complications, 112
Subacromial decompression, 112, 113
"Subcatastrophic capsule or joint failure," 23
Sub-optimal motivation, 314–315
ruling out in neuropsychological tests, 315
Subscapularis muscle, 109
Substance P, 53, 262
actions, 221
depression in MTBI due to changes, 312
inactivation, 262
release
inhibition by ergotamine derivatives, 223
inhibition by opioids, 372
by serotonin, 220
vascular headache, 218
Sudeck's atrophy of bone, 268
Sumatriptan succinate, migraine (vascular headache), 223
Superficial peroneal nerve, 149, 155
entrapment, 51, 258
Superficial radial nerve, 89, 120, 137
course, 137
entrapment, 137, 258
injuries, 137
Superior hypogastric plexus (SHP), 187

Supinator muscle, tenderness, 138
Supinator syndrome *See* Radial tunnel syndrome
Supraclavicular tenderness, 140
Supraspinal impulses, 218–219, 220
Supraspinous ligament, 196
Sural nerve, 149, 151
entrapment, 51
Surgery
Achilles tendon tear/rupture, 160
carpal tunnel syndrome, 130
cervical radiculopathy, 147
cubital tunnel syndrome, 136
epicondylectomy, 103
knee fractures, 171
neurogenic pain management, 263
RSDS after, 269, 270
tarsal tunnel syndrome, 155
Sutures (joints), 48
Sympathectomy, 263, 287–288
chemical or surgical, 287–288
Sympathetically maintained pain (SMP), 267, 280–281
Sympathetic blockade, 261, 264
in RSDS, 271
diagnosis, 275–276
Sympathetic ganglion, 276, 283–284, 285
Sympathetic ganglion blocks, 283–287
Sympathetic nervous system *See also* Stellate ganglion block
abnormalities, examination, 255
efferent, RSDS hypothesis, 277, 278
energy utilization, 276
interruption techniques, 281, 284
overactivity
reflex sympathetic dystrophy, 255, 270
signs/symptoms, 270
underactivity in acute RSDS, 270
Sympathetic reflex, injuries provoking, 276
Sympatholytic medications, 281–282
Symptomatology
in accident or ambulance report, 6
injury chronicity prediction, 28
Symptom Checklist-90 Revised (SCL90-R), 329
Synarthrosis, 48, 196
SynchroMed Infusion Pump, 402, 404, 405
Synovial fluid, 198
Synovial joint, 48, 198
Systemic lupus erythematosus (SLE), diagnostic tests, 73

T

Tarsal tunnel, anatomy, 156, 158
Tarsal tunnel syndrome, 51, 154, 158–159, 258
  examination, 154, 158, 255
  surgery, 155
Taste, sense, alterations, 316–317
Technetium 99M diethylenetriamine pentaacetic acid (DTPA), 79
Technetium 99M dimercaptosuccinic acid (DMSA), 79
Teeth, grinding, 43
Tegretol See Carbamazepine (Tegretol)
Temperature
  reflex sympathetic dystrophy syndrome, 272
  sympathetic nervous system abnormality, 255, 272
  thermography See Thermography
Temporalis muscle, trigger points, 44
Temporal lobe, dysfunction, test results in MTBI, 356–357
Temporomandibular joint dysfunction, 43
  headaches due to, 44, 216–218
Tender spots, myofascial pain syndrome, 236
Tendon(s)
  anatomy, 47
  ankle joint, 156
  hand and wrist, 91, 92
  injuries, pain, 47
  shoulder joint, 105, 107, 108, 109
Tendonitis
  Achilles, 160–161
  bicipital, 111, 113–114
  hand and wrist, 93–94
  knee, 47, 168–169
  rotator cuff, 47, 113
Tenosynovitis, DeQuervain's See DeQuervain's tenosynovitis
Tenovaginectomy, first dorsal compartment, 95
Tenovaginitis, stenosing, trigger finger, 96
TENS
  ankle osteoarthritis, 160
  chronic cervical radiculopathy, 147
  "dashboard knee," 165
  knee bursitis/tendonitis, 169
  knee fractures, 171
  myofascial pain syndrome, 237
  neurogenic pain management, 262
  RSDS treatment and, 288
  thoracic outlet syndrome, 141
Tensile strain, 307

Tensor fascia lata muscle, 171, 175
  spasm, 180
Teres minor, 110
Thalamic nuclei, medial, and lateral, 55, 57
  change associated with time after accident, 59
Thalamus, pain pathway, 54, 55, 219, 254
Thenar eminence, wasting, carpal tunnel syndrome, 127
Thermography, 80–81
  carpal tunnel syndrome, 129
  neurogenic pain, 260–261
  reflex sympathetic dystrophy syndrome, 274
  stress testing, 80–81, 274
Thoracic costochondral joints, injuries, 50
Thoracic nerve roots, 253
Thoracic outlet syndrome, 120, 139–142, 258
  complications, 142
  myogenic, 45, 51, 113, 118, 140
    clinical features and causes, 140
    humeral head fracture complication, 116
    symptoms, 119
  pain, 140, 141
  physical examination/diagnosis, 140–141, 255
  postural maneuvers (test), 140–141, 255
  RSDS due to, 269
  supraclavicular tenderness, 140
  treatment, 141–142
Thoracic spine
  malalignment, thoracic outlet syndrome due to, 140
  vertebrae, 191
Thoraco lumbosacral orthoses (TLSO), 204
Thumb
  anatomy, 89
  hyperextension (at base), 92
  pain, strained ligaments, 97
  tendons, 91
Thurstone Verbal Fluency, 353
Thyroid hormones, evaluation, 74
Thyroid stimulating hormone (TSH), 74
Tibia, 155
Tibialis anterior muscle
  activity linked with posterior head tilt, 70
  innervation, 182
Tibial nerve, 149, 156, 158
  branches, 156
  course, 158, 159
  entrapment, 51, 154
Tibial plateaus, 161, 164

Tinel's sign, 127, 128, 256
  carpal tunnel syndrome, 127, 255
  cubital tunnel syndrome, 136
  Guyon's canal syndrome, 134
  neurogenic pain in foot, 154
  pronator syndrome, 132–133
  radial nerve entrapment at humeral groove, 139
  superficial radial nerve entrapment, 137
  supraclavicular tenderness, 140
  tarsal tunnel syndrome, 154, 158, 255
  thoracic outlet syndrome and, 140, 141, 255
Tinnitus, 303, 316, 344
Tissue damage, in injury potential evaluation, 17
Tissue tolerance to injury, 2–3
Toenails, 150
Tofranil (imipramine), 239
Tolerance to injury (impact injury), 2–3, 28, 30
  definition, 2
  evaluation, stress–strain curve, 18–20
  variability of accidents affecting, 13
Tolerance to opioids See Opioid(s)
Tolerance to pain, reduced in chronic pain, 40
Torque, 8
  axial, lateral bending force effect, 66
Torque (rotational) forces, spinal injury, 198
Torquing injuries, causes, 42
Transcranial magnetic stimulation (TMS), 324
Transcutaneous electrical nerve stimulation See TENS
Transduction, nociceptive stimuli, 53
Transferable skills, assessment after MTBI, 344
Transneuronal degeneration, 309
Transverse carpal ligament, 126, 127
Trapezii, injuries, 45
Trazodone (Desyrel), 239
  sleep disorders in MTBI, 314
Triceps muscle, innervation, 145
Tricyclic antidepressants See also Amitriptyline (Elavil)
  in chronic pain, 238–239, 243
    indications, 243
  in depression after MTBI, 312
  drugs and dosages, 239
  headache prophylaxis, 227, 228
  mechanism of action, 243, 246
  neurogenic pain management, 246, 262
  RSDS treatment, 289
  side effects and contraindications, 228, 246
  for sleep disturbance, 238–239
    in MTBI, 314
Trigeminal nuclear complex, 218–219

Trigger finger, 96–97
Trigger points, 42, 43
  injection therapy, forearm myofascial pain, 102
  myofascial pain syndrome, 42, 236
  pterygoid muscle, 217
  shoulder, 118
Triple-phase bone scanning See Bone scanning, triple-phase
Triptan derivatives, 223, 227
  migraine (vascular headache), 222, 223, 227
Trochanteric bursitis, 173
Two-point discrimination testing, carpal tunnel syndrome, 127–128
Tylenol (acetaminophen), 242

U
Ulnar groove, 120
  anatomy, 100
Ulnar nerve, 89, 90
  anatomy, 135
  course, 101, 120, 135
  at elbow, 100
  injuries, 135
  motor and sensory fibers, 89, 90, 135
  neurolysis, 136
  origin, 135
  tunnel See Guyon's canal
  at wrist, 91
Ulnar nerve entrapment, 86, 91, 133–137, 258
  at elbow, 104, 121, 135–137 See also Cubital tunnel syndrome
  sites, 121
  at wrist, 121, 133–134 See also Guyon's canal
Ultrasound
  ankle osteoarthritis, 160
  aseptic necrosis of hip, 175
  epicondylitis, 103
  knee ligament injuries, 167
  sacroiliac joint dysfunction, 178
  trochanteric bursitis, 173
Uncovertebral joints, 195
Unmyelinated nerve fibers See C-fibers (unmyelinated)
Unrestrained drivers, accidents, pain, 41
Upper extremity See also specific anatomical regions
  dermatomes and myotomes, 143
  electrodiagnostic testing, 145
  fractures, 48
  injuries causing RSDS, 269
  innervation, 257

Upper extremity (Continued)
  joint injuries, 49, 50
  ligament injuries, 46–47
  motor loss, 209
  muscles, nerve root innervation, 143, 144
  nerve entrapments, 51, 86, 119–147, 257–258
    See also Peripheral nerve entrapment
  neurological examination, 143–145
  pain, 89–148
    causes, 42
    elbow, 99–105
    hand and wrist, 89–99
  peripheral nerves, anatomy, 90, 120–122
  reflex testing, 144
  sensory testing, 144, 256
  tendon injuries, 47
Upper extremity bracing (in accidents), 41
  carpal tunnel syndrome, 126
  elbow injuries, 100
  hand and wrist injuries, 93
  ligament injuries, 46–47
  shoulder injuries, 111
  ulnar nerve entrapment, 133
Urinary incontinence, 186
  stress, 180
Urodynamic workup, 180, 186

V
Validity, definition, 2
Valium, 243
Valproate (Depakote)
  migraine headache prophylaxis, 228
  neurogenic pain management, 245
Vascular headache See Migraine (vascular
  headache)
Vascular pain syndrome, 26
Vasoconstriction
  alpha-receptor stimulation causing, 276–277
  norepinephrine causing, 276, 281
  sympathetic overactivity, 270
Vasomotor instability, reflex sympathetic
  dystrophy syndrome, 272
Vastus medialis activity, linked with posterior head
  tilt, 70
Vector, properties, 8
Vehicle(s) See also Headrest; Shoulder harness
  bumpers See Bumpers (car)
  energy-absorbing factors/structures, 13
  mass and injury relationship, 27
  size, effect on kinetic energy and injury,
    27

Vehicle damage
  absence
    impact speeds and acceleration force, 15, 29
    injury potential despite, 10, 12
    kinetic energy increase for occupants and, 15,
      29, 30, 31
  $\triangle t$ increase and injury potential reduced, 13
  injury potential not determined from, 29
  poor evaluation of injury potential, 10, 29
  reduced, low speed not validated, 29
Vehicle speed
  estimation, 10, 12
  injury increased, 27
  maximum, without damage, 12
  prior to skidding, 12
Velocity
  changes (acceleration), 6, 10, 298
    MTBI biomechanics, 305–306
  relative change and interval, 305
Venlafaxine hydrochloride (Effexor)
  depression management, 247–248
  dosage, 248
  mechanism of action, 247–248
Venograms, thoracic outlet syndrome, 141
Verapamil
  contraindications, 228
  high-dose, 228
  migraine (vascular headache), 222, 228
Verbal fluency problem, 317
  testing, 353
Verbal IQ, 337
Vertebrae, 191–193 See also Lumbar vertebrae;
    Spine
  adjacent, movement, 210
  cervical, 142, 191
  fused, 175
Vertebral arch, 181, 191, 193
Vertebral artery, in vascular pain syndrome, 26
Vertebral body, 191, 193
  cervical spine, 142
  fractures, 204–205
  height loss, 204, 205
  lumbar spine, 181
  pain sensitivity, 202
  separation distance, 206
Vertebral compression fractures, 42, 48, 204, 205
  grading, 48, 204
  wedge, 205
Vertebral endplates
  calcification (osteophytes), 207
  microtrauma, 206

Vertigo, cervical, 45
Vestibular-ocular reflex, 71
Vestibular system, 70
    evaluation/treatment, after MTBI, 344–345
    problems after MTBI, 316, 344–345
Vestibulospinal reflexes, 70
Victim, perception as, 234
Video gait analysis, 63–64
    advantages, 63–64
    observational vs, 63
Vioxx (rofecoxib), 242
Vision
    assessment after MTBI, 354
    binocular, deficits after MTBI, 346
    blurred, 319
    deficits, after MTBI, 319–320, 321, 345–347
        case study, 350
    double, 319, 345
    night, decreased, 320
    role in postural stability after whiplash, 71
    role in upside-down standing posture, 70–71
Vistaril, 383
Visual Midline Shift Syndrome (VMSS), 319, 346
Visual orientation problems, after MTBI, 346
Visual scanning problems, 319, 357
Visual system
    ambient, 319, 346
    focal, 346
Vocational losses/impairment *See also*
    Employment
    after MTBI, 343–344, 359–360
    chronic pain syndrome, 233
    neuropsychological test result, 337
Vocational rehabilitation, after MTBI, 343–344
    alternative vocations, 344, 359–360
Vocational status, assessment after MTBI,
    343–344
Volunteer tests, 18
Vomiting
    drug treatment, 223
    opioids causing, 373

W

Waddell signs, 271
Walking *See* Gait
Walking aids
    Achilles bursitis/tendonitis, 161
    ankle sprains, 158
    knee bursitis/tendonitis, 169
    knee fractures, 171
    tarsal tunnel syndrome, 159

Warm-water stress test, 81, 274
Water hammer theory, 25–26
Wechsler Adult Intelligence Scale-III (WAIS-III),
    336, 352
Wechsler Adult Intelligence Scale-Revised
    (WAIS-R), 336, 351, 352
    negative impact of MTBI, 336
Wellbutrin, 248
Whip, definition, 8
Whiplash
    arguments against validity, 32
    definition, 41
    hyperflexion–hyperextension injury, 21,
        22, 41
    translational and rotational accelerations,
        306
    without external trauma, 301
Wide dynamic-range neurons (WDRN), 54, 55
    in nucleus caudalis, 218
    reflex sympathetic dystrophy syndrome, 277,
        278
    RSDS pathophysiology and, 279
    sympathetically maintained pain (SMP), 281
Women
    increased incidence of injury, 27
    neck pain, 16–17
World Health Organization (WHO), analgesic
    ladder, 242, 383
Wrist, 89–99 *See also* Hand and wrist
    anatomical relations, 92
    anatomy, 89–92
    extension pain, 102–103
    flexion pain, 102
    hyperextension, 41, 50
        cubital tunnel syndrome, 135
        forearm muscle strain, 101
        nerve entrapments due to, 258
        RSDS, 269
        sequelae, 93
    immobilization, 103
    injuries *See under* Hand and wrist
    pain
        Guyon's canal syndrome, 133
        strained ligaments, 97
        superficial radial nerve injury, 137
    painless lump on back of,
        95
    range of motion, 49
    splints, 102
Wrist tendons, injuries,
    47

X

X-rays, 74 *See also* Radiography
    tissues absorbing, 76

Y

Yield stress, 8

Z

Zolmitriptan (Zomig), migraine (vascular
    headache), 223
Zoloft (sertraline hydrochloride), 246–247
Zolpidem tartrate (Ambien), in sleep disturbance,
    239